Hypertension Manual

Hypertension Manual

Chief Editor

A Muruganathan MD
Director
Hold Medical Academy
Tirupur, Tamil Nadu, India
Director-Elect, API—Physician Reach Foundation
Chairman, IMA Hypertension Standing Committee
Imm Past Governor, American College of Physicians India Chapter
Dean, Indian College of Physicians (ICP) (2016–2017)
President, Hypertension Society of India (HSI) (2015–2016)
President, Association of Physicians of India (API) (2013–2014)
President, IMA Tamil Nadu State Branch (2002–2003)
Editor, MediBeats

Associate Editors

Bidita Khandelwal
MD (Medicine)
Professor
Department of Medicine
Sikkim Manipal Institute of Medical Sciences
Sikkim Manipal University
Gangtok, Sikkim, India

Sadanand R Shetty
DM (Cardiology) MD (Med) FACC FSCAI FACA (USA)
FCPS FISE FICC FICP FCSI FESC
Director
Department of Cardiology
KJ Somaiya Medical College and Research Center
Mumbai, Maharashtra, India
Emeritus Professor
DY Patil University School of Medicine
Navi Mumbai
CMD and Founder
Sadanand Healthy Living Center Ltd, Mumbai
Founder, Sadanand G2S2 Foundation, Mumbai
Member, American College of Cardiology and
European Society of Cardiology

Foreword

Gurpreet S Wander

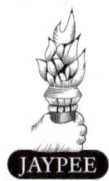

JAYPEE BROTHERS MEDICAL PUBLISHERS
The Health Sciences Publisher
New Delhi | London

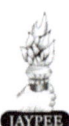 **Jaypee Brothers Medical Publishers (P) Ltd**

Headquarters
Jaypee Brothers Medical Publishers (P) Ltd
EMCA House, 23/23-B
Ansari Road, Daryaganj
New Delhi 110 002, India
Landline: +91-11-23272143, +91-11-23272703
+91-11-23282021, +91-11-23245672
Email: jaypee@jaypeebrothers.com

Corporate Office
Jaypee Brothers Medical Publishers (P) Ltd
4838/24, Ansari Road, Daryaganj
New Delhi 110 002, India
Phone: +91-11-43574357
Fax: +91-11-43574314
Email: jaypee@jaypeebrothers.com

Overseas Office
JP Medical Ltd.
83, Victoria Street, London
SW1H 0HW (UK)
Phone: +44 20 3170 8910
Fax: +44 (0)20 3008 6180
Email: info@jpmedpub.com

Website: www.jaypeebrothers.com
Website: www.jaypeedigital.com

© 2024, Jaypee Brothers Medical Publishers

The views and opinions expressed in this book are solely those of the original contributor(s)/author(s) and do not necessarily represent those of editor(s) or publisher of the book.

All rights reserved. No part of this publication may be reproduced, stored or transmitted in any form or by any means, electronic, mechanical, photocopying, recording or otherwise, without the prior permission in writing of the publishers.

All brand names and product names used in this book are trade names, service marks, trademarks or registered trademarks of their respective owners. The publisher is not associated with any product or vendor mentioned in this book.

Medical knowledge and practice change constantly. This book is designed to provide accurate, authoritative information about the subject matter in question. However, readers are advised to check the most current information available on procedures included and check information from the manufacturer of each product to be administered, to verify the recommended dose, formula, method and duration of administration, adverse effects and contraindications. It is the responsibility of the practitioner to take all appropriate safety precautions. Neither the publisher nor the author(s)/editor(s) assume any liability for any injury and/or damage to persons or property arising from or related to use of material in this book.

This book is sold on the understanding that the publisher is not engaged in providing professional medical services. If such advice or services are required, the services of a competent medical professional should be sought.

Every effort has been made where necessary to contact holders of copyright to obtain permission to reproduce copyright material. If any have been inadvertently overlooked, the publisher will be pleased to make the necessary arrangements at the first opportunity.

Inquiries for bulk sales may be solicited at: jaypee@jaypeebrothers.com

Hypertension Manual

First Edition: **2024**

ISBN: 978-93-5696-834-9

Printed in India

Dedicated to
*My resilient parents, elders, and the COVID warriors among them, who faced
hypertension complications with knowledge and courage.
This manual is crafted with love and dedication,
aiming to empower all navigating the complex terrain of hypertension.
May it serve as a beacon of hope, guiding towards a healthier future
and a hypertension-free world.*

Contributors

A Muruganathan MD
Director
Hold Medical Academy
Tirupur, Tamil Nadu, India
Director Elect, API—Physician Reach Foundation
Chairman, IMA Hypertension Standing Committee
Imm Past Governor, American College of Physicians India Chapter
Dean, Indian College of Physicians (ICP) (2016–2017)
President, Hypertension Society of India (HSI) (2015–2016)
President, Association of Physicians of India (API) (2013–2014)
President, IMA Tamil Nadu State Branch (2002–2003)
Editor, MediBeats

Abhay Narain Rai
MBBS MRCP (UK) FRCP (Glasgow)
Former Professor and Head
Internal Medicine and Cardiology Medicine
Principal
Anugrah Narayan Magadh Medical College and Hospital, Gaya, Bihar, India
Director and Head
Department of Medicine
Abhay Institute of Medical Science
Gaya, Bihar, India

Abhishek Byahut MSc (Med Biotechnology)
PhD Research Scholar
Medical Biotechnology
Sikkim Manipal Institute of Medical Sciences
Sikkim Manipal University
Gangtok, Sikkim, India

Aditi Parimoo MD (Medicine)
Senior Resident
Department of Cardiology
Seth GS Medical College and KEM Hospital
Mumbai, Maharashtra, India

Alladi Mohan
MD (Medicine) (AIIMS, New Delhi) FAMS FRCP (Edin) FCCP (USA) FICP PG Diploma in Epidemiology (PHFI-IIPH)
Dean, Professor (Senior Grade) and Head
Department of Medicine
Sri Venkateswara Institute of Medical Sciences
Tirupati, Andhra Pradesh, India

Alok Kumar Singh MD (Medicine) DM (Cardiology)
Senior Interventional Cardiologist
Alok Heart Clinic and Opal Hospitals Pvt Ltd
Director, Cardiac Cath Lab Cygnus Hospital
Varanasi, Uttar Pradesh, India
Chief Trustee, Heart India Charitable Trust
Vice President, API Varanasi Branch
Editor-in-Chief, Heart India

Ameet G Sattur MBBS MD DM FSCAI
Director
Department of Cardiology
Cath Lab HCG Suchirayu Hospital
KLE Suchirayu (HCG)
Hubballi, Karnataka, India

Anant Ramkishanrao Munde MBBS DNB DM
Assistant Professor
Department of Cardiology
Grant Government Medical College and
Sir JJ Group of Hospitals
Mumbai, Maharashtra, India

Anita Jaiswal Ektate MBBS MD (Med)
ACHD (SAG)
Department of Medicine
BAMH, Central Railway Hospital
Mumbai, Maharashtra, India

Anjan Lal Dutta MD DM FACC
Clinical Director and Head
Department of Cardiology
Peerless Hospital
Kolkata, West Bengal, India

Ankita Kulkarni DM (Cardiology)
Assistant Professor
Department of Cardiology
King Edward Memorial Hospital
Seth Gordhandas Sunderdas Medical College
Mumbai, Maharashtra, India

Arundhati Bag PhD
Associate Professor
Medical Biotechnology
Sikkim Manipal Institute of Medical Sciences
Sikkim Manipal University
Gangtok, Sikkim, India

Bidita Khandelwal MD (Medicine)
Professor
Department of Internal Medicine
Sikkim Manipal Institute of Medical Sciences
Sikkim Manipal University
Gangtok, Sikkim, India

Boudhayan Das Munshi
MBBS DNB (General Medicine) Fellowship in Diabetology (JIPMER) MNAMS FIACM
Associate Professor
Department of General Medicine
All India Institute of Medical Sciences
Kalyani, West Bengal, India

Chamma Gupta MSc (Med Biotechnology)
Tutor
Medical Biotechnology
Sikkim Manipal Institute of Medical Sciences
Sikkim Manipal University
Gangtok, Sikkim, India

Chandrasekhar Valupadas MD FICP
Professor
Department of General Medicine
Kakatiya Medical College/MGM Hospital
Warangal, Telangana, India

Dilip A Kirpalani MD DM (Nephro)
Consultant Nephrologist, Kidney Transplant Physician and Assistant Professor
Department of Nephrology
Bombay Hospital Institute of Medical Sciences
Mumbai, Maharashtra, India

E Cowshik
MBBS MD (Community Medicine) DNB (Community Medicine) Diploma in Public Health
Assistant Professor
Department of Community Medicine
Government Medical College
Tirupur, Tamil Nadu, India

Fraz A Mir BSc MA MBBS FRCP
Consultant Physician
Clinical Pharmacology and Therapeutics
Department of Medicine
Cambridge University Hospitals NHS Trust
Cambridge, UK

Geetha Subramanian
MD DM FISC FCSI FIAE FISE FICC FMMC ISH ICIC
Head (Retd)
Department of Cardiology
Institute of Medical Sciences
Banaras Hindu University
Varanasi, Uttar Pradesh, India
Emeritus Professor
Department of Cardiology
Tamil Nadu Dr MGR Medical University
Chennai, Tamil Nadu, India
Member, ESC, EACVI, ACC, PCSI

J Cecily Mary Majella MD DM FESC FSCAI
Professor
Department of Cardiology
Tamil Nadu Government Multi Super Specialty Hospital
Chennai, Tamil Nadu, India

Kannan Meera Devi MBBS MD (General Medicine)
Senior Resident
Department of Medicine
Karpagam Faculty of Medical Sciences and Research
Coimbatore, Tamil Nadu, India

Karma G Dolma PhD (Microbiology)
Associate Professor
Department of Microbiology
Sikkim Manipal Institute of Medical Sciences
Sikkim Manipal University
Gangtok, Sikkim, India

Keyur R Rathod MD (Medicine) DM (Cardiology)
3rd year Resident
Department of Cardiology
Seth GS Medical College and KEM Hospital
Mumbai, Maharashtra, India

Lydia Rai MBBS
Postgraduate Teacher
Department of Biochemistry
Sikkim Manipal Institute of Medical Sciences
Sikkim Manipal University
Gangtok, Sikkim, India

M Chenniappan MD DM
Consultant Cardiologist
Department of Cardiology
Ramakrishna Medical Center
Tiruchirappalli, Tamil Nadu, India

M Gowri Sankar MD (General Medicine)
Senior Assistant Professor
Department of General Medicine
Government Medical College and ESI Hospital
Coimbatore, Tamil Nadu, India

Madhu Gupta MPharm (Pharmaceutics) PhD
Associate Professor
Department of Pharmaceutics
School of Pharmaceutical Sciences
Delhi Pharmaceutical Sciences and Research University
New Delhi, India

Michaela M Watts RGN NMP
Clinical Pharmacology and Research
RGN, Independent and Supplementary Prescriber
Specialist Nurse for Cardiovascular Medicine and Research Co-ordinator
General Medicine
Addenbrooke's Hospital
(Cambridge University NHS Trust)
West Mersea, Essex England, UK

Minakshi Dhar
MD (Internal Medicine) PGDGM (Geriatric Medicine) ICP FACP (USA)
Additional Professor and Head
Department of Geriatric Medicine
All India Institute of Medical Sciences
Rishikesh, Uttarakhand, India

Mingma Lhamu Sherpa MBBS MD
Professor and Head
Department of Biochemistry
Sikkim Manipal Institute of Medical Sciences
Sikkim Manipal University
Gangtok, Sikkim, India

Mritunjay Kumar Singh MBBS MD (Medicine)
Consultant Physician and Head
Department of Nephrology
Abhay Institute of Medical Sciences
Gaya, Bihar, India

N Vimal Kumar MS (Ophthalmology)
Senior Assistant Professor
Department of Ophthalmology
Government Medical College and ESI Hospital
Coimbatore, Tamil Nadu, India

Neeta Narang
MD (Dermat) Special Fellowship in HIV and STD
Online Consultant
Dermatologist

NN Anand MBBS MD FRCP (Glasgow) FACP (USA)
Head
Department of General Medicine
Sree Balaji Medical College and Hospital
Chennai, Tamil Nadu, India

NR Rau
MBBS (JIPMER, Puducherry) MD (Medicine, PGI Chandigarh)
Professor and Head
Department of Medicine
Adarsha Super Specialty Hospital
Udupi, Karnataka, India

P Deepa MS MD
Senior Assistant Professor
Department of General Surgery
Government Medical College and ESI Hospital
Coimbatore, Tamil Nadu, India

Parvati Nandy MD (Medicine) FICP
Head
Department of Medicine
Sikkim Manipal Institution of Medical Sciences
Sikkim Manipal University
Gangtok, Sikkim, India

Contributors

Pavni Agrawal MD
Senior Resident
Department of Medicine
Sri Aurobindo Medical College and PG Institute
Indore, Madhya Pradesh, India

PK Krishnapriya DGO
Senior Divisional Medical Officer (Retd)
Department of Obstetrics and Gynecology
Southern Railways
Coimbatore, Tamil Nadu, India

Rajesh Kumar Jha MD (Medicine)
Professor and Head
Department of Medicine
Sri Aurobindo Medical College and PG Institute
Indore, Madhya Pradesh, India

Rajib Ratna Chaudhary
MBBS MD (General Medicine)
Professor and Head (Retd)
Department of Medicine
Nalanda Medical College and Hospital
Patna, Bihar, India

Reeta James MBBS MD (General Medicine)
Associate Professor
Department of General Medicine
KMCT Medical College
Kozhikode, Kerala, India

Rohit Kapoor MD FACC FACP FRCP
Medical Director
Department of Medicine
Carewell Heart and Super Specialty Hospital
Amritsar, Punjab, India

Rojana Tamang MBBS
Postgraduate Teacher
Department of Biochemistry
Sikkim Manipal Institute of Medical Sciences
Sikkim Manipal University
Gangtok, Sikkim, India

Rubi Dey MBBS MSc (Medical Physiology) PhD
Professor
Department of Physiology
Sikkim Manipal Institute of Medical Sciences
Sikkim Manipal University
Gangtok, Sikkim, India

S Prema MS (Ophthalmology) FVRS
Medical Consultant
Department of Ophthalmology
Aravind Eye Hospital
Coimbatore, Tamil Nadu, India

Sadanand R Shetty
DM (Cardiology) MD (Med) FACC FSCAI FACA (USA)
FCPS FISE FICC FICP FCSI FESC
Director
Department of Cardiology
KJ Somaiya Medical College and Research Center
Mumbai, Maharashtra, India
Emeritus Professor
DY Patil University School of Medicine
Navi Mumbai
CMD and Founder
Sadanand Healthy Living Center Ltd, Mumbai
Founder, Sadanand G2S2 Foundation, Mumbai
Member, American College of Cardiology and
European Society of Cardiology

Sarath Bhaskar S MD (General Medicine) CCEBDM
ACS Medical College and Hospital
Chennai, Tamil Nadu, India

Shahid Abbas MD
Professor
Department of General Medicine
Sri Aurobindo Medical College and
Postgraduate Institute
Indore, Madhya Pradesh, India

Shivam Kapoor MBBS MRCP
Medicine Specialist
Department of Medicine
Carewell Heart and Super Specialty Hospital
Amritsar, Punjab, India

Shivashankara KN MD FICP FIACM FIMSA
Professor
Department of Medicine
Kasturba Medical College
Manipal, Karnataka, India

Soumik Chaudhuri MD DM FSCAI
Clinical Lead and In-charge ICCU
Department of Cardiology
Peerless Hospital
Kolkata, West Bengal, India

Srishti Jha
PG Student
Department of Obstetrics and Gynecology
Sri Aurobindo Medical College and
Postgraduate Institute
Indore, Madhya Pradesh, India

Subhajeet Dey MBBS MS (Surgery)
Professor
Department of General Surgery
Nagaland Institute of Medical Sciences
and Research
Kohima, Nagaland, India

Toshi Tiwari MD
Assistant Professor
Department of Medicine
Sri Aurobindo Medical College and
Postgraduate Institute
Indore, Madhya Pradesh, India

Upasana Mohanty MBBS DNB (General Medicine)
Divisional Medical Officer
Department of General Medicine
Dr Babasaheb Ambedkar Memorial Hospital
Mumbai, Maharashtra, India

V Padma MD (Medicine) FRCP FACP
Professor
Department of Medicine
Sree Balaji Medical College
Chennai, Tamil Nadu, India

Vasili Pradeep MD
Assistant Professor
Department of General Medicine
ACSR Government Medical College and Hospital
Nellore, Andhra Pradesh, India

Viknesh Prabu Anbalagan
MD MRCP (London) MRCP (Edinburgh, UK)
Assistant Professor
Department of General Medicine
Sree Balaji Medical College
Chennai, Tamil Nadu, India

Virendra Chauhan 3rd year DrNB Nephrology
Resident Nephrology
DNB General Medicine
Institute of Renal Sciences
Global Hospitals
Mumbai, Maharashtra, India

Foreword

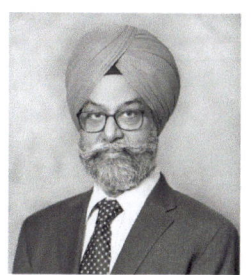

This is the best time to have a new *Hypertension Manual* from India since we have large amount of data from our own country in the last few years. We all know hypertension effects 28% of Indian adults. The disease is different in many aspects since it starts early and only 20% of urban and 10% of rural individuals have their blood pressure controlled. The book will inspire physicians of South Asia to break the inertia to treat patients effectively. There is greater emphasis on engaging patients in the care process. Home monitoring of blood pressure is being emphasized more and more. Dr A Muruganathan is the torch bearer in our country who has devoted a lot of time and effort in propagating the virtues of home monitoring. He has been spearheading hypertension control programs in many states and has a vast experience in management of hypertension and the processes by which we can make patients compliance better.

The recent developments and messages from some of the latest guidelines have been incorporated in this excellent manual and will update those who read this manual regarding the latest evidence base on this most common public health problem. The topics are very practical and reflect the focus on better management. The authors are some of the bests in the country on management of hypertension and I would like to congratulate each one of them for their excellent scientific contribution. The publisher of the book M/s Jaypee Brothers Medical Publishers (P) Ltd, New Delhi, India is the best in the country and as usual it has done an excellent job of editing and publishing this book. My best wishes to each and every reader of this manual and I hope that this book will go a long way to improve hypertension control statistics in our country.

Gurpreet S Wander
DM FACC FAMS
Professor
Department of Cardiology
Hero DMC Heart Institute, Ludhiana
Chairman, Research and Development Centre
Dayanand Medical College and Hospital
Ludhiana, Punjab, India
Director, Physicians Research Foundation—API)
Past President, Association of Physicians of India

Preface

As the landscape of cardiovascular health continues to evolve, so does the knowledge and understanding of hypertension—a condition of paramount significance in the realm of global public health.

Hypertension Manual has been a labor of love and commitment, aiming to bridge the gap between the ever-expanding body of research and the practical needs of healthcare professionals.

Hypertension as a Major Health Concern: This book underscores the significant impact of hypertension in India affecting millions of individuals and posing a substantial risk factor for various diseases.

Prevention and Control: Proper control of hypertension is emphasized as a crucial strategy to prevent a considerable number of deaths associated with the condition.

Awareness and Access to Health Care: We acknowledge the challenges related to awareness, treatment, and control of hypertension in India.

Updates and Changes: This book aims to provide updates and changes in the field of hypertension, reflecting the dynamic nature of medical knowledge. It continues to cover a broad-spectrum of topics, including epidemiology, pathophysiology, molecular basis, guidelines, evaluation, target organ damage, special conditions, therapeutic aspects, genetics, and meta-analysis. We continue our commitment to excellence, incorporating the latest advancements in hypertension research, diagnostic techniques, and therapeutic interventions. The global burden of hypertension persists, affecting millions of lives, and this book seeks to empower healthcare professionals in the fight against this silent epidemic.

May this book be a valuable companion to postgraduate students, junior doctors, seasoned clinicians, and all those dedicated to advancing the understanding and management of hypertension.

A Muruganathan
Bidita Khandelwal
Sadanand R Shetty

Acknowledgments

Acknowledgment of Contributors: I extend my heartfelt gratitude to the esteemed contributors—experts in the field, whose meticulous work ensures the content remains both comprehensive and accessible. Their unwavering support has been instrumental in the evolution of this manual.

My gratitude extends to the efforts of all contributors who have provided new information, making the manual a valuable reference for healthcare professionals, including Postgraduate Students, Junior Doctors, Clinicians, and Hypertension Specialists. My special thanks to Dr Sadanand R Shetty and Professor (Dr) Bidita Khandelwal.

Call to Action for Hypertension Specialists: There is a call for hypertension specialists to contribute to hypertension registries and conduct research suitable for the Indian context.

I also emphasized the need for more Hypertension clinics, Hypertension specialty centers and Hypertensionologists.

As hypertension specialists, educators, and researchers, I recognize the evolving nature of my field. It is my hope that this book serves as a dynamic resource, fostering a deeper understanding of hypertension, encouraging ongoing research, and ultimately contributing to improved patient outcomes.

Appreciation for the publishing team, special thanks is also due to the publishing team at M/s Jaypee Brothers Medical Publishers (P) Ltd, New Delhi, India, whose commitment to excellence has been evident at every stage of this project. Personal thanks are given to Shri Jitendar P Vij (Group Chairman), Mr Ankit Vij (Managing Director), Mr MS Mani (Group President), Ms Chetna Malhotra (Senior Director—Professional Publishing, Marketing, and Business Development), Ms Pooja Bhandari [Director—Production (Books and Journals)], and Ms Asmi Bharati (Development Editor).

Contents

SECTION 1: History and Epidemiology

1. **Historical Aspects of Hypertension** 3
   M Gowri Sankar, P Deepa, PK Krishnapriya

SECTION 2: Etiological and Pathophysiological Aspects (Pathogenesis)

2. **Overview of Various Pathogenic Mechanisms in Essential Hypertension** 13
   NN Anand, Viknesh Prabu Anbalagan
3. **Renin-Angiotensin-Aldosterone System in Hypertension** 27
   Rubi Dey, Bidita Khandelwal

SECTION 3: Molecular Basis of Hypertension

4. **Role of Cell Membrane (Red Blood Cells and Platelets) in Essential Hypertension** 35
   Arundhati Bag, Bidita Khandelwal, Abhishek Byahut
5. **Matrix Metalloproteinases and the Extracellular Matrix** 42
   Bidita Khandelwal, Chamma Gupta
6. **Role of Calcium Channels in Hypertension** 52
   Arundhati Bag, Bidita Khandelwal, Abhishek Byahut
7. **Role of Cytokines and Inflammation in Hypertension** 57
   Mingma Lhamu Sherpa, Lydia Rai, Bidita Khandelwal
8. **Natriuretic Peptides in Hypertension** 64
   Rubi Dey, Bidita Khandelwal
9. **Multiple Roles of Eicosanoids in Blood Pressure Regulation** 68
   Mingma Lhamu Sherpa, Rojana Tamang, Bidita Khandelwal

SECTION 4: Accuracy of Blood Pressure Measurement

10. **Correct Methodology of Blood Pressure Measurements** 77
    Boudhayan Das Munshi

11. **Home Blood Pressure Monitoring** 87
    A Muruganathan, E Cowshik

12. **Ambulatory Blood Pressure Monitoring** 94
    Parvati Nandy

13. **Central Aortic Blood Pressure: An Overview** 98
    Rohit Kapoor, Shivam Kapoor

SECTION 5: Evaluation of Hypertension

14. **Hypertension: Clinical Approach** 109
    M Chenniappan

15. **Hypertension: Electrocardiogram in Decision Making** 118
    M Chenniappan

SECTION 6: Target Organ Damage: Evaluation and Clinical Importance

16. **Hypertensive Retinopathy** 137
    N Vimal Kumar, S Prema

SECTION 7: Special Conditions and Situations

17. **Hypertensive Crisis** 145
    Reeta James

18. **Difficult to Control Hypertension (Resistance, Pseudoresistance, and Malignant Hypertension)** 151
    Ameet G Sattur, Sadanand R Shetty

19. **Hypertension in Pregnancy** 161
    Abhay Narain Rai, Mritunjay Kumar Singh

20. **Metabolic Syndrome and Hypertension** 167
    Chamma Gupta, Abhishek Byahut, Karma G Dolma

21. **White Coat Hypertension and Masked Hypertension** 174
    V Padma, Sarath Bhaskar S

22. **Perioperative Hypertension** 179
    Subhajeet Dey

23. **Blood Pressure Variability and Target Organ Damage** 184
    NR Rau, Shivashankara KN

24. Exercise and Hypertension 197
    Kannan Meera Devi, V Padma

25. Air Pollution and Hypertension 202
    Minakshi Dhar

26. Isolated Nocturnal Hypertension 206
    Geetha Subramanian, J Cecily Mary Majella

27. Resistant Hypertension 213
    NN Anand

28. Hypertension in Elderly 224
    Karma G Dolma, Chamma Gupta, Madhu Gupta

SECTION 8: Secondary Hypertension

29. Coarctation of Aorta 237
    Ankita Kulkarni, Sadanand R Shetty

30. Sleep Apnea and Hypertension 246
    Vasili Pradeep, Alladi Mohan

SECTION 9: Therapeutic Aspects: Pharmacologic and Nonpharmacologic Interventions

31. Angiotensin-converting Enzyme Inhibitors: What is New? 255
    Rajesh Kumar Jha, Toshi Tiwari, Srishti Jha

32. Angiotensin II Receptor Blockers: What is New? 260
    Rajesh Kumar Jha, Pavni Agrawal, Srishti Jha

33. Calcium Channel Blockers and Hypertension 267
    Rajesh Kumar Jha, Shahid Abbas, Srishti Jha

34. Diuretics and Hypertension 273
    Anita Jaiswal Ektate, Neeta Narang, Virendra Chauhan, Upasana Mohanty

35. Beta-blockers in Hypertension 278
    Chandrasekhar Valupadas

36. Alpha-blockers: Role in Hypertension 286
    Dilip A Kirpalani

37. Direct Vasodilators in Hypertension 290
    Rajib Ratna Chaudhary

38. Hypertensive Heart Disease 295
    Keyur R Rathod, Sadanand R Shetty

39. Emerging Antihypertensive Drugs 303
    Anant Ramkishanrao Munde, Sadanand R Shetty

40. Combination Therapy in Hypertension 325
    A Muruganathan

SECTION 10: Genetics and Hypertension

41. Genetic Approaches to Hypertension: Reverence to
    Human Hypertension 339
    Chamma Gupta, Abhishek Byahut, Bidita Khandelwal

SECTION 11: Interventional Interventions in Hypertension

42. Baroreceptor Stimulation and Hypertension 349
    Anjan Lal Dutta, Soumik Chaudhuri

SECTION 12: Guidelines and Meta-analysis

43. Comparison of Various Guidelines in Hypertension:
    Which is Best for India? 361
    Anant Ramkishanrao Munde, Sadanand R Shetty

SECTION 13: Miscellaneous

44. Lipid and Hypertension 381
    Aditi Parimoo, Sadanand R Shetty

45. Role of Vitamin D_3 and Hypertension 384
    Rajesh Kumar Jha, Srishti Jha

46. Telemedicine and Its Role in the Management of Resistant Hypertension 388
    Anant Ramkishanrao Munde, Sadanand R Shetty

47. Adherence to the Treatment for Hypertension 404
    Michaela M Watts, Fraz A Mir

48. Navigating Dilemmas in the Management of Hypertension:
    A Perpetual Challenge 416
    Alok Kumar Singh, Sadanand R Shetty

49. Hypertension Clinic and Hypertension Center 421
    A Muruganathan

Index *429*

PLATE 1

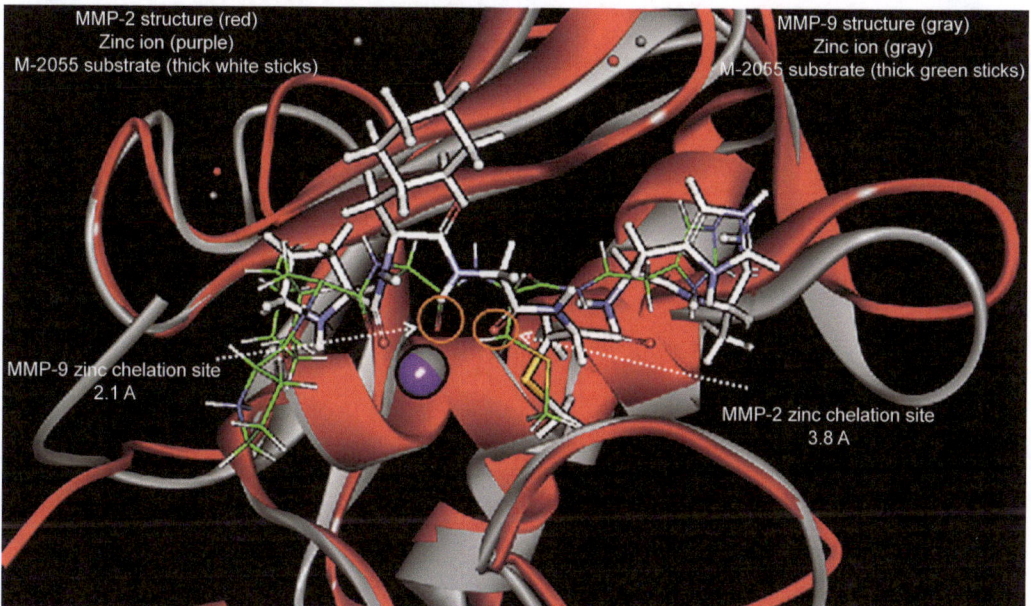

Fig. 1: Docked complexes of 1 substrate and the catalytic domain of human MMP-2 (PDB code, 1QIB) and MMP-9 (PDB code, 1GKC). The MMP-substrate docked complexes are merged with zinc as the same point of view. The MMP-2 structure is shown in red, zinc as purple, and 1 substrate (white sticks) docked within MMP-2 active site; MMP-9 is shown in gray, zinc as green and 1 substrate (thin green sticks) is docked within its active site. (Bottom) Schematic representation of 1 substrate: Active site binding interaction in human MMP-2 and MMP-9. MMP-2 and MMP-9 enzyme binding pockets are shown in red and green, respectively. The substrate's chemical structure and its scissile bond are shown in black. The zinc ion is indicated in blue. *(Chapter 5)*

PLATE 2

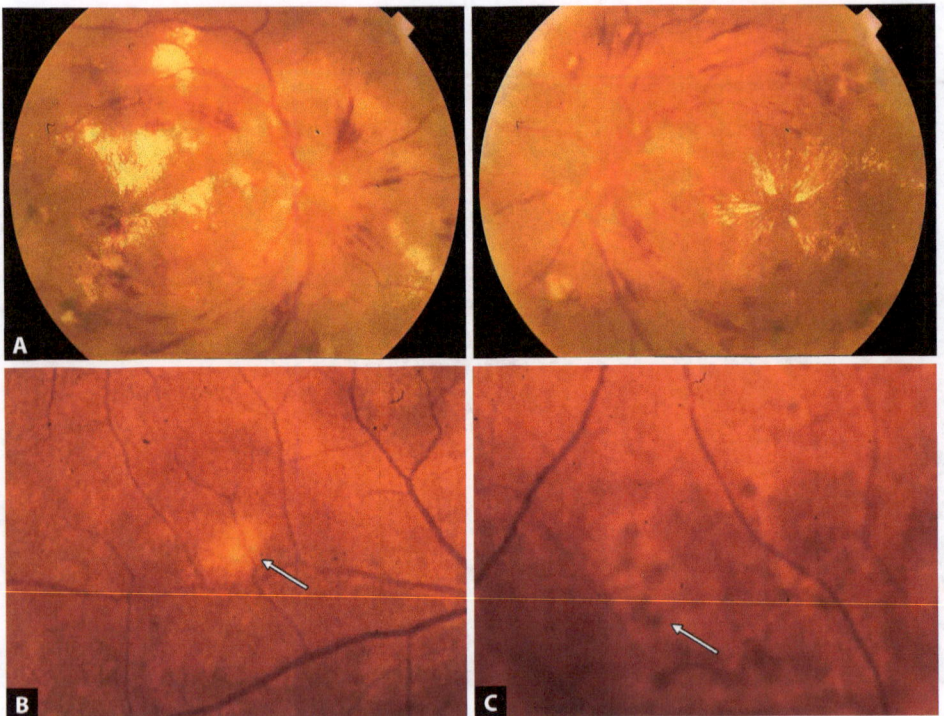

Figs. 1A to C: (A) Papilledema; (B) Elschnig's spots; (C) Siegrist's streak. *(Chapter 16)*

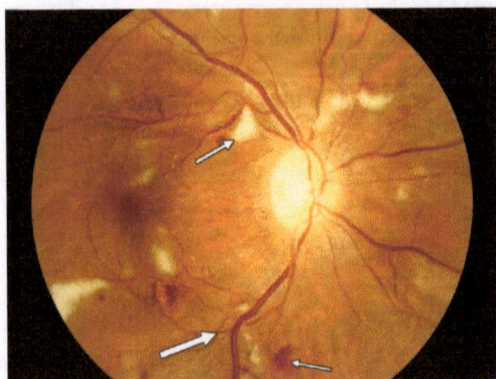

Fig. 2: Group 3 – white arrow points to exudates, bold white arrow points to AV crossing changes and the white arrow show retinal hemorrhages. *(Chapter 16)*

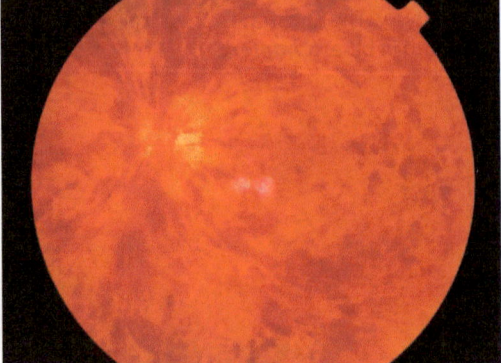

Fig. 3: Retinal vein occlusion. *(Chapter 16)*

PLATE 3

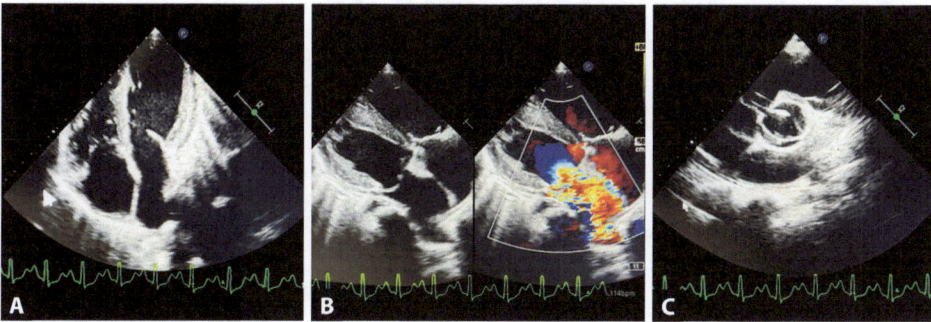

Figs. 1A to C: (A) and (B) Echocardiography of a 27-year-old male with coarctation of aorta and associated parachute mitral valve with severe mitral regurgitation; and (C) Bicuspid aortic valve. *(Chapter 29)*

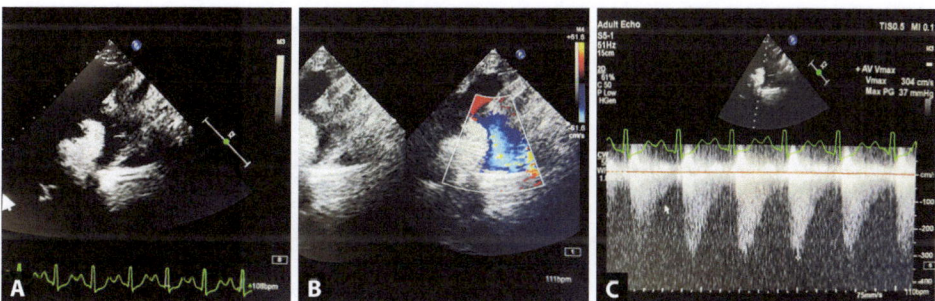

Figs. 2A to C: *Echocardiography*: (A) Suprasternal view showing a long segment coarctation; (B) Color Doppler across the narrowed segment showing turbulence across the coarctation segment; (C) Continuous Doppler across coarct segment. *(Chapter 29)*

PLATE 3

Figs. 1A to C(a) and (b) Photomicrographs of a 77 year old male with co-existence of adenoma and associated carcinoid of stomach (Ca) with severe atrophic gastritis (G) and IM (see inset – also, Chapter 23).

Figs. 2A to C. Photomicrographs (A) – upper half view showing glandular communication (arrow). (B) Colonic adenoma containing carcinoid fragments showing transition across the basement membrane (CT neoplasia) (inset). More on this in Chapter 23.

SECTION 1
History and Epidemiology

1. **Historical Aspects of Hypertension**
   M Gowri Sankar, P Deepa, PK Krishnapriya

SECTION

1

History and Epidemiology

1. Historical Aspects of Hypertension
   Through Human Disease, Harriet Dustan

CHAPTER 1

Historical Aspects of Hypertension

M Gowri Sankar, P Deepa, PK Krishnapriya

"Study the past if you would define the future"
—**Confucius (Chinese philosopher)**

◼ INTRODUCTION

History is an amalgamation of huge sacrifices, sufferings, trials, and failures. Also, it tells the tale for the next generations to analyze and explore science and its roots. Hypertension is an age-old disease, which has crossed a distant way and has challenged even the most famous medical practitioners for centuries. Moreover, there is a long list of physicians and experimenters who have spent their entire lives advancing blood pressure (BP) measuring techniques. As of now, the management of hypertension has become the astounding medical achievement anecdote of the twentieth century. Presently, BP instruments are feasible everywhere in the world but this instrument was invented in the late 19th century and it has taken around 200 years to get an accurate measurement of BP.

◼ HISTORICAL PERSPECTIVES ON HYPERTENSION[1,2]

The historical feature of hypertension goes back a long way from sage Maharishi Sushruta, who was the fundamental figure of Indian medicine and considered the "Father of Indian Medicine". He composed a book called *Sushruta Samhita*. This was one of the age-old treatises and the source of wisdom about medicine in ancient India. He elucidated medicine in a broader sense and displayed his extraordinary surgical skills and methods. He further advanced many special and practical techniques in dissections and studied the anatomy of the human body including the structure of the heart and its function in circulation. Moreover, he cited and narrated hritshoola (meaning heart pain), circulation of body fluids (blood as rakta dhatu, lymph as rasa dhatu), madhumeha (diabetes), obesity (medoroga) and hypertension as sira-kunchan and rakta-poornata and its symptom as vatarakta. Outstandingly, Sushruta characterized these conditions a few centuries before the Greek physician Hippocrates.

The sage Maharishi Patanjali, who lived in the second century BCE, authored the treatise on living tradition entitled Pathanjali's Yoga Sutra which is a foundation text of classical yoga philosophy. His discipline describes asanas (stretching exercises and body postures), pranayama (deep breathing exercises), and meditation. In the modern era, yoga appears to be a cost-effective complementary intervention for controlling prehypertension and hypertension.

HARD PULSE DISEASE[1-3]

In the ancient period, hypertension was identified only by the quality of the pulse. The traditional Tamil system of Siddha medicine also called "Siddha Vaidyam" originated between 10,000 and 4,000 BCE. The Siddhar saintly persons who attained eight supernatural powers laid the foundation for this traditional medicine. Subsequently, a wrist pulse reading called the Naadi method was developed by the Siddha practitioners of the past which became the window for the cardiovascular system. They named hard pulse disease "Kuruthi azhal noi" and described its clinical presentation and complications. Also, advocated salt and sour diet restrictions, asanas, meditation, and some compound preparations by using medicinal plants to treat the illness.

Furthermore, the early history related to hypertension was portrayed in the textbook *Classics in Arterial Hypertension*, which was published in 1956 by Professor Dr Arthur Ruskin, University of Texas. In his book, he highlighted the ancient Chinese medical textbook called *Yellow Emperor's Classic of Medicine* dated as early as 2,600 BCE which stated that "The consumption of excess salt in food will harden the pulse". Also, the relationship between hypertension and congestive heart failure was stated "When the pulse is abundant but tense and hard like a cord there are dropsical swellings (severe generalized edema)".

Earlier, the ancient Egyptian physicians in the Ebers Papyrus (1,550 BCE) described the relationship between the palpated pulse and the development of heart and brain disease. In addition, Hippocrates (460–370 BCE) revealed that sudden death occurred more commonly in obese people than in the lean.

Subsequently, the Roman patrician Cornelius Celsus (25 BC–50 AD) was much concerned with the pulse in his days and he explained that "The increase in heart rate and tense pulse with exercise, emotion, and even physician's arrival (which we call 'White-coat effect' today)".

In ancient times, the hard pulse disease was treated by venesection, bleeding by leeches, and acupuncture methods. These methods were advocated by the Yellow Emperor of China, Hippocrates, Celsus, and Galen.

However, the modern history of hypertension began with the work of English physician William Harvey (1578–1657), who described the fundamentals of circulation that blood circulates in the body in one direction. In 1628, he published a book titled *On the Motion of the Heart and Blood in Animals*, which explained the above-stated fundamentals through his scientific and experimental methods which later became a remarkable milestone in medicine.

EVOLUTION OF BLOOD PRESSURE MEASUREMENTS[3-5]

Stephen Hales (1677–1761), an English clergyman, gave the first description of measurement of the force of the blood (BP) in the modern era. In 1733, he carried out the catheterization of a live horse by inserting fine tubes into the carotid artery and measured the BP by assessing the rise in a column of blood in a glass tube of 9' 6" in height initially and which gradually fell. Thus, he demonstrated that the amount of pressure generated by the heart could be measured through the displacement of blood.

Jean Louis Poiseuille (1797–1869), a French physiologist, dedicated himself to research during the early 17th century with the invention of the U-tube mercury manometer. He called the mercury instrument as hydrodynamometer. By using this, he greatly reduced the height of the column needed for measuring BP. Thereupon, he measured the pressures in the arteries of horses and dogs by inserting a hollow tube into the artery and attaching it to a manometer on another end. He then identified the BP by measuring the amount of mercury displacement. Moreover, he was the first one who introduced the "mm Hg" units and explained the physics of blood flow in small vessels by Poiseuille's equation in 1846.

Karl von-Vierordt (1818-1884), a German physiologist, was the first to develop a noninvasive technique to estimate BP by using his newly invented sphygmograph in 1854. His instrument was made up of weights and levers through which he postulated that "To measure the BP accurately, it is necessary to stop the pulse". He did this by applying weight (counter pressure) on an artery and obliterated the radial arterial pulse. Furthermore, he published his investigation titled *A Treatise on the Arterial Pulse*.

Etienne Jules Marey (1830-1904), a French physiologist, upgraded the von Vierordt cumbersome sphygmograph to a wearable sphygmograph to measure BP. He refined the technique to measure BP by enclosing the arm in a water-filled glass chamber and increasing the water pressure until no circulation occurred.

Karl Samuel Ritter von Basch (1837-1905), an Austrian physiologist, created a new device called the sphygmomanometer and further introduced the aneroid manometer for the measurement of BP. Here, he placed a rubber bag around a manometer bulb and inflated it with water. As the water pressure increased, the mercury in the manometer was displaced enabling the measurement of the pressure. The bag was placed over the distal pulse and inflated until the pulse stopped being felt and the pressure at that point was noted as the systolic pressure.

Pierre Potain (1825-1901), a French cardiologist, contributed enormously to the field of cardiology. He was also credited for his significant modifications done in the sphygmomanometer by using air rather than water in the compressed bag.

Scipione Riva-Rocci (1863-1937), an Italian physician, is best known for his invention and initiation of an easy-to-use upper arm cuff-based mercury sphygmomanometer for measuring brachial BP in 1896. He developed the apparatus by using copper pipes, bicycle tubes, and a mercury barometer and he also designed an inflatable rubber cuff to encircle the arm. He further did palpation of the radial artery and measured the peak systolic BP by observing the cuff pressure at which there was a disappearance of the radial pulse on palpation. During 1896 and 1897, he published a series of four articles regarding his new method of BP measurement. Sir Harvey Cushing, an American neurosurgeon, was an early adopter of the Riva-Rocci mercury sphygmomanometer. He successfully used his apparatus to monitor his patients during anesthesia and surgery at Johns Hopkins Hospital, Baltimore, MD, USA.

Heinrich von Recklinghausen (1867-1942), a German physician, popularized the aneroid manometer which had a double cuff, the upper 5 cm cuff overlapping the lower 10 cm cuff encircling the arm connected to a single bulb to measure the BP.

Nikolai Korotkoff (1874-1920), a Russian surgeon, further proceeded to improvise the Riva-Rocci–von Recklinghausen inflatable cuff by attaching it to a stethoscope. In 1905, he invented the auscultatory technique for BP measurement. By applying a cuff on the upper arm and slowly deflating it, he described both the appearance and disappearance of sounds over the brachial artery and it is measured as systolic and diastolic BP. Since this method was found to be easy and accurate, it was considered as a "gold standard" for BP measurement.

GROWTH OF KNOWLEDGE IN HYPERTENSION[3-5]

In the 18th and 19th Century

Thomas Young (1773-1829), a British polymath and a physician, made a significant contribution to hemodynamics by measuring the fall in BP in dogs from the aorta to mesenteric arteries. Subsequently, he derived a formula for the wave speed of the pulse and stated that the quality of the arterial pulsation depended on the force of the heart. He further presented his experimental research, the *"Functions of the Heart and Arteries"*, in the Croonian lecture in 1808.

Richard Bright (1789-1858), a British physician who was known as the "Father of Nephrology", brought his various observations such as albuminuria, hardening of the pulse, and dropsy (severe generalized edema) with hardening of the kidneys, together named as "Bright's disease". In 1836, he further observed and linked the hypertrophy of the left ventricle with advanced kidney disease.

Additionally, a British physician, Sir Samuel Wilks (1824-1911), correlated both clinical and pathological findings and described the cases of hardening of arteries with contracted kidney (Bright's disease) and also hardening of arteries with cardiac hypertrophy without the presence of kidney disease in 1853. In 1872, two British physicians, Sir William Gull and Dr HG Sutton, proposed the pathological findings of Bright's disease by observing the generalized hyaline fibrinoid deposits in arterioles and capillaries.

Dr Frederick Akbar Mahomed (1849-1884), an Indian-origin Irish physician, was strongly influenced by the previous work of Richard Bright. Moreover, he modified the device sphygmograph while he was a medical student. By using his quantitative sphygmogram, he measured the arterial tension in "Troy ounces" and published his modified instrument in 1872. Subsequently, he was the first to report the elevation of BP in a patient without evidence of kidney disease, which he assessed by measuring proteins in urine. Furthermore, he was the first one who correlated the pathological effects of elevated BP and its postmortem changes such as cardiac hypertrophy, thickening of the arterial wall, aneurysm formation, and arteriocapillary fibrosis. He then described it as "high-pressure diathesis". Additionally, he explained the characteristics of pulse in patients with elevated BP and in persons with arteriosclerosis consequent on aging.

William Gowers (1845-1915), a British neurologist, was the greatest clinical neurologist of all time and an early adopter of the ophthalmoscope for systemic diseases. He gave a clear description of the constricted retinal vessels in relation to hypertension in 1876.

Sir Thomas Clifford Allbutt (1836-1925), an English physician, who was well known for his invention of the clinical thermometer. He also disclosed the concept of hypertensive disease as a generalized circulatory disease in 1896 and he called the disease "hyperpiesia" a term that continued to use in England until 1930. In his textbook *Diseases of the Arteries, Including Angina Pectoris* (1915), he exhibited the role of excessive salt, stress, and anxiety in elevating BP.

In the Early 20th Century[3-6]

The term "essential hypertension" (Essentielle Hypertonie) was coined by German physician Eberhard Frank in 1911. He was the first one to describe that "Hypertension occurs without any other obvious cause".

Theodore Caldwell Janeway (1872–1917), an American physician, was the first full-time professor of medicine in the United States. He collaborated with Sir Harvey Cushing, who was one of the supporters of the sphygmomanometer. They both researched together about hypertension and mainly focused on determining the accurate apparatus and a range of normal values for BP. In 1913, they described the varied course of hypertension and called the disorder as "Hypertensive Cardiovascular Disease".

In 1928, another term named "malignant hypertension" was coined by Mayo Clinic physicians, who described that high BP causes organ damage and eventually death.

Even in the early 20th century, physicians have not recognized the need for aggressive management of hypertension. Dr Paul Dudley White (1886–1973) who was an American cardiologist and a prominent advocate of preventive medicine said that "Hypertension may be an important compensatory mechanism that should not be tampered with, even where it is certain that we could control it ..." which has been proved by his quote.

However, the impact of untreated hypertension came to public attention only after the ill effect on American President Franklin D Roosevelt. The President Roosevelt's physician gave a clean chit of health with documented BP of 200/100. While at the Yalta conference held in Russia in February 1945, Winston Churchill's physician recorded President Roosevelt's BP of 260/150 and further noted his signs and symptoms of cardiac failure. Unfortunately, on 12 April, 1945, President Roosevelt had a severe occipital headache followed by loss of consciousness with a BP of 300/190 and ultimately had a fatal hemorrhagic stroke. Finally, his death brought hypertension as a deadly malady to the limelight.[5]

Three years later from President Roosevelt's death, American President Harry S Truman signed the "National Heart Act" which created a new path for several cardiac studies including Framingham Heart Study. Before Framingham's studies, nothing was known about the epidemiology of hypertension or atherosclerotic cardiovascular disease. Consequently, this study introduced the term "risk factor" which clearly showed that hypertension and hyperlipidemia are risk factors associated with cardiovascular morbidities and lead to premature deaths and also the need for therapeutic intervention.

Low-salt Diets

The nonpharmacological methods to treat hypertension came to light through Ambard and Beaujard, who were medical students from France. They discovered the direct relationship between sodium chloride retention and hypertension in 1904 and they both were credited for the salt and BP hypothesis. Later in 1922, Allen and Sherrill's case report suggest that patients with hypertension had a clinical benefit from a salt-restricted diet. However, the use of a low-salt diet in the treatment of hypertensive patients became popular in 1940.

Surgical Sympathectomy

In 1923, the first surgical sympathectomy for hypertension was done by the surgeon Fritz Bruening based on the hypothesis that a reduction of sympathetic outflow will lead to a reduction in BP. The experience with surgical sympathectomy paved the way for the development of drugs causing chemical sympathectomy by ganglion-blocking agents such as tetraethylammonium chloride, hexamethonium pentaquine, bretylium, and others.

■ BEGINNING OF THE DRUG ERA[3-8]

Before the Second World War, there were no effective antihypertensive drugs. Sodium thiocyanate was the first chemical used by two German scientists, Gustav Adolph Treupel and Albert Edinger, in 1900. However, the drug was poorly tolerated due to its toxicity.

In 1927, Professor Salimuzzaman Siddiqui, after completing his PhD at Frankfurt University, Germany started his research career at the Ayurvedic and Unani Tibbia College and Hospital in Delhi. He successfully extracted nine distinct alkaloids from the dried root of Rauwolfia serpentina (Indian snakeroot) which was known as "Sarpaganda" in the ancient Indian medicine. This root has been used for centuries in India for the treatment of insanity as well as for fever and snakebites. At the same time, the two Calcutta physicians, Dr Kartick Chandra Bose and Dr Gananath Sen, have independently reported on the use of Rauwolfia alkaloid extract in treating hypertension. They also collaborated with Dr RN Chopra, who was the father of Indian Pharmacology, and published an article titled "Rauwolfia serpentine, a New Indian Drug for Insanity and Blood Pressure", in 1931.

Thereafter, Dr Rustom Jal Vakil, who earned his medical degree from the University of London in 1938 returned to India and undertook clinical research on patients with hypertension by using alkaloid extracts of Rauwolfia. After 10 years of research, he published his historical case study on the use of Rauwolfia therapy in hypertension which appeared in the *British Heart Journal* in 1949. Based on his work, in 1952, the pure crystalline form of reserpine was isolated from Rauwolfia by the scientists of the Swiss Pharmaceutical Company and it became the first effective antihypertensive drug. Dr Vakil's epoch-making discovery was widely recognized in the Western medicine and he the first Indian to be awarded the "International Albert Lasker Award" in 1959.

Also, a breakthrough in the treatment of hypertension occurred after the introduction of chlorothiazide in 1958, which was achieved by the scientists of the American pharmaceutical company Merck & Co. In 1964, a landmark first multicentric trial was organized by America's health research named "Veterans Administration Study Group", which compared the active treatment group (hydrochlorothiazide plus reserpine and hydralazine) versus placebo in treating hypertensive patients. The study reported that "Antihypertensive drugs were found more beneficial in lowering moderate-to-severe hypertension with a remarkable decrease in the incidence of mortality and cardiovascular events". To honor their remarkable work, the "Lasker Special Public Health Award" was presented to the team in 1975.

At the same time, the Scottish physician Dr James Black showed interest in finding the effects of adrenaline on the heart and initiated the development of beta (β) blockers. The drug propranolol was introduced into clinical practice for angina and then turned out to lower the BP. Eventually, β-blockers heralded a new era in pharmacology and his groundbreaking work was honored with the "Albert Lasker Award" in 1976 and with the most prestigious "Nobel Prize in Medicine" in 1988. In addition, the English scientists Prichard and Gillam were the first one to demonstrate the effectiveness of β-blockers in hypertension.

Dr Albrecht Fleckenstein was a German pharmacologist who contributed to the discovery of calcium channel blockers.

He described that the drug verapamil acts as a calcium antagonist in 1964. He further coined the term calcium antagonist and its inhibitory actions of excitation-contraction coupling. He subsequently identified nifedipine, a dihydropyridine to lower the BP.

Development of Angiotensin-converting Enzyme Inhibitors[6,7]

The first step in the development of angiotensin-converting enzyme (ACE) inhibitors was started with the serendipitous discovery of ACE in plasma by the American Biochemist Leonard T Skeggs in 1956. In 1967, Kevin KF Ng and John Vane (Nobel Prize winner in 1982 for his work on Aspirin) showed plasma ACE is too slow to account for the conversion of angiotensin I to angiotensin II (a potent vasoconstrictor) in vivo. Subsequently, their investigation showed that rapid conversion occurs during its passage through the pulmonary circulation. Further, in 1968, John Vane proved that the vasoactive properties of peptides isolated from the venom of Brazilian pit viper (Bothrops jararaca) inhibits the activity of ACE and thereby it blocks the conversion of angiotensin I to angiotensin II. Then, John Vane suggested ACE as a target for hypertension research.

Furthermore, the American chemist Dr David Cushman, Dr Miguel Ondetti, and his colleagues at The Squibb Institute for Medical Research, United States advanced their studies on venom peptide analogs and created the first ACE Inhibitor captopril in 1975. The drug captopril was approved by the United States Food and Drug Administration in 1981 and entered into the antihypertensive armamentarium. Later in 1995, another class of drugs angiotensin II receptor blocker (ARB) named Losartan was launched followed by Renin Inhibitor named Aliskiren was introduced into the clinical practice in 2000 to control hypertension.

World Hypertension League

The World Hypertension League, an umbrella to organizations of 85 national hypertension societies and leagues, was launched in 2005 to create a global awareness campaign. It has been declared on 17 May of each year as "World Hypertension Day".

■ CONCLUSION

Noi naadi noi mudhal naadi athuthanikkum Vai naadi vaippachcheyal
—**Tamil saint Thiruvalluvar**

The meaning of which is as follows:
"Diagnose the disease, detect its root cause, Seek the proper remedy and apply it with skill"

Hypertension, an ancient disease with a long journey has been challenging the physicians for centuries and many physicians and scientists have invested their whole life in its research. The management strategies keep evolving continuously over time. Nowadays, BP apparatus are feasible everywhere in the world but it has taken around 200 years to get an accurate measurement of BP. Today, it will take less than 2 minutes for the measurement of BP and it needs no excuse for not measuring it.

■ REFERENCES

1. Sankar MG, Historical aspects of hypertension. In: Muruganathan BA (Ed). Manual of Hypertension, 2nd edition, New Delhi: Jaypee Brothers Medical Publishers (P) Ltd; 2020. pp. 3-9.
2. Bansal A. India's contribution to medical science. [online] Available from: https://indiamedicalscience.blogspot.com/ [Last accessed November, 2023].

3. Harold JG. (2017). Historical perspectives on hypertension. Cardiology Magazine. [online] Available from: https://www.acc.org/latest-in-cardiology/articles/2017/11/14/14/42/harold-on-history-historical-perspectives-on-hypertension [Last accessed November, 2023].
4. Freis ED. Historical development of antihypertensive treatment. In: Laragh JH, Brenner BM (Eds). Hypertension: Pathophysiology, Diagnosis, and Management, 2nd edition. New York: Raven Press Ltd; 1995, pp. 2741-51.
5. Wikipedia (online) Available from www.wikipedia.com [Last Accessed December 2023]
6. Saklayen MJ, Deshpande NV. Timeline of history of hypertension treatment. Front Cardiovasc Med. 2016;3:3.
7. Bryan J. From snake venom to ACE inhibitor: The discovery and rise of captopril. Pharma J. 2009; 282(7548):455-56.
8. Roy P. Global pharma and local science: The untold tale of reserpine. Indian J Psychiatry. 2018;60(6):277-83.

SECTION 2
Etiological and Pathophysiological Aspects (Pathogenesis)

2. **Overview of Various Pathogenic Mechanisms in Essential Hypertension**
   NN Anand, Viknesh Prabu Anbalagan

3. **Renin-Angiotensin-Aldosterone System in Hypertension**
   Rubi Dey, Bidita Khandelwal

CHAPTER 2

Overview of Various Pathogenic Mechanisms in Essential Hypertension

NN Anand, Viknesh Prabu Anbalagan

■ INTRODUCTION

Hypertension [persistent elevation of arterial blood pressure (BP)] is one of the leading causes of the following diseases:[1-3]
1. Global burden of diseases (GBDs)
2. Preventable causes of cardiovascular diseases (CVDs)

The definition and classification of hypertension have been evolving over the years.[1] Epidemiological (observational) studies have shown that in adults, the risk for CVD, stroke, and renal disease is continuous and incremental across levels of systolic blood pressure (SBP) and diastolic blood pressure (DBP).[2,4] In a meta-analysis of 61 studies, the mortality due to ischemic heart disease (IHD) and stroke was directly related to the height of the BP, from a value of 115/75 mm Hg, in subjects aged 40–89 years; no threshold level of BP was noted.[2,5]

> The risk for CVD increases 2-fold with every 20 mm Hg rise in SBP and 10 mm Hg rise in DBP.[2]

In another study involving 1.25 million patients aged ≥30 years, and initially free from CVD (one-fifth of these patients were receiving BP-lowering treatments), the lowest risk for CVD was noted in subjects with SBP of 90–114 mm Hg and DBP of 60–74 mm Hg, with no evidence of a J-shaped increased risk at lower BP levels.[5]

From a clinical viewpoint, hypertension is defined as the level of BP at which treatment of BP (either with lifestyle interventions or drugs) reduces the BP-related mortality risk.[2,6]

From the foregoing, it can be seen that it is difficult to delineate a distinction between normotension and hypertension, based on cut-off values of BP.[6]

■ DEFINING HYPERTENSION

Despite the existence of a linear relationship between BP and CVD risk, it is necessary to establish different categories of BP levels to facilitate clinical and public health decision making.[4] Previously, all the guidelines defined hypertension as SBP ≥140 mm Hg and/or DBP ≥90 mm Hg. Currently, the American guidelines have defined hypertension as SBP values of 130 mm Hg or more and/or DBP >80 mm Hg **(Table 1)**.[1,2,4] This categorization was arrived at based on observational data related to the association between SBP/DBP and CVD risk as well as findings from randomized controlled trials (RCTs) of lifestyle modification to lower BP, and RCTs of treatment with antihypertensive medication to prevent CVD.[4]

The European guidelines, Indian guidelines, as well as the guidelines by the International Society of Hypertension have, however, recommended the cut-off values of ≥140/90 mm Hg **(Table 1)** for defining hypertension.[6-9] The terminologies used to categorize BP and hypertension in various guidelines vary substantially, as can be seen in **Table 1**.

SECTION 2: Etiological and Pathophysiological Aspects (Pathogenesis)

TABLE 1: Categorization of BP in adults: Defining cut-offs for hypertension in different guidelines.[4,6,8,9]

BP category	BP (mm Hg)	ACC/AHA (2017)[4]	ESC/ESH (2018)[6,*,†]	Indian (2019)[8]	ISH (2020)[9]
Optimal	SBP	NA	<120	<120	NA
	DBP		<80	<80	
Normal	SBP	<120	120–129	<130	<130
	DBP	<80	80–84	<85	<85
High normal[¶]	SBP	NA	130–139	130–139	130–139
	DBP		85–89	85–89	85–89
Elevated	SBP	120–129	NA	NA	NA
	DBP	<80			
Hypertension Stage[ǁ] 1/Grade 1	SBP	130–139	140–159	140–159	140–159
	DBP	80–89	90–99	90–99	90–99
Hypertension Stage 2/Grade 2	SBP	≥140	160–179	160–179	≥160
	DBP	≥90	100–109	100–109	≥100
Hypertension Stage 3/Grade 3	SBP	NA	≥180	≥180	NA
	DBP		≥110	>110	
Isolated systolic hypertension	SBP	≥160[§]	≥140	140–159[‡]	≥140
	DBP	≤90, ≤95, or ≤110	<90	<90	<90

(ACC: American College of Cardiology; AHA: American Heart Association; BP: blood pressure; SBP: systolic blood pressure; DBP: diastolic blood pressure; ESC: European Society of Cardiology; ESH: European Society of Hypertension; ISH: International Society of Hypertension; NA: not applicable in the selected guideline; RCTs: randomized controlled trials)
*Seated clinic BP.
†Isolated systolic hypertension is graded 1, 2, or 3 according to SBP values in the ranges indicated.
‡Grade 1; Grade 2 is SBP ≥160 and DBP <90.
§As defined in RCTs.
ǁISH guidelines, hypertension is classified as Grades 1, 2, etc.
¶High-normal BP helps identify individuals who could benefit from lifestyle interventions and in whom pharmacological treatment is needed if compelling indications are present.

EPIDEMIOLOGY OF HYPERTENSION

Fast Facts on Hypertension[10]
- About 46% of adults with hypertension are unaware that they have high BP.
- About two-thirds of the people with hypertension belong to the low- and middle-income countries.
- Less than half of the adults (42%) with hypertension are diagnosed and treated.
- Only about 1 in 5 adults (21%) with hypertension have their BP under control.

Global Scenario

Hypertension, defined as BP ≥140/90 mm Hg and/or current use of antihypertensive

CHAPTER 2: Overview of Various Pathogenic Mechanisms in Essential Hypertension

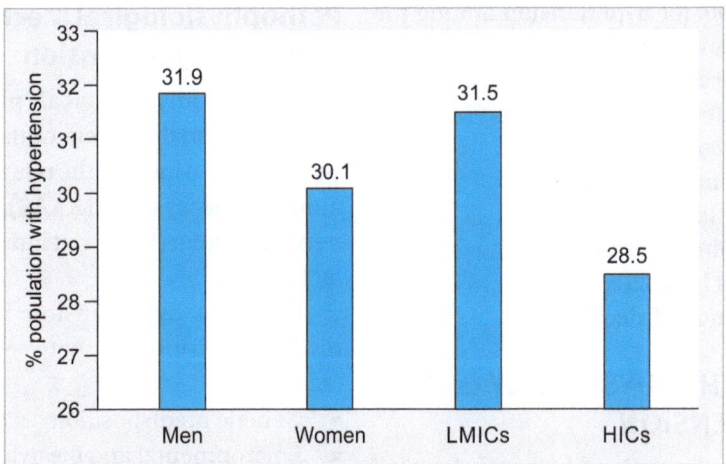

Fig. 1: Age-standardized prevalence of hypertension in population-based studies.[3*]
*Based on analysis of data from 135 population-based studies, n = 968,419 adults from 90 countries. (LMICs: low- and middle-income countries; HICs: high-income countries)

medication, was reported to affect 1.39 billion adults, equivalent to 31.1% of the global adult population as per 2010 statistics. The prevalence of hypertension was slightly higher among men compared to women and higher in low- and middle-income countries (LMICs) compared to high-income countries (HICs, **Fig. 1**). Between 2000 and 2010, the global age-standardized prevalence of hypertension in adults aged ≥20 years increased by 5.2%, with the LMICs showing a rise and HICs showing a decline in the prevalence of hypertension.[3]

There is a general rise in the prevalence of hypertension globally, consequent to the rise in the aging population; unhealthy lifestyle (increased salt intake, low potassium intake, sedentary lifestyle, etc.).[3]

Indian Scenario

In India, hypertension imposes a significant public health impact on cardiovascular health and healthcare systems.[11]

A systematic review and meta-analysis of studies evaluating the prevalence, awareness, and control of hypertension among Indian patients was undertaken. The findings of this analysis are summarized in **Table 2**.[11]

TABLE 2: Prevalence of hypertension in India.[11]

Population	Prevalence (%)	
Overall prevalence	29.8	
Rural population	27.6	
Urban population	33.8	
Regional prevalence data (%)		
Region	Rural	Urban
East	31.7	34.5
West	18.1	35.8
North	14.5	28.8
South	21.1	31.8
Estimated prevalence of awareness, treatment, and control of BP (%)		
Parameter	Rural	Urban
Awareness	25.3	42
Treatment	25.1	37.6
BP control	10.7	20.2

(BP: blood pressure)

The risk factors for hypertension among the Indian population were:[11]
- Advancing age
- Smoking and oral consumption of khaini and tobacco
- Extra salt intake in food
- Sedentary lifestyle
- Central obesity and body mass index (BMI) of at least 25 kg/m^2
- Consumption of alcohol

ETIOPATHOPHYSIOLOGY OF HYPERTENSION

Depending on the etiology, hypertension may be classified into the following categories:[12,13]
- *Essential or primary hypertension:* There is no clearcut etiological factor to explain the raised BP—seen in 95% of the patients with hypertension.
- *Secondary hypertension:* Specific identifiable causes **(Table 3)** are noted in these patients, who account for 5% of all patients with hypertension.

Pathophysiological Mechanisms of Essential Hypertension

Numerous physiological processes that regulate normal BP were outlined in the last section. These include the renin-angiotensin-aldosterone system (RAAS), sympathetic nervous system (SNS), salt intake, endothelial factors, etc.

Essential hypertension is believed to result from an interplay between the following factors:[12]
- Genetic predisposition
- Environmental and lifestyle factors
- Derangement in normal BP regulatory mechanisms

Essential hypertension is characterized by an inappropriate increase in peripheral vascular resistance (PVR) relative to the cardiac output (CO). Raised PVR is a consequence of the remodeling of small arteries (arterioles), characterized by an increase in their media/lumen ratio. Stiffness of

TABLE 3: Causes of secondary hypertension.[13]

Renal	*Endocrine*	*Medications*
• Parenchymal kidney disease • Polycystic kidney disease • Systemic sclerosis (scleroderma) • Page kidney • Mutations in the genes encoding ion-transport proteins	• Conn's syndrome (hyperaldosteronism) • Cushing's syndrome (hypercortisolism) • Pheochromocytoma • Thyroid disease • Acromegaly • Hypercalcemia • Intake of licorice • Mutations in steroid gene regulatory domains	• NSAIDs • Corticosteroids • Calcineurin inhibitors • Stimulants • Decongestants • Tyrosine kinase inhibitors • Angiogenesis inhibitors • Estrogens • Alcohol • Cocaine • Gemcitabine • MAO inhibitors • Atypical antipsychotics • Erythropoietin
Vascular	*Autonomic*	*Others*
• Renal artery stenosis • Coarctation of aorta	• Stress • Neurogenic	• Obstructive sleep apnea • Pregnancy

(MAO: monoamine oxidase; NSAIDs: nonsteroidal anti-inflammatory drugs)

the large conduit arteries (i.e., the aorta) leads to the development of systolic hypertension.[12]

The role of RAAS, SNS activation, salt intake, and metabolic factors such as obesity and insulin resistance in essential hypertension have been investigated thoroughly.[12,14] Other aspects that have been examined in recent years include genetics, endothelial dysfunction [as seen in alterations in endothelin (ET) and nitric oxide (NO)], low birth weight and intrauterine nutrition, and neurovascular abnormalities **(Box 1)**.[14]

BOX 1: Physiological mechanisms involved in the development of essential hypertension.[14]

- Cardiac output (CO)
- Peripheral resistance
- Renin-angiotensin-aldosterone system (RAAS)
- Autonomic nervous system
- Other factors:
  – Bradykinin
  – Endothelin (ET)
  – Endothelial-derived relaxing factor (EDRF) or nitric oxide (NO)
  – Atrial natriuretic peptide (ANP)
  – Ouabain

Cardiac Output and Peripheral Resistance

Elevated CO, PVR, or both together can cause high BP. While PVR is regulated by smooth muscle cells from small arteries and arterioles, CO is influenced by stroke volume and heart rate **(Fig. 2)**. Activation of SNS (e.g., by drop in BP) causes the release of adrenal medullary hormones noradrenaline and adrenaline and stimulation of the SNS. This results in increased PVR and CO (due to enhanced cardiac contractility), which raises BP.[15]

The contraction of smooth muscle cells may be related to an increase in intracellular calcium concentration. This mechanism may explain the vasodilatory impact of calcium channel-blocking medications. Prolonged smooth muscle constriction induces structural changes, presumably mediated by angiotensin, that result in an irreversible increase in PVR. In very early hypertension, the increase in BP is driven by an increase in CO, which is related to sympathetic overactivity. The ensuing increase in PVR may emerge as a compensatory mechanism to prevent the

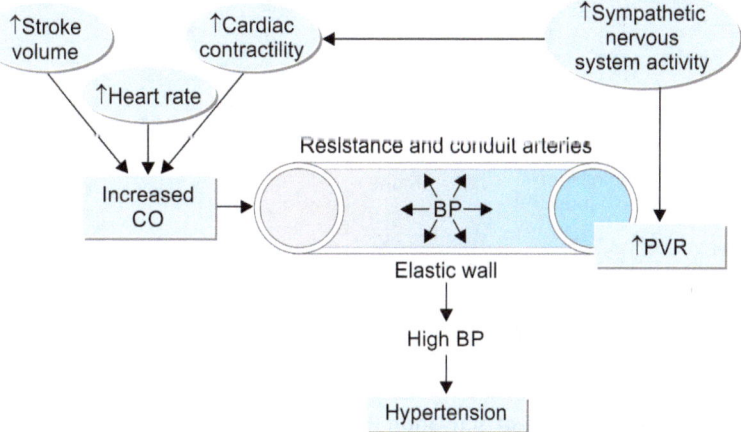

Fig. 2: Relationship of BP to CO and PVR.[15]
(BP: blood pressure; CO: cardiac output; PVR: peripheral vascular resistance)

increased pressure from being conveyed to the capillary bed, where it would significantly impact cell homeostasis.[14]

Renin-Angiotensin System

The RAAS, whose primary effector molecules are angiotensin 2 and aldosterone, is vital in BP control **(Fig. 3)**.[16] The RAAS is active locally in tissues as well as throughout the circulation. Also, the angiotensin 1 receptor (AT_1) and angiotensin 2 receptor (AT_2) are the two main angiotensin receptors. Angiotensin 2 primarily acts through the AT_1 receptor. The AT_2 receptor is less widely expressed than the AT_1 receptor, and its activation appears to cause consequences that contradict those of AT_1 activation.[2,12]

Angiotensin 2

Angiotensin 2 causes an increase in BP by several different mechanisms **(Fig. 4)**. Angiotensin 2 causes end-organ damage

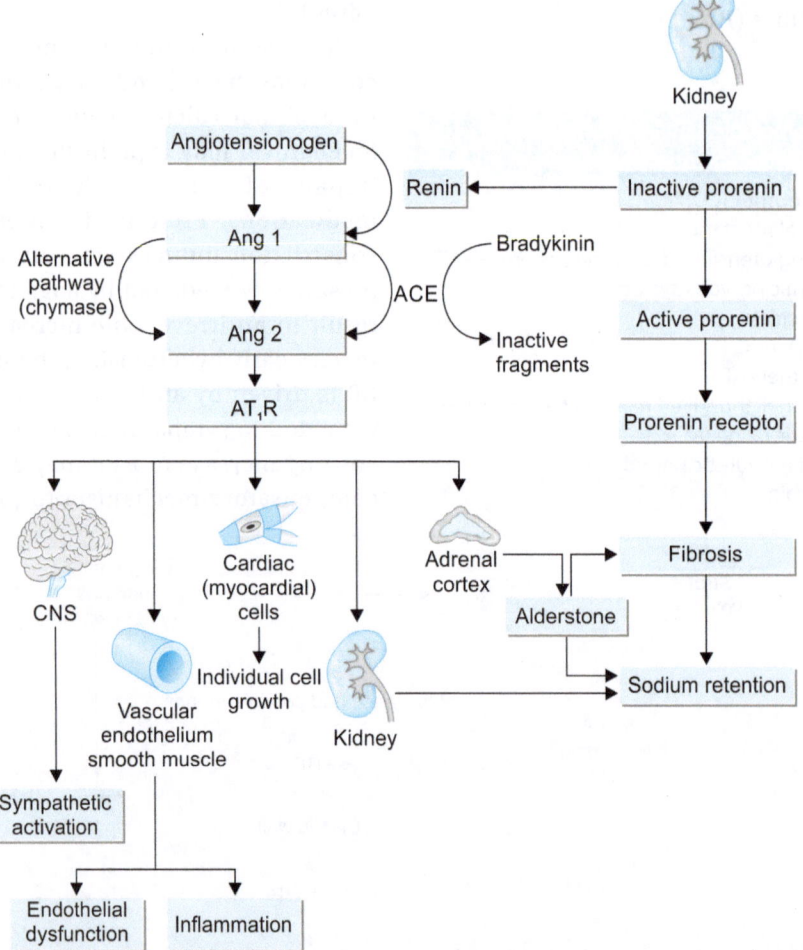

Fig. 3: Pathological consequences of activation RAAS.[16] (ACE: angiotensin-converting enzyme; Ang: angiotensin; AT_1R: angiotensin 1 receptor; CNS: central nervous system; RAAS: renin-angiotensin-aldosterone system)

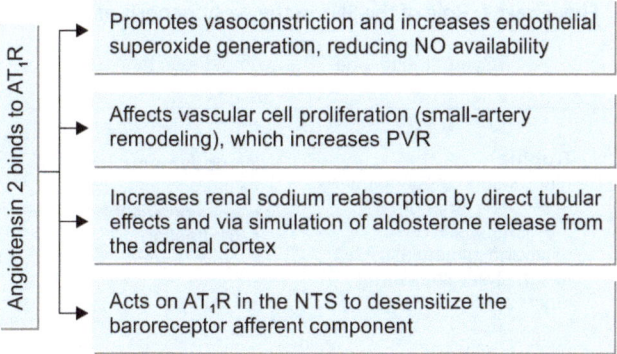

Fig. 4: Mechanisms by which angiotensin 2 raises the BP.[12] (AT$_1$R: angiotensin 1 receptor; NO: nitric oxide; PVR: peripheral vascular resistance; NTS: nucleus tractus solitarius)

through trophic effects on the myocardium, resulting in left ventricular hypertrophy (LVH); glomerular hypertension, albuminuria, and interstitial fibrosis, leading to chronic renal disease; and pro-oxidant actions, contributing to atherosclerosis. Consequently, the RAAS has become a popular target for drug therapy to lower BP and limit its cardiovascular consequences.[12]

Aldosterone

Aldosterone is the other RAAS effector molecule. The adrenal cortex produces it in response to sodium and volume depletion, angiotensin 2, excess potassium, trauma, and stress. It promotes salt absorption in the distal tubule of the kidney in exchange for potassium. Increased aldosterone can cause hypertension.[12]

Autonomic Nervous System

Increased SNS activity elevates BP *via* stimulating the heart, peripheral vasculature, and kidneys, resulting in increased CO, PVR, and fluid retention.[17]

Hypertension causes complicated changes in baroreflex and chemoreflex circuits. Hypertension resets arterial baroreceptors to a higher pressure, suppressing sympathetic inhibition. This baroreflex reset seems to be mediated by angiotensin 2. Angiotensin 2 enhances sympathetic activation by facilitating norepinephrine release. Chronic sympathetic stimulation produces vascular remodeling and LVH, likely via direct and indirect effects of norepinephrine on its own receptors and on the release of other trophic factors, including transforming growth factor-β, insulin-like growth factor 1, and fibroblast growth factors. Thus, sympathetic pathways lead to organ damage and hypertension **(Flowchart 1)**.[17]

Endothelial Dysfunction

Evidence suggests a link between the level of endothelial dysfunction and the severity of hypertension. The main underlying reason for endothelial dysfunction in hypertension is a decrease in NO availability as a result of elevated oxidative stress in these patients. A decrease in NO alters endothelium-dependent vasorelaxation, contributing to hypertension. Thus, endothelial dysfunction may be a contributing factor to hypertension.[18]

Several other vasoactive agents (besides NO), including arachidonic acid metabolites, reactive oxygen species (ROS), vasoactive

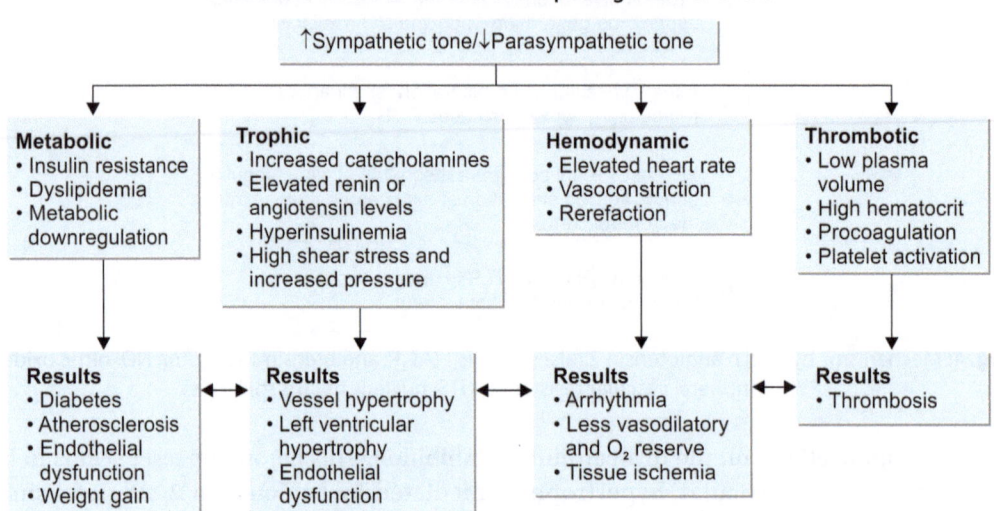

Flowchart 1: Role of the SNS in the pathogenesis of CVDs.[17]

(SNS: sympathetic nervous system; CVDs: cardiovascular diseases)

peptides, and microparticles of endothelial origin contribute to excessive vascular oxidative stress and inflammation, which leads to endothelial dysfunction. Endothelial progenitor cells (EPCs) that develop into mature endothelial cells have been implicated in the maintenance of arterial stiffness in recent years, and as such are now considered endothelial function determinants. Endothelial dysfunction is implicated in causing structural and functional changes within the arteries. Therapies that target key pathways involved in the process have been shown to reduce vascular remodeling, improve vascular function, and reduce the overall cardiovascular risk.[18]

Vasoactive Substances

Many other vasoactive systems and mechanisms affecting sodium transport and vascular tone are involved in the maintenance of a normal BP **(Table 4)**.[18,19] It is not clear, however, what part these play in the development of essential hypertension.[14]

CONSEQUENCES AND COMPLICATIONS OF HYPERTENSION

The consequences of hypertension are a function of its severity. There is no threshold for the occurrence of problems, as high BP is related to higher morbidity over the whole BP range **(Table 5)**.[20,21]

Two major cardiac consequences of hypertension include LVH and coronary artery disease (CAD) **(Fig. 5)**. Stroke may be caused by thrombosis, thromboembolism, or cerebral bleeding. Effect of hypertension on the kidney may initially manifest as microalbuminuria, which may progress to chronic kidney disease in the later years.[20]

CHALLENGES IN MANAGING HYPERTENSION IN INDIA

In India, hypertension is one of the most serious public health issues. India is a vast developing country with a diverse population and economic conditions. Some regions of the nation, particularly rural India,

TABLE 4: Vasoactive substances involved in the pathogenesis of hypertension.[18,19]

ET[18]	• A vasoconstrictor, maintains vascular tone • Secreted by endothelial cells • Exerts paracrine or autocrine effects on vascular smooth muscle cells and counteracts vasorelaxing function of NO • ET-1 infusion raises the BP in animals and humans, whereas antagonists reverse the effect • Mainly implicated in salt-sensitive and renal hypertension
Natriuretic peptides[18]	• ANP belongs to a family of structurally and functionally, related peptide hormones with cardiorenal functions • ANP mediates its functions via membrane-bound guanylate cyclase-linked receptor (NPR-A), which further activates intracellular cGMP-mediated processes • Released from the atria in response to atrial distention stemming from hemodynamic overload, ANP causes natriuresis and diuresis resulting in modest reductions in BP, with concomitant decreases in plasma renin and aldosterone • Thus, the natriuretic peptide system, by decreasing PVR, balances the activity of the SNS and the RAAS in maintaining the BP
Bradykinin[18]	• A product of kallikrein–kinin system • Vasodilatory peptide with autocrine and paracrine function • Stimulates the release of other vasoactive substances like prostaglandins • Reduces BP by vasodilation as well as by enhanced natriuresis and diuresis (via increased renal blood flow mediated by NO and prostaglandin release)
Arginine–vasopressin (AVP)[19]	• One of the body's most effective vasoconstrictor peptides • Acts on renal V2 receptors, determines the fluid balance • Vasopressin regulates BP in physiological and pathological situations such as posture, dehydration, bleeding, adrenal insufficiency, and heart failure • Recent studies have linked vasopressin to the pathogenesis of various kinds of hypertension
Dopamine[19]	• Abnormalities in dopamine production or dopamine receptor signaling can increase BP and salt sensitivity • GRK4, a G protein-coupled receptor kinase subfamily that alters dopamine receptor function, is found to promote renal sodium reabsorption, which is linked to essential hypertension

(ANP: atrial natriuretic peptide; BP: blood pressure; cGMP: cyclic guanosine monophosphate; ET-1: endothelin-1; NO, nitric oxide; PVR: peripheral vascular resistance; RAAS: renin-angiotensin-aldosterone system; SNS: sympathetic nervous system)

TABLE 5: Complications of hypertension.[21]

Affected organ	Complications
Cardiovascular system	Cardiac hypertrophy, heart failure, angina pectoris, coronary heart disease, and myocardial infarction
Artery	Atherosclerosis and aneurysms
Brain	Stroke (ischemic or hemorrhagic), hypertensive encephalopathy, cognitive decline, and dementia
Eye	Retinopathy
Kidney	Hypertensive nephropathy and chronic kidney disease

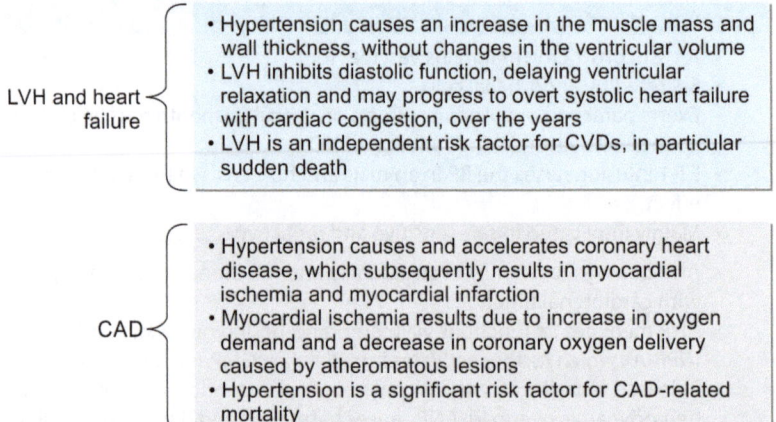

Fig. 5: Cardiac consequences of hypertension.[20] (CAD: coronary artery disease; LVH: left ventricular hypertrophy)

are developing, whereas the urban areas are developed. A rise in cardiovascular and cerebrovascular disorders that cause early death and morbidity, especially in young Indians, is a result of growing urbanization and unhealthy lifestyle changes. Diversity is a significant barrier to accurate epidemiological studies of the whole Indian population.[22]

Other challenges in managing hypertension, especially in the Indian context are summarized below.

High Incidence

Hypertension is a growing problem in India and causes a significant burden on the health-care system. Data from the GBD study of 2016 reported 1.63 million deaths in India attributable to hypertension in the year 2016 alone. GBD data also showed that over half of the deaths due to IHD (54.2%), stroke (56.2%), and chronic kidney disease (54.5%) were attributable to high SBP.[23]

India has also been experiencing an increase in the prevalence of hypertension. A cross-sectional, population-based study on a large nationally representative sample of 1.3 million individuals carried out between 2012 and 2014 revealed that the crude prevalence of hypertension in India was 25.3%.[23]

Earlier Onset of Hypertension

High BP among young Indians is rising, which increases the risk of premature mortality. In the recently published "REAL YOUNG (hypertension) study," it has been discussed that Indians have a higher chance of acquiring hypertension in early life than Western cohorts, and initial heart attacks and strokes occur a decade sooner on an average.[24]

Ramakrishnan et al. reported the findings from an Indian BP study conducted across 24 states and union territories. The prevalence of hypertension was 55.3% in persons aged 20–44 years. This changing and fast-rising epidemic of hypertension among young Indians is a grave situation warranting early diagnosis and treatment.[24]

Comorbidities

In India, hypertension and its associated comorbidities are important health concerns among young individuals. The "REAL YOUNG (hypertension) study" was a retrospective, multicentric, real-world analysis of risk factors and comorbidities in young Indian individuals with hypertension. The study revealed that diabetes mellitus was the most prevalent comorbidity in the overall population.[24]

The significant association between hypertension and diabetes, along with a higher incidence of kidney damage and CVD, necessitates vigorous BP control for diabetic hypertensive patients. This is reflected in guideline recommendations, which advocate aggressive targets of 130/80 mm Hg. However, BP is difficult to regulate in this patient population, and these objectives are frequently missed in daily practice.[25]

Lack of Awareness

Hypertension is a persistent, chronic, and often asymptomatic condition. In India, the majority of patients with hypertension are uninformed of their illness. This is a result of low levels of awareness and a lack of systematic programs or opportunistic tests to screen for hypertension in individuals during visits to healthcare providers. Only a quarter of rural and two-fifths of urban Indians are aware of their hypertension, and only a quarter and a third of those identified in rural and urban India receive treatment for it.[26]

Low Therapeutic Response Rates

Patients with hypertension frequently receive inappropriate care or fail to adhere to therapy, resulting in uncontrolled hypertension. Only about 10% of the patients in rural areas and 20% of those in urban areas have their hypertension under control. Misdiagnosis of hypertension is a problem in India, adding to the burden of undiagnosed, uncontrolled hypertension. This is due to poorly standardized BP measurement techniques, poorly calibrated devices, and reliance on single readings for diagnosis rather than multiple readings confirmed by elevated readings on follow-up.[26]

Need for Treatment Up-titration

Most patients with hypertension require multiple classes of BP-lowering medications to achieve adequate BP control. Medication titration and adding multiple drug classes require multiple doctor visits, which can lead to poor medication adherence and missed appointments. The need to take multiple medications in complex regimens results in poor medication adherence. The need for repeatedly up-titrating or adding medications can be limited due to physician inertia, resulting in inadequate BP control. Dual combination therapy accelerates antihypertensive treatment and lowers the final target. This may also improve patient adherence without escalating the side effect profile. Simplifying up-titration regimes may also result in additional benefits in BP control.[27]

Need for Primary Care Screening

Screening is an important tool for increasing the detection of and awareness of hypertension. All adults should have opportunistic BP screenings at every visit to the healthcare system. Screening can be accomplished during routine medical consultations and by nonphysician healthcare workers.[28]

Early diagnosis and optimal management is associated with significant reductions in cardiovascular mortality and morbidity. Nonphysician healthcare workers can be trained to provide lifestyle advice, initiate low doses of safe medications, and reinforce adherence in addition to screening. This task-shifting strategy is likely to be cost-effective in controlling hypertension, a condition affecting a third of the adult population, in a large and resource-constrained country like India.[28]

> **KEY POINTS**
> - There has been a steady increase in the prevalence of hypertension, both globally as wel as in India.
> - Numerous physiological processes regulate normal blood pressure, and their dysfunction may contribute to the emergence of essential hypertension.
> - In very earlystages of hypertension, the increase in BP is driven by an increase in CO, which is related to sympathetic overactivity.
> - The RAAS, whose primary effector molecules are angiotensin 2 and aldosterone, is vital in BP control.
> - Hypertension has two cardiac consequences: left ventricular hypertrophy and CAD.
> - A rise in cardiovascular and cerebrovascular disorders that cause early death and morbidity, especially in young Indians, is a result of growing urbanization and unhealthy lifestyle changes.
> - All adults should have opportunistic BP screenings at every visit to the healthcare system.

■ CONCLUSION

In conclusion, hypertension remains a global health challenge with profound implications for cardiovascular diseases, stroke, and renal disorders. The evolving definitions and classifications reflect the complex relationship between blood pressure and associated risks. While guidelines differ in defining hypertension thresholds, the linear correlation between elevated blood pressure and cardiovascular risk underscores the need for effective management. The etiopathophysiology of hypertension involves intricate mechanisms, including genetic predisposition, environmental factors, and dysregulation in blood pressure regulatory systems. The renin-angiotensin-aldosterone system, autonomic nervous system, and endothelial dysfunction contribute significantly to its pathogenesis. The consequences of hypertension, ranging from cardiac hypertrophy to renal and cerebral complications, emphasize the importance of early diagnosis and optimal management. In India, the challenges in hypertension management, including lack of awareness, early onset among the population, and comorbidities like diabetes, warrant a comprehensive and proactive healthcare approach. Understanding these pathophysiological mechanisms is crucial for developing effective strategies for the diagnosis, management, and prevention of hypertension. Targeting key components, such as the RAAS and SNS, has become a cornerstone in drug therapy to lower blood pressure and mitigate cardiovascular consequences. The complexity of hypertension underscores the importance of personalized and multidimensional approaches to its management, addressing both lifestyle modifications and pharmacological interventions tailored to individual patient needs.

■ REFERENCES

1. Iqbal AM, Jamal SF. Essential hypertension. In: StatPearls. [Online]. Treasure Island (FL): StatPearls Publishing; 2023. Available from https://www.ncbi.nlm.nih.gov/books/NBK539859/ [Last accessed November, 2023].

2. Kotchen TA. Hypertension. In: Loscalzo J, Fauci AS, Kasper DL, et al (Eds). Harrison's Principles of Internal Medicine, 21st edition. New York: McGraw-Hill; 2022. pp. 7631-88.
3. Mills KT, Stefanescu A, He J. The global epidemiology of hypertension. Nat Rev Nephrol. 2020;16(4):223-37.
4. Whelton PK, Carey RM, Aronow WS, Casey DE Jr, Collins KJ, Himmelfarb CD, et al. 2017 ACC/AHA/AAPA/ABC/ACPM/AGS/APhA/ASH/ASPC/NMA/PCNA Guideline for the Prevention, Detection, Evaluation, and Management of High Blood Pressure in Adults: A Report of the American College of Cardiology/American Heart Association Task Force on Clinical Practice Guidelines. Hypertension. 2018;71(6):e13-15.
5. Rapsomaniki E, Timmis A, George J, Pujades-Rodriguez M, Shah AD, Denaxas S, et al. Blood pressure and incidence of twelve cardiovascular diseases: Lifetime risks, healthy life-years lost, and age-specific associations in 1.25 million people. Lancet. 2014;383(9932):1899-911.
6. Williams B, Mancia G, Spiering W, Rosei EA, Azizi M, Burnier M, et al. 2018 ESC/ESH Guidelines for the management of arterial hypertension Eur Heart J. 2018;39(33):3021-104.
7. Ramakrishnan S, Zachariah G, Gupta K, Rao JS, Mohanan PP, Venugopal K, et al. Prevalence of hypertension among Indian adults: Results from the great India blood pressure survey. Indian Heart J. 2019;71(4):309-13.
8. Shah SN, Munjal YP, Kamath SA, Wander GS, Mehta N, Mukherjee S, et al. Indian guidelines on hypertension-IV (2019). J Hum Hypertens. 2020;34(11):745-58.
9. Unger T, Borghi C, Charchar F, Khan NA, Poulter NR, Prabhakaran D, et al. 2020 International Society of Hypertension Global Hypertension Practice Guidelines. Hypertension. 2020;75(6):1334-57.
10. World Health Organization. (2022). Hypertension. [Online]. Available from https://www.who.int/news-room/fact-sheets/detail/hypertension [Last accessed November, 2023]
11. Anchala R, Kannuri NK, Pant H, Khan H, Franco OH, Angelantonio ED, et al. Hypertension in India: A systematic review and meta-analysis of prevalence, awareness, and control of hypertension. J Hypertens. 2014;32(6):1170-77.
12. Williams B, Firth JD. Essential hypertension: Definition, epidemiology, and pathophysiology. In: Firth JD, Conlon CP, Cox TM (Eds). Oxford Textbook of Medicine, 5th edition, Vol III. Oxford: United Kingdom; 2020. pp. 3735-53.
13. Sutters M. Systemic Hypertension. In Papadakis MA, McPhee SJ, Rabow MW (Eds). Current Medical Diagnosis & Treatment. 61st edition. New York: McGraw-Hill; 2022. pp. 463-94.
14. Beevers G, Lip GY, O'Brien E. ABC of hypertension: The pathophysiology of hypertension. BMJ 2001;322(7291):912-16.
15. Nemecz M, Alexandru N, Tanko G, Georgescu A. Role of miRNA in endothelial dysfunction and hypertension. Curr Hypertens Rep. 2016;18(12):87.
16. Ram CV. Hypertension: A Clinical Guide, 1st edition. Florida: CRC Press; 2014, pp. 27-37.
17. Oparil S, Zaman MA, Calhoun DA. Pathogenesis of hypertension. Ann Intern Med. 2003;139(9):761-76.
18. Delacroix S, Chokka RG, Worthley SG. Hypertension: Pathophysiology and treatment. J Neurol Neurophysiol. 2014;5(6):1-8.
19. Burnier M, Wuerzner G. Pathophysiology of Hypertension. In: Jagadeesh G, Balakumar P, Maung-U K (Eds). Pathophysiology and Pharmacotherapy of Cardiovascular Disease. New York: Springer International Publishing; 2015. pp. 655-84.
20. Foëx P, Sear JW. Hypertension: Pathophysiology and treatment. Continuing Education in Anaesthesia Critical Care & Pain. 2004;4(3):71-75.
21. Lin SR, Lin SY, Chen CC, Fu YS, Weng AF. Exploring a new natural treating agent for primary hypertension: Recent findings and forthcoming perspectives. J Clin Med. 2019;8(11):2003.

22. Sogunuru GP, Mishra S. Asian management of hypertension: Current status, home blood pressure, and specific concerns in India. J Clin Hypertens (Greenwich). 2020;22(3):479-82.
23. Jose AP, Prabhakaran D. World Hypertension Day: Contemporary issues faced in India. Indian J Med Res. 2019;149(5):567-70.
24. Desai N, Unni G, Agarwala R, Salagre S, Godbole S, Dengra A, et al. Risk factors and comorbidities in young Indian patients with hypertension: REAL YOUNG (hypertension) study. Integr Blood Press Control. 2021;14:31-41.
25. Schmieder RE, Ruilope LM. Blood pressure control in patients with comorbidities. J Clin Hypertens (Greenwich). 2008;10(8):624-31.
26. Ministry of Health & Family Welfare, Government of India. (2016). Standard treatment guidelines. Hypertension—screening, diagnosis, assessment, and management of primary hypertension in adults in India [Online]. Available from https://nhm.gov.in/images/pdf/guidelines/nrhm-guidelines/stg/Hypertension_QRG.pdf [Last accessed November, 2023].
27. Vedanthan R, Bernabe-Ortiz A, Herasme OI, Joshi R, Lopez-Jaramillo P, Thrift AG, et al. Innovative approaches to hypertension control in low- and middle-income countries. Cardiol Clin. 2017;35(1):99-115.
28. Gupta R, Yusuf S. Towards better hypertension management in India. Indian J Med Res. 2014;139(5):657-60.

CHAPTER 3

Renin-Angiotensin-Aldosterone System in Hypertension

Rubi Dey, Bidita Khandelwal

■ INTRODUCTION

Kidneys are one of the major organs that are instrumental in providing the physiological means for the maintenance of blood pressure and electrolyte homeostasis. Blood pressure has a direct relation to the body's tissue perfusion. The two most important etiologic factors of BP include sodium-volume factor and vascular tonality. These factors reside in the kidney and therefore kidney plays an important role in the regulation of BP. The kidney has the capability of controlling arterial BP mainly through the various changes in the extracellular fluid and by the renin-angiotensin-aldosterone system (RAAS).

Tigerstedt and Bergman in the year 1889 reported the vasopressor effect of renal extract—Renin—which was found to cause a sustained rise in arterial pressure.[1] This formed the stepping stone in the discovery of the RAAS, although this finding was criticized for quite a long period before it got recognition. Goldbaltt et al. validated the rise in arterial pressure following renal ischemia.[2] Within a short period after this, it was found that along with renin, the ischemic kidney also released a short-lived pressor substance called angiotensinogen.

The RAAS is a complex multiorgan hormonal cascade that plays an important role as a critical regulator of BP, vascular resistance, and tone. The RAAS has a direct impact on systemic BP by regulating sodium concentration and water absorption in the kidney. The monitoring and controlling of the arterial tone by RAAS helps in maintaining the physiological perfusion, in spite of the constantly changing internal and external influences on the BP. A short-term decrease in arterial pressure is a function of the baroreceptor reflex whereas the RAAS is responsible for chronic alterations in arterial pressure. Long-term activation of RAAS is maladaptive and adversely affects the heart, vessels, and kidneys. The RAAS activation affects every organ along with the resultant hypertension, cell proliferation, inflammation, and fibrosis. An overwhelming number of chronic and acute diseases are because of the imbalance of renin and angiotensin II.

The primary function of RAAS is the regulation of BP by modulating blood volume, sodium reabsorption, potassium secretion, water reabsorption, and vascular tone. Apart from this, other functions of RAAS include inflammation, apoptosis, and fibrosis.[3] The various organs involved in RAAS include the kidneys, lungs, systemic vasculature, and brain.[4] The main players in the RAAS are renin, angiotensin II, and aldosterone which act as a series of designed reactions. They are responsible for elevation of the arterial BP in response to a decrease in renal BP, a decrease in salt delivery to the distal convoluted tubule, and β-agonism.[5-7]

MECHANISM OF RENIN-ANGIOTENSIN-ALDOSTERONE SYSTEM

Juxtaglomerular (JG) cells, present within the afferent arterioles of the kidney, contain prorenin. Prorenin is in its inactive form and activation of JG cells causes the cleavage of prorenin to renin which is the active form and is released into the blood. The JG cell activation occurs in response to decreased BP, β-activation, or activation by macula densa cells in response to a decreased sodium load in the distal convoluted tubule.[8,9]

Renin released into the blood acts on the target angiotensinogen which is produced by the liver and is present continuously circulating in the blood. Renin then causes the cleaving of angiotensinogen into angiotensin I **(Flowchart 1)**. Angiotensin I which is physiologically inactive is the precursor for the active form—angiotensin II.[4] The angiotensin-converting enzyme (ACE) is found primarily in the vascular endothelium of the lungs and kidneys and catalyzes the conversion of angiotensin I to angiotensin II. Angiotensin II causes a diverse set of RAAS-induced physiological and pathophysiological actions by acting on its target organs. So far, four subsets of angiotensin receptors have been described.[10] Type 1 angiotensin (AT1) receptor—most of the physiological function of angiotensin II is mediated by the AT1 receptor widely distributed in many cells of the target organs. The main physiological actions mediated by the AT1 receptor include vasoconstriction; a rise in BP, increased cardiac contractility; vascular and cardiac hypertrophy; Na^+ reabsorption by renal tubules; and stimulation of aldosterone synthesis. Other actions mediated by the AT1 receptor are cell growth and proliferation, inflammatory responses, and oxidative stress. (2) Type 2 angiotensin (AT2) receptor are more present abundantly during fetal life mainly in the kidneys and brain and the levels of the same decreases markedly in the postnatal period. The actions mediated by the AT2 receptor in adults are uncertain but it is thought to cause vasodilation, antiproliferative, and apoptotic

Flowchart 1: Renin-angiotensin-aldosterone system.

```
Kidney secretes renin ──▶ Angiotensinogen (secreted from the liver)
                                   │
                                   ▼
• Lungs secretes              Angiotensin I
• ACE                              │
                                   ▼
                              Angiotensin II ◀── AT receptors
         ┌──────────────┬──────────┴──────────┬──────────────┐
         ▼              ▼                     ▼              ▼
   Adrenal gland     Kidney          Posterior pituitary  Blood vessel    Hypothalamus
         │              │                     │              │               │
         ▼              ▼                     ▼              ▼               ▼
   • Zona         Constriction of        ADH secretion   Vasoconstriction  Increase in thirst
   • Glomerulosa  efferent arteriole
     secretes     and increase in
   • Aldosterone  sodium Na⁺/H⁺
                  exchanger
                  activity
```

(ACE: angiotensin-converting enzyme; AT: angiotensin; ADH: antidiuretic hormone)

effects in the vascular smooth muscles. (3) Type 3 angiotensin (AT3) receptor action is still not fully ascertained. (4) Type 4 angiotensin (AT4) receptor is to be instrumental in mediating the release of plasminogen inhibitor I. Angiotensin II then has its effects on the kidney, adrenal cortex, arterioles, and brain by binding to angiotensin II type 1 (AT1) and type 2 (AT2) receptors.[11] Angiotensin II has a half-life of 1–2 min and at this point, the peptidases in the plasma degrades it to angiotensin III and IV. Angiotensin III has been found to have 100% of the aldosterone stimulating effect as angiotensin II but it has only 40% of the pressor effects. Angiotensin IV further decreases the systemic effect **(Flowchart 1)**.

Angiotensin II acts in the proximal convoluted tubule of the kidney to increase sodium–hydrogen (Na^+/H^+) exchange and to increase sodium reabsorption. Increased levels of Na in the body lead to an increase in the osmolarity of the blood which causes a shift of fluid into the blood volume and extracellular space (ECF) thereby increasing the arterial pressure.

Angiotensin II also acts specifically on the zona glomerulosa of the adrenal cortex and stimulates the release of aldosterone. Aldosterone being a steroid hormone enacts change by binding to nuclear receptors and altering gene transcription as a result of which the effect of aldosterone takes hours to days to begin. Effects of aldosterone include sodium reabsorption and potassium excretion at the distal tubule and collecting duct of the nephron by stimulating the insertion of luminal Na channels and basolateral sodium–potassium (Na^+/K^+) adenosine triphosphatase (ATPase) proteins.

Angiotensin II has influences on renal epithelial cells, phosphorylation of mineralocorticoid receptors (MRs) in the intercalated cells of the distal nephron, and inhibition of potassium secretion by altering kinase activity, specifically WNK family kinases.[12] The vasoconstrictive effect of angiotensin II takes place in systemic arterioles. Angiotensin II binds to G protein-coupled receptors which causes a secondary messenger cascade that results in potent arteriolar vasoconstriction leading to an increase in the total peripheral resistance and a subsequent increase in BP.

The final effect of angiotensin II is on the brain; initially, it binds to the hypothalamus, stimulating thirst and increasing water intake. Subsequently, it stimulates the release of antidiuretic hormone (ADH) by the posterior pituitary which thereafter acts to increase water reabsorption in the kidney by inserting aquaporin channels at the collecting duct. Angiotensin II also decreases the sensitivity of the baroreceptor reflex thus diminishing the baroreceptor response to an increase in BP. The net effect of these interactions is an increase in total body sodium, total body water, and vascular tone causing an increase in BP.

DYSREGULATED RENIN-ANGIOTENSIN-ALDOSTERONE SYSTEM: EFFECTS AND MANAGEMENT (FLOWCHART 2)

The RAAS helps to manage long-term basis of blood volume and arteriolar tone. Inappropriate activation of the RAAS in various conditions causes the development of hypertension and cardiovascular disorders. The baroreceptor reflex manages minor and rapid shifts whereas the RAAS has the capability to alter blood volume chronically. Dysregulated RAAS is an essential factor in essential hypertension.[13] In young male patients with essential hypertension around

15% have mild-to-moderate rise in plasma renin activity which can be due to sympathetic overactivity and mild volume depletion. Apart from hypertension, RAAS plays a pivotal role in several nonhypertensive conditions, especially in congestive heart failure (CHF) **(Flowchart 2)**.

The RAAS is a frequently manipulated system in the management of several diseases like heart failure, hypertension, diabetes mellitus, and acute myocardial infarction. Renin is the first step in the RAAS cascade and the inhibition of renin decreases the levels of renin, angiotensin I, angiotensin II, aldosterone, and subsequent decrease in BP. This can be thought to be a logical therapeutic target for RAAS blockade. Aliskiren—a renin inhibitor is available for use but because of its side effects especially in combination with ACE inhibitors or ARBs it is not advocated.[14] Drugs such as ACE inhibitors (e.g., enalapril) inhibit the action of ACEs, thus decreasing the production of angiotensin II and inhibiting the progression of the RAAS cascade and the physiological effects of angiotensin II. The physiological actions of angiotensin II are mediated by its receptors present in target organs. Angiotensin receptor blockers (ARBs; e.g., losartan) inhibit the action of ARBs to block AT receptors, thus inhibiting angiotensin's effect while maintaining normal levels of the compound. Aldosterone antagonists have two specific varieties. The first (e.g., spironolactone or eplerenone) group acts as an aldosterone antagonist by preventing the binding of aldosterone to binding sites in the kidney thus preventing insertion of Na channels and the second

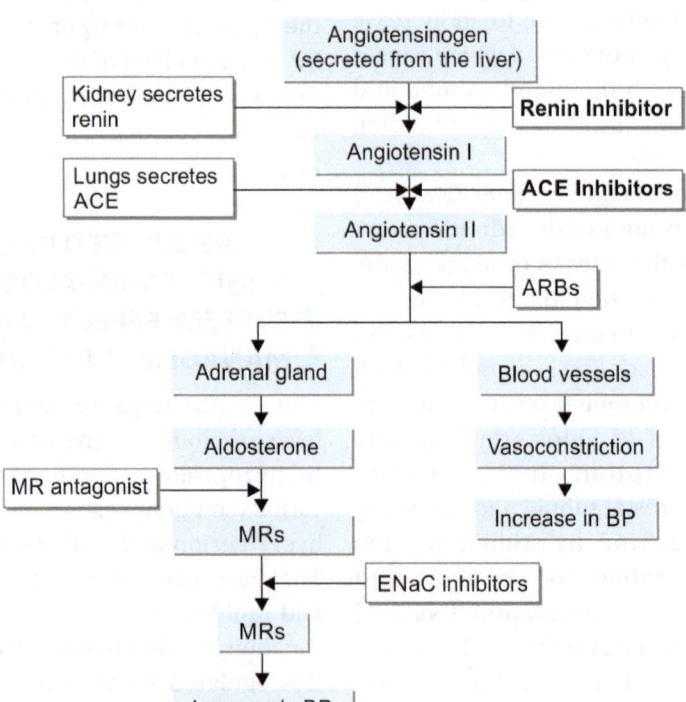

Flowchart 2: Pharmacological modulation of dysregulated RAAS.

(ACE: angiotensin-converting enzyme; ARBs: angiotensin receptor blockers; MRs: mineralocorticoid receptors)

(e.g., amiloride or triamterene) group acts by blocking the inserted Na channels in the distal convoluted tubule. These drugs act by decreasing the effect of the RAAS. The ACE inhibitors or ARBs are commonly used in the management of hypertension by decreasing sodium and water reabsorption, leading to a reduction in blood volume, and decreasing arteriolar tone.

The renin-angiotensin-aldosterone pathway is mainly regulated by the mechanisms that stimulate renin release. However, it is also found to be modulated by natriuretic peptides released by the heart and acts as an important counterregulatory system.

■ FUTURE PROSPECTS

The ACE inhibitors and the ARBs have shown promising results in improving the survival of the high-risk group of patients. They are currently advocated in the management of hypertension, diabetic nephropathy, left ventricular dysfunction, and chronic cardiac failure. Though treatment modalities with the present drugs have shown promising results, more targeted therapies including molecular approaches like antisense gene therapy, and parallel intervention at various sites of the RAAS cascade could help slow the progression of cardiovascular and renal diseases.

■ REFERENCES

1. Tigerstedt R, Bergman PG. Niere and Kreislauf. Skand Arch Physiol. 1898; 8: 223.
2. Goldblatt H. Studies on experimental hypertension: I. The production of persistent elevation of systolic blood pressure by means of renal ischemia. J Exp Med 1934; 59:347.
3. Laghlam D, Jozwiak M, Nguyen LS. Renin-angiotensin-aldosterone system and immunomodulation: A State-of-the-art review. Cells. 2021;10(7):1767.
4. Santos RAS, Oudit GY, Verano-Braga T, Canta G, Steckelings UM, Bader M. The renin-angiotensin system: Going beyond the classical paradigms. Am J Physiol Heart Circ Physiol. 2019;316(5):H958-70.
5. Liu J, Zhou Y, Liu Y, Li L, Chen Y, Liu Y, et al. (Pro)renin receptor regulates lung development via the Wnt/β-catenin signaling pathway. Am J Physiol Lung Cell Mol Physiol. 2019;317(2):L202-11.
6. Hall JE, do Carmo JM, da Silva AA, Wang Z, Hall ME. Obesity, kidney dysfunction and hypertension: Mechanistic links. Nat Rev Nephrol. 2019;15(6):367-85.
7. Drummond GR, Vinh A, Guzik TJ, Sobey CG. Immune mechanisms of hypertension. Nat Rev Immunol. 2019;19(8):517-32.
8. Ren L, Lu X, Danser AHJ. Revisiting the brain renin–angiotensin system: Focus on novel therapies. Curr Hypertens Rep. 2019;21(4):28.
9. Nehme A, Zouein FA, Zayeri ZD, Zibara K. An Update on the tissue renin angiotensin system and its role in physiology and pathology. J Cardiovasc Dev Dis. 2019;6(2):14.
10. Stanton, A. Therapeutic potential of renin inhibitors in the management of cardiovascular disorders. Am J Cardiovasc Drugs. 2003;3:389-94.
11. Bernstein KE, Khan Z, Giani JF, Cao DY, Bernstein EA, Shen XZ. Angiotensin-converting enzyme in innate and adaptive immunity. Nat Rev Nephrol. 2018;14(5):325-36.
12. Shibata S, Arroyo JP, Castañeda-Bueno M, Puthumana J, Zhang J, Uchida S, et al. Angiotensin II signaling via protein kinase C phosphorylates Kelch-like 3, preventing WNK4 degradation. Proc Natl Acad Sci U S A. 2014;111(43):15556-61.
13. Laragh J. Laragh's lessons in pathophysiology and clinical pearls for treating hypertension. Am J Hypertens. 2001;14(2):186-94.
14. Staessen JA, Li Y, Richart T. Oral renin inhibitors. Lancet 2006;368(9545):1449-56. Erratum in: Lancet 2006;368(9553):2124.

SECTION 3: Molecular Basis of Hypertension

4. **Role of Cell Membrane (Red Blood Cells and Platelets) in Essential Hypertension**
   Arundhati Bag, Bidita Khandelwal, Abhishek Byahut

5. **Matrix Metalloproteinases and the Extracellular Matrix**
   Bidita Khandelwal, Chamma Gupta

6. **Role of Calcium Channels in Hypertension**
   Arundhati Bag, Bidita Khandelwal, Abhishek Byahut

7. **Role of Cytokines and Inflammation in Hypertension**
   Mingma Lhamu Sherpa, Lydia Rai, Bidita Khandelwal

8. **Natriuretic Peptides in Hypertension**
   Rubi Dey, Bidita Khandelwal

9. **Multiple Roles of Eicosanoids in Blood Pressure Regulation**
   Mingma Lhamu Sherpa, Rojana Tamang, Bidita Khandelwal

CHAPTER 4

Role of Cell Membrane (Red Blood Cells and Platelets) in Essential Hypertension

Arundhati Bag, Bidita Khandelwal, Abhishek Byahut

■ INTRODUCTION

Essential or primary hypertension is the most common type of hypertension and it affects approximately 90–95% of hypertensive cases. It is followed by secondary hypertension which includes approximately 5–10% of the hypertensive population.[1] Essential hypertension (EH) is associated with disability, significant morbidity, and mortality. However, its underlying causes are not understood very well. Current literature suggests an involvement of genetic and environmental factors which interplay and give rise to this condition.[1] Research in the last few decades reveals that changes in the physical properties of cell membranes may be a key factor in developing EH.[2] The cell-membrane changes or abnormalities may take place in different cell types including red blood cells (RBCs), and platelets. Various abnormalities in membranes of these cell types in relation to EH are discussed in this chapter.

■ RED BLOOD CELL MEMBRANE IN ESSENTIAL HYPERTENSION

Altered physiological and functional properties of RBCs have been suggested to play an important role in the development of hypertension. It is known that EH is associated with increased vascular resistance and blood viscosity.[3] Altered rheological properties of RBCs, for example, reduced deformability can be responsible for the increased blood viscosity.[3,4] Different factors may be responsible for the reduced deformability of RBCs including changed membrane–lipid composition, increased ATPase activity, or altered Na^+-K^+ transport system.[3]

Red Blood Cell Membrane

The lipid bilayer of the RBC membrane is interspersed with integral membrane proteins, namely, band-3, glycophorin A, B, and C, and transporters **(Fig. 1)**. The cytoskeleton consists of spectrin tetramers (two α- and two β-spectrins), which is tethered to the lipid bilayer either through actin and glycophorin or through ankyrin and band-3 proteins. The cytoskeleton maintains the integrity of the cell membrane.

Alteration in Membrane Deformability

Deformability is a characteristic feature of RBCs for which they can travel through the smallest passages of blood capillary in our body.[5] Reduction in deformability of RBC can affect microcirculatory blood flow and oxygen transport to the tissues. It also increases the viscosity of blood and impairs the perfusion of blood into the tissues. Deformability is determined by surface-to-volume ratio, intracellular viscosity, and membrane fluidity.[6]

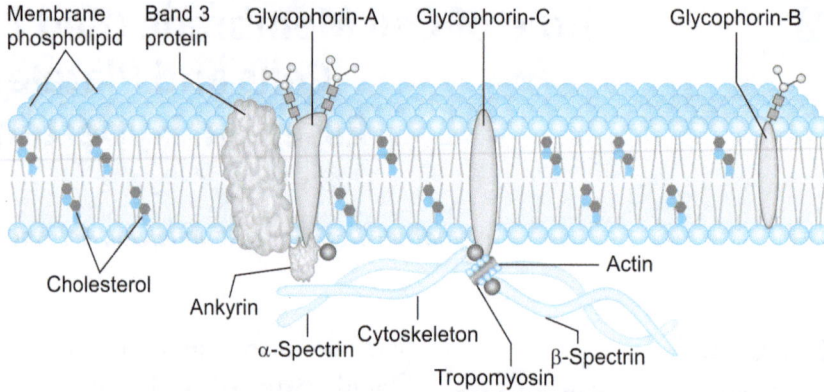

Fig. 1: Structure of RBC membrane.

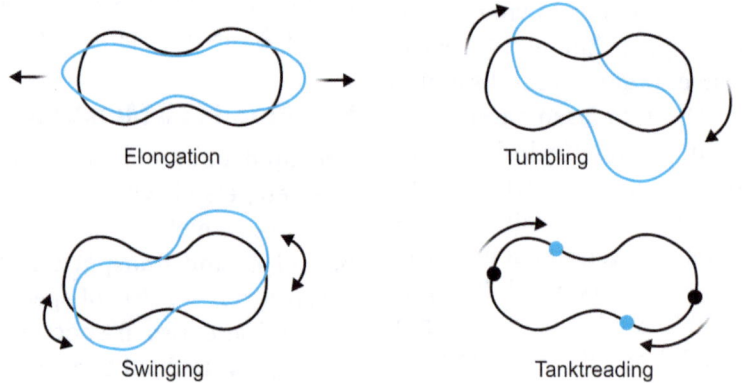

Fig. 2: Red blood cell deformability.

Elongation of the principal ellipsoid axis of RBC, end-over-end tumbling, periodic swinging, and membrane tanktreading enable cell deformability **(Fig. 2)**. Tanktreading involves points on the membrane traverse around the discoid without changing cell shape.[7] Deformability is dependent on cytoskeletal proteins, the interaction between the cytoskeleton and integral membrane processes, ion channels, and intracellular viscosity.[5] While reduced RBC deformability is a common phenomenon in hereditary anemia, it is also associated with EH. Deformability may be highly dependent on the membrane's sodium–potassium pump as the activity of membrane Na^+-K^+ adenosine triphosphatase (ATPase) contributes in intracellular viscosity and surface-to-volume ratio.[6,8]

Membrane Transporters and Red Blood Cell Deformability in Essential Hypertension

Essential hypertension is characterized by alterations in cation transporters, especially for Na^+-K^+ATPase, Na^+-K^+ cotransport, and sodium–lithium (Na–Li) counter transport of RBC membrane.[9] Role of Na^+-K^+ATPase has been understood most well **(Fig. 3)**. Less number of Na^+-K^+-ATPase were reported for

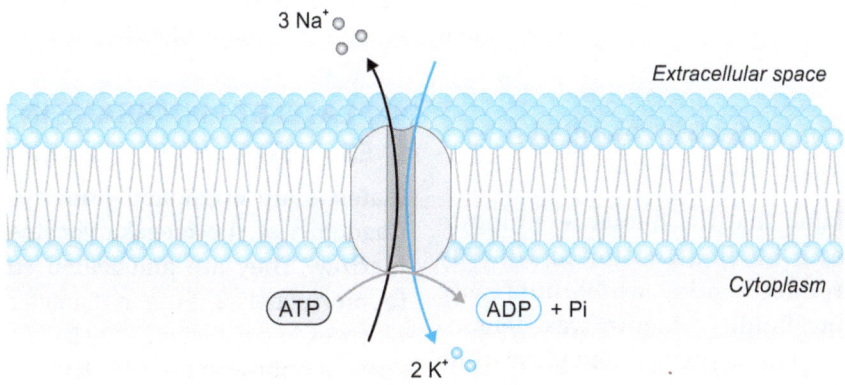

Fig. 3: Schematic diagram of Na^+-K^+ pump.

familial EH.[9] This pump is present in the cell membrane, maintains the electrochemical gradient across the membrane, and influences transepithelial transport. This enzyme transports Na^+ outside the cell and K^+ inside, thus maintaining cell volume and water homeostasis. A lowered activity of this pump causes increased intracellular sodium ion concentration, which has been found to be associated with hypertension.[6] It is hypothesized that accumulated intracellular Na^+, in turn, raises the cellular Ca^{2+} concentration via the Na^+-Ca^{2+} exchanger. This results in increased contraction in vascular smooth muscle or heart muscle leading to hypertension.

Role of Cytoskeleton in Changed Deformability

The basic triangular network of spectrin–band 3, ankyrin, and protein 4.1 of RBC membrane creates a dynamic scaffold, supports integral membrane proteins, and provides integrity of the cells under stress. Connectivity of the skeletal proteins with the membrane proteins through junctional or ankyrin complexes has been found to be altered in the erythrocytes of the individuals with EH.[10]

Altered Membrane Fluidity

The cell membrane is a complex of proteins and lipids, and is fluidic in nature, that is, lipids and proteins move laterally in the plane of the plasma membrane. Fluidity is essential for cell growth, signaling, function, and reproduction. It has been shown that membrane fluidity is also essential for maintaining cell shape and motility in bacterial cells.[11] Membrane fluidity plays a key role in changing the rheologic behavior of cells. Membrane fluidity or reciprocal value of membrane microviscosity may affect membrane permeability, transport, and receptor functions.[2] This property can be affected by various factors including the state of membrane lipids, proteins, cytoskeletal members, intracellular ion contents, and neurohumoral molecules.[2] It was found that fluidity was significantly decreased with increased membrane microviscosity in the RBCs of EH patients than normotensives, and it was not observed for secondary hypertension.[2] Thus, it can be said that this abnormality is genetically inherited and is not a consequence of high blood pressure. Deformability of RBCs as well as oxygen perfusion in microcirculation would be reduced if membrane fluidity is decreased, which would contribute to the development of EH.

Effect of Nitric Oxide on Red Blood Cell Membrane Fluidity

It was found that the human erythrocyte possesses a binding site for the obesity gene product leptin, which increases membrane fluidity.[2] Leptin was demonstrated to increase plasma[2] and nitric oxide can enhance membrane fluidity.[12] RBC membrane possesses endothelial nitric oxide synthase (eNOS),[13] is a key enzyme in the production of NO, a vasodilator. NO also inhibits platelet aggregation and adhesion.[14]

Effect of Intracellular Calcium (Ca^{2+}) on Red Blood Cell Membrane Fluidity

Intracellular Ca^{2+} is usually elevated in different cell types in hypertension, including smooth muscle cells, RBCs, and platelets. Intracellular calcium (Ca^+) may also regulate the size, and shape thus fluidity of the cells.[2] It is proposed that Ca^{2+} may induce precipitation or cross-linkage of the membranous proteins, which confer rigidity to the erythrocytes.[15] Membrane fluidity of erythrocytes decreased markedly in the case of EH than in the normotensive control individuals when cells were exposed to calcium ionophore and calcium.[2]

Role of Insulin on Red Blood Cell Membrane Fluidity

Interestingly, insulin can affect fluidity as it influences several ionic membrane transporters such as Na, K-ATPase, Ca-ATPase, and sodium–calcium (Na-Ca) exchange mechanism, etc., and can enhance intracellular Ca^{2+} in vascular smooth muscle cells, RBCs, and platelets. Higher plasma insulin level has been found to be associated with decreased membrane fluidity of RBCs.[2]

PLATELET MEMBRANE IN ESSENTIAL HYPERTENSION

Platelets are originated from cytoplasmic fragments of the megakaryocytes in bone marrow. They are anucleated small cells (approximately 2–3 µm in diameter) and are biconvex in circulation. They have a short life span of approximately 10 days in humans. They are metabolically active cells containing intracellular organelles. The cell surface typically has a diverse type of receptors, and adhesion molecules and interior contain numerous granules.[16] While blood platelets account for two-thirds of available platelets, the remaining one-third are found in the spleen. When required, they move out from the spleen to the blood, are activated, and become irregular and sticky. They extend pseudopods adhere to the damaged blood vessels, and bind to other platelets to form aggregates resulting in the formation of thrombi and preventing excessive bleeding.[17]

Platelet Membrane

A platelet membrane is a standard lipid bilayer with cholesterol distributed asymmetrically. Neutral phospholipids are predominant in the lipid bilayer. Anionic or polar phospholipids including phosphatidylinositol, and phosphatidylserine are also present in the membrane. Upon activation, polar phosphatidylserine flips to the extracellular side of the membrane and helps in the binding of coagulation factors.[17]

The plasma membrane of a platelet has unique invaginations forming a canalicular system, that twists through the platelet and connects with the exterior through small pores. Remnants of rough endoplasmic

CHAPTER 4: Role of Cell Membrane (Red Blood Cells and Platelets) in Essential Hypertension

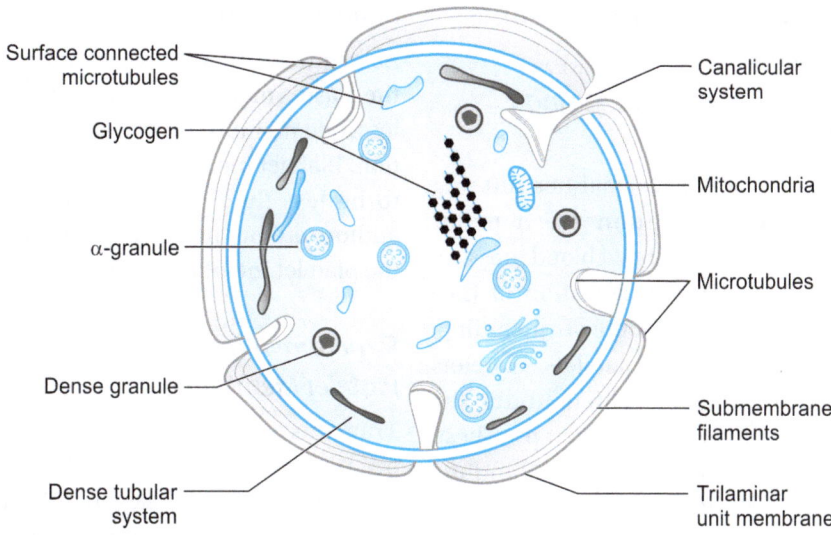

Fig. 4: Platelet cell structure.
Source: Mohan SP, Jaishangar N, Devy S, Narayanan A, Cherian D, Madhavan SS. Platelet-rich plasma and platelet-rich fibrin in periodontal regeneration: A review. J Pharm Bio Sci. 2019;11(Suppl. 2):S126-30.

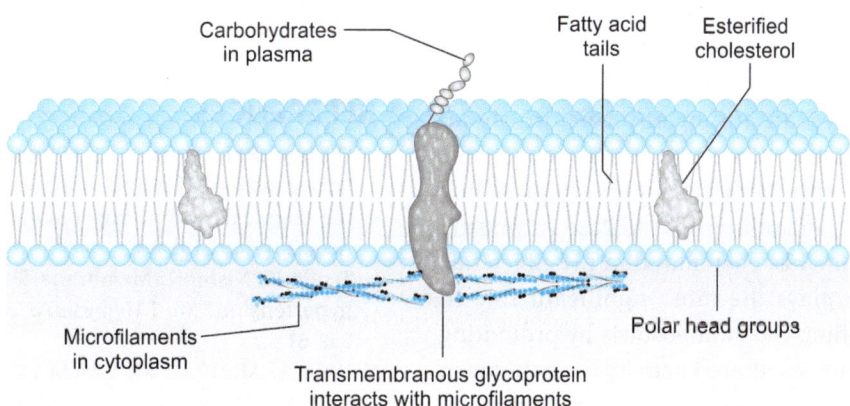

Fig. 5: General diagram of a platelet lipid bilayer.
Source: Fritsma GA.[17]

reticulum form a dense tubular system located close to the plasma membrane and store Ca^{2+} and enzymes required for platelet activation **(Figs. 4 and 5)**. The membrane is characterized by the presence of more than 50 categories of receptors including different cell adhesion molecules (CAM), which bind with a wide range of ligands; for example, collagen, fibronectin, fibrinogen, laminin, von Willebrand factor, etc.[17]

Platelets have a strong networking of cytoskeleton; a bundle of microtubules along with the circumference maintains the platelet's discoid shape and provides rigidity to the pseudopods. Between the microtubules and the membrane lies meshwork of actin microfilaments, which is contractile in nature. Intermediate filaments connect microtubules and actin microfilaments to maintain platelet shape.[17]

Platelet Membrane in Essential Hypertension

Membrane Ca^{2+} Binding Causing Ca^{2+} Influx

Platelet membrane abnormalities altering cellular Ca^{2+} concentration are a major underlying cause of enhanced blood pressure in EH. Intracellular concentration of Ca^{2+} is elevated in various blood cells including, RBCs, lymphocytes, and platelets. Platelets have intrinsic defects, which limits the outcome of antihypertensive therapy. These defects may be in membrane Ca^{2+} binding, Ca^{2+} influx, Ca^{2+} efflux/sequestration, and hormone responsiveness.[18] A decreased Ca^{2+} binding to the plasma membrane can cause partial depolarization of plasma membrane resulting in increased Ca^{2+} influx, and intracellular Ca^{2+} concentration. Calmodulin is a cytoplasmic calcium-binding protein that plays an important role in signal transduction. Changed interaction of this protein with its target protein in signaling pathway, including Ca^{2+}-ATPase in plasma membrane has been found in EH. Since this enzyme plays the most significant role in maintaining Ca^{2+} homeostasis by promoting Ca^{2+} efflux, its altered activity contributes in elevating intracellular Ca^{2+} concentration. A phosphoinositide-mediated Ca^{2+} release from ER store can also add to intracellular Ca^{2+} concentration.[18]

Alteration in the function of membrane-bound adenylate cyclase that synthesizes cyclic AMP from ATP has also been implicated with EH. Low intracellular Ca^{2+} concentration in platelets activates this enzyme and the resulting increase in cAMP promotes Ca^{2+} efflux. Thus, increased concentration in platelets inhibits adenylate cyclase and further Ca^{2+} efflux.[18]

Platelet Membrane Fluidity

As mentioned earlier, structural alteration in the plasma membrane can result in stiffer and less fluid membranes that affect cellular function. Platelet membrane has also been found to be less fluidic in EH.[19] However, some authors did not find any change in fluidity in the platelet membrane of hypertensives.[20]

Structural Alterations of Platelet Membrane

Transmission electron microscopic study on platelet ultrastructural morphology has shown that platelet membrane, when activated, undergoes morphological changes resulting in six forms, discoid, pseudotubular, saccular, membranous, pseudopodal, and hyaline, which correlated with the severity of hypertension.[21]

■ REFERENCES

1. O'Shea PM, Griffin TP, Fitzgibbon M. Hypertension: The role of biochemistry in the diagnosis and management. Clin Chim Acta. 2017;465:131-43.
2. Tsuda K, Nishio I. Membrane fluidity and hypertension. Am J Hypertens. 2003;16(3):259-61.
3. Vayá A, Martínez M, Garcia J, Labios M, Aznar J. Hemorheological alterations in mild essential hypertension. Thromb Res. 1992;66(2-3):223-9.
4. Cherubini P, Bozzoni M, Agosti R, Clivati A, Somazzi R, Longhini E. Red blood cell filterability in essential hypertension: Role of transmembranary ions fluxes. Clin Hemorheol. 1989;9(1):89-100.
5. Huisjes R, Bogdanova A, van Solinge WW, Schiffelers RM, Kaestner L, van Wijk R. Squeezing for life—properties of red blood cell deformability. Front Physiol. 2018;9:656.
6. Radosinska J, Vrbjar N. The role of red blood cell deformability and Na,K-ATPase function in selected risk factors of cardiovascular

diseases in humans: focus on hypertension, diabetes mellitus and hypercholesterolemia. Physiol Res. 2016;65(Suppl. 1):S43-54.
7. Kuhn V, Diederich L, Keller TCS IV, Kramer CM, Lückstädt W, Panknin C, et al. Red blood cell function and dysfunction: Redox regulation, nitric oxide metabolism, anemia. Antioxid Redox Signal. 2017;26(13):718-42.
8. Tsuda K. Red blood cell abnormalities and hypertension. Hypertens Res. 2020;43(1):72-3.
9. Canestrari F, Gallia F, Boschib S, Gheller G, Crescentini SD, Bossú M. Erythrocyte Na^+,K^+-ATPase properties and adenylate energy charge in normotensives and in essential hypertensives. Clinica Chimica Acta. 1994;224(2):167-79.
10. Kaczmarska M, Fornal M, Messerli FH, Korecki J, Grodzicki T, Burda K. Erythrocyte membrane properties in patients with essential hypertension. Cell Biochem Biophys. 2013;67(3):1089-102.
11. Kurita K, Kato F, Shiomi D. Alteration of membrane fluidity or phospholipid composition perturbs rotation of MreB complexes in *Escherichia coli*. Front Mol Biosci. 2020;7:582660.
12. Tsuda K, Kimura K, Nishio I, Masuyama Y. Nitric oxide improves membrane fluidity of erythrocytes in essential hypertension: An electron paramagnetic resonance investigation. Biochem Biophys Res Commun. 2000;275(3):946-54.
13. Kleinbongard P, Schulz R, Rassaf T, Lauer T, Dejam A, Jax T, et al. Red blood cells express a functional endothelial nitric oxide synthase. Blood. 2006;107:2943-51.
14. Kleinert H, Forstermann U, Endothelial nitric oxide synthase. In: Enna SJ, Bylund DB (Eds). xPharm: The Comprehensive Pharmacology Reference, Elsevier, Amsterdam;2007. pp. 1-8.
15. Kuettner JF, Dreher KL, Rao GHR, Eaton JW, Blackshear PL Jr, White JG. Influence of the ionophore A23187 on the plastic behavior of normal erythrocytes. Am J Pathol. 1977;88(1):81-94.
16. Gremmel T, Frelinger AL III, Michelson AD. Platelet physiology. Semin Thromb Hemost 2016;42(3):191-204.
17. Fritsma GA. Platelet structure and function. Clin Lab Sci. 2015;28(2):125-31.
18. Bühler FR, Resink TJ. Platelet membrane and calcium control abnormalities in essential hypertension. Am J Hypertens. 1988;1(1):42-6.
19. Naftilan AJ, Dzau VJ, Loscalzo J. Preliminary observations on abnormalities of membrane structure and function in essential hypertension. Hypertension. 1986;8(6 Pt 2):II174-9.
20. Caimi G, Presti RL, Montana M, Contorno A, Canino B, Catania A, et al. Platelet membrane fluidity and platelet membrane lipid pattern in essential hypertension. Am J Hypertens. 1995;8:82-6.
21. Pande I, Bajpai VK, Chandra M, Singh BN. Platelet ultrastructural morphology and its relevance in essential hypertension. Int J Cardiol 1993;41(1):13-20.

CHAPTER 5

Matrix Metalloproteinases and the Extracellular Matrix

Bidita Khandelwal, Chamma Gupta

■ INTRODUCTION

The multifaceted nature of complications that accompany hypertension (HTN) makes it challenging to develop a molecular model for HTN and its target organ damage. Cardiac and vessel remodeling; atherosclerosis; and diabetes mellitus (DM) are present in patients with a family history of HTN even before they develop HTN. The varied pathophysiological phenomenon has not been conclusively defined under a common molecular basis. However, extracellular matrix (ECM) and its regulation by matrix metalloproteinases (MMPs) have been documented extensively in the pathogenesis of HTN. There are still unanswered questions pertaining to MMPs being involved in the early stages of HTN and whether they are mediators of HTN and associated complications.

▍VASCULAR REMODELING IN HYPERTENSION

Both large (conductance) arteries (i.e., aorta and large arteries) and small (resistance) arterioles are involved in the pathophysiology of HTN. The structure of the conductance arteries helps in serving as a blood reservoir and to stretch or recoil corresponding with the contractile activity of the heart. The arterioles, which are the major site of resistance have more smooth muscle cells and less elastic fibers in their walls. Minor changes in the caliber of the arterioles lead to large changes in the total peripheral resistance. Several types of remodeling, that is, eutrophic, hypertrophic, and hypertrophic are identified in the vasculature depending on the decrease or increase of cellular components of the wall or in its absence.

Thickening of the medial layer leads to a reduction of the lumen of the vessel and an increased ratio of wall/lumen of the vessel. This is known as eutrophic inward remodeling. This is observed in the initial stage of mild HTN. An increase in the lumen of the vessel without alteration of its cross-sectional area is characteristic of eutrophic outward remodeling. An increased ratio of wall/lumen of the vessel caused by the thickening of the medial layer is observed in hypertrophic inward remodeling. This has been observed in renovascular HTN and in well-established HTN. Hypotrophic outward remodeling is characterized by an increase in the lumen of the vessel wall with a decrease in its cross-sectional area. Increased intravascular pressure or reduced blood flow results in concentric (inward) vascular remodeling while increased blood flow leads to eccentric (outer) remodeling. However, multiple factors may work simultaneously in a patient and so the effect of antihypertensive drugs on the remodeling of the medial layer is also variable.

Rearrangement of the existing cellular and extracellular components of the arterial wall leads to remodeling.[1] Hypertension-induced maladaptive remodeling is improved by inhibition of ECM proteolysis by MMPs. The hypertrophic remodeling mainly in conductance arteries is associated with increased proliferation of vascular smooth muscle cells (VSMCs), thickening of arterial media, and resynthesis of many ECM components. Resistance arteries undergo eutrophic modeling due to the rearrangement of VSMC. Moreover, MMP-2 degrades collagen type IV, thus facilitating migration, proliferation, vascular wall thickening, and thus further remodeling. There is a rise in the synthesis of collagen type I, tenascin, and elastin in VSMC as compensation for MMP-2 degradation of collagen IV, leading to a further increase in the vascular wall thickening. The cleavage products of collagen degradation bind to different integrins in VSMC leading to the synthesis of new ECM components. Increased apoptosis and/or atrophy of some layers of vascular wall further contribute to the remodeling.[2]

CARDIAC REMODELING IN HYPERTENSION

The increased wall pressure in the heart results in increase in wall tension and stress leading to excess accumulation of ECM components which in turn raises myocardial stiffness, thus compromising diastolic function. Further accumulation impairs myocardial contraction and systolic function. In postmortem of human hearts and endomyocardial human biopsies, an increase in the amount of fibrillar collagen in the myocardium of patients with hypertensive heart disease was observed.[3] An increase in the proteoglycan biglycan, and the adhesive proteins fibronectin and laminin are also reported.[4] The increase in wall stress itself is the initial stimulus for excessive collagen deposition which starts as a physiological process but later becomes maladaptive and leads to fibrosis.

MATRIX METALLOPROTEINASES

The MMPs are members of metzincins, a ubiquitously expressed family of multidomain zinc (II)—dependent endopeptidases. The MMPs are initially produced as zymogen (nonfunctional) as propeptide sequence by a wide range of tissues and cells. It is divided into six major classes based on their structural and substrate specificity as listed in the following:[5]

1. Collagenases—MMP-1 (collagenase-1), MMP-8 (collagenase-2), MMP-13 (collagenase-3), and MMP-18 (collagenase-4).
2. Gelatinases—MMP-2 (gelatinase-A and type IV collagenase) and MMP-9 (gelatinase-B and type IV collagenase).
3. Stromelysins—MMP-3 (stromelysin-1), MMP-10 (stromelysin-2), and MMP-11 (stromelysin-3).
4. Matrilysins—MMP-7 (matrilysin-1) and MMP-26 (matrilysin-2).
5. Membrane type—MMP-14, MMP-15, MMP-16, MMP-17, MMP-24, and MMP-25 (MT1-MMP and MT6-MMP, respectively).
6. Other MMPs—MMP-12 (metalloelastase), MMP-19 (RASI-1), MMP-20 (enamelysin), MMP-21 (xenopus-MMP), MMP-22 (chicken-MMP), MMP-23 (CA-MMP), MMP-27 (human MMP-22 homolog), and MMP-28 (epilysin).

The first MMP, interstitial collagenase was identified in 1962 as the protease responsible for the degradation of fibrillar collagen in tadpole tail during metamorphosis which was subsequently named as MMP-1 after identification of similar collagenase in human skin.[5] The versatile MMP family with wide physiological functions consists of 23 distinct proteases which share structural domains but have variable substrate specificity, cellular sources, tissue localization, membrane binding and transcriptional regulation. There are several conserved domains in the excreted MMPs. The prodomain shields the catalytic domain in the inactive form of the enzyme. The gelatinases (MMP-2 and MMP-9) additionally contain a series of three fibronectin type II inserts in the catalytic domain, which helps binding of gelatin and collagen **(Fig. 1)**.[6]

■ EXTRACELLULAR MATRIX

Extracellular matrix is broadly classified into three major types—structural proteins such as collagen and elastin, specialized and adhesive proteins such as fibronectin and laminin,

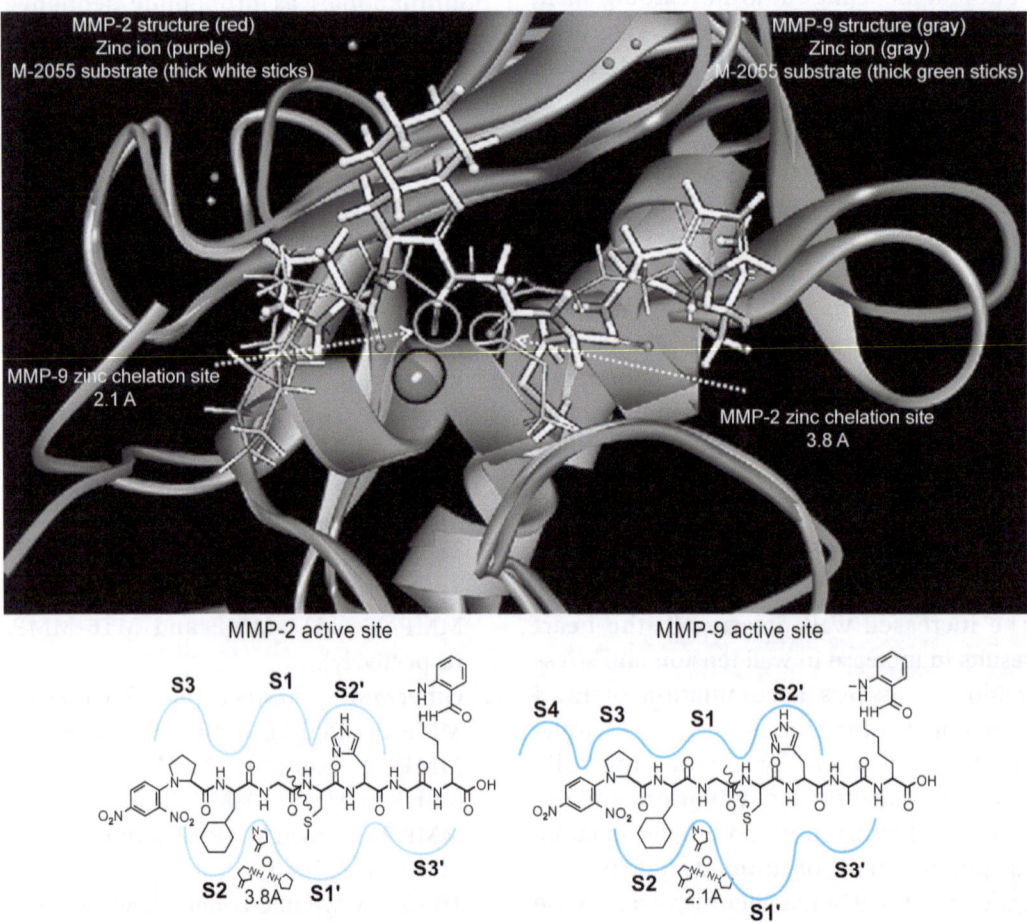

Fig. 1: Docked complexes of 1 substrate and the catalytic domain of human MMP-2 (PDB code, 1QIB) and MMP-9 (PDB code, 1GKC). The MMP-substrate docked complexes are merged with zinc as the same point of view. The MMP-2 structure is shown in red, zinc as purple, and 1 substrate (white sticks) docked within MMP-2 active site; MMP-9 is shown in gray, zinc as green and 1 substrate (thin green sticks) is docked within its active site. (Bottom) Schematic representation of 1 substrate: Active site binding interaction in human MMP-2 and MMP-9. MMP-2 and MMP-9 enzyme binding pockets are shown in red and green, respectively. The substrate's chemical structure and its scissile bond are shown in black. The zinc ion is indicated in blue. *(For color version, see Plate 1)*

and proteoglycan and glycosaminoglycan. Type I and type III collagens form 60 and 30% of vascular collagens, respectively, and are found in intima, media and adventitia. They are the major source of tensile strength. Elastin in the ECM provides elasticity and is present in the large arteries as well as the resistance arteries **(Fig. 2)**.[7]

Matrix Metalloproteinases Regulation

Regulation of MMPs is mediated through gene transcription, zymogen activation, post-translational modification, and tissue inhibitors of metalloproteinase (TIMP) inhibition. The TIMPs, four distinct ones, have broad MMP inhibitory activities. They are unique with some similar characteristics. The binding of N-terminal region of TIMP to the catalytic domain of MMPs leads to inhibition of their activity. The inhibitory complex is stabilized by the binding of C-terminal to the hemopexin domain of MMPs. The TIMP-1 predominantly inhibits MMP-9, TIMP-2 inhibits MMP-2, TIMP-3 inhibits almost all MMPs in ECM and is an important marker of cardiac hypertrophy. Also, TIMP-4 inhibits MMP-2 and MTI-MMP.[8,9] Furthermore, TIMP-4 is present inside the cardiomyocytes as well as in the ECM. There are speculations that MMP synthesis and activity may be time dependent. The MMP system is activated in early phase of HTN to allow smooth muscle cells migration and vessel wall restructuring. With disease progression, there is suppression of MMP system causing ECM deposition and fibrosis **(Figs. 3A and B)**. In the case of a blade (IV) of MMP9 and CD44, it is unknown whether the interaction is associated with zymogen activation or inhibition. However, CD44-bound MMP-9 was shown to be in the active state.[10]

Extracellular Matrix Regulation

Extracellular matrix metabolism is regulated by MMP and natural tissue endogenous inhibitors. Interstitial collagenase MMP-1 degrades structural and fibrillar collagens (types I–III). Gelatinase-A (MMP-2) and MMP-9 are two enzymes that mainly digest denatured collagen (gelatins), elastin, fibronectin, laminin as well as collagens types IV and V (found predominantly in the subendothelial basement membrane of the vessel wall). Proteoglycans also indirectly regulate ECM synthesis and degradation. Apart from fibroblasts, other cellular components of cardiovascular system and infiltrative cells may also synthesize ECM components.

Matrix Metalloproteinases and Hypertension

Regulation and modulation of ECM by direct proteolytic degradation of the ECM proteins (e.g., collagen, proteoglycans, and fibronectin) are the principal physiological function. MMPs are not just ECM modeling protease. Major complications of HTN also have alterations in their levels.[11,12] All members of MMP family have been linked to disease development ranging from chronic inflammation, HTN, other cardiovascular disease and neurological disorders to cancer metastasis. Several mechanisms including the elevated level of vasoactive peptides, catecholamine, oxidative stress, inflammation, endothelial dysfunction, and altered MMPs level are responsible for the persistently increased BP values. Through the induction of theses mechanism, it favors changes in MMPs/TIMPs activity and/or level. This occurrence is probably going to lead to a vicious cycle where altered MMPs are in charge of altering the ECM, VSMCs,

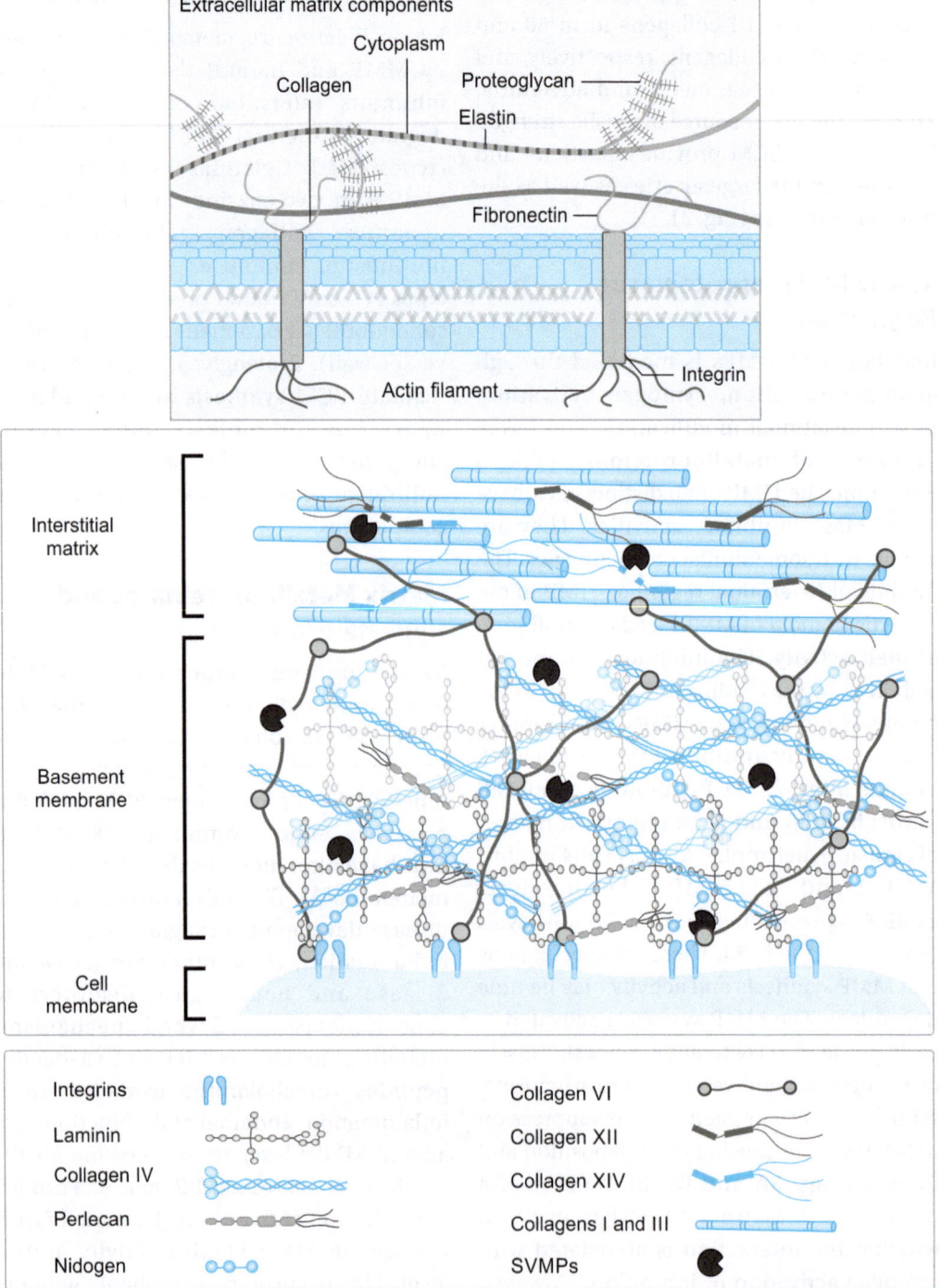

Fig. 2: Extracellular matrix and its component. (SVMPs: snake venom metalloproteinases) [7]

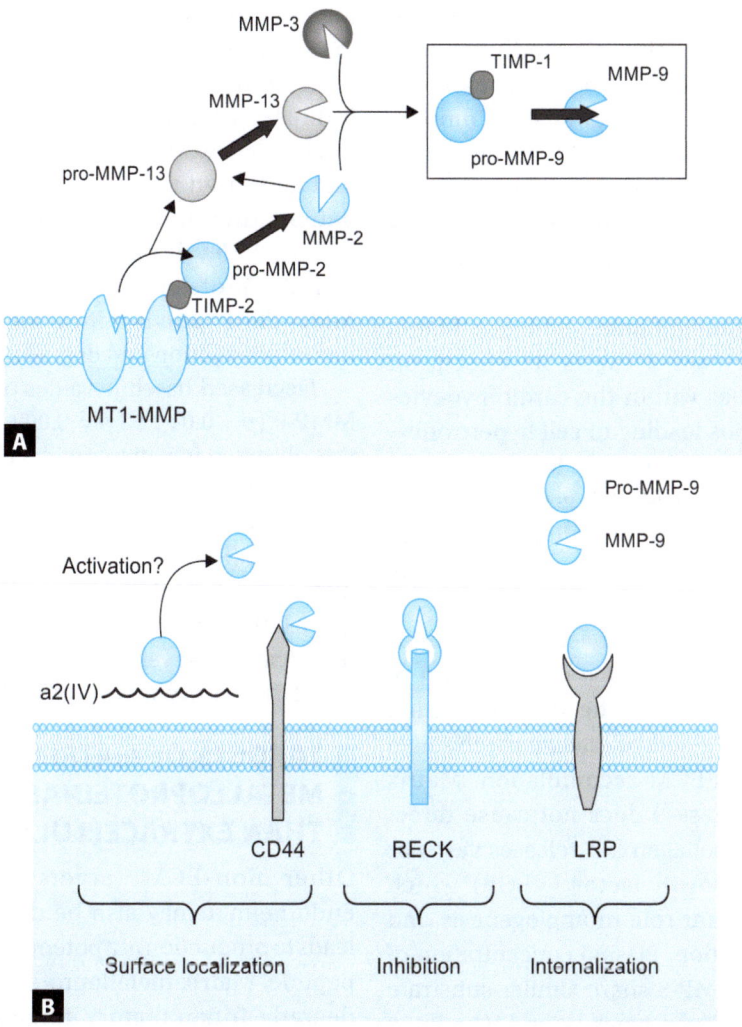

Figs. 3A and B: (A) Matrix metalloproteinase cascade of zymogen activation involved in pro-MMP-9 activation. The pro-MMP-9 can be activated by several MMPs including MMP-3, MMP-2, and MMP-13. This cascade of zymogen activation is initiated by MT1-MMP at the cell membrane and requires the action of TIMP-2. It culminates with the generation of MMP-2 and MMP-13, which in turn can activate pro-MMP-9. Matrix metalloproteinase-3 is another pro-MMP-9 activator, probably the most efficient, but is activated by plasmin via uPAR and uPA on the cell surface (not depicted here). Pro-MMP-9 can be found in a complex with TIMP-1 but the role of this complex on activation is unknown. How pro-MMP-9 can be in proximity to this potential activation cascade is also unknown; (B) Reported proteins involved in pro-MMP-9/MMP-9 cell surface association. These diverse proteins play distinct roles in MMP-9 function including surface localization, inhibition, and internalization.

and cardiomyocytes, causing organ damage, and sustenance of high blood pressure.[13,14]

Matrix metalloproteinase-2 is a neutral endopeptidase and its inhibitors may help in maintaining local adrenomedullin (AM) levels and in mitigating HTN.[15,16] Adrenomedullin is a fragment peptide resulting from the degradation of the vasodilator peptide by

MMP-2 and has vasoconstrictive properties. AM, apart from being a vasodilator also inhibits myocardial fibrosis expressed in endothelium and vascular smooth muscle. Due to both the properties, it has direct impact on the vascular tone in arteries and arterioles.[17] Whether MMP-2-mediated HTN has differential signaling in the arterial wall of angiotensin 2-induced HTN and cardiac remodeling has conflicting evidence. Matrix metalloproteinase-2 exerts its effects on ECM as well as within the cardiomyocytes and VSMC thus leading to cell hypertrophy, proliferation and migration. It was observed that expression of MMP-9 is greatly increased in MMP-2 null mice which led to the hypothesis that MMP-2 function may be interchangeable with other MMPs.[18]

Matrix metalloproteinase-7 also modulates cardiac hypertrophy via activation of MMP-2. The increase in the MMP expression and activity is a compensatory mechanism to limit excess ECM accumulation. Matrix metalloproteinase-9 does not cause direct proteolysis of collagen I. It releases vascular endothelial growth factor (VEGF) which has an important role in angiogenesis and neovascularization. Plasma concentration of MMP-2 and MMP-9 share similar substrate specificity (collagen types IV and V) related to vascular remodeling and are depressed in essential HTN. Matrix metalloproteinase-2 due to its ability to cleave ECM and other intracellular targets in the cardiomyocytes affects the contractile ability and contributes to structural changes also. Other vasoactive peptides, cytokines, and growth factors such as transforming growth factor-β (TGF-β) also mediate the process.

Portik–Dobos AEV, et al. reported decrease in MMP-1, MMP-2, and MMP-9 activity in the internal mammary artery specimens of hypertensive patients undergoing coronary artery bypass grafting surgery. Matrix metalloproteinase activator protein (MTI-MMP), extracellular matrix metalloproteinase inducer (EMMPRIN) protein and tissue inhibitors of MMPs (TIMP-1 and TIMP-2), all had decreased tissue levels in hypertensive patient thus indicating that in HTN not only MMP levels but also their inducer and activator proteins are downregulated. Thus, MMP/TIMP ratio is critical for coordinating matrix production and degradation.[19]

Decreased baseline values of MMP-2 and MMP-9 ($p = 0.01$ and $p = 0.002$, respectively) was observed in patients with HTN compared to normotensives. Among the hypertensive patients also, those with systemic vascular resistance (SVR) less than 1440 dyn s/cm had higher values of MMP-2 ($p = 0.005$) and MMP-9 ($p = 0.001$) compared to those with SVR > 1440 dyn s/cm.[5] However, the study did not evaluate the plasma concentration of TIMP.[1]

TARGETS OF MATRIX METALLOPROTEINASES OTHER THAN EXTRACELLULAR MATRIX

Other non-ECM targets such as big endothelin-1 may also be degraded which leads to production of a potent vasoconstrictor peptide. Matrix metalloproteinases can also degrade inflammatory targets. Increased MMPs activate cytokines and in turn increased cytokines and oxidative stress increase the MMP activity and the proteolytic actions in the vasculature.

EXTRACELLULAR MATRIX AND HYPERTENSION

Hypertension-related accumulation of ECM proteins in the myocardium and arteries is modulated by altered MMP and/or TIMP activity. Cytoskeletal rearrangement of the vessel wall also occurs (via integrin-mediated signaling) due to ECM modulation by MMP.

Abnormal degradation of collagen type I (the major form of collagen in hypertensive myocardial fibrosis) is observed in patients with essential HTN. The three-dimensional spatial arrangement responsible for the metabolic function and integrity of the tissue in extracellular space is dependent on the ECM. Alterations in the density of ECM components, ECM architecture and cell ECM attachments (both in myocardium and vessel) are evident in HTN. ECM requires constant synthesis and degradation.

Vasoactive hormones and mediators, together with local growth factors and cytokines play a key intermediary role in converting changes in blood pressure to the adaptive changes in the ECM. Multiple systemic and local factors such as vasoactive substances (angiotensin 2, aldosterone, adrenergic stimuli, natriuretic peptides, endothelin, AM, prostanoids nitric oxide), growth factors, cytokines, and other mediators (TGF-β, platelet-derived growth factor, fibroblast growth factor, insulin-like growth factor 1, bone morphogenetic proteins, tumor necrosis factor-α, connective tissue growth factor hepatocyte growth factor, interleukins, interferons, and plasminogen activator inhibitor-1) may be involved in the processes of ECM remodeling in HTN.

Structural changes involving myocyte hypertrophy and excessive accumulation of ECM are important components of cardiac remodeling which is associated with arterial HTN. Accumulation of ECM leads to fibrosis thus influencing myocardial stiffness and promoting arrhythmias.

Serum Markers of Cardiovascular Extracellular Matrix Regulation in Hypertension

New noninvasive assays have been used for collagen fragment peptides by several groups for assessment of cardiovascular collagen synthesis and degradation in hypertensive patients. The type 1 procollagen carboxy-terminal peptide (PIP) and type III collagen amino-terminal peptide (PIIIP) produced during the synthesis of collagen fibrils and the carboxy-terminal telopeptide of collagen type I (CITP) is a marker of degradation of type I collagen. Increased levels of PIP, PIIIP, CITP, and TIMP-1a and reduced MMP-1 have been reported in hypertensive patients compared to normotensives.[20-23] Whether the changes seen in the serum accurately reflect the situation in the heart and vessel needs further evidence. In future they could be potential serum markers for ECM metabolism.

■ CONCLUSION

The role of ECM and MMP in the pathogenesis of HTN and its comorbidities have ample evidence but unexplored domains still exist. Other MMP—specific signaling cascades; for example, MMP-14 (MT-1 MMP) is involved in cell migration (through ECM) and in fibroblast proliferation. Matrix metalloproteinase not only contributes to the maladaptive vascular and cardiac alterations in HTN by ECM degradation but also affects the non-ECM and inflammatory components in cardiomyocytes and VSMC thus having intracellular effects leading to cell hypertrophy and associated dysfunction. As MMPs are a major contributor to tissue repair and their activity and endogenous inhibitors are not only member specific but also organ specific, hence a broader understanding of the genetic as well as environmental cause of MMP activation is a necessity before therapeutic interventions can be targeted towards it as a molecular culprit with certainty. However, the fact that ECM has a pivotal role in vascular, cardiac and renal remodeling, which results in deterioration of tissue structure, function, and perfusion and thus to the morbidity and mortality related to HTN makes it an important target.

■ REFERENCES

1. Zervoudaki A, Economou E, Stefanadis C, Pitsavos C, Tsioufis K, Aggeli C, et al. Plasma levels of active extracellular matrix metalloproteinases 2 and 9 in patients with essential hypertension before and after antihypertensive treatment. J Hum Hypertens. 2003;17(2):119-24.
2. Page-McCaw A, Ewald AJ, Werb Z. Matrix metalloproteinases and the regulation of tissue remodelling. Nat Rev Mol Cell Biol. 2007;8(3):221-33.
3. Grimm D, Kromer EP, Böcker W, Bruckschlegel G, Holmer SR, Riegger GA, et al. Regulation of extracellular matrix proteins in pressure-overload cardiac hypertrophy: Effects of angiotensin-converting enzyme inhibition. J Hypertens. 1998;16(9):1345-55.
4. López-Jaramillo P, Camacho PA, Forero-Naranjo L. The role of environment and epigenetics in hypertension. Expert Rev Cardiovasc Ther. 2013;11(11):1455-7.
5. Gross J, Lapiere CM. Collagenolytic activity in amphibian tissues: A tissue culture assay. Proc Natl Acad Sci USA. 1962;48(6):1014-22.
6. Brinckerhoff CE, Matrisian LM. Matrix metalloproteinases: A tail of a frog that became a prince. Nat Rev Mol Cell Biol. 2002;3(3):207-14.
7. Gutiérrez JM, Escalante T, Rucavado A, Herrera C, Fox JW. A comprehensive view of the structural and functional alterations of extracellular matrix by snake venom metalloproteinases (SVMPs): Novel perspectives on the pathophysiology of envenoming. Toxins (Basel). 2016;8(10):304.
8. Nagase H, Visse R, Murphy G. Structure and function of matrix metalloproteinases and TIMPs. Cardiovasc Res. 2006;69(3):562-73.
9. Schulze CJ, Wang W, Suarez-Pinzon WL, Sawicka J, Sawicki G, Schulz R. Imbalance between tissue inhibitor of metalloproteinase-4 and matrix metalloproteinases during acute myocardial (correction of myocardial) ischemia-reperfusion injury. Circulation. 2003;107(19):2487-92.
10. Melendez-Zajgla J, Pozo LD, Ceballos G, Maldonado V. Tissue inhibitor of metalloproteinases-4. The road less traveled. Mol Cancer. 2008;7:85.
11. Rosell A, Lo EH. Multiphasic roles for matrix metalloproteinases after stroke. Curr Opin Pharmacol. 2008;8(1):82-9.
12. Rodriguez JA, Orbe J, de Lizarrondo SM, Calvayrac O, Rodriguez C, Martinez-Gonzalez J, et al. Metalloproteinases and atherothrombosis: MMP-10 mediates vascular remodeling promoted by inflammatory stimuli. Front Biosci. 2008;13:2916-21.
13. Bisogni V, Cerasari A, Pucci G, Vaudo G. Matrix metalloproteinases and hypertension-mediated organ damage: Current insights. Integr Blood Press Control. 2020;13:157-69.
14. Wang X, Khalil RA. Matrix metalloproteinases, vascular remodeling, and vascular disease. Adv Pharmacol. 2018;81:241-330.
15. Nawarskas J, Rajan V, Frishman WH. Vasopeptidase inhibitors, neutral endopeptidase inhibitors, and dual inhibitors of angiotensin-converting enzyme and neutral endopeptidase. Heart Dis. 2001;3(6):378-85.
16. Corti R, Burnett JC, Rouleau JL, Ruschitzka F, Lüscher TF. Vasopeptidase inhibitors: A new therapeutic concept in cardiovascular disease? Circulation. 2001;104(15):1856-62.
17. Martínez A, Oh HR, Unsworth EJ, Bregonzio C, Saavedra JM, Stetler-Stevenson WG, et al. Matrix metalloproteinase-2 cleavage of adrenomedullin produces a vasoconstrictor out of a vasodilator. Biochem J. 2004;383 (Pt. 3):413-8.
18. Esparza J, Kruse M, Lee J, Michaud M, Madri JA. MMP-2 null mice exhibit an early onset and severe experimental autoimmune encephalomyelitis due to an increase in MMP-9 expression and activity. FASEB J. 2004;18(14):1682-91.
19. Ergul A, Portik-Dobos V, Hutchinson J, Franco J, Anstadt MP. Downregulation of vascular matrix metalloproteinase inducer and activator proteins in hypertensive patients. Am J Hypertens. 2004;17(9):775-82.

20. Laviades C, Varo N, Fernández J, Mayor G, Gil MJ, Monreal I, et al. Abnormalities of the extracellular degradation of collagen type I in essential hypertension. Circulation. 1998;98(6):535-40.
21. Díez J, Laviades C, Mayor G, Gil MJ, Monreal I. Increased serum concentrations of procollagen peptides in essential hypertension. Relation to cardiac alterations. Circulation. 1995;91(5):1450-6.
22. Timms PM, Wright A, Maxwell P, Campbell S, Dawnay AB, Srikanthan V. Plasma tissue inhibitor of metalloproteinase-1 levels are elevated in essential hypertension and related to left ventricular hypertrophy. Am J Hypertens. 2002;15(3):269-72.
23. Lindsay MM, Maxwell P, Dunn FG. TIMP-1: A marker of left ventricular diastolic dysfunction and fibrosis in hypertension. Hypertension. 2002;40(2):136-41.

Role of Calcium Channels in Hypertension

Arundhati Bag, Bidita Khandelwal, Abhishek Byahut

■ INTRODUCTION

Calcium channels are transmembrane ion channels that selectively permit calcium ions (Ca^{2+}) to pass through them. Located in the cell membrane and lipid bilayers of some intracellular compartments, calcium channels play a critical role in the regulation of cellular concentration of Ca^{2+}. These ions are crucial for almost every aspect of cellular functions including muscle contraction, cell growth, gene transcription, enzyme activities, secretions of neurotransmitters, and other essential cellular activities. Also, Ca^{2+} ions are unique in their function, as they not only contribute in generating membrane potential but also play an important role in signal transduction acting as a second messenger. Due to its chemical structure, Ca^{2+} can bind sites with irregular shapes, which makes it a more efficient ligand than the other abundant cations such as Na^+, K^+, and Mg^{2+}.[1] At rest, in general, calcium channels maintain extremely low Ca^{2+} concentration in the cytosol, which is about 1,000 times lower than those in the extracellular environment.[2] As an imbalance in this concentration may lead cells to apoptosis and can cause other deleterious effects, Ca^{2+} concentration is tightly regulated by calcium channels. A disturbed regulation of Ca^{2+} can develop hypertension and influence its treatment because smooth muscle cells, platelets, heart, juxtaglomerular apparatus, neural synapses, and adrenal glomerulosa as an intracellular messenger.[3]

■ CALCIUM CHANNELS

Calcium channels can be gated ion channels, either voltage-gated or ligand-gated. Voltage-gated ion channels open due to depolarization of the membrane whereas ligand-gated channels open due to conformational changes following a ligand-receptor binding. Voltage-gated channels are major types of calcium channels present in plasma membranes. In response to a change in the voltage across the plasma membrane due to an electrochemical gradient, these channels cause a rapid influx of Ca^{2+}. Other than gated calcium channels, some channels on the plasma membrane may be calcium adenosine triphosphatase (ATPase) pumps. They send Ca^{2+} outside the cell through energy-dependent active transport to maintain a steep electrochemical gradient of Ca^{2+} across the plasma membrane. Another kind of calcium channel on the plasma membrane include sodium-calcium exchanger. Na^+/Ca^{2+} exchangers cause efflux of Ca^{2+}. Mostly the Na^+/Ca^{2+} exchanger transports one Ca^{2+} per three Na^+.

Ligand-gated calcium channels include IP3 receptors, and ryanodine receptors (in some plants) on membranes of endoplasmic reticulum (ER) or sarcoplasmic reticulum (SR) in muscle cells, and two-pore channels on endosomal or lysosomal membranes.

Both ER and SR act as large reservoirs of Ca^{2+}. Inositol 1,4,5-trisphosphate (IP3) receptors (IP3Rs) mediate Ca^{2+} release from ER thereby increasing cytosolic calcium concentration to help in necessary calcium-dependent cell functions. The binding of IP3 ligands to IP3R receptors initiates this calcium release. Again, To maintain low calcium concentration, ATP-dependent active pumps; for example, SR calcium ATPase transport [sarcoplasmic/endoplasmic reticulum Ca^2-ATPase (SERCA)] transport Ca^{2+} from the cytosol to ER/SR against the electrochemical gradient. Two-pore channels span the membrane of endosomes and lysosomes. They act as receptors for nicotinic acid adenine dinucleotide phosphate (NAADP) release from lysosomes or endosomes to perform some essential cellular functions such as trafficking of receptor proteins, and viruses, stabilizing junctions with other cellular organelles, etc.[4] Plasma membrane of neurons also hosts some special types of ligand-gated calcium channels, where calcium channels open in response to binding of neurotransmitters.

Structure of Voltage-gated Calcium Channels

Among all the calcium transporters voltage-gated calcium channels are of particular interest as they are the main transducers of membrane potential. The altered function of these channels is commonly have been associated with cardiovascular diseases.

Ion channels are usually composed of different combinations of subunits that interact with one another to form a channel those are selectively permeable to a specific ion. Calcium ion channels are multimeric proteins with pore-forming α subunit and three ancillary subunits, β, δ, and γ (**Fig. 1**). The α subunit has two subunits, α1 and α2. The α1 is the largest subunit, which forms transmembrane pore, sensitive to voltage-gating, and incorporates sites to interact with second messengers, drugs, and toxins.[5] β subunit constitutes the cytosolic part of the pore complex and takes an essential role in signal transduction by interacting with intracellular domains of α1 subunit and downstream proteins. Transmembrane α2δ complex and a γ subunit interact with the

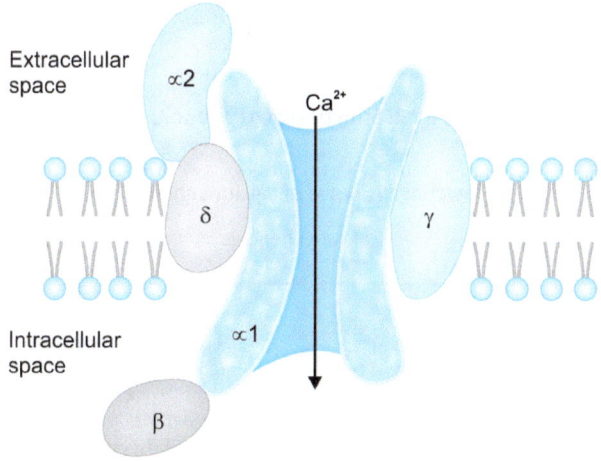

Fig. 1: Generalized structure of calcium channels.
Source: Shah et al.[5]

α1 subunit to regulate voltage gating and membrane trafficking.[5]

The α1 subunit is composed of about 2,000 amino acid residues,[6] which are arranged in four repeated domains I–IV, each containing six transmembrane segments, S1–S6 **(Fig. 2)**. Three large loops, with both amino- and carboxyl-terminal ends in the cytosol, connect the segments together.[7] The S5 and S6 segments of the repeats take part in channel formation while S1–S4 segments of each domain form the voltage sensor.[5] Repeats act as selectivity filters also.

Types of Voltage-gated Channel

Six classes of calcium channels have been identified, L, T, N, P, Q, and R types. Among them, L and T-types are major types of calcium channels found in cardiomyocytes whereas N, P, Q, and R are predominant types in the nervous system.[5]

Calcium channels can be broadly grouped into high- and low-voltage-activated types depending on their voltage sensitivities **(Flowchart 1)**. The L (long-lasting), N, P, Q, and R types are high-voltage-activated calcium channels, which differ from one another based on their pharmacological and biophysical features.[8] The low-voltage channels include T-type (transient) channels.

So far, 10 different α1 subunits have been reported which are encoded by 10 different genes. There are four L-type channels with four different α1 subunits (Cav1.1—Cav1.4). Cav1.1, 1.2, 1.3, and 1.4 possesses α1S, α1C, α1D, and α1F, respectively. Both P- and Q-types have Cav2.1, N-type has Cav2.2, and R-type has Cav2.3 α1 subunit. Furthermore, T-types include Cav3.1, Cav3.2, or Cav3.3 α1 subunits. Amino acid sequences of α1 subunits are more than 70% similar within the members of a channel type but they are only

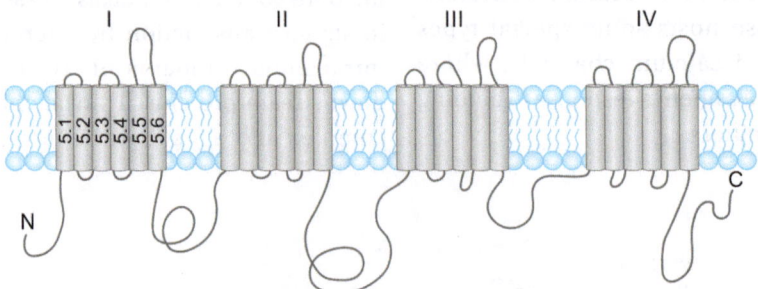

Fig. 2: Structure of α1 subunit.

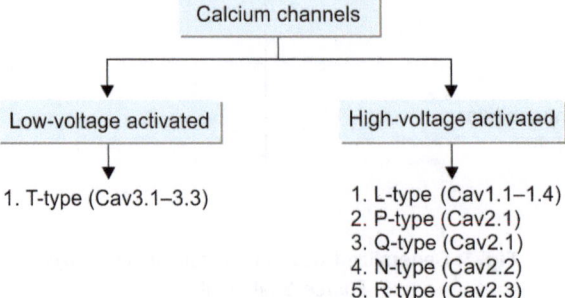

Flowchart 1: Types of calcium channels.

less than 40% similar between the channel types.[9]

Generalized Function of Calcium Channels

Calcium channels work by generating brief pulses of Ca^{2+} on their opening.[2] These calcium pulses generate different types of calcium signals. Short pulses mediate exocytosis of neurotransmitters, hormones, etc. by creating rapid calcium fluxes. Whereas repeated activation of brief pulse-generating calcium channels may generate comparatively longer, more robust signals in the form of "waves" essential for muscle contraction that can last for seconds to minutes. Further, repeated generation of waves over an extended period can cause calcium "oscillations," which can exist for minutes to hours and are involved in cellular functions such as cell proliferation, migration etc.[2] In response to the increased intracellular concentration of Ca^{2+}, calmodulin, a ubiquitous cytosolic protein binds to Ca^{2+} and undergoes conformational changes, and activate calmodulin-dependent protein kinase. The kinase, in turn, phosphorylate target proteins and transduce signal for specific cellular functions.

Calcium Channel and Hypertension

Calcium channels play a key role in membrane excitation in vascular muscles and develop voltage sensitivity to the small arteries and arterioles. Evidences suggest that calcium channel malfunction is associated with hypertension. Vascular tone or the contractile activity of vascular smooth muscle cells of resistance vessels determines arterial blood pressure. Peripheral vascular resistance is increased in hypertension

Remarkably, Ca^{2+} influx through L-type voltage-gated channels is a hallmark event.[10] Also, Ca^{2+} influx through Cav1.2 L-type calcium channels is the predominant type of Ca^{2+} influx mechanism and is responsible for the regulation of the diameter of small arteries and arterioles and thus controls the myogenic tone of the resistance vessels.[11] The resistance vessels cause increased peripheral resistance thus resulting in increased blood pressure. Alteration in resistance vessel function can play an important role in hypertension pathogenesis.[12] Contraction of vascular smooth muscles is regulated by various factors including increased intracellular Ca^{2+} concentration, altered membrane potential, and also on calcium-independent mechanisms. An increase in intracellular Ca^{2+} concentration either by Ca^{2+} influx or by Ca^{2+} release from intracellular stores leads to Ca^{2+}/calmodulin-dependent signal transduction resulting in phosphorylation of regulatory myosin light chain.[13]

It is known that L-type channels are upregulated in hypertension, and abnormality of this channel is a common mechanism in the pathogenesis of different forms of hypertension.[10] However, the mechanisms that cause upregulation of arterial Cav1.2 L-type channels in hypertension are not fully understood.

During the past decades, several drugs have been developed to treat hypertension. Among them, calcium channel blockers (CCBs) reduce cellular calcium influx by inhibiting voltage-gated L-type calcium channels, which are potent vasodilators and are used as a first-line or second-line drugs.[14] Mostly the drug of choice in treating hypertension is Cav1.2 blockers.

■ REFERENCES

1. Fedrizzin L, Lin D, Canafoli E. Calcium and signal transduction. Biochem Mol Biol Educ. 2008;36(3):175-80.

2. Cooper D, Dimri M. Biochemistry, Calcium Channels. 2022. In: StatPearls. Treasure Island (FL): StatPearls Publishing; 2022.
3. Bühler FR, Resink TJ. Platelet membrane and calcium control abnormalities in essential hypertension. Am J Hypertens. 1988;1(1):42-6.
4. Patel S. Two-pore channels open up. Nature. 201556(7699):38-40.
5. Shah K, Seeley S, Schulz C, Fisher J, Rao SG. Calcium channels in the heart: disease states and drugs. Cells. 2022;11(6):943.
6. Catterall WA. Voltage-gated calcium channels Cold Spring Harb Perspect Biol. 2011;3(8):a003947.
7. Rossier MF. T-Type calcium channel: A privileged gate for calcium entry and control of adrenal steroidogenesis. Front Endocrinol (Lausanne). 2016;7:43.
8. Zamponi GW. A crash course in calcium channels. ACS Chem. Neurosci. 2017;8(12):2583-5.
9. Catterall WA. Calcium channels. In: Squire LR (Ed). Encyclopedia of Neuroscience. Elsevier Ltd, Amsterdam, the Netherlands; 2009, pp. 543-50.
10. Sonkusare S, Palade PT, Marsh JD, Telemaque S, Pesic A, Rusch NJ. Vascular calcium channels and high blood pressure: Pathophysiology and therapeutic implications. Vascul Pharmacol. 2006;44(3):131-42.
11. Pesic A, Madden JA, Pesic M, Rusch NJ. High blood pressure upregulates arterial L-type Ca^{2+} channels: Is membrane depolarization the signal? Circ Res. 2004;94(10):e97-104.
12. Mulvany MJ. Structure and function of resistance vessels in hypertension. In: Bruschi G, Borghetti A (Eds). Cellular Aspects of Hypertension. Berlin, Heidelberg: Springer;1991, pp. 3-11.
13. Moosmang S, Schulla V, Welling A, Feil R, Feil S, Wegener JW, et al. Dominant role of smooth muscle L-type calcium channel Cav1.2 for blood pressure regulation. EMBO J 2003;22(22):6027-34.
14. Ozawa Y, Hayashi K, Kobori H. New generation calcium channel blockers in hypertensive treatment. Curr Hypertens Rev. 2006;2(2):103-11.

CHAPTER 7

Role of Cytokines and Inflammation in Hypertension

Mingma Lhamu Sherpa, Lydia Rai, Bidita Khandelwal

INTRODUCTION

Hypertension is one of the leading causes of cardiovascular risk and a major burden of mortality and morbidity worldwide.[1] Despite a large number of available medical treatments, both in terms of lifestyle modification and antihypertensive formulations, a large portion of the hypertensive population has still not achieved the desired blood pressure (BP) control.[1,2] According to the American Heart Association (AHA),[3] blood pressure in adults is categorized as listed in **Table 1**.

Genetic and environmental factors play important roles in the prevalence of hypertension. Obesity and weight gain, dietary sodium chloride intake, alcohol intake, psychosocial stress, less physical activity and a decrease in dietary intake of calcium and potassium are known risk factors seen among hypertensive patients.[2]

The complex network of specialized cells with type-specific roles with interorgan interaction between lymphoid organs, humoral factors, and cytokines are responsible for the broad effect of inflammation in response to stimuli.[4]

Inflammation plays a vital role in preserving the normal physiological function (homeostasis) of an organism, during the repair process and during protection against xenogeneic agents such as toxins, bacteria, and viruses. Both innate and acquired immune responses are known to result in changes in vascular tone. There is adequate scientific evidence that has demonstrated the association of inflammation with hypertension. However, despite many known secondary causes of hypertension, primary and essential hypertension biology is still not elucidated and there are still 8–12% of hypertensive patients with uncontrolled hypertension despite better therapy alternatives.[1]

TABLE 1: Blood pressure in adults according to AHA*.

Category	Systolic BP (mm Hg)		Diastolic BP (mm Hg)
Normal	<120	and	<80
Elevated	120–129	and	<80
Hypertension (stage 1)	130–139	or	80–89
Hypertension (stage 2)	≥140	or	≥90

*Persons with systolic BP and diastolic BP in two different categories will be allocated to the higher BP category. The BP is based on average on two different readings that are obtained on two different occasions. (AHA: American Heart Association; BP; blood pressure)

IMMUNE SYSTEM AND HYPERTENSION

Inflammation is the rapid, generalized reaction to toxins, invading organisms, foreign objects, necrotic cells, irritants, or cancerous cells. It is a coordinated effect of interaction between immune cells, the vascular wall, and chemical and humoral mediators' results in an innate immune response. Vascular responses include enhanced permeability and modifications to endothelial characteristics that encourage the rolling, adhesion, and diapedesis of different immune cells.

Both the innate and adaptive immune systems affect renal sodium balance, blood flow, and the functions of the vasculature and epithelial cells in the kidney, both of which contribute to the pathogenesis of hypertension. Also, T lymphocytes and monocytes/macrophages play a crucial role in facilitating hypertensive responses, while dendritic cells and B lymphocytes indirectly control BP by stimulating T lymphocyte activation. Tumor necrosis factor-α (TNF-α), interleukin-1 (IL-1), interleukin-17 (IL-17), and interferon (IFN) are examples of proinflammatory cytokines that can aggravate renal dysfunction or BP elevation.

The immune (innate and adaptive) response leads to hypertension as there is infiltration of adaptive immune cells into the kidneys, blood vessel wall, and the area surrounding the blood vessels that takes place simultaneously with the stages of the inflammatory process, such as an increase in cytokine release, reactive oxygen species (ROS) production, and the emergence of adhesion molecules. This immune cell infiltration also stimulates the intrarenal angiotensin system. In addition, there is endothelial activation due to inflammation. High BP results from the combined effects of inflammation-induced impairment in the pressure natriuresis relationship, dysfunctional vascular tone, and overactivity of the sympathetic nervous system. Furthermore, the imbalances between proinflammatory effector responses and anti-inflammatory responses of regulatory T cells to a large extent determine the severity of inflammation.[5-7]

The renal system is affected during inflammation and the immune response leads to disturbance of the natriuretic regulation in the renal medulla leading to increased risk for hypertension as revealed by the animal studies. There is also the effect of the perfusion of the immune cells in the renal system and the sympathetic stimulation effect on the kidneys. The inflammatory response due to the production of ROS under oxidative stress within the kidney causes impairment in the renal blood flow as well as distortion in the absorption of sodium across the renal tubules is a key feature of the development of hypertension. The presence of inflammatory cells in the kidneys of autopsy findings of hypertensive patients supports the role of immune cells in the causation and sustenance of hypertension.[2]

There are reports from different parts of the world which state that there are increased levels of inflammatory markers such as C-reactive protein and interleukin-6 (IL-6) in hypertensive patients. The levels of inflammatory markers, oxidative stress, and end-organ damage in hypertension are correlated positively. The thymus is an organ where T cells responsible for cellular immune response are generated. Some animal model studies in mice with the thymus removed have reported protection from BP elevation. Immune-mediated response in vascular endothelium not only results in a change in vascular tone but also results in the genesis of atherosclerosis which is one of the precursors of hypertension.

CYTOKINES AS MEDIATORS OF HYPERTENSIVE ACTION OF IMMUNE RESPONSE

Immune cells enter the area of local inflammation during the inflammatory process through a variety of chemokines, such as monocyte chemotactic protein-1 (MCP-1). Immune cells that have been localized in the kidney release proinflammatory cytokines such as TNF-α, IL-6, IL-1β, IL-17, and IFN-γ, which leads to an increase in proinflammatory cytokines in the kidneys and to local tissue damage. Proinflammatory cytokines have been cited as mediators of the hypertensive effects of immune response.[8]

Both structural alterations and arterial stiffening are a result of inflammatory cellular activity and changes can be a result of the activation of immune cells and proinflammatory cytokines resulting in dysfunctional vascular resistance leading to hypertension.

Cytokines are proteins released from a large group of cells and are responsible for the inflammatory response by influencing the interaction between inflammatory cells, lymphoid cells, and hematopoietic cells. They are secreted by white blood cells. They act by binding to the target cells receptors activating/inhibiting the pathways of signal transduction resulting in various gene alterations.

Cytokines act through an amplifying cascade of reactions that release other cytokines and induce the activation of enzymes such as inducible nitric oxide synthase (iNOS) and cycloxigenase 2 (COX-2) which generate chemical messengers to affect vascular dysfunction through endothelial activation as an inflammatory response **(Fig. 1)**.[9]

Following are the six major cytokine families that take part in BP regulation:
1. Interferon family.
2. Chemokine family.
3. Interleukin family.
4. Tumor necrosis factor family.
5. Transforming growth factor family.
6. Hematopoiesis.

Interferon-γ

It is an inflammatory cytokine which is produced by white blood cells like macrophages and T lymphocytes. Interferons

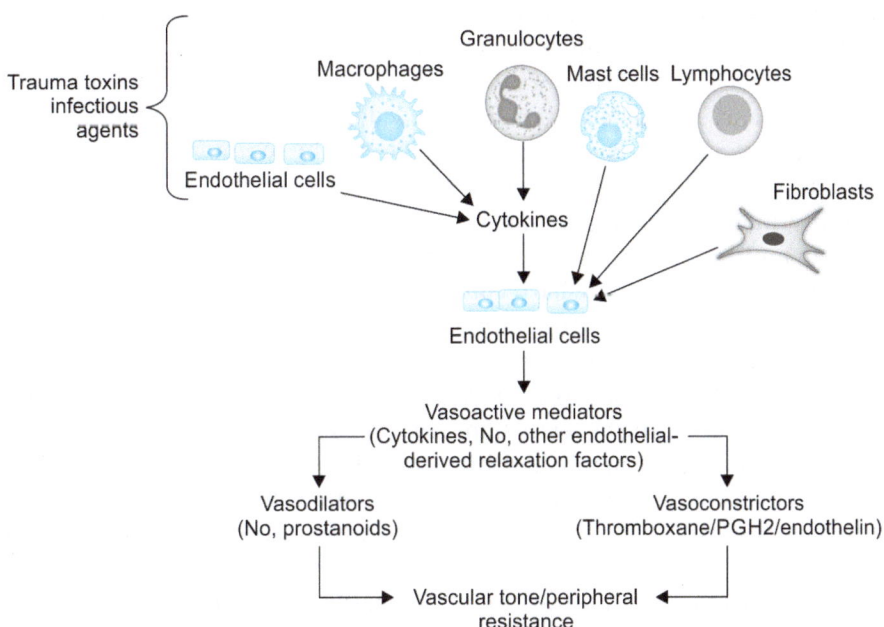

Fig. 1: Role of cytokines and their effect on the renal system in hypertension.

can also be manufactured in the laboratory and commercial formulations are now used for cancer therapy. There are three types of IFNs: Interferon alpha (IFN-α), interferon beta (IFN-β), and interferon gamma (IFN-γ). It helps in diverting the differentiation of T cell toward a proinflammatory T helper cell subtype. It enhances the transport of sodium via the NHE3 transporter in the proximal tubule and through NCC and NKCC2 in the distal nephron.[10]

Chemokine Family

The chemokines (or chemotactic cytokines) are a large family of small, secreted proteins that signal through cell surface G protein-coupled hepta-helical chemokine receptors. They are best known for their ability to stimulate the migration of cells, most notably white blood cells (leukocytes). Consequently, chemokines control both the development and homeostasis of the immune system and are involved in all protective or destructive immune and inflammatory responses. They induce the chemotactic migration of immune cells to stimuli and also stimulate a variety of other types of directed and undirected migratory behavior, such as haptotaxis, chemokinesis, and hypokinesis, in addition to inducing cell arrest or adhesion. Their guidance of mononuclear motility and migration are concentration gradient dependent based on their ligation to their receptors and initiating a cascade of chemical signaling. Immune cell infiltration of kidney, vasculature, and central nervous system during hypertension following tissue damage is medicated by elevation of chemokines. Furthermore, chemokine receptor expression in immune cells is enhanced during hypertension leading to dysfunctional immune cell infiltration of the cardiac control centers. T lymphocytes and monocytes/macrophages are the most important mediators of hypertensive inflammation, and these cells migrate in response to several chemokines. Chemokines are potent drivers of diapedesis (the passage of blood cells through the intact walls of the capillaries,), especially the chemokines CCL2 and CCL5 that are associated with hypertension; however, experimental data highlight divergent, context-specific effects of these chemokines on BP and tissue injury.

Interleukins

Interleukins are a type of inflammatory cytokines, which were first thought to be expressed by leukocytes alone and are currently known to be produced by many other body cells. They are essential in the activation and differentiation of immune cells, and also for proliferation, maturation, migration, and adhesion. They exhibit both proinflammatory and anti-inflammatory properties. The primary function of ILs is, therefore, to modulate growth, differentiation, and activation during inflammatory and immune responses. Interleukins consist of a large group of proteins that can elicit many reactions in cells and tissues by binding to high-affinity receptors in cell surfaces. They exert their actions in both paracrine and autocrine manner. To date, 40 types of ILs have been identified (from IL-1 to IL-40).

Interleukin-1

Interleukin-1 is secreted by macrophages, large granular lymphocytes, B cells, endothelium, fibroblasts, and astrocytes. T cells, B cells, macrophages, endothelium, and tissue cells are the principal targets of ILs. Furthermore, IL-1 causes activation of lymphocytes, stimulation of macrophages, increased leukocyte/endothelial adhesion, hypothalamus stimulation leading to fever, and release of acute phase proteins by the liver.

It has also been known to cause apoptosis in many cell types and cachexia.[11,12,14,15]

IL-1 is also known to enhance sympathetic outflow causing systemic vasoconstriction which impairs renal sodium excretion thereby potentiating hypertension.[16,17]

Interleukin-10

It is an anti-inflammatory cytokine that is secreted by T helper 2 (Th2) cells, mast cells, and monocytes. Administration of interleukin-10 (IL-10) in experimental rats with pregnancy-induced hypertension has reduced BP along with decreased levels of urinary proteins and endothelial dysfunction. Various studies have revealed the protective characteristic of IL-10 on the vasculature in preclinical hypertensive patients.[18]

The Th2 cells produce IL-10. Its principal targets are Th1 cells. It causes inhibition of IL-2 and IFN gamma. It decreases the antigen presentation, and MHC class II expression of dendritic cells, and costimulatory molecules on macrophages and it also downregulates pathogenic Th17 cell responses. It inhibits IL-12 production by macrophages.[19-21]

Interleukin-17

This cytokine is produced by Th-17. It acts on epithelial and endothelial cells. IL-17 main effects are the release of IL-6 and other proinflammatory cytokines. It enhances the activities of antigen-presenting cells. It stimulates chemokine synthesis by endothelial cells.[22,23]

Interleukin-17A (IL-17A) which is a member of the IL-17 family causes damage to smooth muscle cells by increasing the production of ROS, IL-6, and IL-8. Studies have revealed that the serum levels of IL-17 are markedly increased in patients with hypertension compared to the normotensive patients.[24,25]

Tumor Necrosis Factor-α

Tumor necrosis factor-α are pleiotropic cytokines mainly secreted by macrophages during chronic inflammatory states, such as diabetes and hypertension. It causes decreased filtration by vasoconstriction of renal vessels and also inhibits the transport of sodium in the distal renal tubule.[26]

There are bidirectional changes seen during hypertension. Elevated levels of TNF-α decrease BP, whereas moderate increases in TNF-α have been associated with increased NaCl retention and hypertension. These bidirectional effects are not clear but could be due to different concentrations of TNF-α within the kidney, the physiological state of the subject, or the type of inflammatory stimulus and response. Renal hemodynamics and nephron transport are altered by TNF-α, affecting both the activity and expression of transporters. It also mediates organ damage by stimulating immune cell infiltration and cell death.

Similarly, TNF-α mediated inhibition endothelial nitric oxide synthase (eNOS) has been seen in in vitro cell culture. Furthermore, eNOS is responsible for the synthesis of endothelial nitric oxide which is known for its endothelial activity as an endothelial-derived relaxation factor. These studies stated that inflammation decreases the bioavailability of endothelial NO and thus impairs vascular smooth muscle relaxation and subsequent vasodilatations, thereby affecting the vascular tone and pressure.

Transforming Growth Factor-β

Transforming growth factor beta (TGF-β), another pleiotropic cytokine, is expressed by most tissues and it performs a wide range of biological functions including senescence
1. Cell proliferation
2. Apoptosis

3. Tumor suppression
4. Differentiation
5. Migration
6. Immunity
7. Osteogenesis
8. Adipogenesis
9. Wound healing.

It also plays a major role in fibrosis of the kidney, specifically during activation of renin-angiotensin-aldosterone system (RAAS) and in the pathogenesis of hypertension. The fibrosis in the kidney is attributed to inhibitory action on matrix metalloproteinases and increased deposition of extracellular matrix proteins accumulation. It is also known to cause epithelial/endothelial mesenchymal transformation and this leads to end-organ damages. Also, TGFβ1 has been implicated as a cause in the development of cardiovascular-renal complications diseases. Patients with chronic diseases such as diabetes mellitus, hypercholesterolemia, and hypertension, develop end-organ damage (e.g., cardiac dysfunction, and chronic renal failure) leading to substantial morbidity and mortality. Prior studies show that TGFβ1 is an important cause of fibrosis.

The RAAS induced by TGFβ1 is important for the regulation of BP and RAAS blocking is effective in treating hypertension and diabetes-induced cardiovascular and renal complications. The role of TGFβ1 as a regulator of BP without RAAS has not been clarified yet despite recent information on its role in BP regulation. It is known that TGFβ1 suppresses the adrenal production of corticosteroids.[26-28]

■ HEMATOPOIETINS

Hematopoietins (hematopoietic cytokines) belong to the family of cytokines which are polypeptide products of activated cells. They are extracellular ligands that stimulate hematopoietic cells to differentiate into eight types of blood cells. This is a tightly regulated process and these hematopoiesis have a hormone-like action with specific receptor binding leading to pleiotropic and overlapping effects across different organ functions including a two-way relationship with hypertension and cardiovascular disease.

■ CONCLUSION

The immune system, cytokines, and hypertension are all related to one another. The immune system activation and increased cytokines may either be a cause or effect of hypertension. Cytokines are intrinsic to the chemical cascade and chemical messenger network that alter BP. Although a lot has been elicited for the role of inflammation, the role of cytokines in hypertension. There is still some clarity required in the exact pathways for its relation with hypertension control. In vitro studies and animal studies are ongoing to map out the specific control network.[29-31]

■ REFERENCES

1. NCD Risk Factor Collaboration (NCD-RisC). Worldwide trends in blood pressure from 1975 to 2015: A pooled analysis of 1479 population-based measurement studies with 19.1 million participants. Lancet. 2017; 389(10064):37-55.
2. Loscalzo J, Dennis K, Dan LL, Anthony F, Stephan HL, Larry JL. Harrison's Principle of Internal Medicine, 21st edition. New York: McGraw Hill; 2022.
3. Unger T, Borghi C, Charchar F, Khan NA, Poulter NR, Prabhakaran D, et al. 2020 International Society of Hypertension Global Hypertension Practice Guidelines. Hypertension. 2020;75(6):1334-57.
4. Parkin J, Cohen B. An overview of the immune system. Lancet. 2001;357(9270):1777-89.
5. Caillon A, Paradis P, Schiffrin EL. Role of immune cells in hypertension. Br J Pharmacol. 2019;176:1818-28.

6. Loperena R, Harrison DG. Oxidative stress and hypertensive diseases. Med Clin North Am. 2017;101(1):169-93
7. Arisya A, Alsagaff MT. Inflammation, immunity and Hypertension. Acta Med Indones. Indones J Intern Med. 2017;49(2):158-65.
8. Wen Y, Crowley SD. Renal effects of cytokines in hypertension. Adv Exp Med Biol. 2019;1165:443-54.
9. Denise FR, Ritu S, Rajeev G. Lippincott Illustrated Reviews Biochemistry South Asian Edition, 7th edition. New Delhi: Wolters Kluwer; 2021.
10. https://www.cancer.gov
11. Zhu Z, Wang D, Jiao W, Chen G, Cao Y, Zhang Q, et al. Bioinformatics analyses of pathways and gene predictions in IL-1α and IL-1β knockout mice with spinal cord injury. Acta Histochem 2017;119(7):663-70.
12. Boraschi D, Bossu P, Macchia G, Ruggiero P, Tagliabue A. Structure-function relationship in the IL-1 family. Front Biosci. 1996;1:d270-308.
13. Arend WP, Malyak M, Guthridge CJ, Gabay C. Interleukin-1 receptor antagonist: Role in biology. Annu Rev Immunol. 1998;16:27-55.
14. Dinarello CA. Overview of the IL-1 family in innate inflammation and acquired immunity. Immunol Rev. 2018;281(1):8-27.
15. Sims JE, Smith DE. The IL-1 family: Regulators of immunity. Nat Rev Immunol. 2010;10(2):89-102.
16. Krishnan SM, Dowling JK, Ling YH, Diep H, Chan CT, Ferens D, et al. Inflammasome activity is essential for one kidney/deoxycorticosterone acetate/salt-induced hypertension in mice. Br J Pharmacol. 2016;173(4):752-65.
17. Rodriguez-Iturbe B, Pons H, Johnson RJ. Role of the immune system in hypertension. Physiol Rev. 2017;97(3):1127-64.
18. Dinarello CA. Overview of the IL-1 family in innate inflammation and acquired immunity. Immunol Rev. 2018;281(1):8-27.
19. Couper KN, Blount DG, Riley EM. IL-10: The master regulator of immunity to infection. J Immunol. 2008;180(9):5771-7.
20. Vaillant AAJ, Qurie A. Interleukin. In: StatPearls [Online]. Treasure Island (FL): StatPearls Publishing; 2022. [Last accessed November, 2023].
21. Dhaouadi T, Chahbi M, Haouami Y, Sfar I, Abdelmoula L, Ben Abdallah T, et al. IL-17A, IL-17RC polymorphisms and IL17 plasma levels in Tunisian patients with rheumatoid arthritis. PLoS One. 2018;13(3):e0194883.
22. Guerra ES, Lee CK, Specht CA, Yadav B, Huang H, Akalin A, et al. Central role of IL-23 and IL-17 producing eosinophils as immunomodulatory effector cells in acute pulmonary aspergillosis and allergic asthma. PLoS Pathog. 2017;13(1):e1006175.
23. Chen K, Kolls JK. Interluekin-17A (IL17A). Gene. 2017;614:8-14.
24. Eid RE, Rao DA, Zhou J, Lo SL, Ranjbaran H, Gallo A, et al. Interleukin-17 and interferon-gamma are produced concomitantly by human coronary artery-infiltrating T cells and act synergistically on vascular smooth muscle cells. Circulation. 2009;119:1424-32.
25. Ramseyer VD, Garvin JL. Tumor necrosis factor-alpha: Regulation of renal function and blood pressure. Am J Physiol Renal Physiol. 2013;304(10):F1231-42.
26. Schreiner GF, Kohan DE. Regulation of renal transport processes and hemodynamics by macrophages and lymphocytes. Am J Physiol. 1990; 258:F761-7.
27. Kagami S, Border WA, Miller DE, Noble NA. Angiotensin II stimulates extracellular matrix protein synthesis through induction of transforming growth factor-beta expression in rat glomerular mesangial cells. J Clin Invest. 1994;93(6):2431-7.
28. Kamat NV, Thabet SR, Xiao L, Saleh MA, Kirabo A, Madhur MS, et al. Renal transporter activation during angiotensin-II hypertension is blunted in interferon-gamma–/– and interleukin-17A–/– mice. Hypertension. 2015;65(3):569-76.
29. Kelso A. Cytokines: Principles and prospects. Immunol Cell Biol. 1998:76(4):300-17.
30. Caillon A, Paradis P, Schiffrin EL. Role of immune cells in hypertension. Br J Pharmacol. 2019;176(12):1818-28.
31. Mertelsmann R. Hematopoietins: Biology, pathophysiology, and potential as therapeutic agents. Ann Oncol. 1991;2(4):251-63.

CHAPTER 8

Natriuretic Peptides in Hypertension

Rubi Dey, Bidita Khandelwal

INTRODUCTION

The study of natriuretic peptides (NPs) started over 50 years ago.[1] The family of NPs consists of three members, namely, atrial natriuretic peptide (ANP), brain natriuretic peptide (BNP), and C-type natriuretic peptide (CNP). They are structurally related to hormone and paracrine factors. Natriuretic peptides are instrumental in the regulation of fluid volume and blood pressure. They have the ability to counter the effects of volume overload or sympathetic activation of the cardiovascular system. NPs are known to cause vasodilatations, diuresis and natriuresis. Apart from these actions they also reduce the activity of the renin–angiotensin–aldosterone system (RAAS) and the sympathetic nervous system. The characteristics of the NPs have made them the biomarker of choice in heart failure. Essential hypertension being the major determining factor of cardiovascular disease, needs more effective treatment options and the role of NPs can be of vital importance. Natriuretic peptides have low chemical synthetic efficiency, expensive fabrication cost, and vulnerability to degradation in vivo and this has made its clinical application limited.[2,3] More extensive investigation of the role of NPs in hypertension is the need of the hour and can be an excellent example of translational medicine.

NATRIURETIC PEPTIDES: STRUCTURES AND RECEPTORS

Natriuretic peptides were discovered in mammalian tissues mainly in the heart and brain. They consist of three major polypeptides atrial (ANP), brain (BNP), and C-type (CNP). All three members are similar in primary amino acid structure, containing a 17-residue disulfide ring, and are the products of separate genes. They all exist as a pro-hormone which is then cleaved into an N-terminal peptide and C-terminal active hormone.[4] The NP family system constitutes ANP, BNP, and CNP, the NP receptors (NPRA, NPRB, and NPRC), and the protease convertases such as furin, corin, and PCSK6. This system represents relevant protective mechanisms toward the development of hypertension and associated conditions like atherosclerosis, stroke, myocardial infarction, heart failure, and renal injury. The molecular mechanisms underlying the physiological and pathological impact of NPs on blood pressure regulation and hypertension development are mediated by the specific biological receptors whereas the clearance receptors influence their plasma levels.

Atrial natriuretic peptide was found in cardiac atrial cells in the early 1980s by Adolpho de Bold and consists of 28 amino acids.[5,6] Brain natriuretic peptide was discovered in 1988 from the ventricular myocardium in response to stretch and CNP was isolated from the porcine brain in 1990.[7,8] C-type natriuretic peptide plays an important role in ossification process, vasoreactivity, vascular smooth muscle proliferation, endothelial cell migration and also acts as a neurotransmitter by virtue of its paracrine and autocrine functions.[9,10] CNP also acts as a local mediator potentially serving protective functions for the blood vessels. From the venom of the green mamba in 1992, *Dendroaspis* natriuretic peptide (DNP) was identified.[11] Urodilatin and ventricle natriuretic peptides are other peptides identified from the distal tubules of the kidney or ventricles of rainbow trout and eel and have been shown to exhibit the same cardiovascular effects.[12,13] Natriuretic peptides have a very short circulating half-life. The circulating half-life of ANP is only 3–5 minutes, that of BNP is approximately 23 minutes, and CNP has a half-life of only 2–3 minutes.

To date, three kinds of NP receptors have been detected. They include natriuretic peptide receptor A (NPR-A), natriuretic peptide receptor B (NPR-B), and natriuretic peptide receptor C (NPR-C). They all contain a relatively large (~450 amino acid) extracellular ligand binding domain and a single membrane-spanning region of about 20 residues. NPR-B is biologically least active, and the major effects are carried out by NPR-A and NPR-C. Both NPR-A and NPR-B are guanylyl cyclase receptors with cyclic guanosine monophosphate as the second messenger. Also, NPR-A is a stimulatory receptor and regulates the action of both ANP and BNP whereas NPR-C causes the destruction of both. The clearance function of NPR-C is mainly due to receptor-mediated endocytosis and subsequent lysosomal hydrolysis. NPR-C along with renal excretion and plasma-neutral endopeptidase helps in the removal of NPs from circulation.[4,9] All NP receptors are found in cardiovascular tissues, renal tissues, central nervous system, bone, and other tissues.[14] Binding to NPR-A results in diuresis, natriuresis, vasodilatation, and RAAS inhibition, and that leads to blood pressure lowering.[6] The antiproliferative effect of the peptides on cardiac and vascular myocyte growth has also been documented. It has been proved that NPR-A knock-out mice exhibit hypertension, cardiac hypertrophy, and fibrosis.[10,14] It has also been documented that apart from NPR-C the destruction and neutralization of the NPs are also done by an endopeptidase system called neprilysin. Therefore, both NPR-C and neprilysin together by controlling the degradation of NPs play a vital role in various disease conditions.[15-17]

NATRIURETIC PEPTIDES AND BLOOD PRESSURE

A diverse group of physiologic effects ranging from blood pressure control to endochondral ossification are mediated by NPs and their receptors. Blood pressure regulation is mediated by volume change, sodium retention, sympathetic nervous system tone, and the RAAS and NPs have been shown to have an effect on all the above factors.[18] In hypertension, NPs have been found to reduce the RAAS activity and sympathetic nervous system tone, causing vasorelaxation and have antiatherosclerotic effects. Natriuretic peptides have also been found to counterbalance the RAAS activity in the controlling of blood pressure. Blood pressure reduction is found to be better with angiotensin receptor neprilysin inhibitor therapy as compared to RAAS inhibition alone.[19] In hypertensive patients' upregulation of ANP gene transcription is considered to be a protective factor in the long term. Studies have shown that the levels of NPs in early hypertension are reduced as compared to late hypertension, which shows an increase in the NP levels.[20] Natriuretic peptides are considered as an important predictor of neurovascular ischemic events because the high NP levels detected in these events show a positive correlation.[21] Natriuretic peptides are known to have effects on the target organs in hypertension. ANP has physiological effects on the kidney, heart, and blood vessels and acts as a tool for supporting the delicate cardiorenal balance whereas BNP is activated in pathological conditions like myocardial stress. Natriuretic peptides cause increased lipolysis and energy utilization in the adipose tissues. Natriuretic peptides can alter lipolysis very efficiently by causing browning of the white fat and making it more energy efficient. Such alterations modify the sympathetic tone and improve the cardiovascular status making it beneficial.[22] The cardiovascular effects of NPs are good and favorable for the cardiovascular system. They include vasodilation that causes volume reduction, decreases atherosclerosis, myohypertrophy, and myocardial interstitial fibrosis, and improves myocardial relaxation which improves the myocardial function in cardiac failure.

THERAPEUTIC ROLE OF NATRIURETIC PEPTIDES

Natriuretic peptides not only have a profound effect in lowering blood pressure but also alleviate hypertensive organ damage. In this context, multiple attempts are being undertaken to develop therapeutic agents for hypertension by utilizing the NP family. Inhibitors of neprilysin, the enzyme degrading NPs, are an option for treating hypertension by enhancing the actions of endogenous peptides. Recently, angiotensin receptor and neprilysin were approved for cardiac failure patients. The role of neprilysin inhibition has also shown promising results in treating patients with hypertension.

FUTURE PROSPECTS

Natriuretic peptides have shown a promising role in the clinical arsenal. Natriuretic peptides are used as diagnostic markers as well as for the treatment of cardiac failure. The physiological effect of NPs on the cardiovascular system and in the maintenance of blood pressure is very complex. Elevated NP levels have deleterious effects on the heart in the presence of hypertension. Also, NPR-C blockers and drugs for long-term modulation of the NPs can be challenging and promising for the future.

REFERENCES

1. Woodard GE, Rosado JA. Recent advances in natriuretic peptide research. J Cell Mol Med. 2007;11(6):1263-71.
2. Burger AJ, Horton DP, LeJemtel T, Ghali JK, Torre G, Dennish G, Koren M, et al. Effect of nesiritide (B-type natriuretic peptide) and dobutamine on ventricular arrhythmias in the treatment of patients with acutely decompensated congestive heart failure: the PRECEDENT study. Am Heart J. 2002; 144(6):1102-8.
3. Park YH, Park HJ, Kim BS, Ha E, Jung KH, Yoon SH, et al. BNP as a marker of the heart failure in the treatment of imatinib mesylate. Cancer Lett. 2006;243(1):16-22.
4. Nakao K, Ogawa Y, Suga S, Imura H. Molecular biology and biochemistry of the natriuretic peptide system. II: Natriuretic peptide receptors. J Hypertens. 1992;10(10):1111-4.
5. De Bold AJ, Borenstein HB, Veress AT, Sonnenberg H. A rapid and potent natriuretic response to intravenous injection

of atrial myocardial extract in rats. Life Sci. 1981;28(1):89-94.
6. Levin ER, Gardner DG, Samson WK. Natriuretic peptides. N Engl J Med. 1998; 339(5):321-8.
7. Sudoh T, Kangawa K, Minamino N, Matsuo H. A new natriuretic peptide in porcine brain. Nature1988;332(6159):78-81.
8. Sudoh T, Minamino N, Kangawa K, Matsuo H. C-type natriuretic peptide (CNP): a new member of natriuretic peptide family identified in porcine brain. Biochem Biophys Res Commun. 1990;168(2):863-70.
9. Kone BC. Molecular biology of natriuretic peptides and nitric oxide synthases. Cardiovasc Res. 2001;51(3):429-41.
10. Vanderheyden M, Bartunek J, Goethals M. Brain and other natriuretic peptides: Molecular aspects. Eur J Heart Fail. 2004; 6(3):261-8.
11. Schweitz H, Vigne P, Moinier D, Frelin C, Lazdunski M. A new member of the natriuretic peptide family is present in the venom of the green mamba (*Dendroaspis angusticeps*). J Biol Chem. 1992;267(20):13928-32.
12. Takei Y, Takano M, Itahara Y, Watanabe TX, Nakajima K, Conklin DJ, et al. Rainbow trout ventricular natriuretic peptide: Isolation, sequencing, and determination of biological activity. Gen Comp Endocrinol. 1994;96(3):420-6.
13. Forssmann WG, Richter R, Meyer M. The endocrine heart and natriuretic peptides: histochemistry, cell biology, and functional aspects of the renal urodilatin system. Histochem Cell Biol. 1998;110(4): 335-57.
14. Maack T. The broad homeostatic role of natriuretic peptides. Arq Bras Endocrinol Metabol. 2006;50:198-207.
15. Waldman SA, Rapoport RM, Murad F. Atrial natriuretic factor selectively activates particulate guanylate cyclase and elevates cyclic GMP in rat tissues. J Biological Chem. 1984;259(23):14332-4.
16. Schlueter N, de Sterke A, Willmes DM, Spranger J, Jordan J, Birkenfeld AL. Metabolic actions of natriuretic peptides and therapeutic potential in the metabolic syndrome. Pharmacol Ther. 2014;144(1):12-27.
17. Mukoyama M, Nakao K, Hosoda K, Suga S, Saito Y, Ogawa Y, et al. Brain natriuretic peptide as a novel cardiac hormone in humans. Evidence for an exquisite dual natriuretic peptide system, atrial natriuretic peptide and brain natriuretic peptide. J Clin Invest. 1991;87(4):1402-12.
18. Heymsfield SB, Wadden TA. Mechanisms, pathophysiology, and management of obesity. New Eng J Med. 2017;376(3):254-66.
19. Ruilope LM, Dukat A, Böhm M, Lacourcière Y, Gong J, Lefkowitz MP. Blood-pressure reduction with LCZ696, a novel dual-acting inhibitor of the angiotensin II receptor and neprilysin: A randomised, double-blind, placebo-controlled, active comparator study. Lancet. 2010;375(9722):1255-66.
20. Macheret F, Heublein D, Costello-Boerrigter LC, Boerrigter G, McKie P, Bellavia D, et al. Human hypertension is characterized by a lack of activation of the antihypertensive cardiac hormones ANP and BNP. J Am Coll Cardiol 201216;60(16):1558-65.
21. Folsom AR, Nambi V, Bell EJ, Oluleye OW, Gottesman RF, Lutsey PL, et al. Troponin T, N-terminal pro-B-type natriuretic peptide, and incidence of stroke: The Atherosclerosis Risk in Communities Study. Stroke. 2013;44(4):961-7.
22. Sarzani P, Dessi-Fulgheri P, Paci VM, Espinosa E, Rappelli A. Expression of natriuretic peptide receptors in human adipose and other tissues. J Endocrinol Invest. 1996;19(9):581-5.

CHAPTER 9

Multiple Roles of Eicosanoids in Blood Pressure Regulation

Mingma Lhamu Sherpa, Rojana Tamang, Bidita Khandelwal

■ INTRODUCTION

Eicosanoids are a family of potent biological signaling molecules, with physiological and pharmacological actions characterized by their paracrine hormone-like actions (act locally) and short half-life. The four types of eicosanoids are prostaglandins (PGs), thromboxane (TX), leukotrienes (LTs), and lipoxins (LXs). They are majorly synthesized from the diet and from arachidonate from phospholipids of plasma membranes via the cyclooxygenase (COX) pathway and lipoxygenase pathway. Physiologically eicosanoids exert their actions through the G-protein coupled transmembrane protein receptors (GPCRs), inositol 1,4,5-phosphate (IP) cascade. Eicosanoids are named according to the functional group on the ring and the numbers indicate the number of double bonds in the hydrocarbon.[1] Many of the eicosanoid analogs are being used for the treatment.

■ EICOSANOIDS

The 20 carbon-containing eicosanoids are a group of compounds derived from essential, polyunsaturated fatty acid (PUFA) such as arachidonic acid (AA) and other 20 carbon-containing eicosapentaenoic acid, the basis of their Greek origin ("eikosi" means 20 in Greek). They act locally in a paracrine fashion and have a short half-life. Their synthesis is induced in a need-based manner. Eicosanoids can be classified as autocrine/paracrine hormones that exert regulatory activity at the site of production. Most eicosanoid metabolites are excreted in urine.[1]

■ TYPES OF EICOSANOIDS, THEIR SOURCES, SYNTHESIS AND FUNCTIONS

There are four different types of eicosanoids in three groups, and they are PGs, TX (both of which are collectively called prostanoids), LTs, and LXs. Eicosanoids are synthesized from 20 carbon (eicosa), essential PUFA such as linoleate and arachidonate. Linoleate is majorly from the diet and arachidonate is derived from the breakdown of phospholipids present in the plasma membrane. Synthesis of eicosanoids is either through the COX pathway or the lipoxygenase pathway.

The three groups of eicosanoids (prostanoids and LTs) are formed via the COX and lipoxygenase pathways. Prostaglandins are found in all mammalian tissues, they have both pharmacologic and physiologic properties. Prostanoids include various types of PGs and TX. The number reflects the double bonds and the alphabet is the series labeled A, B, E, and F, etc. are based on the substituent group attached giving rise to a series of PGs and TXs.[2]

"Group 1" prostanoids such as prostaglandin E_1 (PGE$_1$), prostaglandin F_1 (PGF$_1$), and thromboxane A_1 (TXA$_1$); leukotrienes

A_3 (LTA$_3$), leukotrienes C_3 (LTC$_3$), and leukotrienes D_4 (LTD$_4$) are derived from dietary linoleate. Furthermore, 5,8,11,14-eicosatetraenoate (arachidonate) is formed from this pathway along with the group 1 prostanoids and LTs.

Arachidonate could be dietary or derived from membrane phospholipids, the latter being more common. This is a result of the action of the membrane bound to phospholipase A_2 (PLA$_2$, which is inhibited by angiotensin 2, bradykinin, epinephrine, and thrombin). Arachidonate further gives rise to "group 2" prostanoids through the COX pathway. These include the prostaglandin D_2 (PGD$_2$), prostaglandin E_2 (PGE$_2$), prostaglandin F_2 (PGF$_2$), and prostaglandin I_2 (PGI$_2$); thromboxane A_2 (TXA$_2$). Through the lipoxygenase pathway, arachidonate gives rise to group 2 LTs and LXs. The LTs of group 2 are LTs, A_4, B_4, C_4, D_4, and E_4 (LTA$_4$, LTB$_4$, LTC$_4$, LTD$_4$, and LTE$_4$) and LXs synthesized are LXs, A_4, B_4, C_4, D_4, and E_4 (LXA$_4$, LXB$_4$, LXC$_4$, LXD$_4$, and LXE$_4$), respectively.

Group 3 prostanoids are formed from dietary eicosapentaenoate which is also derived from dietary linoleate. Prostaglandin D_3 (PGD$_3$), prostaglandin E_3 (PGE$_3$), prostaglandin F_3 (PGF$_3$), and prostaglandin I_3 (PGI$_3$), and thromboxane A_3 (TXA$_3$) are synthesized through the COX pathway and the LTs, A_5, B_5, and C_5 (LTA$_5$, B_5, and C_5) are synthesized via the lipoxygenase pathway.

Cyclooxygenase, also known as prostaglandin H (PGH) synthase, has COX and peroxidase activities. There are two known isoenzymes of COX; COX-1 and COX-2. Aspirin, indomethacin, and ibuprofen act by inhibiting the COX enzymes.

Arachidonate is converted to prostaglandin G_2 *(PGG$_2$)* by COX enzyme consuming two molecules of oxygen. This PGG$_2$ is converted to PGH$_2$ by peroxidase; PGH$_2$ is further converted to PGI$_2$ by prostacyclin synthase, PGE$_2$, and PGD$_2$ by isomerase. Isomerase also converts TXA$_2$ to thromboxane B$_2$ (TXB$_2$). Furthermore, malondialdehyde (MDA), hydroxyheptadecatrienoate (HHT), and TXA$_2$ are synthesized by TX synthase from PGG$_2$. Both PGH$_2$ and PGE$_2$ are reduced to PGF2α by reductase enzyme.

Cyclooxygenase-1 isoenzyme, a dominant source of prostanoids in cells that are cytoprotective and maintain homeostasis such as gastric epithelial cells. Inflammatory stimuli triggered by hormones and growth factors induced by COX-2 action serve as an important source of prostanoids (PGs and TX) during inflammation and cancer. Both COX-1 and COX-2 contribute to prostanoid release during homeostasis and autoregulatory requirements during inflammation.

Functions of Important Eicosanoids (Prostanoids and Leukotrienes) and their Role in Regulating Peripheral Resistance

Eicosanoids and their derivatives are responsible for important physiological and pathological responses such as inflammation, fever, and pain associated with injury or disease, smooth muscle contraction, functions of reproduction, maintaining platelets hemostasis, renal function and the regulation of blood pressure (BP), in gastric acid secretion maintain gastric functions roles in Intestine, blood vessels, uterus and various other functions in the human body. The inflammatory response consists of the following two phases: Initiation and resolution, which can be triggered by any insult by pathogens or irritants (air pollution, tobacco smoke).[1]

Prostaglandins have a range of varied physiologic functions in vivo. Vasodilatation

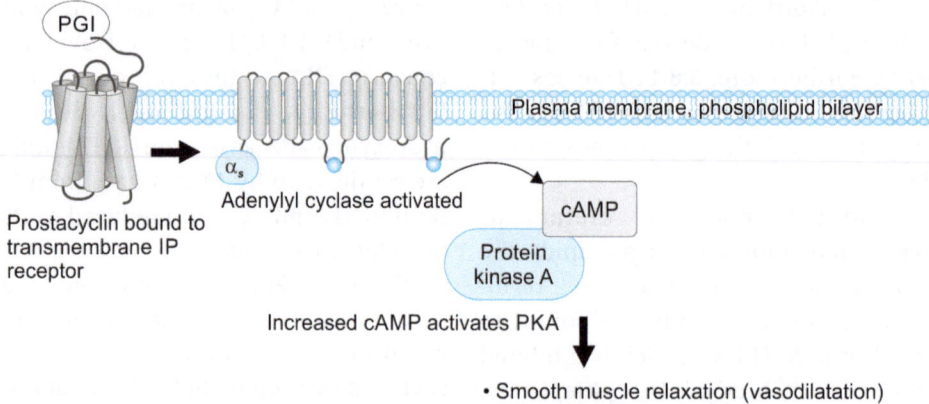

Fig. 1: Cascade of reactions to mediate actions of prostacyclin through IP-cAMP cascade to mediate vasodilation and regulation of peripheral vascular pressure. (cAMP: cyclic adenosine 3′,5′-monophosphate; IP: inositol 1,4,5-phosphate; PGI: prostaglandin; PKA: protein kinase A)

and vascular leakages are mediated by PGE_2, while PGD_2 is responsible for the maturation of mast cells and recruitment of eosinophils. Also, PGD_2 is majorly responsible for the allergic response while PGF_2 causes the contraction of smooth muscles of vessels and the respiratory system. Prostacyclin, PGI_2, is responsible for inhibiting platelet aggregation. It is also produced endogenously by endothelial cells and acts as a tonic vasodilatory stimulus under physiologic conditions in vivo. This is responsible for maintaining the vascular tone and the peripheral resistance. Contraction of smooth muscles is seen with as little as 1 ng/mL of plasma PGs in animals. The biochemical actions of eicosanoids are mediated through the transmembrane G protein receptors **(Fig. 1)**.

PROSTANOIDS AND THEIR ROLE IN VASCULAR TONE

Thromboxane A_2 (TXA_2) synthesized by COX-1 enzyme which is formed within the platelets promotes platelets aggregation and thrombus formation, resulting in disturbances in the blood flow leading to vasoconstrictions leading to increased vascular tone and pressure. Such contractions of smooth muscle lead to the mobilization of intracellular calcium and an increase in Ca^{2+}. Intracellular calcium is important in the regulation of cardiovascular functions: Muscular tone of smooth muscles of the vessel is increased due to an increased influx of calcium leading to a rise in BP due to increased vascular resistance.

Prostacyclin, PGI_2, is synthesized through the COX-2 enzymes, its action is opposite to that of TXA_2. Cyclooxygenase is also known as suicide enzymes and it switches off of PG activity. Blocking the action of cyclooxygenase can prolong the half-life of PG in our body. Nonsteroidal anti-inflammatory drugs inhibit COX-1 and COX-2 and inhibit prostanoid synthesis by blocking only the cyclooxygenase activity. It does not affect the peroxidase activity of this enzyme.[4] Prostacyclin, PGI_2 produced in the vascular endothelium have a dual action of inhibiting platelet aggregation and vasodilatation. Prostaglandin $F_{2\alpha}$

($PGF_{2\alpha}$) is produced by most of the tissues, contraction of smooth muscles, vasoconstriction, stimulate uterine muscle contraction. Prostaglandins E_2 has a role in fever, produced by most tissues, especially kidneys, relaxes smooth muscles; vasodilatation is used for induction of labor.[5]

Prostaglandin I_2 is among the more important prostanoids responsible for regulating cardiovascular homeostasis. Endothelial cells, endothelial progenitor cells (EPCs), and vascular smooth muscle cells (VSMCs) are the major source of prostacyclin.[4] Both prostacyclin and COX are found in the Endoplasmic reticulum, plasma membrane, and nuclear membrane. Thromboxane receptor (TP) and prostaglandin I synthase (PGIS) are expressed in endothelial cells and they bind with COX-1 for action. Prostaglandin I_2, which is released as described, then acts locally on the circulating platelets and nearby VSMCs in an autocrine manner. Prostacyclin metabolized by hydrolysis to 6-keto-PGF1α.

Prostaglandin actions are mediated via the IP receptor which is found in the kidney, liver, lung, platelets, heart, and aorta.[6] There is a classical IP-cyclic adenosine 3′,5′-monophosphate (cAMP) signaling cascade along with the cascade through the PPAR δ pathway.[7]

In an animal model, IP-knockout mice matured normally without an event of spontaneous thrombosis despite thrombogenic stimuli and vascular injury-induced VSMC proliferation.[8]

This study demonstrated that IP deficiency led to sensitivity to dietary salt-induced hypertension[9] and accelerated atherogenesis with enhanced platelet activation and increased adhesion of leukocytes on the vessel walls.[10,11]

Prostaglandin E_2, under physiological conditions, is an important mediator of many biological functions, such as the regulation of immune responses, BP, gastrointestinal integrity, and fertility, however, more is known about its contrasting role as an inflammatory and anti-inflammatory agent.

THROMBOXANE AND HYPERTENSION

Thromboxane A_2, an unstable AA metabolite has a half-life of about 30 s, and it is synthesized from PGH2 via TXs as shown in **Figure 2**. It is degraded non-enzymatically into biologically inactive TXB2. Also, TXA2 is synthesized predominantly from platelet COX-1, but it can also be produced by other cell types, such as macrophage COX-2.[12,13] Mice that are thromboxane receptor (TP) deficient are normotensive but their vascular responses to TP agonists is blunted and they show a tendency to bleeding.

The deletion of TP decreases both vascular proliferation and platelet activation in response to vascular injury. It also delays atherogenesis and prevents angiotensin II- and L-NAME-induced hypertension and the associated cardiac hypertrophy.[3]

When 5-lipoxygenase enzyme acts on AA, it forms 5-hydroxyperoxyeicosatetraenoic acid (5-HPETE) which is an intermediate for the synthesis of LTs, LTA_4. Leukotrienes A_4 (LTA_4) are produced by mast cells, in leukocytes, platelets, and heart and lung vascular tissue. They also play important roles during inflammation.

They are also known as cysteinyl-containing LTs because cysteine is not removed from these LTs. Leukotrienes are substances of anaphylaxis. There are different LTs, namely, leukotriene C_4, D_4, and T_4 that cause contraction of smooth muscles,

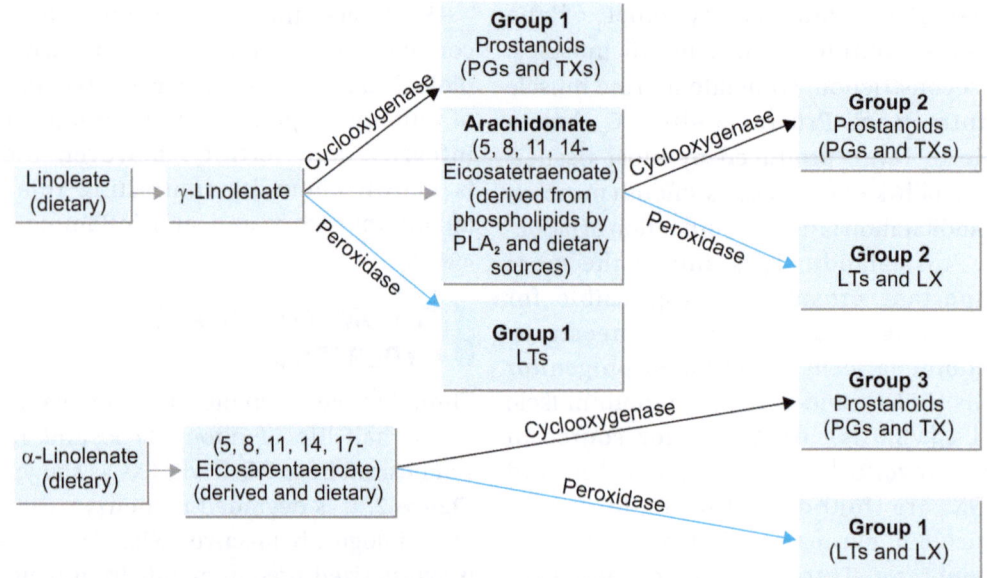

Fig. 2: Precursor and pathway for different groups of prostanoids and LTs with mention of important intermediates (parenthesis is indicative of the sources). (LTs: leukotrienes; LX: lipoxin; PGs: prostaglandins; PLA2: phospholipase A2; TX: thromboxane)
Source: Figure 23.11 of *Harpers Illustrated Biochemistry*, 31st edition.[3]

bronchoconstriction, vasoconstriction, an increase in vascular permeability, and have a role pathophysiology of asthma.[2]

Leukotrienes A_4 directly leads to the formation of leukotrienes B_4 (LTB_4), which increases the chemotaxis of polymorph nuclear leukocytes, lysosomal enzymes release, and adhesions of white blood cells. Furthermore, 5-lipoxygenase is found in the arterial wall; LTs are vasoactive and LXs perform anti-inflammatory and immunoregulatory functions.[4]

ROLE OF CYTOCHROME P450 IN EICOSANOIDS AND BLOOD PRESSURE REGULATION

Eicosanoids are produced by oxidation of AA and other PUFAs, function both as systemic inflammatory activity activators and suppressors. Eicosanoids have a major role in controlling the inflammatory activity in the human body.[14]

Inflammatory activity initiation in humans is controlled by substrates and products of polyunsaturated ω-3 and ω-6 20-carbon fatty acids. Cytochrome P450 (CYP) pathway eicosanoids affect the regulation of renal function, vascular tone, and the development of hypertension.[14]

The renin-angiotensin-aldosterone system (RAAS), renal disease, renal vascular tone, urine salt excretion, peripheral resistance, and endothelial function are some of the essential components of BP regulation.

The CYP pathway metabolizes AA to several eicosanoids, including 20-hydroxyeicosatetraenoic acid (20HETE) and epoxyeicosatrienoic (EET) acid. These metabolites regulate BP and provide cardioprotective and renoprotective effects in chronic kidney disease.[15]

Cyclooxygenase pathway-produced proteinoids are involved in BP homeostasis and short-lived TXA_2 (half-life, 30 s) has an important role in various cardiovascular diseases through action on platelet aggregation, vasoconstriction, and proliferation. Thromboxane A_2 is metabolized to inactive TXB_2, which is degraded through two major pathways (dehydrogenation and β-oxidation).[4]

Cytochrome P450 enzymes of the 4A and 4F families metabolize AA to 20-hydroxyeicosatetraenoic acid (20HETE). Both CYP2C and CYP2J pathways metabolize AA to EET.[6] Both 20HETE and EET affect BP since they affect renal tubular transport; renal and peripheral vascular pressure. Epoxyeicosatrienoic acids are endothelium-derived relaxing factors (EDRFs) that mediate the dilatation of the tiny arterioles and affect the sodium transport in the proximal tubules and the collecting duct of a kidney. They are natriuretic in nature and cause vasodilatation which further decreases the BP.

The role of 20HETE as a powerful vasoconstrictor is known to inhibit sodium transport in the proximal tubule and thick ascending loop of Henle in the kidney. Their vasoconstrictor action increases the BP. Furthermore, 20HETE contains both prohypertensive and antihypertensive properties, decreases salt transport as well as raises renal and peripheral vascular tone.[6]

Both EETs and 20HETE are components of renal vascular and transport mechanism that affects BP control mechanism. Angiotensin II enzyme activates the release of renal 20HETE by stimulating the synthesis of 20HETE in the kidney.[16] Furthermore, 20HETE is crucial for controlling vascular tone. The renal and cerebral arteries produce 20HETE, a strong vasoconstrictor. It blocks the large conductance calcium-sensitive channel, it activates the protein kinase C (PKC), mitogen-activated protein kinases (MAPKs), tyrosine kinase, and rho kinase pathways to promote Ca^{2+} entry through depolarization of VSMCs.[5]

Prostaglandin has a well-established role in the renin–angiotensin system, sympathetic nervous system, and vasopressin. Cyclooxygenase enzyme inhibition leads to an increase in vascular resistance increasing the responses of angiotensin 2 enzymes and other constrictor hormones. Cyclooxygenase 2 enzymes have a role in activating RAAS, action I preglomerular microvessels, metabolizing, and moderating the activity of 20HETE, which is the important product of CYP, the pathway of AA metabolism.[17]

Twenty-hydroxyeicosatetraenoic acid is vasoactive and regulates renal circulation, autoregulates tubule-glomerular feedback, electrolyte excretion cotransporter inhibition of Na^+ pump which has an overall effect on the regulation of BP.[17]

PROSTAGLANDINS AND THROMBOXANE POLYMORPHISM AND HYPERTENSION

Single nucleotide polymorphism (SNPs) in prostaglandin E receptors (PGER) have been associated with hypertension. Like polymorphism in the 3′-untranslated region (UTR) region of PGER; intron icrs2268062 variant in PTGER3 with hypertension the inhibition of sodium and water reabsorption in the kidney.[18-20]

CONCLUSION

Increased prostacyclin formation appears to be a response to the elevated BP, mediated by mechanical stimulation of the VSMCs in the blood vessel wall. Thromboxane A2 rise is responsible for the development and maintenance of hypertension. Since TXA_2 causes vasoconstriction and stimulates

VSMCs growth and vascular hypertrophy are seen in hypertension. This increases the total peripheral resistance and contributes to hypertension.

REFERENCES

1. Nelson DL, Cox MM, Aaron AH. Lehninger's Principles of Biochemistry, 8th edition, New York: Macmillan Learning; 2021.
2. Palmu J, Watrous JD, Mercader K, Havulinna AS, Lagerborg KA, Salosensaari A, et al. Eicosanoid inflammatory mediators are robustly associated with blood pressure in the general population. J Am Heart Assoc. 2020;9(19):e017598.
3. Rodwell VW, Bender DA, Botham KM, Kennelly PJ, Weil PA. Harper's Illustrated Biochemistry, 31st edition. USA: McGraw Hill Education; 2018.
4. Smyth EM, FitzGerald GA. Human prostacyclin receptor. Vitam Horm. 2002;65:149-65.
5. Kawabe J, Ushikubi F, Hasebe N. Prostacyclin in Vascular Diseases. Circ J. 2010;74(5):836-43.
6. Lim H, Dey SK. A novel pathway of prostacyclin signaling-hanging out with nuclear receptors. Endocrinology. 2002;143(9):3207-10.
7. Cheng Y, Austin SC, Rocca B, Koller BH, Coffman TM, Grosser T, et al. Role of prostacyclin in the cardiovascular response to thromboxane A2. Science. 2002;296(5567):539-41.
8. Francois H, Athirakul K, Howell D, Dash R, Mao L, Kim HS, et al. Prostacyclin protects against elevated blood pressure and cardiac fibrosis. Cell Metab. 2005;2(3):201-7.
9. Egan KM, Lawson JA, Fries S, Koller B, Rader DJ, Smyth EM, et al. COX-2-derived prostacyclin confers atheroprotection on female mice. Science. 2004;306(5703):1954-7.
10. Kobayashi T, Yamashita JK, Katagiri H, Majima M, Yokode M, Kita T, et al. Roles of thromboxane A(2) and prostacyclin in the development of atherosclerosis in apoE-deficient mice. J Clin Invest. 2004;114(6):784-94.
11. Funk CD, FitzGerald GA. COX-2 inhibitors and cardiovascular risk. J Cardiovasc Pharmacol. 2007;50(5):470-9.
12. Félétou M, Verbeuren TJ, Vanhoutte PM. Endothelium-dependent contractions in SHR: A tale of prostanoid TP and IP receptors. Br J Pharmacol. 2009;156(4):563-74.
13. Félétou M, Vanhoutte PM, Verbeuren TJ. The TP-receptor: the common villain. J Cardiovasc Pharmacol. 2010;55:317-32.
14. Denise FR, Singh R, Goyal R, Lippincott Illustrated Reviews Biochemistry South Asian Edition, 7th edition. New Delhi: Wolters Kluwer; 2021.
15. Fan F, Muroya Y, Roman RJ. Cytochrome P450 eicosanoids in hypertension and renal disease. Curr Opin Nephrol Hypertens. 2015;24(1):37-46.
16. Minuz P, Jiang H, Fava C, Turolo L, Tacconelli S, Ricci M, et al, Altered release of cytochrome P450 metabolites of arachidonic acid in renovascular disease. Hypertension. 2008;51(5):1379-85.
17. Quilley J, McGiff JC. Multiple roles of eicosanoids in blood pressure regulation. In: Lipp GYH, Hall J (Eds). Comprehensive Hypertension. Philadelphia, PA: Mosby Elsevier; 2007. pp. 377-95.
18. Dorris SL, Peebles RS Jr. PGI_2 as a regulator of inflammatory diseases. Mediators Inflamm. 2012;2012:926968. doi: 10.1155/2012/926968. Epub 2012 Jul 18. PMID: 22851816; PMCID: PMC3407649.
19. Sato M, Nakayama T, Soma M, Aoi N., Kosuge K, Haketa A, et al. Association between prostaglandin E_2 receptor gene and essential hypertension. Prostaglandins Leukot Essent Fatty Acids. 2007;15–20. doi: 10.1016/j.plefa.2007.04.004.
20. Sõber S, Org E, Kepp K, Juhanson P, Eyheramendy S, Gieger C, et al. Targeting 160 candidate genes for blood pressure regulation with a genome-wide genotyping array. PLoSONE 2009;4:e6034. doi:10.1371/journal.pone.0006034.

SECTION 4

Accuracy of Blood Pressure Measurement

10. **Correct Methodology of Blood Pressure Measurements**
    Boudhayan Das Munshi

11. **Home Blood Pressure Monitoring**
    A Muruganathan, E Cowshik

12. **Ambulatory Blood Pressure Monitoring**
    Parvati Nandy

13. **Central Aortic Blood Pressure: An Overview**
    Rohit Kapoor, Shivam Kapoor

CHAPTER 10

Correct Methodology of Blood Pressure Measurements

Boudhayan Das Munshi

■ INTRODUCTION

Blood pressure (BP) measurement is an art and science that needs to be perfected by health care professionals (HCPs) to achieve optimum cardiovascular goals in the patient. The diagnosis, treatment, and follow-up of hypertension require accurate BP measurements. Hence, the several factors that can affect the techniques involved in BP measurement need to be reviewed at periodic intervals.

Blood pressure can be measured using one of the following three acceptable techniques:
1. Ambulatory blood pressure monitoring (ABPM)
2. Home blood pressure monitoring (HBBPM)
3. Office-based BP measurements, which can be manual or automated office BP (AOBP). Screening for hypertension is done by the HCPs in the office.[1,2]

However, for confirmation of the diagnosis ABPM or home blood pressure monitoring (HBPM) is preferred.[3,4] Home blood pressure monitoring and ABPM measurements are lower than the routine office BP measurements by 5–10 mm Hg.[5,6]

Ambulatory BP monitoring is considered the gold standard technique for BP assessment. Details about ABPM will be noted in a subsequent chapter.

■ MANUAL BLOOD PRESSURE MONITORING

Blood pressure is traditionally measured with auscultation for the Korotkoff's sounds. This method utilizes a sphygmomanometer, a device comprised of an inflatable cuff that is connected to a pressure gauge. The classical mercury sphygmomanometers are gradually being discarded due to environmental hazards related to mercury.[7] The deflated cuff is placed around the arm and inflated sufficiently to occlude arterial flow. When the pressure of the cuff exceeds the systolic pressure auscultation over the brachial artery reveals no sound due to complete obstruction of flow. For auscultatory determinations, use a palpated estimate of radial pulse obliteration pressure to estimate systolic blood pressure (SBP). Inflate the cuff 20–30 mm Hg above this level for an auscultatory determination of the BP level deflate the cuff pressure to 2 mm Hg/s and listen for Korotkoff sounds. The cuff is then gradually deflated while continuing the auscultation. When the pressure in the cuff falls to the level of the systolic pressure, pulsatile blood flow begins to re-establish. The resulting turbulence produces characteristic tapping sounds known as Korotkoff sounds. As the cuff continues to deflate to the level of the diastolic pressure, Korotkoff sounds disappear due to pulsatile blood flow. Thus, the systolic pressure is indicated by the origination of Korotkoff sounds, and the diastolic pressure is indicated by their disappearance.

The Korotkoff sounds heard when measuring BP are as follows:[8,9]
- *Phase 1:* Faint but clear tapping sound, that gradually increases in intensity.
- *Phase 2:* Dampening of this sound, that may be heard like blowing or swishing.
- *Phase 3:* Sharper sounds return that does not have the intensity of phase one.
- *Phase 4:* Well-defined muffled sound, that progresses to become soft and blowing.
- *Phase 5:* Disappearance of sounds.

Auscultatory Gap

Premature Recording of the Diastolic Pressure

It is important to continue to auscultate over the brachial artery even when Korotkoff sounds disappear to eliminate the possibility of an auscultatory gap. Only the final disappearance of Korotkoff sounds should be used for recording the diastolic pressure. Korotkoff sounds can temporarily fade but then reappear as the cuff continues to deflate especially in those patients with wide pulse pressure.[10]

Hybrid Sphygmomanometer

A hybrid sphygmomanometer uses an auscultatory approach. The mercury column is replaced by an electronic pressure gauge. A liquid display liquid column or light-emitting diode screen moves smoothly like a mercury column or aneroid-like display. The frequency of its calibration is unknown.[11]

Automated Devices

They measure BP by measuring oscillations in blood flow as the cuff is deflated. Device-specific algorithms are then used to calculate BP indirectly. They require little user knowledge and can be used by laypersons.

In patients with arrhythmias, the newer automated devices have in-built systems and programs to give near-accurate BP readings. During the use of former-generation devices in patients with arrhythmias, measurement of BP was done manually using direct auscultation over the brachial artery.

Invasive Monitoring

The most accurate method is with the use of an invasive probe that is inserted directly into the lumen of an artery. An advantage of invasive monitoring is the ability to display BP variations with each heartbeat. Its use is limited to critical care or operative settings because of its invasive nature and associated risks.

Key Components for Training in Blood Pressure Measurement[8]

- Assess physical and cognitive competencies to perform auscultatory BP measurement.
  - *Vision:* The observer must be able to see the dial of the manometer at eye level without straining and read the sphygmomanometer no further than 3 ft away.
  - *Hearing:* The observer must be able to hear the Korotkoff sounds.
  - *Eye/hand/ear coordination:* The observer must be able to conduct the cuff deflation, listen to Korotkoff sounds, and read the sphygmomanometer simultaneously.
- The evaluation of observers should include an assessment of their knowledge of the following:
  - The different types of observer bias, especially if measurements are made manually.

- General techniques and the interpretation of the measurements.
- Understanding of BP variability by time of day, exercise, and timing of antihypertensive medication consumption.
■ Observers should be aware of the need to do the following:
  - Use only validated devices that are well maintained (including regular recalibration).
  - Choose a quiet location with adequate room temperature (≈72°F).
  - Correctly position the person whose BP is being measured.
  - Ensure that the person does not talk or move during the rest and measurement periods.
  - Ensure that the person does not have a full bladder when BP is measured.
■ The skills of the technician or provider should be demonstrated by assessing the following:
  - Positioning the patient.
  - Selecting the appropriate size cuff.
  - Obtaining a valid and reliable measurement.
  - Recording the measurement accurately.
  - Reporting of abnormal levels.
■ Observers should also know how to interpret and how and when to communicate BP readings to healthcare providers and patients.
■ Questionnaires or interviews can be used to assess knowledge of the BP measurement methodology.
■ Retraining of healthcare professionals every 6 months to 1 year should be considered.

Selection of Cuff Sizes for Blood Pressure Measurement[8]

■ Arm circumference should be measured at the midpoint of the acromion and olecranon.
■ Blood pressure cuff bladder length should be 75–100% of the patient's measured arm circumference.
■ Blood pressure cuff bladder width should be at 37–50% of the patient's arm circumference (a length-to-width ratio of 2:1).
■ Blood pressure cuff should be placed on bare skin.
■ Shirtsleeves should not be rolled up because this may create a tourniquet effect.
■ The most frequent error in measuring office BP is "miscuffing," with undercuffing large arms accounting for 84% of the miscuffings.
■ There is variation in the BP cuff bladder length for adult and large adult cuffs (i.e., the bladder size for large cuff may differ between manufacturers).
■ Individual cuffs should be labeled with the ranges of arm circumferences; lines should be added that show whether the cuff size is appropriate when it is wrapped around the arm.

Cuff size	Arm circumference (cm)	Bladder dimension (width × length) (cm)
Small adult	22–26	12 × 22
Adult	27–34	16 × 30
Large adult	35–44	16 × 36
Extra large adult	45–52	16 × 42

Body Position and Blood Pressure Measurement

■ Systolic BP has been reported to be 3–10 mm Hg higher in the supine than in the seated position.
■ Diastolic blood pressure (DBP) is ≈1–5 mm Hg higher when measured supine versus seated.

- In the supine position, if the arm is resting on the bed, it will be below heart level.
- When BP measurements are taken in the supine position, the cuffed arm should be supported with a pillow.
- In the seated position, the right atrium level is the midpoint of the sternum or the fourth intercostal space.
- If a patient's back is not supported (e.g., the patient is seated on an examination table), SBP and DBP may be increased by 5–15 and 6 mm Hg, respectively.
- Having legs that are crossed during BP measurement may raise SBP by 5–8 mm Hg and DBP by 3–5 mm Hg.
- If the upper arm is below the level of the right atrium (e.g., when the arm is hanging down while in the seated position), the readings will be too high.
- The cuffed arm should be held up by the observer or resting on a table at heart level. If the arm is held up by the patient, BP will be raised.

PROPERLY SEATED OFFICE BLOOD PRESSURE MEASUREMENT[8] (FIG. 1)

- Properly prepare the patient
  - Patient should relax, sitting in a chair with feet flat on the floor and back supported. The patient should be seated for 3–5 minutes without talking or moving around before recording the first BP reading. A shorter wait period is used for some AOBP devices.
  - Avoid caffeine, exercise, and smoking for at least 30 minutes before measurement.
  - Bladder to be emptied.
  - Patient and HCP should avoid talking during the rest period or during the measurement.
  - Clothing covering the location of cuff placement should be removed.
  - Measurements made while the patient is sitting on an examining table do not fulfill these criteria.

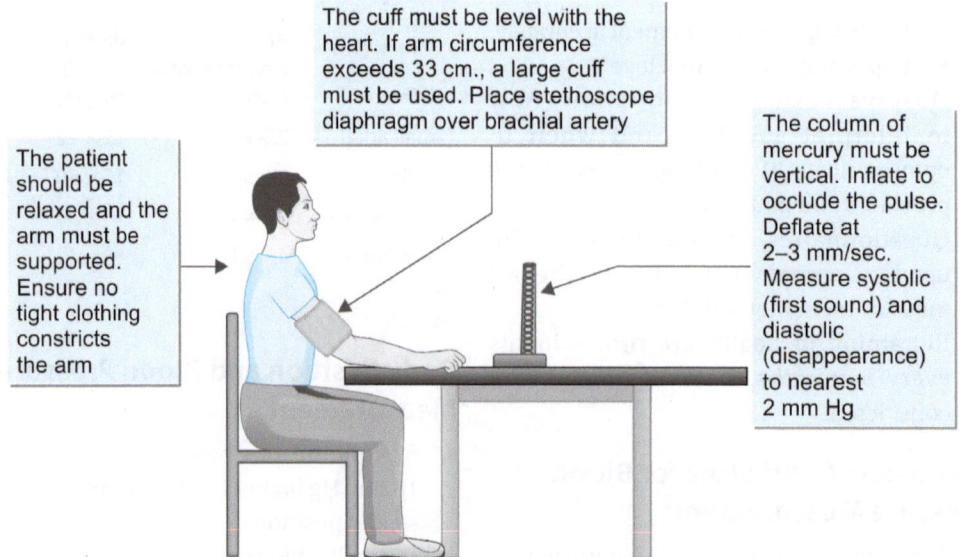

Fig. 1: Technique for BP measurement.[19]

- Use proper technique for BP measurements.
  - Validated upper-arm cuff BP measurement device is used. The device should be periodically calibrated.
  - Patient's arm should be rested/supported on the desk. The patient should not be holding his/her arm because isometric exercise will affect the BP levels.
  - Position the middle of the cuff on the patient's upper arm at the level of the right atrium (midpoint of the sternum).
  - Correct cuff size should be used.
  - Stethoscope diaphragm or bell should be used for auscultatory readings.
- Take the proper measurements needed for diagnosis and treatment of elevated BP/hypertension.
  - First visit—record BP in both arms.; Subsequent visits—arm with higher reading to be used.
  - Separate repeated measurements by 1-2 min.
- Accurate BP readings should be documented to the nearest even number and timing of antihypertensives in relation to the BP measurement should be noted.
- Average the readings—an average of ≥2 readings obtained on ≥2 occasions to estimate the BP.
- Provide BP readings (SBP/DBP) to the patient verbally and in writing.

Need for Multiple Measurements

In the absence of end-organ damage, the diagnosis of hypertension should not be made until the BP has been measured on at least "three visits," spaced over a period of 1 week or more.[12] The "proper measurement" of office-based BP requires attention to all of the following: (1) Time of measurement; (2) type of measurement device; (3) cuff size; (4) patient position; (5) cuff placement; (6) technique of measurement; and (7) number of measurements.

AMBULATORY BLOOD PRESSURE MONITORING[8]

- Medical staff or provider training.
  - Provide knowledge about the BP measures that can be obtained with ABPM.
  - Provide training in the specialized equipment, techniques, and devices used to conduct ABPM and to prepare patients for ABPM.
  - Train staff to prepare/initialize the device for a recording, to fit the device, cuff, and tubing on the patient in the ABPM software, and downloading data.
- Devices and cuffs and equipment.
  - Use validated upper-arm cuff oscillometric devices.
  - Use a cuff that is an appropriate size for the nondominant arm; the nondominant arm is used because movement may interfere with BP measurement.
  - Use new or recharged batteries.
- Patient preparation.
  - May disrupt sleep.
  - Provide instruction to avoid showering or swimming and not to remove the ABPM device, cuff, and tubing (unless showering or swimming).
  - Provide instruction for patients to follow their usual daily activities but to keep their body, especially their arm, still during each BP measurement.
  - Provide a summary of ABPM procedures to the patient on a card that can be referred to during the procedure.
  - Provide instruction on how to refit the cuff if it migrates from its ideal position.

- Provide instruction on placing the device on the bed or beneath a pillow during sleep.
- Provide instructions on how to turn off the device if it is malfunctioning.
- Provide instruction on filling out a diary to document sleep and awakening times, as well as the time of antihypertensive medication intake, the occurrence of symptoms (e.g., dizziness), and meals (if requested by provider).
- Frequency and number of readings.
  - Every 15–30 min during the 24-h period (48–96 total readings).
- Duration of monitoring.
  - Preferred period is 24 h of monitoring.
- Analyzing readings.
  - There are no strong empirical data on the minimum number of readings needed for defining a complete ABPM. Commonly recommended criteria are ≥20 readings during the daytime period and ≥7 readings during the nighttime period. However, an ABPM recording with fewer daytime and/or nighttime readings may still be valid.
  - For each period (daytime, nighttime, and 24 h), the average of all readings should be calculated to determine mean daytime BP, mean nighttime BP, and mean 24-h BP, respectively, and other BP measures (e.g., dipping).

HOME BLOOD PRESSURE MONITORING[8]

1. Patient training provided by healthcare staff or providers.
   a. Provide information
      i. About hypertension diagnosis and treatment;
      ii. On the proper selection of a device.
   b. Provide instruction
      i. On how patients can measure their own BP (if possible, demonstrate the procedure);
      ii. That the HBPM device and BP readings should be brought to healthcare visit;
      iii. That individual BP readings may vary greatly (high and low) across the monitoring period.
2. Preferred devices and cuffs
   a. Use an upper-arm cuff oscillometric device that has been validated.
   b. Use a device that can
      i. Automatically store all readings;
      ii. Print results or send BP values electronically to the healthcare provider;
      iii. Appropriately sized for the patient's arm circumference.
3. Best practices for the patient
   a. Preparation
      i. Have an empty bladder.
      ii. Rest quietly in seated position for at least 5 minutes.
      iii. Do not talk or text.
   b. Position
      i. Sit with back supported.
      ii. Keep both feet flat on the floor.
      iii. Legs should not be crossed.
      iv. Blood pressure cuff should be placed on a bare arm (not over clothes).
      v. Blood pressure cuff should be placed directly above the antecubital fossa (bend of the arm).
      vi. The center of the bladder of the cuff (commonly marked on the cuff by the manufacturer) should be placed over the arterial pulsation of the patient's bare upper arm.
      vii. The cuff should be pulled taut, with comparable tightness at the

CHAPTER 10: Correct Methodology of Blood Pressure Measurements

top and bottom edges of the cuff, around the bare upper arm.

viii. The arm with the cuff should be supported on a flat surface such as a table.

4. *Number of readings:* Take two readings at least 1 min apart in the morning before taking antihypertensive medications and 2 readings at least 1 min apart in the evening before going to bed.

5. Duration of monitoring
   a. Preferred monitoring period is ≥7 days (28 readings or more scheduled readings), a minimum period of 3 days (i.e., 12 readings) may be sufficient, ideally in the period immediately before the next appointment with the provider.
   b. Monitoring conducted over consecutive days is ideal, however readings taken on nonconsecutive days may provide valid data.

Analyzing Readings (Table 1)

For each monitoring period, the average of all readings should be obtained. Some guidelines and scientific statements recommend excluding the first day of readings. If the first day of readings is excluded, the minimum and preferred periods of HBPM should be 4 and 8 days, respectively.

Clinical Indications for the Use of Home Blood Pressure Monitoring

- Masked hypertension/Whit-coat hypertension assessment **(Fig. 2 and Flowcharts 1 and 2)**.
- Efficacy monitoring of antihypertensive use.

SPECIAL BLOOD PRESSURE MEASUREMENT TECHNIQUES

Alternative sites for measurement include the following:
- *Wrist:* Used in obese people and in patients with breast cancer who have had axillary

TABLE 1: Corresponding values of SBP/DBP for the clinic, HBPM, daytime, nighttime, and 24-h ABPM measurements.[13-15]

Clinic	HBPM	Daytime ABPM	Nighttime ABPM	24-h ABPM
120/80	120/80	120/80	100/65	115/75
130/80	130/80	130/80	110/65	125/75
140/90	135/85	135/85	120/70	130/80
160/100	145/90	145/90	140/85	145/90

(ABPM: ambulatory blood pressure monitoring; DBP: diastolic blood pressure; HBPM: home blood pressure monitoring; SBP: systolic blood pressure)

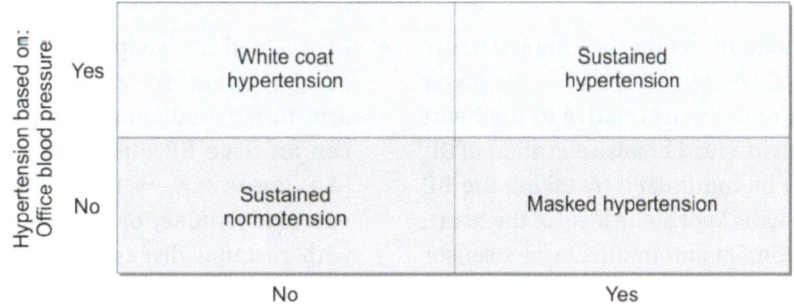

Fig. 2: Cross-classification of office and out-of-office hypertension.[8]

Flowchart 1: Detection of white coat effect or masked uncontrolled hypertension in patients on drug therapy.[16]

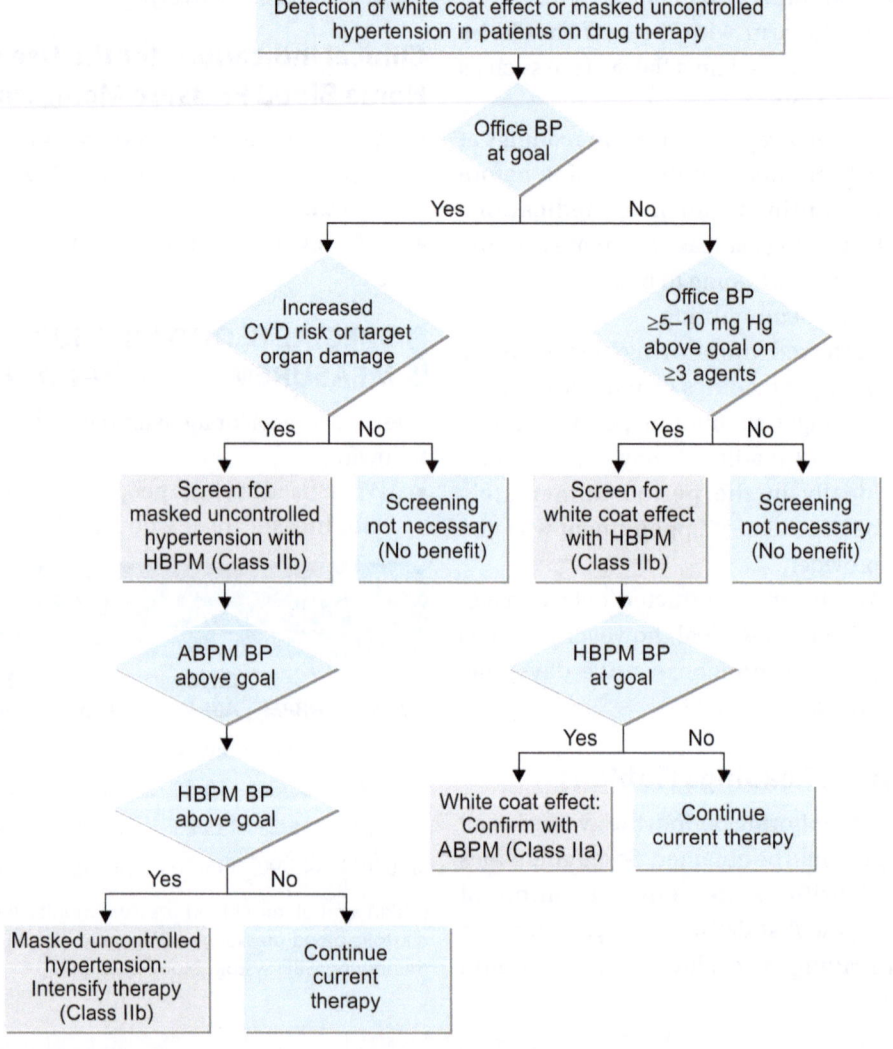

lymph node resection.[17] At the wrist, the hydrostatic pressure related to the lower position of the wrist relative to the heart can result in a further false elevation of BP. This can be minimized by taking the BP with the wrist kept at the level of the heart. In addition, an automatic device's sensor must remain directly over the radial artery for an accurate reading, and wrist flexion may interfere with appropriate sensor positioning.[8]

- Leg: Used in suspected coarctation of the aorta in which there is an arm-to-leg gradient and in patients who cannot have BP measured in the arms (e.g., due to surgery, indwelling catheters, vascular fistulae, or grafts). In patients with vascular disease, SBP at the ankle is often lower than the BP in the arm.[18] No oscillometric BP monitors have been validated for lower extremity BP measurements.

Flowchart 2: Detection of white coat hypertension or masked hypertension in patients not on drug therapy.[16]

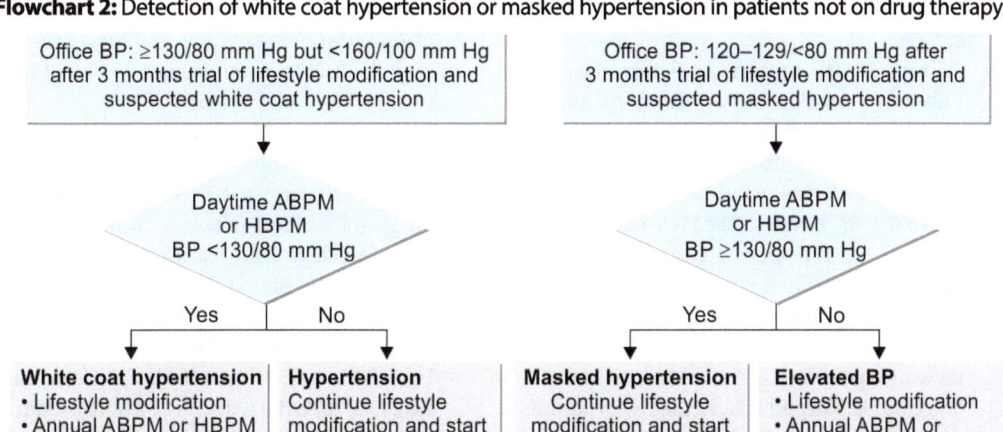

■ SUMMARY

- Blood pressure can be monitored in an ambulatory status, at home, or in the office.
- Appropriate technique for BP measurement requires attention to the time of measurement, type of measurement devices, cuff size, patient position, cuff placement, measurement technique, and number of measurements.

■ REFERENCES

1. Guirguis-Blake JM, Evans CV, Webber EM, Coppola EL, Perdue LA, Weyrich MS, et al. Screening for hypertension in adults: Updated evidence report and systematic review for the US Preventive Services Task Force. JAMA. 2021;325(16):1657-69.
2. Piper MA, Evans CV, Burda BU, Margolis KL, O'Connor E, Whitlock EP, et al. Diagnostic and predictive accuracy of blood pressure screening methods with consideration of rescreening intervals: a systematic review for the U.S. Preventive Services Task Force. Ann Intern Med. 2015;162(3):192-204.
3. Stergiou GS, Palatini P, Parati G, O'Brien E, Januszewicz A, Lurbe E, et al. 2021 European Society of Hypertension practice guidelines for office and out-of-office blood pressure measurement. J Hypertens. 2021;39(7):1293-302.
4. Viera AJ, Yano Y, Lin FC, Simel DL, Yun J, Dave G, et al. Does this adult patient have hypertension? The rational clinical examination systematic review. JAMA. 2021;326(4):339-47.
5. Roerecke M, Kaczorowski J, Myers MG. Comparing automated office blood pressure readings with other methods of blood pressure measurement for identifying patients with possible hypertension: a systematic review and meta-analysis. JAMA Intern Med. 2019;179(3):351-62.
6. Wohlfahrt P, Cífková R, Krajčoviechová A, Šulc P, Bruthans J, Linhart A, et al. Comparison of three office blood pressure measurement techniques and their effect on hypertension prevalence in the general population. J Hypertens. 2020;38(4):656-62.
7. Pickering TG, Hall JE, Appel LJ, Falkner BE, Graves J, Hill MN, et al. Recommendations for blood pressure measurement in humans and experimental animals. Circulation. 2005;111(5):697-716.
8. Muntner P, Shimbo D, Carey R, Charleston J, Gaillard T, Misra S, et al. Measurement of blood pressure in humans: A scientific statement from the American Heart

Association. Hypertension. 2019;73(5): e35-66.
9. Campbell M, Sultan A, Shumway KR, Pillarisetty LS. Physiology, Korotkoff sound. In: StatPearls [Onlinet]. Treasure Island (FL): StatPearls Publishing; 2022. Available from https://www.ncbi.nlm.nih.gov/books/NBK539778/ [Last accessed November 2023]
10. Beevers G, Lip GY, O'Brien E. ABC of hypertension: Blood pressure measurement. Part II—conventional sphygmomanometry: Technique of auscultatory blood pressure measurement. BMJ. 2001;322(7293):1043-7.
11. Stergiou GS, Karpettas N, Kollias A, Destounis A, Tzamouranis D. A perfect replacement for the mercury sphygmomanometer: the case of the hybrid blood pressure monitor. J Hum Hypertens. 2012;26(4):220-7.
12. U.S. Preventive Services Task Force. Screening for high blood pressure: U.S. Preventive Services Task Force reaffirmation recommendation statement. Ann Intern Med. 2007;147(11):783-6.
13. Uhlig K, Balk EM, Patel K, et al. Self-measured blood pressure monitoring: comparative effectiveness. Comparative Effectiveness Review No. 45. (Prepared by the Tufts Evidence-based Practice Center under Contract No. HHSA 290-2007-10055-I.) AHRQ Publication No. 12-EHC002-EF. Rockville, MD: Agency for Healthcare Research and Quality, US Dept of Health and Human Services; 2012. Available from http://www.effectivehealthcare.ahrq.gov/ehc/products/193/893/CER45_SMBP_20120131.pdf [Last accessed November, 2023].
14. Margolis KL, Asche SE, Bergdall AR, Dehmer SP, Groen SE, Kadrmas HM, et al. Effect of home blood pressure telemonitoring and pharmacist management on blood pressure control: A cluster randomized clinical trial. JAMA. 2013;310(1):46-56.
15. McManus RJ, Mant J, Haque MS, Bray EP, Bryan S, Greenfield SM, et al. Effect of self-monitoring and medication self-titration on systolic blood pressure in hypertensive patients at high risk of cardiovascular disease: The TASMIN-SR randomized clinical trial. JAMA. 2014;312(8):799-808.
16. Whelton PK, Carey RM, Aronow WS, Casey DE, Collins KJ, Himmelfarb CD, et al. 2017 ACC/AHA/AAPA/ABC/ACPM/AGS/APhA/ASH/ASPC/NMA/PCNA guideline for the prevention, detection, evaluation, and management of high blood pressure in adults: A report of the American College of Cardiology/American Heart Association Task Force on Clinical Practice Guidelines. Hypertension. 2018;71(6):e13-115.
17. Palatini P, Asmar R, O'Brien E, Padwal R, Parati G, Sarkis J, et al. Recommendations for blood pressure measurement in large arms in research and clinical practice: Position paper of the European society of hypertension working group on blood pressure monitoring and cardiovascular variability. J Hypertens. 2020;38(7):1244-50.
18. Sheppard JP, Albasri A, Franssen M, Fletcher B, Pealing L, Roberts N, et al. Defining the relationship between arm and leg blood pressure readings: a systematic review and meta-analysis. J Hypertens. 2019;37(4):660-70.
19. Victor R, Kaplan NM. Kaplan's Clinical Hypertension, 10th edition. Philadelphia: Wolters Kluwer Lippincott Williams & Wilkins Health; 2010.

CHAPTER 11

Home Blood Pressure Monitoring

A Muruganathan, E Cowshik

INTRODUCTION

As the primary preventable risk factor for the global burden of cardiovascular (CV) disease, hypertension raises the risk of heart attack, stroke, renal disease, and heart failure.[1,2] For people between the ages of 40 and 69 years, the baseline death rate from cardiovascular disease (CVD) more than doubles with every 20-mm Hg increase in systolic blood pressure (BP).[3] However, few clinical investigations have focused on the topic of BP measurement and its validity, even though the impact of BP on CV risk is supported by one of the largest sets of clinical trial data in medicine.[4]

This chapter aims to discuss the advantages and limitations of home BP monitoring (HBPM).

USE OF HOME BLOOD PRESSURE MONITORING

Office BP monitoring (BPM) has a number of drawbacks. Clinical trials and primary care settings have both found high levels of variability in office BP readings. In a study, differences in BP as high as 30 mm Hg were seen without any changes in medication throughout a 2-week period of repeated measurements conducted under research study circumstances.[5] In a recent observational study, primary care physicians (PCPs) had to take the BP of 10 volunteers. The measurements were redone right after the PCPs by two skilled research assistants. Next, the PCPs were randomized to either group 1 (which had comprehensive training documents on standardized BP measurement) or group 2 (which included information regarding high BP). A few weeks later, the BP readings were taken once more, and the PCPs' readings were compared to the average of the four readings taken by the research assistants (the gold standard). At baseline, there were mean BP disparities of 23.0 mm Hg for systolic and 15.3 mm Hg for diastolic BP between PCPs and the gold standard. The mean difference persisted to be high after PCP training (Group 1: 22.3 and 14.4 mm Hg; Group 2: 25.3 and 17.0 mm Hg). Due to the inaccurate BP reading, 24–32% of participants had false diagnoses of systolic hypertension and 15–21% of diastolic hypertension.[6]

There are two different methods for determining BP while away from the workplace. Ambulatory BP monitoring (ABPM) devices are the gold standard for BP measurement; patients wear them for repeated measures over the course of a 24-hour period.[5] When comparing many measures taken at home to those taken after surgery, the average is typically lower and more repeatable than when taking measurements at a clinic. It also has the benefit of detecting an attenuated dip in BP during the night by measuring nocturnal BP. Unfortunately, ABPM monitors are pricey and impractical for long-term BP monitoring, even though they are economical for diagnosing hypertension.[5]

Over the last 10 years, HBPM has become a practical, efficient, and reasonably priced method of screening for hypertension.[7,8] Noninvasive techniques for measuring BP include tonometry, oscillometric, auscultatory, and pulse wave recording and analysis. Although individuals can check their BP as often as they would like, HBPM monitors use the same technology as ABPM monitors. While ABPM provides BP data at multiple points throughout a given day while engaging in unrestricted daily activities, HBPM provides BP data collected over an extended period of time under fixed times and conditions; as a result, HBPM has been demonstrated to be just as reliable as ABPM in terms of providing stable readings with high reproducibility.[9]

HOME BLOOD PRESSURE MONITORING: RECOMMENDATIONS

The National Institute for Clinical Excellence (NICE) guidelines[10] for HBPM state that the following must be followed when using HBPM to confirm a diagnosis of hypertension: BP should be recorded twice a day, ideally in the morning and evening; two consecutive measurements should be taken for each recording, with the subject seated, and at least 1 minute apart; and the BP is recorded for a minimum of 4 days, but preferably for 7 days.

The average value of the days that remain after the first day is deleted should be used instead of the measurements that were made on that day. The use of auscultatory equipment (mercury, aneroid, or other) for HBPM is not advised unless there are exceptional circumstances (such as patients with arrhythmias trained in auscultatory BP monitoring).[11] Guidelines have been put in place to guarantee that monitoring equipment are accurate.

A comprehensive agreement on recommendations for HBPM has been created by the European Society of Hypertension Working Group on Blood Pressure Monitoring.[11] It suggests that the best options for HBPM are semiautomated (manual cuff inflation) or automated electronic devices that measure BP at the upper arm. These gadgets prevent observer bias and are simpler to operate. Patients should not be able to record their BP incorrectly if their monitors have an automated memory feature. Unless brachial measures are extremely difficult or impossible to collect, finger and wrist devices are less accurate and should be avoided (e.g., in persons with very large arm circumference or excessive obesity).

ADVANTAGES OF HOME BLOOD PRESSURE MONITORING

The advantages of HBPM are as follows:
- Telemonitoring enables healthcare professionals to monitor patients remotely
- Prevents white-coat reaction to BP measurements
- Detects increased BP variability
- Is reproducible
- Diagnoses white-coat and masked hypertension
- Diagnoses CV morbidity and mortality better than office BP
- Helps patients better understand hypertension management.

LIMITATIONS OF HOME BLOOD PRESSURE MONITORING

The limitations of HBPM are as follows:
- Device-related errors
- Positioning of a cuff can impact accuracy
- Potentially causes anxiety and overmonitoring

- Lack of nocturnal recording
- Patients' might alter their course of treatment based on home measurements without consulting their doctors
- Insurance companies have not yet paid for these services in many countries.

It has been discovered that 24-hour ABPM average BP values are more closely aligned with HBPM readings, which are frequently lower than office readings. HBPM offers better correlations with measurements of target organ damage, permits more readings, and produces more repeatable readings than office readings. The quality and accuracy of automated office BP measurement were found to be significantly greater than those of manual office BP measurement in a randomized controlled experiment ($n = 555$) that compared the two methods.[12] The within-patient variability of the various BP measurement techniques for at least 6 weeks was evaluated in a retrospective study of a clinical trial ($n = 163$), and coefficients of variation for office BPM, ABPM, and HPBM were determined to be 8.6%, 5.5%, and 4.2%, respectively. The study found that the most accurate way to measure BP was to self-monitor for a week.[13] A different study ($n = 133$) discovered that HBPM is more reproducible than both office BPM and ABPM.[14]

WHITE-COAT HYPERTENSION AND MASKED HYPERTENSION

Case Scenario 1

A 35-year-old individual, without a known history of hypertension, visits the doctor's office for a routine checkup. During previous clinic visits, the BP readings consistently ranged around 150/90 mm Hg. However, at home, the person has been monitoring their BP using a home BP monitor and consistently records readings of around 120/80 mm Hg.

This is a case of white-coat hypertension. Extremely high clinic readings may indicate the white-coat effect, which is characterized by increased office and low ambulatory or home BP. In primary care settings, this effect has been considerably mitigated by the introduction of automated BP monitors.

Case Scenario 2

A 45-year-old individual with no known history of hypertension visits the doctor's office for a routine checkup. During clinic visits, the BP readings consistently fall within the normal range, around 120/80 mm Hg. However, the person has been monitoring their BP at home using a home BP monitor and consistently records readings of around 140/90 mm Hg.

This is a case of masked hypertension and is linked to an increased risk of CVD. It is normal clinic BP and elevated out-of-clinic BP. While some studies imply that ABPM has more sensitivity, others find that HBPM is more convenient and as effective as ABPM in the diagnosis of this phenomenon.[5,10]

According to a meta-analysis, HPBM is especially helpful for risk stratification in cases of concealed hypertension.[15] Although these occurrences are somewhat common, occurring in 10–15% of hypertensive patients, diagnosis necessitates doctors being aware of the possibility, especially in cases with masked hypertension. It is advised that ABPM or HBPM be used to diagnose both masked and white-coat hypertension.

BLOOD PRESSURE VARIABILITY

Types of BP variability include both short-term variability and long-term variability. The factors influencing blood pressure variability include circadian rhythm, physical activity, emotional stress, medications, and autonomic nervous system. In the autonomic nervous system, the balance between the sympathetic and parasympathetic nervous systems plays a role in BP regulation and variability.

PREDICTION OF CARDIOVASCULAR AND STROKE MORBIDITY AND MORTALITY

Five thousand and eight individuals with home and conventional BP measures who were not using antihypertensive medication that could affect their prognosis result were included in a meta-analysis. Participants were stratified into five categories of BP:

1. *Optimal:* 120/80 mm Hg.
2. *Normal:* 120–129/80–84 mm Hg.
3. *High normal:* 130–139/85–89 mm Hg.
4. *Mild hypertension:* 140–159/90–99 mm Hg.
5. *Severe hypertension:* ≥160/ ≥100 mm Hg.

The best category was 120/80 mm Hg. The extra measurements from HBPM enhanced risk stratification at all BP levels less than severe hypertension, hence bolstering the use of HBPM in routine risk assessment.[15] This discovery may improve risk assessment in individuals who are not receiving traditional medical care yet have optimum, normal, or high-normal BP. In terms of outcomes such as heart attack, stroke, renal failure, and/or all-cause mortality, a recent systematic review compared HBPM with ABPM and found that HBPM promotes patient-centered treatment and enhances BP control and patient outcomes.[16]

Nowadays, extensive research is looking at the best way to employ HBPM to avoid CV outcomes. A computer algorithm that automatically generated treatment recommendations based on HBPM was used in the multicenter Hypertension Objective Treatment Based on Measurement by Electrical Devices of Blood Pressure (HOMED-BP; 2001–2010; $n = 3,518$) trial to demonstrate the feasibility of adjusting antihypertensive drug treatment. The algorithm suggested that a safe and achievable target for systolic HBPM should be 130 mm Hg.[17] Morning BP should be regulated to <145 mm Hg, according to the Home Blood Pressure Measurement With Olmesartan Naive Patients to Establish Standard Target Blood Pressure (HONEST) research, a prospective observational trial ($n = 21,591$).[18]

COMPLIANCE AND IMPROVEMENT OF BLOOD PRESSURE CONTROL

Improved BP control may result from routinely managing individuals with uncontrolled hypertension using HBPM. The use of HBPM is linked to significant reductions in systolic and diastolic BP when compared to usual care, as well as in antihypertensive medication and therapeutic inertia—defined as continuing treatment despite elevated BP.[19] While the majority of research has concentrated on White populations, other studies have examined ethnically diverse adults with uncontrolled BP and high-risk patients from clinics in low-income, medically underserved communities who have a history of stroke, coronary heart disease, diabetes, or chronic kidney disease (CKD) and whose baseline BP is at least 130/80 mm Hg.[20]

Home BP monitoring works best when combined with input from a medical professional. One such method is telemonitoring, in which readings taken at home are immediately transmitted to a PCP. This allows the physician to guide treatment along a predefined algorithm so that readings obtained can affect treatment more directly.[20,21]

The use of telemonitoring and HBPM has been supported by numerous studies.[20-24] By using telemonitoring, patients can avoid travel and the medical staff can save time. Additionally, it has been postulated that patients may be more willing to adhere to medical therapy in the long run, even if the medication does not seem to be improving their condition, if they are able to comprehend their own BP readings and recognize the effects of the treatment. Data from clinical trials are required to validate this theory.[22-24]

Home BP monitoring as a good and useful companion:
- Accurate and comprehensive monitoring
- Identification of white-coat and masked hypertension
- Longitudinal assessment of BP trends
- Early detection and management
- Enhanced medication management
- Patient engagement and empowerment
- Improved adherence to treatment plans
- Telehealth integration
- Cost-effective and convenient
- Individualized treatment plans
- Proactive health management
- Useful in CKD and dialysis patients
- Useful to change from two to three drugs.

HOME BLOOD PRESSURE MONITORING AND TELEMEDICINE

Advantages of HBPM and telemedicine include:
- Remote monitoring
- Visual consultations
- Data sharing
- Treatment adjustments
- Reducing clinic visits
- Improving adherence
- Health education
- Monitoring trends and patterns
- Addressing white-coat hypertension
- Remote follow-ups.

COST-EFFECTIVENESS OF HOME BLOOD PRESSURE MONITORING

Home BP monitoring is less labor- and capital-intensive than ABPM and is more successful than traditional clinic BP monitoring in the diagnosis and treatment of hypertension. It is also simpler to adopt. The application of HBPM as a supplement to traditional office management is also encouraged by various standards.

RECOMMENDATIONS TO IMPROVE THE UTILITY OF HOME BLOOD PRESSURE MONITORING IN INDIA

- *Public awareness campaigns:* Launch public awareness campaigns to educate the general population about the importance of monitoring BP at home. Disseminate information through various channels, including television, radio, social media, and community events.
- *Healthcare professional training:* Train healthcare professionals, including general practitioners, nurses, and pharmacists, on the benefits and proper utilization of HBPM.
- *Affordability and accessibility:* Promote the availability of affordable and reliable home BP monitors in the market. Collaborate with manufacturers to develop cost-effective devices suitable for the diverse socioeconomic backgrounds in India.
- *Government initiatives:* Collaborate with government health agencies to integrate HBPM into national health programs. Consider subsidizing home BP monitors for individuals with limited financial means.
- *Community outreach programs:* Conduct community outreach programs to provide hands-on training on using home BP monitors. Create partnerships with local community centers, clinics, and pharmacies to facilitate access to monitors and educational resources.
- *Digital health platforms:* Leverage digital health platforms to provide online resources, tutorials, and support for

individuals using home BP monitors. Develop mobile applications that can assist in monitoring, recording, and interpreting BP readings.
- *Cultural sensitivity:* Tailor educational materials to be culturally sensitive, considering diverse linguistic and cultural backgrounds in India. Involve community leaders and influencers to promote the importance of HBPM.
- *Integration with telehealth:* Integrate HBPM into telehealth initiatives, allowing patients to share their readings with healthcare professionals remotely. Encourage healthcare providers to include home BP data in virtual consultations.
- *Regular follow-ups:* Emphasize the importance of regular follow-ups with healthcare providers based on home BP readings. Implement systems for healthcare professionals to review and adjust treatment plans based on the data provided by patients.
- *Research and data collection:* Encourage research studies to assess the impact of HBPM on hypertension management in the Indian population. Collect data to understand the effectiveness of home monitoring in improving patient outcomes.

CONCLUSION

The use and accessibility of HBPM devices have increased due to the rising prevalence of hypertension. Since HBPM offers comprehensive BP data collected over an extended period of time under predetermined settings and time frames, the mean values of HBP are highly reproducible and stable. Compared to clinic BP monitoring, the use of HBPM devices is more cost-effective and provides a greater predictive value in terms of CV risk. With the use of telemonitoring, HBPM facilitates remote consultations and is simple to integrate into everyday routines. It can also effectively assess response to hypertensive therapy.

REFERENCES

1. George J, MacDonald T. Home blood pressure monitoring. Eur Cardiol. 2015;10(2):95-101.
2. Parati G, Stergiou GS, Bilo G, Kollias A, Pengo M, Ochoa JE, et al.; Working Group on Blood Pressure Monitoring and Cardiovascular Variability of the European Society of Hypertension. Home blood pressure monitoring: Methodology, clinical relevance and practical application: A 2021 position paper by the Working Group on Blood Pressure Monitoring and Cardiovascular Variability of the European Society of Hypertension. J Hypertens. 2021;39(9):1742-67.
3. Tran K, Padwal R, Khan N, Wright MD, Chan WS. Home blood pressure monitoring in the diagnosis and treatment of hypertension in pregnancy: A systematic review and meta-analysis. CMAJ Open. 2021;9(2):E642-50.
4. Shimbo D, Artinian NT, Basile JN, Krakoff LR, Margolis KL, Rakotz MK, et al.; American Heart Association and the American Medical Association. Self-Measured Blood Pressure Monitoring at Home: A Joint Policy Statement from the American Heart Association and American Medical Association. Circulation. 2020;142(4):e42-63.
5. Padfield PL. Self-monitored blood pressure: A role in clinical practice? Blood Press Monit. 2002;7(1):41-4.
6. Sebo P, Pechere-Bertschi A, Herrmann FR, Haller DM, Bovier P. Blood pressure measurements are unreliable to diagnose hypertension in primary care. J Hypertens. 2014;32(3):509-17.
7. Imai Y, Obara T, Asamaya K, Ohkubo T. The reason why home blood pressure measurements are preferred over clinic or ambulatory blood pressure in Japan. Hypertens Res. 2013;36(8):661-72.
8. Arrieta A, Woods JR, Qiao N, Jay SJ. Cost-benefit analysis of home blood pressure

monitoring in hypertension diagnosis and treatment: an insurer perspective. Hypertension. 2014;64(4):891-6.
9. McManus RJ, Little P, Stuart B, Morton K, Raftery J, Kelly J, et al. Home and Online Management and Evaluation of Blood Pressure (HOME BP) using a digital intervention in poorly controlled hypertension: Randomised controlled trial. BMJ. 2021;372:m4858.
10. National Clinical Guideline Centre (UK). Hypertension: Clinical management of primary hypertension in adults: Update of Clinical Guidelines 18 and 34 [Internet]. London: Royal College of Physicians (UK); 2011.
11. Parati G, Stergiou GS, Asmar R, Bilo G, de Leeuw P, Imai Y, et al. European Society of Hypertension practice guidelines for home blood pressure monitoring. J Hum Hypertens. 2010;24(12):779-85.
12. Myers MG, Godwin M, Dawes M, Kiss A, Tobe SW, Grant FC, et al. Conventional versus automated measurement of blood pressure in primary care patients with systolic hypertension: Randomised parallel design controlled trial. BMJ. 2011;342:d286.
13. Warren RE, Marshall T, Padfield PL, Chrubasik S. Variability of office, 24-hour ambulatory, and self-monitored blood pressure measurements. Br J Gen Pract. 2010;60(578):675-80.
14. Stergiou GS, Baibas NM, Gantzarou AP, Skeva II, Kalkana CB, Roussias LG, et al. Reproducibility of home, ambulatory, and clinic blood pressure: Implications for the design of trials for the assessment of antihypertensive drug efficacy. Am J Hypertens. 2002;15:101-4.
15. Asayama K, Thijs L, Brguljan-Hitij J, Niiranen TJ, Hozawa A, Boggia J, et al. Risk stratification by self-measured home blood pressure across categories of conventional blood pressure: a participant-level meta-analysis. PLoS Med. 2014;11:e1001591.
16. Breaux-Shropshire TL, Judd E, Vucovich LA, Shropshire TS, Singh S. Does home blood pressure monitoring improve patient outcomes? A systematic review comparing home and ambulatory blood pressure monitoring on blood pressure control and patient outcomes. Integr Blood Press Control. 2015;8:43-9.
17. Asayama K, Ohkubo T, Metoki H, Obara T, Inoue R, Kikuya M, et al. Cardiovascular outcomes in the first trial of antihypertensive therapy guided by self measured home blood pressure. Hypertens Res. 2012;35(11):1102-10.
18. Kario K, Saito I, Kushiro T, Teramukai S, Ishikawa Y, Mori Y, et al. Home blood pressure and cardiovascular outcomes in patients during antihypertensive therapy: Primary results of HONEST, a large-scale prospective, real-world observational study. Hypertension. 2014;64(5):989-96.
19. Agarwal R, Bills JE, Hecht TJ, Light RP. Role of home blood pressure monitoring in overcoming therapeutic inertia and improving hypertension control: a systematic review and meta-analysis. Hypertension. 2011;57(1):29-38.
20. Kario K. Management of hypertension in the digital era: Small wearable monitoring devices for remote blood pressure monitoring. Hypertension. 2020;76(3):640-50.
21. Kario K, Tomitani N, Iwashita C, Shiga T, Kanegae H. Simultaneous self-monitoring comparison of a supine algorithm-equipped wrist nocturnal home blood pressure monitoring device with an upper arm device. J Clin Hypertens. 2021;23(4):793-801.
22. McManus RJ, Mant J, Bray EP, Holder R, Jones MI, Greenfield S, et al. Telemonitoring and self management in the control of hypertension (TASMINH2): a randomised controlled trial. Lancet 2010;376(9736):163-72.
23. Margolis KL, Asche SE, Bergdall AR, Dehmer SP, Groen SE, Kadrmas HM, et al. Effect of home blood pressure telemonitoring and pharmacist management on blood pressure control: The hyperlink cluster randomized trial. JAMA. 2013;310(1):46-56.
24. Mengden T, Ewald S, Kaufmann S, vor dem Esche J, Uen S, Vetter H. Telemonitoring of blood pressure self measurement in the OLMETEL study. Blood Press Monit. 2004;9(6):321-5.

CHAPTER 12

Ambulatory Blood Pressure Monitoring

Parvati Nandy

INTRODUCTION

Screening for hypertension and monitoring of treated hypertension are typically performed by obtaining blood pressure (BP) measurements in a clinician's office. However, office-based BP readings may not always accurately represent an individual's blood pressure. Many individuals with elevated office BP will not have hypertension upon further testing (i.e., white coat hypertension). Consequently, the use of out-of-office BP measurement is appropriate to confirm the diagnosis of hypertension and to monitor patients on therapy.

IMPORTANCE OF AMBULATORY BLOOD PRESSURE MONITORING[1]

Ambulatory blood pressure monitoring (ABPM) is important for the information it provides after measuring the BP of a person as he goes about his daily life activities including the period he is sleeping, for a span of 24–48 h.

Ambulatory BP monitoring evolved into a tool of BP monitoring for a certain subset of people, and although it has some disadvantages, in being costly and cumbersome to wear at times, it provides useful prognostic information about hypertension patients.

Thus, this tool is crucial in the identification of white coat and masked hypertension. White coat hypertension refers to elevated BP in the clinic setup, masked hypertension refers to elevated BP in the out-of-the-office situation. The white coat effect is present in patients who are already being treated with antihypertensive medications, yet office BP is above the threshold.

Ambulatory BP monitoring also helps to demonstrate the effect of antihypertensive drugs and drug-related low BP. Ambulatory BP monitoring also predicts fatal and nonfatal myocardial infarction, and stroke better than routine BP measurement. It is also the only method whereby one can estimate nocturnal BP.

Ambulatory BP monitoring gives average BP readings over a defined period—usually 24–48 h. Readings will be recorded as per the instrument's settings—usually at 24–48 h intervals. To define hypertension, at least 14 readings of the ABPM is needed.

Blood pressure varies according to many external and internal factors. Behavioral factors also have an important role in diurnal BP variation. Blood pressure rises sharply on waking in the morning and falls during sleep at night, these changes are closely related to other behavioral factors, mental and physical activities such as food consumption and obesity, dietary intake of salt, drinking and smoking habits, consumption of coffee, and bathing. Appropriate lifestyle modifications may improve both the level and rhythm of

BP in these patients. Ideal 24-h BP control consists of not only control of average daily BP but also its diurnal and nocturnal variability.[2]

Most hypertension patients are monitored by clinic-based BP measurement and their daily BP variability is not available. However, studies have shown that office BP measurement is not an ideal method for representing 24-h BP compared to ABPM which can give ample data about the patient's 24-h BP variability.

Mental and physical stress elevates BP in the morning and during the daytime. Sleep irregularities may also cause elevated night-time BP.

SOME IMPORTANT DEFINITIONS RELATED TO AMBULATORY BLOOD PRESSURE MONITORING (TABLE 1)[1]

- *Nocturnal dipping of blood pressure:* Dipping is the proportional decrease in night-time compared with daytime BP (reported as the percentage decline). The normal dip in systolic blood pressure (SBP) is 10–20%. Failure of the BP to fall by at least 10% during sleep is called "nondipping." The underlying mechanisms of nondipping are unknown, but intrinsic kidney defects may contribute. Nondipping is a risk factor for the development of heart failure and other cardiovascular complications. In one large cohort, e.g., the risk of heart failure among nondippers was more than twice that of dippers even after controlling office BP.
- *Morning surge:* Morning surge is the difference between the night-time BP and the average early morning BP. The average BP from the first 2 h after awakening minus the average night-time BP may be most reproducible. Patients who have a larger surge from night-time to early morning BP may have a greater risk of future cardiovascular events.
- *Systolic blood pressure load:* This is the proportion of time during the day in which the SBP is above the threshold for elevated daytime BP. This value provides insight into the duration and lability of elevated BP. A patient whose SBP is above the threshold for more than 40% of daytime measurement is generally considered to have an excessively high SBP load.
- *Diastolic blood pressure (DBP) load:* This is the proportion of time during the day in which the DBP is above the threshold for elevated daytime BP.
- *Ambulatory arterial stiffness index (AASI):* The AASI is determined by plotting a regression of all the DBP values with simultaneous SBP values during a period of ABPM and subtracting the slope of this line from 1. Higher values generally correspond to stiffer blood vessels and a higher risk of cardiovascular disease.[4]

TABLE 1: Definitions of hypertension according to office ambulatory and home blood pressure levels.[3]

Category	SBP (mm Hg)		DBP (mm Hg)
Office BP	>140	and/or	>90
Ambulatory BP			
Daytime/awake mean	>135	and/or	>85
Night-time/asleep mean	>120	and/or	>70
24-h mean	>130	and/or	>80
Home BP mean	>135	and/or	>85

(DBP: diastolic blood pressure; SBP: systolic blood pressure)

Indications to Measure BP by Ambulatory BP Monitoring[3]

- Prehypertension or grade-I hypertension.
- Increase in BP in the office without target organ damage.
- Normal office BP in patients with target organ damage or with high cardiovascular risk.
- Evaluation of resistant hypertension.
- When there are symptoms and signs of hypotension during antihypertensive therapy.
- Postural and postprandial hypotension in patients with or without antihypertensive medications.
- Patients with autonomic dysfunction.
- Patients with endocrine hypertension
- Patients with sleep apnea and raised BP.

Performance and Interpretation of Ambulatory BP Monitoring[1]

- *Performing ABPM:* Ambulatory blood pressure monitoring can be arranged in the clinician's office. Appropriate devices have to be procured, which are identified by online validated listings, such as "Hypertension Canada" and "STRIDE BP."
- *Patients preparation and instruction:* patients should arrive ready for having the monitor applied, wear short sleeved shirts. They have to wear the monitor for 24 h. The patients should be instructed to relax their arms and stay still as each timed measurement starts.
- *Configuring the monitor before use:* Clinicians are required to manually enter measurement timings.
- *Applying the monitor:* The cuff should be applied to the nondominant arm with the attached inflation/recording unit worn on the opposite hip using a belt or a strap.

At least two inflations of ABPM unit should be obtained in the office so that the patients become comfortable with how the device works.

Ambulatory BP Monitoring Report

The major data provided by the ABPM report include the following:
- Average 24-h BP.
- Average daytime (awake) BP.
- Average night-time (asleep) BP.
- Nocturnal dipping of BP.
- Morning surge.
- Systolic BP load.
- Diastolic BP load.
- Ambulatory arterial stiffness index.

In the study by Najafi MT et al.,[5] "Ambulatory BP monitoring and diabetes complications: Targeting morning BP surge and nocturnal dipping," they demonstrated that diabetic neuropathy was associated with morning blood pressure surge (MBPS) and abnormal nocturnal dipping status. Loss of nocturnal dipping was a risk factor for cardiovascular disease and retinopathy in patients with type 2 DM. These findings highlight the importance of ABPM and targeted antihypertensive therapy directed toward restoration of normal circadian BP in patients with type 2 DM **(Table 2)**.

In the study by Gorostidi et al.,[3] "Abnormalities in ambulatory blood pressure monitoring, in hypertensive patients with diabetes," it was found that 50% of the subjects had daytime BP uncontrolled, circadian rhythm was blunted, and nocturnal BP rise was seen, especially in type 2 DM patients as compared to diabetes-free patients. About 52% of diabetic patients had daytime BP above 135/85 mm Hg. The prevalence of white coat hypertension was 33% in this study. Hypertensive patients with diabetes

TABLE 2: Comparison between ABPM and home BP monitoring.[3]

S. no.	ABPM	Home BP monitoring
1.	Can identify white coat and masked HTN	Can identify white coat and masked HTN
2.	Stronger prognostic evidence	Measurement in home setting which is more relaxed than doctor's office
3.	Night-time readings	Nonnocturnal reading
4.	Measurement in real-life settings	Patient's engagement in BP measurement
5.	Additional prognostic BP phenotypes	Easily repeated and used over longer periods to assess day to day BP variability
6.	Abundant information from a single measurement session, including short-term BP variability	Only static BP is available
7.	Expensive and sometime limited availability	Cheap and widely available
8.	Can be uncomfortable	Potential for measurement error

(ABPM: ambulatory blood pressure monitoring; HTN: hypertension)

showed a remarkably high prevalence of alterations in ABPM.[6]

CONCLUSION

Ambulatory BP monitoring with advanced techniques, and low-cost, effective instruments will provide clinicians with important data regarding BP and its circadian pattern. This is especially important in patients with comorbidities like diabetes.

However, as of now, ABPM is costly, available in limited places, and needs technical expertise to operate it.

REFERENCES

1. Shimbo D, Abdalla M, Falzon L, Townsend RR, Muntner P, et al. Out of office blood pressure measurement: Ambulatory and self-measured blood pressure monitoring. J Am Soc Hypertens. 2016;10(3):224.
2. Kawano Y. Diurnal BP variation and related behavioural factors. Hypertens Res. 2011; 34(3):281-5.
3. Bansode BR. Prognostic Value of Ambulatory BP Monitoring, API Medicine Update; 2022, Vol. 32, Chapter 6.
4. Williams B, Marcia G, Spicring W, Rosei EA, Azizi M, Burnier M, et al. 2018 ESC/ESH Guidelines for management of arterial hypertension. Eur Heart J. 2018;39(33):3021-104.
5. Najafi MT, Khaloo P, Alemi H, Jaafarinia A, Blaha MJ, Mirbolouk M, et al. Ambulatory BP monitoring and diabetes complications: Targeting morning blood pressure surge and nocturnal dipping. Medicine (Baltimore). 2018;97(38):e12185.
6. Gorostidi M, de la Sierra A, González-Albarrán O, Segura J, de la Cruz JJ, Vinyoles E, et al. Abnormalities in ambulatory blood pressure monitoring in hypertensive patients with diabetes. Hypertens Res. 2011;34(11): 1185-9.

Central Aortic Blood Pressure: An Overview

Rohit Kapoor, Shivam Kapoor

■ INTRODUCTION

In the realm of blood pressure (BP) measurement, the traditional approach has revolved around assessing the brachial artery using the time-honored sphygmomanometer. For over a century, this method has been a cornerstone for evaluating hypertension and gauging the efficacy of its treatment. This conventional brachial BP measurement has demonstrated its ability to predict cardiovascular (CV) morbidity and mortality. However, recent advancements in technology and understanding have paved the way for novel devices capable of automatic BP measurement, both for around-the-clock monitoring and self-assessment at home. Despite these innovations, the focus remains on brachial BP assessment, although there is an emerging body of evidence advocating for the measurement of central (aortic) BP.[1-3]

Central BP refers to the pressure exerted directly on critical organs such as the brain, heart, and kidneys. Distinguished from peripheral (arm) BP measurement, central BP experiences an amplification effect, known as pulse pressure (PP) amplification, as it travels through the circulatory system. This amplification leads to a disparity between systolic blood pressure (SBP) measured in the brachial artery and in the aorta **(Fig. 1)**. The growing body of research indicates that central SBP might serve as a more robust predictor of future CV events than its brachial counterpart.

While the convenience and wide array of available devices have made brachial BP measurement a mainstay, studies reveal that it inadequately represents aortic pressure, which generally registers lower than corresponding brachial values. Furthermore,

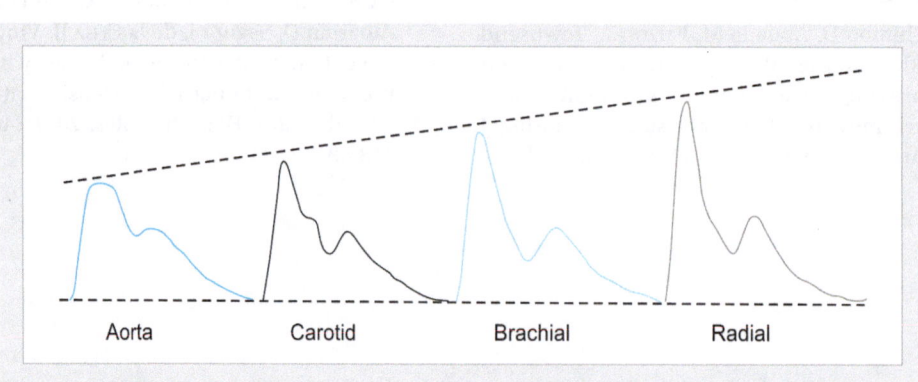

Fig. 1: Amplification of the pressure waveform moving from the aorta to the radial artery.

central pressure has demonstrated differential responses to certain medications and holds a stronger correlation with future CV events.[4,5] Despite the noninvasive accessibility of central pressure assessment, clinicians are cautious about abandoning brachial cuff sphygmomanometers without solid evidence that central pressure measurements offer superior CV risk stratification and treatment monitoring.

In this comprehensive review, is the author aims to delve into the contemporary comprehension of central BP measurements. We will explore the current methodologies available for assessing central aortic pressure, and the clinical implications associated with their use. Specifically, we will address their potential for enhancing the diagnostic and prognostic stratification of hypertension, as well as their ability to provide a more accurate evaluation of the impact of treatment on BP. Through this exploration, we seek to shed light on the evolving landscape of BP measurement and its implications for CV health.[6]

The physiological basis for measuring central BP lies in the intricate dynamics of the CV system, particularly in individuals with hypertension. In hypertensive patients, there is a notable reduction in the caliber and number of small peripheral arteries, accompanied by an elevation in mean arterial pressure. This mean arterial pressure is determined by the interplay between cardiac output and peripheral vascular resistance. It is important to note that peripheral arteries are characterized by a muscular composition and collagen fibers, rendering them less distensible. On the contrary, larger arteries such as the aorta and carotid arteries are predominantly comprised of elastin fibers.[7,8]

The unique properties of elastic arteries enable them to function as pressure reservoirs. During systole, these arteries undergo distension, allowing them to accommodate blood being ejected from the left ventricle. Then, during diastole, the elastic recoil of the arterial wall propels blood forward in a continuous flow. This property results in the lowest arterial stiffness in elastic arteries such as the ascending and thoracic aorta and higher stiffness in distal arteries such as the tibial artery.

A key phenomenon that occurs in the arterial system is the generation and propagation of pressure waves. When the left ventricle contracts, it generates a pressure wave that travels down the arterial tree. At the junction between large arteries and arterioles, this pressure wave is reflected centrally. As a consequence, the pressure waveform in the aorta becomes a composite of the forward-traveling wave from the left ventricle and the backward-reflected wave from the peripheral muscular and stiffer arteries.[9]

The impact of this reflected wave is significant. It leads to an increase in central peak SBP and a subsequent augmentation of PP. This phenomenon, termed "augmentation pressure," contributes to an elevated PP. This increase is quantified as a percentage of the total pressure and is represented by the augmentation index (AIx). The AIx offers insight into the interaction between the forward and reflected waves in the arterial system and is a valuable parameter for assessing central BP.[10]

In summary, the physiological concept of measuring central BP revolves around the differences in arterial properties and wave dynamics between peripheral and central arteries. The unique characteristics of elastic arteries and the interactions between pressure waves underscore the importance of evaluating central BP to gain a more comprehensive understanding of CV health, particularly in hypertensive individuals.[11]

The continuous variation in arterial pressure throughout the cardiac cycle is a fundamental aspect of CV physiology. However, in clinical practice, only the traditional sphygmomanometric measurements of systolic and diastolic pressures are routinely reported. These measurements are typically taken in the brachial artery using cuff sphygmomanometry, a method that has remained largely unchanged for decades. However, the shape of the pressure waveform undergoes continuous changes as it travels through the arterial tree. While diastolic and mean arterial pressures tend to remain relatively stable, systolic pressure can differ significantly between different locations along the arterial tree.[12]

This phenomenon is known as systolic pressure amplification and is primarily attributed to the increasing arterial stiffness as one moves away from the heart. As the pressure wave propagates from the highly elastic central arteries towards the stiffer brachial artery, the upper portion of the wave becomes narrower, causing the systolic peak to become more pronounced and leading to an elevation in systolic pressure.

Various techniques have been developed to assess central BP, each with its own advantages and limitations. One direct but invasive method involves cardiac catheterization, wherein a pressure-sensing catheter is used to measure BP in the ascending aorta.[13] However, this approach is highly invasive, necessitates specialized training, and is not suitable for routine population screening.

Noninvasive methods have also been devised, involving the recording of pressure waveforms from sites distal to the aorta, such as the carotid, radial, or brachial arteries. These waveforms are then calibrated to BP measurements obtained through cuff sphygmomanometry. Each noninvasive approach has its strengths and drawbacks, and these methods include the following:

- *Carotid artery:* Pressure waveforms can be recorded from the carotid artery, which is easily accessible. However, factors such as anatomical variations and local changes in arterial properties may affect the accuracy of measurements.
- *Radial artery:* The radial artery, located at the wrist, is another site for noninvasive pressure waveform recording. While convenient, the radial artery's distance from the aorta may lead to distortions in the pressure waveform.
- *Brachial artery:* Pressure waveforms can also be obtained from the brachial artery, similar to traditional cuff sphygmomanometry. This approach benefits from its ease of use and familiarity but may still have limitations due to differences between central and brachial pressures **(Figs. 2A to D)**.

It is important to note that each method has its own set of strengths and limitations, and the choice of technique depends on various factors including the clinical context, available equipment, and patient characteristics. While noninvasive methods offer valuable insights into central BP, further research is needed to refine their accuracy and establish their clinical utility.[14,15]

Central pressures are derived from noninvasive techniques that measure radial or carotid pulses. These techniques involve applanation tonometry, where pressure waveforms are obtained using transcutaneous pressure transducers. The carotid or radial waveform is then used to estimate the central aortic waveform. Another method involves a mathematical description of the charge from input to output signals to derive an aortic waveform from measurements at the radial artery. Computerized programs adjust for factors such as heart rate, height, and age to obtain central SBP, diastolic BP, PP, and arterial stiffness indices such as AIx and pulse wave velocity (PWV).[16]

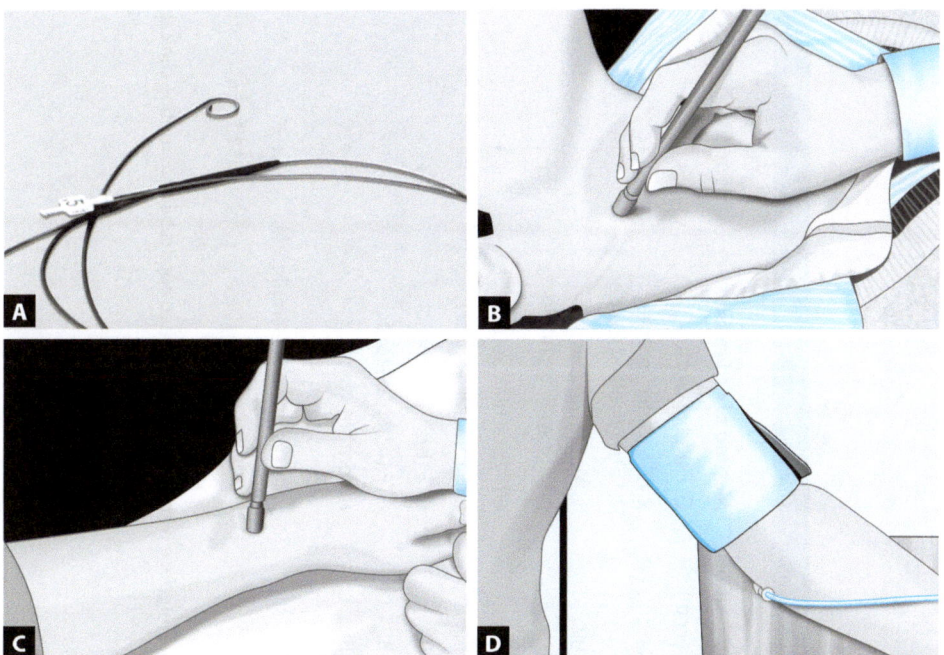

Figs. 2A to D: Techniques for assessing central blood pressure: (A) Invasive cardiac catheterization—This method involves inserting a pressure-sensing catheter into the ascending aorta to directly measure central BP. It provides highly accurate data but is invasive and not suitable for routine screening; (B) Direct applanation tonometry of the carotid artery: Transcutaneous pressure transducers are placed over the carotid artery to obtain pressure waveforms, which are then used to estimate central pressures. The carotid waveform is used as a surrogate for the aortic waveform; (C) Applanation tonometry of the radial artery: Similar to the carotid approach, pressure waveforms are obtained from the radial artery using transcutaneous pressure transducers. The radial waveform is calibrated to estimate central pressures; (D) Cuff-based oscillometry at the brachial artery: This technique utilizes cuff-based oscillometry at the brachial artery, similar to traditional BP measurement. Central pressures are estimated based on a validated generalized transfer function.

The general transfer functions of applanation tonometry have some error, which is typically lower than that of standard brachial cuff pressure measurements. Variations in measurements between different instruments and operators can occur. AIx, a reflection of arterial wave reflection on total BP, can vary with heart rate, cardiac contractility, and age. Pulse wave velocity, a measurement of aortic pulse velocity, is calculated by dividing the distance between two arteries (e.g., carotid and femoral) by transit time. Pulse wave velocity has emerged as a reliable marker of arterial stiffness and is influenced by factors such as age, BP levels, heart rate, and diabetes.[17]

Studies have shown the clinical relevance of arterial stiffness assessment. Aortic PWV has been identified as a strong predictor of future CV events and all-cause mortality, independent of classic CV risk factors. The Reference Values for Arterial Stiffness Collaboration group in Europe has published reference values for PWV, indicating normal ranges for different age groups.

Overall, measuring central BP and arterial stiffness provides valuable insights into CV

TABLE 1: Indirect noninvasive methods for measuring central BP.

Method of waveform recording	Device	Company	Method of calibration	Method of estimation	Clinical applicability[†]
Radial tonometry	BPro	Health STATS	Brachial–radial cuff BP	GTF (radial–aortic)	++
	SphygmoCor	Cor Medical	Brachial–radial cuff BP	2. GTF (radial–aortic) 2. Late systolic shoulder	++
	HEM9000AI	Omron	Brachial cuff BP	1. Algorithm 2. Late systolic shoulder	++ ++
Brachial cuff PVP	*ARC solver		Brachial cuff BP	GTF (brachial–aortic)	+++
	Centron cBP301	Centron Diagnostics	Brachial cuff BP	GTF (brachial–aortic)	++++
	Vicorder	Skidmore Medical	Brachial cuff BP	GTF (brachial–aortic)	+++
	XCEL	Cor Medical	Brachial cuff BP	GTF (brachial–aortic)	+++
	Method by Sung et al.		Brachial cuff BP	Algorithm	++
Suprasystolic brachial cuff PVP	Arteriograph	Tens ioMed	Brachial cuff BP	Late systolic wave amplitude	+++
	Cardoscope II	Pulsecor	Brachial cuff BP	Algorithm	++++

*Incorporated in Mobil-O-Graph FWA device (IEH GmbH).
[†]Personal view based on experience, operator dependency, and need for computer/software interface with "+" indicating limited applicability to routine clinical practice and "+++" indicating high applicability.
(GTF: generalized transfer function; PVP: pulse volume plethysmography)

risk and can aid in risk stratification and prognosis.

Table 1 illustrates various indirect noninvasive methods for measuring central BP. These methods involve obtaining pressure waveforms from peripheral arteries, such as the carotid or radial arteries, and then using validated techniques to estimate central aortic pressure. The carotid or radial waveform is calibrated to obtain central SBP, diastolic BP, PP, and arterial stiffness indices such as AIx and PWV **(Table 1)**.

IMPLICATIONS OF CENTRAL BLOOD PRESSURE ON THERAPY

Central BP plays a crucial role in CV health, as it directly influences vital organs such as the heart, kidneys, and brain, which receive blood from major arteries exposed to aortic pressure. Numerous studies conducted over the past decade have highlighted the strong connection between central pressure and both surrogate markers of CV risk and actual CV events.[18]

Cross-sectional studies have shown that central pressure is more closely linked to surrogate measures of CV risk, such as carotid intima–media thickness (CIMT) and left ventricular mass (LVM), compared to brachial pressure. Regression of LVM was found to be more strongly related to changes in central pressure, and the reduction in CIMT due to antihypertensive treatment correlated better with the fall in central pressure.

It was previously believed that BP reduction itself was the primary factor, regardless of the choice of antihypertensive agent.[19] However, studies have demonstrated that different antihypertensive drug classes exert varying effects on brachial vs central pressure. Notably, β-blockers such as atenolol were found to be inferior to other major antihypertensive drug classes in preventing CV events. This discrepancy between brachial and central pressure effects provides insight into the outcomes seen with specific drugs and supports the hypothesis that agents that lower central pressure more effectively are likely to be more beneficial in reducing CV risk. This observation underscores the importance of considering central BP in the choice of antihypertensive therapy.[21,21]

CONCLUSION

In conclusion, central BP measurement offers valuable insights into CV health and risk assessment beyond traditional brachial BP measurements. The core BP to which vital organs such as the heart, brain, and kidneys are exposed, central BP holds promise as a better prognostic indicator for target organ damage and CV events. Arterial stiffness, a key factor in central BP assessment, has emerged as an established CV risk marker, providing valuable information about inherent atherosclerotic risk and predicting incident hypertension in high-risk individuals.

Years of research have revealed that antihypertensive drugs, particularly β-blockers, have varying effects on brachial and central pressure. This observation highlights the potential benefits of future treatment strategies based on central BP measurements, which could have significant implications for the diagnosis and management of hypertension.[22]

While central BP measurement offers exciting prospects, cuff measurements for brachial BP will continue to be the cornerstone of clinical practice. It remains essential for appropriately powered clinical trials to demonstrate that preferential lowering of central pressure translates into improved outcomes. Only then will central pressure become widely accepted as a surrogate marker for CV risk and play a significant role in guiding clinical decisions.

■ REFERENCES

1. Trudeau L. Central Blood Pressure as an Index of Antihypertensive Control: Determinants and Potential Value. Can J Cardiol 2014;30:S23-S28.
2. Muiesan ML, Salvetti M, Bertacchini F, Agabiti-Rosei C, Maruelli G, Colonetti E. et al. Central blood pressure assessment using 24-hour brachial pulse wave analysis. J Vascular Diagnostic Interventions 2014:2;141-148.
3. McEniery MC, Cockroft JR, Roman MJ, Franklin SS, Wilkinson IB. Central blood pressure: current evidence and clinical importance. Eur Heart J 2014;35:1719-25.
4. Siebenhofer A, Kemp CR, Sutton AJ, Williams B. The reproducibility of central aortic blood pressure measurements in healthy subjects using applanation tonometry and sphygmocardiography. J Hum Hypertens 1999;13:625-9.
5. Kelly R, Hayward C, Avolio A, O'Rourke M. Noninvasive determination of age-related changes in the human arterial pulse. Circulation 1989;80:1652-9.
6. Mancia G, De Backer G, Dominniczak A, Cifkova R, Fagard R, Germano G, et al. 2007 Guidelines for the management of arterial hypertension: the Task Force for the Management of Arterial Hypertension of the European Society of Hypertension (ESH) and of the European Society of Cardiology (ESC). J Hypertens 2007;25:1105-87.
7. O'Brien E, Waeber B, Parati G, Staessen J, Myers MG. Blood pressure measuring devices: recommendations of the European Society of the European Society of Hypertension. BMJ 2001;322:531-6.
8. Mancia G, Fagard R, Narkiewicz K, Redón J, Zanchetti A, Böhm M et al.ESH/ESC Task Force for the Management of Arterial Hypertension. 2013 Practice guidelines for the management of arterial hypertension of the European Society of Hypertension and the European Society of Cardiology. J Hypertens 2013;31:1925-38.
9. Mitchell GF, Hwang SJ, Vasan RS, Larson MG, Pencina MJ, Hamburg NM, et al. Arterial stiffness and cardiovascular events; the Framingham Heart Study. Circulation 2010; 121: 505-11.
10. Vlachopoulos C, Aznaouidis K, Stefanadis C. Prediction of cardiovascular events and all-cause mortality with arterial stiffness. J Am Coll Cardiol 2010; 55:1318-27.
11. The Reference Values for Arterial Stiffness' Collaboration. Determinants of pulse wave velocity in healthy people and in the presence of cardiovascular risk factors: 'establishing normal and reference values'. Eur Heart J 2010; 31:2338-50.
12. Laurent S, Cockcroft JR, van Bortel LM, Boutouyrie P, Giannattasio C, Hayozet D et al. Abridged version of the expert consensus document. Artery Res 2007;1:2-12.
13. Boutouyrie P, Bussy C, Lacolley P. Girerd X, Laloux B, Laurent S. Association between local pulse pressure, mean blood pressure, and large-artery remodeling. Circulation 1999; 100:1387-93.
14. Wang KL, Cheng HM, Chuang SY, Spurgeon HA, Ting CT, Lakatta EG, et al. Central or peripheral systolic or pulse pressure: which best relates to target organs and future mortality? J Hypertens 2009;27:461-7.
15. de Luca N, Asmar RG, LondonGM, O'Rourke MF, Safar ME. Selective reduction of cardiac mass and central blood pressure on low-dose combination perindopril/ indapamide in hypertensive subjects. J Hypertens 2004; 22:1623–1630.
16. Manisty CH, Zambanini A, Parker KH, Davies JE, Francis DP, Mayet J, et al. Differences in the magnitude of wave reflection account for differential effects of amlodipine- versus atenolol-based regimens on central blood pressure: an Anglo-Scandinavian Cardiac Outcome Trial sub study. Hypertension 2009;54:724-30.

17. Major outcomes in high-risk hypertensive patients randomized to angiotensin converting enzyme inhibitor or calcium channel blocker vs diuretic: The Antihypertensive and Lipid-Lowering Treatment to Prevent Heart Attack Trial (ALLHAT). JAMA 2002;288:2981-97.
18. Carlberg B, Samuelsson O, Lindholm LH. Atenolol in hypertension: is it a wise choice?. Lancet 2004;364:1684-9.
19. Lindholm LH, Carlberg B, Samuelsson O. Should beta blockers remain first choice in the treatment of primary hypertension? A Meta-Analysis. Lancet 2005; 366:1545-53.
20. Medical Research Council trial of treatment of hypertension in older adults: principal results. MRC Working Party. BMJ 1992; 304:405-12.
21. Dahlof B, Devereux RB, Kjeldsen SE, Julius S, Beevers G, de Faire U, et al. Cardiovascular morbidity and mortality in the Losartan Intervention for Endpoint reduction in hypertension study (LIFE): a randomized trial against atenolol. Lancet 2002; 359: 995-1003.
22. Dahlof B, Sever PS, Poulter NR, Wedel H, Beevers DG, Caulfield M, et al. Prevention of cardiovascular events with an antihypertensive regimen of amlodipine adding perindopril as required versus atenolol adding bendroflumethiazide as required, in the Anglo-Scandinavian Cardiac Outcomes Trial- Blood Pressure Lowering Arm (ASCOT-BPLA): a multicentre randomised controlled trial. Lancet 2005;366: 895-906.

SECTION 5
Evaluation of Hypertension

14. **Hypertension: Clinical Approach**
    M Chenniappan

15. **Hypertension: Electrocardiogram in Decision Making**
    M Chenniappan

CHAPTER 14

Hypertension: Clinical Approach

M Chenniappan

■ INTRODUCTION

The incidence, prevalence, and complications of hypertension (HT) are increasing in India. This is primarily due to uncontrolled HT. However, the complications are also due to late diagnosis, failure to identify secondary causes, missing hypertension-mediated organ damage (HMOD), and ignoring other risk factors as well as comorbidities and their drugs.[1] Most often, we rely upon investigations such as echocardiogram (ECG) and laboratory investigations to diagnose the above conditions. A good clinical approach which includes good history taking and meticulous physical examination will help us in identifying all the abnormalities mentioned above at the earliest with little or no cost to the patient. In this article, we are aiming at exploring this possibility.

■ CLINICAL APPROACH

1. History
2. Physical examination

In both these segments, we should concentrate on:
- Identifying secondary causes,
- Other risk factors,
- Recognition of HMOD, and
- Comorbidities and their drugs.

History

History Identifying Secondary Causes

Identifying secondary causes in HT is very crucial in the management of HT because most of the secondary HT is curable whereas essential HT is only controllable.

In any new or uncontrolled HT, the following factors may indicate the possibility of secondary HT **(Box 1)**:
- Any difficult to control HT
- Onset of HT before 30 years
- New onset of diastolic HT after 65 years
- Abrupt onset of HT
- Sudden out of control of blood pressure (BP)
- Unprovoked or excessive hypokalemia after diuretics

BOX 1: History clues to secondary HT.

History regarding the specific cause:
- Family history of renal disease (polycystic kidney)
- Renal disease, UTI, hematuria, and analgesic abuse (parenchymal renal disease)
- Oral contraceptives (HT due to drugs)
- Episodes of sweating, headache, and anxiety (pheochromocytoma)
- Episodes of muscle weakness and tetany (hyperaldosteronism)
- Intermittent claudication in young (coarctation of aorta)
- Intermittent episodes of sudden acute dyspnea requiring hospitalization (flash acute pulmonary edema due to renal artery stenosis)
- Snoring and acute breathlessness at night with daytime sleepiness (sleep apnea)
- Increased weight and striae (Cushing's syndrome)
- Weight gain or weight loss with HT (thyroid disorders)

(HT: hypertension; UTI: urinary tract infection)

- Acclerated or malignant HT or any hypertensive crisis
- Dispropotionate HMOD to the degree of HT
- Claudication in young patients
- Unexplained anemia in HT
- Daytime sleepiness or tiredness
- Drugs (other allopathic or other system medicines).

History to Identify Other Risk Factors

- Family and personal history of HT, CVD, stroke, or renal disease
- Family and personal history of associated risk factors (e.g., familial hypercholesterolemia)
- Tobacco use in any form including passive smoking
- Dietary history and salt intake
- Alcohol consumption
- Lack of physical exercise/secondary lifestyle
- History of erectile dysfunction
- Sleep history, snoring, and sleep apnea (information also from partner)
- Polyuria and polydipsia of diabetes mellitus (DM)

History Suggestive of Hypertension-mediated Organ Damage

- *Brain and eyes:* Headache, vertigo, syncope, impaired vision, transient ischemic attack (TIA), sensory or motor deficit, stroke, carotid revascularization, cognitive impairment, or dementia (in elderly people).
- *Heart:* Coronary artery disease (CAD)—exertional and rest angina, history of revascularization; heart failure—dyspnea, paroxysmal nocturnal dyspnea, and orthopnea for left heart failure; neck pulsation, right hypochondrial tenderness, swelling of the abdomen, pedal edema for right heart failure; arrhythmias–palpitation and syncope.
- *Kidney:* Thirst, polyuria, nocturia, hematuria, and UTIs.
- *Peripheral arteries:* Cold extremities, intermittent claudication, pain-free walking distance, pain at rest, and peripheral revascularization.

History Regarding Comorbidities and Drugs

- History of bronchial asthma and intake of drugs such as sympathomimetic and steroids
- History of orthopedic diseases and intake of non-steroidal anti-inflammatory drugs (NSAIDs) and cyclooxygenase 1 (COX-2) inhibitors
- History of anemia of renal disease and erythropoietin
- History of malignancy and chemotherapeutic drugs
- History of psychiatric diseases and antipsychiatric drugs
- Routine use of drugs such as ginseng and herbal medicines.

■ PHYSICAL EXAMINATION

Physical examination in HT is divided into general examination and specific examination to identify secondary causes, other risk factors, HMOD, and comorbidities. General examination includes an examination of the pulse (arterial and venous), BP, pallor, edema, obesity (general or mid-segment), and features suggestive of endocrine disorders (thyroid and Cushing's syndrome).

Examination of Arterial Pulse in Hypertension

All pulses should be palpated. The absence of lower limb pulse and brachiofemoral delay is suggestive of coarctation, asymmetry of pulse in a hypertensive emergency is suggestive of aortic dissection, asymmetry of pulse in chronic situations is indicative of peripheral arterial disease, absence of upper limb pulse is suggestive of Takayasu's disease and absence of individual pulse is suggestive of embolism in a case of atrial fibrillation (AF).

The rate may be fast, slow, regular, or irregular. Tachycardia with HT may occur in hyperthyroidism, pheochromocytoma, and heart failure. Slow pulse with HT is suggestive of hypothyroidism, drugs induced or sinus node or atrioventricular (AV) conduction disorder. Irregular pulse is likely to be due to premature beats or AF.

Volume of the pulse is to be checked which has to be correlated with pulse pressure. The pulse volume is normal if the pulse pressure is normal (30–50 mm Hg). The volume of the pulse can be normal, high, or low in HT. Whenever pulse volume is high, aortic regurgitation (AR), hyperthyroidism, anemia, pregnancy, and high pulse pressure HT should be suspected. In high pulse pressure HT, the systolic blood pressure (SBP) is high, and diastolic blood pressure (BP) is low due to aortic stiffening and high pulse wave velocity which is the most dangerous HT. The low-volume pulse in HT is rare and if present it is suggestive of arterial disease and end-stage hypertensive heart disease due to severe left ventricular (LV) dysfunction.

The character of the pulse can give some clues regarding the basic disease. Collapsing pulse or Corrigan's pulse indicates AR which may produce systolic HT Bisferiens pulse is a sign of chronic severe AR or aortic stenosis (AS) with AR. Change in volume of pulse for alternate beats, pulsus alternans occurs in LV failure.

Examination of Venous Pulse

Jugular venous pressure (JVP) and pulse should be examined in HT. Elevated JVP and prominent 'a' wave are the signs of associated pulmonary HT which may coexist with systemic HT. The JVP is elevated in all volume-overloaded conditions which may produce HT such as chronic kidney disease (CKD) and iatrogenic fluid overload. Flat JVP even in a lying position is indicative of dehydration which can also produce HT due to increased renin release secondary to hyponatremia which happens in the polyuric phase of CKD. Intermittent cannon waves with bradycardia may happen in isolated systolic HT due to complete heart block (CHB).

Measurement Blood Pressure

The first and foremost important prerequisite for correct management of HT is the proper recording of BP **(Fig. 1)**.

Measurement of Blood Pressure (European Society of Cardiology Guidelines 2018)

Steps to record the BP correctly is listed in **Box 2**.

Blood Pressure Apparatus, Cuff Size, and Lowering of Column[2]

Mercury BP apparatus has been replaced by an aneroid in recent days which should be calibrated every year. As there are no proper calibrating methods in India it is preferable to get a new BP apparatus every year. The width of the cuff should be 40% of the arm circumference and the length of the cuff is 80% of the arm circumference. The cuff width and length for proper measurement of BP are shown in **Table 1**.

A large cuff for the small arm will underestimate SBP and a small cuff for the large arm overestimates SBP. Lowering of the

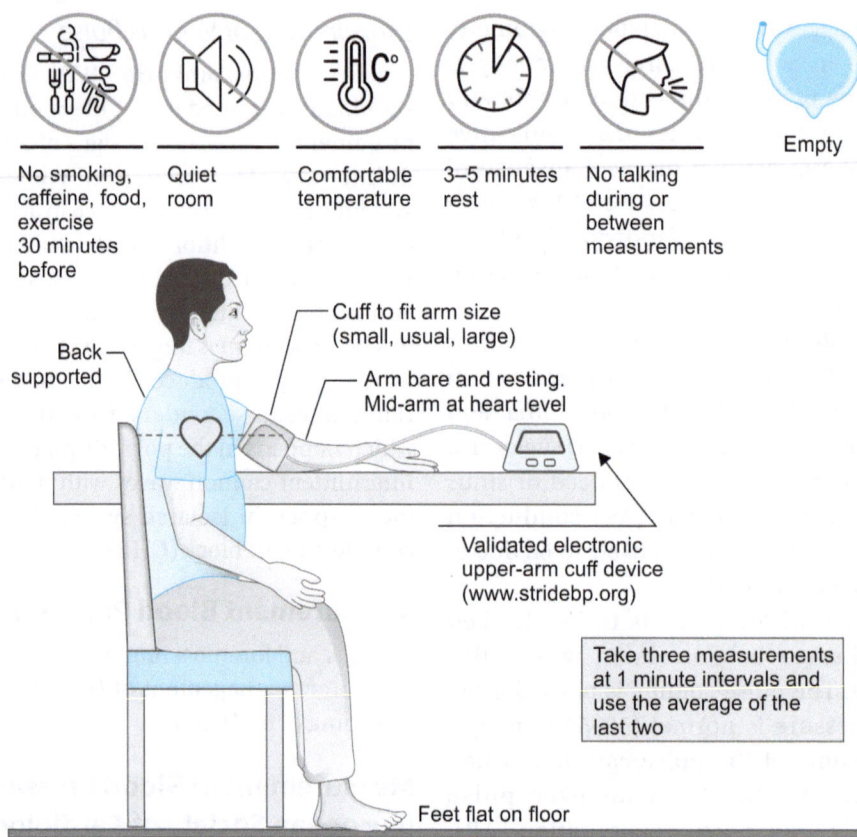

Fig. 1: Steps to be followed for proper recording of BP at office and home.
Source: International Society of Hypertension (ISH) guidelines.

BOX 2: Steps that should be followed for correct recording of BP.

Recommendations:
- Office BP should be measured in both arms at least at the first visit because a between-arm SBP difference of >15 mm Hg is suggestive of atheromatous disease and is associated with an increased CV risk
- If a between-arm difference in BP is recorded, then it is recommended that all subsequent BP readings use the arm with the higher BP reading
- It is recommended to base the diagnosis of HT on repeated office BP measurements on more than one visit, except when HT is severe (e.g., grade 3 and especially in high-risk patients). At each visit, three BP measurements should be recorded, 1–2 min apart, and additional measurements should be performed if the first two readings differ by >10 mm Hg. The patient's BP is the average of the last two BP readings or out-of-office BP measurement with ABPM and/or HBPM, provided that these measurements are logistically and economically feasible
- When using auscultatory methods, use phases I and V (sudden reduction/disappearance) Korotkoff sounds to identify SBP and DBP, respectively
- Measure BP in both arms at the first visit to detect possible between-arm differences. Use the arm with the higher value as the reference

Contd...

Contd...

- Measure BP 1 minute and 3 minutes after standing from a seated position in all patients at the first measurement to exclude orthostatic hypotension. Lying and standing BP measurements should also be considered in subsequent visits in older people, in people with diabetes, and in other conditions in which orthostatic hypotension may frequently occur
- Record heart rate and use pulse palpation to exclude arrhythmia
- Because individual BP measurements tend to vary in an unpredictable or random fashion, a single reading is inadequate for clinical decision-making. An average of two to three BP measurements obtained on two to three separate occasions will minimize random error and provide a more accurate basis for the estimation of BP

(ABPM: ambulatory blood pressure monitoring; BP: blood pressure; CV: cardiovascular; DSP: diastolic blood pressure; HBPM: home blood pressure monitoring; HT: hypertension; SBP: systolic blood pressure)

TABLE 1: Table showing required cuff width and length in various groups.

Cuff denomination	Arm circumference (cm)	Cuff width (cm)	Bladder length (cm)
Small adult	22–26	10	24
Adult	27–34	13	30
Large adult	35–44	16	38
Thigh	45–52	20	42

mercury column or the numbers in aneroid BP apparatus is about 2-3 mm Hg/s. Rapid lowering results in the overestimation of diastolic blood pressure.

Blood Pressure Measurement Methods[3]

- Office [attended, office blood pressure monitoring (OBPM)]-oscillometric (electronic)-preferred method; auscultatory (mercury, aneroid).
- Office automated [unattended, automated office blood pressure (AOBP)]-oscillometric (electronic)
- Ambulatory blood pressure monitoring (ABPM)
- Home blood pressure monitoring (HBPM).

Grade of Hypertension

Once the BP is recorded correctly, the classification of HT is done based on numbers into various grades. The grades of HT vary according to different guidelines **(Table 2)**.

Specific Physical Examination to Identify Secondary Causes

- Features of Cushing's syndrome (obesity, striae, and facies)
- Skin stigmata of neurofibromatosis (pheochromocytoma)
- Palpation of enlarged kidneys (polycystic kidney)
- Auscultation of abdominal murmurs (renovascular HT)
- Auscultation of precordial or chest murmurs (aortic coarctation)
- Diminished and delayed femoral pulses and reduced leg BP (aortic coarctation)
- Short neck and obesity (sleep apnea)
- Edema, pallor, and facial puffiness (CKD)
- Typical hypothyroid features with bradycardia (hypothyroidism)
- Tachycardia and sweating (pheochromocytoma and hyperthyroidism).

Specific Physical Examination to Diagnose Other Risk Factors[4,5]

Features of metabolic syndrome—Waist circumference >90 cm in men; >80 cm in women with other laboratory features—Prediabetic, prehypertensive, and precardiovascular disease status

TABLE 2: Classification of HT according to recent American and European guidelines.

ESC/ESH vs. ACC/AHA HT guideline

	ESC/ESH 2018 (June)			ACC/AHA 2017 (November)			
Category	Systolic (mm Hg)		Diastolic (mm Hg)	Category	Systolic (mm Hg)		Diastolic (mm Hg)
Optimal	<120	And	<80	Normal	<120	And	<80
Normal	120–129	And	80–84	Elevated BP	120–129	And	<80
High Normal	130–139	And/or	85–89	Stage 1	130–139	Or	80–89
Grade 1	140–159	And/or	90–99	Stage 2	≥140	Or	≥90
Grade 2	160–179	And/or	100–109	Hypertensive crisis	≥180	Or	≥120
Grade 3	≥180	And/or	≥110				

Isolated systolic HT: Systolic >140, diastolic <90

(ACC/AHA: American College of Cardiology/American Heart Association; BP: blood pressure; ESC/ESH: European Society of Cardiology/European Society of Hypertension; HT: hypertension)

- External features of DM—Acanthosis nigricans, foot ulcers, and features of metabolic syndrome
- External features of hypercholesterolemia—Xanthelasma
- Tar staining of fingers—Chronic smoker

Specific Physical Examination to Identify Hypertension-mediated Organ Damage

- *Brain:* The presence of previous cerebrovascular accident (CVA) such as hemiplegia or paresis; focal neurological deficit; carotid bruit; and motor or sensory defects indicate chronic HMOD. Acute ischemic or hemorrhagic stroke and hypertensive encephalopathy indicate a hypertensive emergency.
- *Eye:* There may be various grades of hypertensive retinopathy and objective visual disturbances as HMOD in the eye. The presence of grade 3 retinopathy indicates accelerated HT and the presence of papilledema is malignant HT. Papilledema with loss of vision is a hypertensive emergency.
- *Heart:* The abnormalities in arterial pulse and venous pulse indicative of cardiac HMOD are already explained.[6,7]

Left ventricular hypertrophy (LVH) is indicative of chronic pressure overload due to HT which is an important HMOD determining the prognosis. Left ventricular hypertrophy can be diagnosed clinically by the presence of heaving apical impulse where the duration of apical thrust is prolonged without much altering the position of the apical impulse. Sometimes there may be palpable fourth heart sound in addition to heaving apical impulse. The presence of clinical evidence of LVH and palpable or auscultatory LV fourth heart sound indicate diastolic dysfunction which is the earliest manifestation of cardiac HMOD. In all patients with HT clinical evidence for LVH should be looked for clinically.[8]

Auscultation of the heart includes abnormalities of heart sounds, the presence of additional heart sounds, and murmurs.

S_1 and S_2–S_1 may be soft due to increased end-diastolic pressure of LV. In HT, A_2 is loud due to high diastolic pressure in the aorta. Hypertension produces paradoxical splitting of S_2 due to prolonged LV systole **(Figs. 2A and B)**.

- *Presence of additional sounds (Fig. 3):* Left-sided third and fourth sounds are low-pitched sounds heard with bell of stethoscope lightly applied to the apex and they give valuable information regarding LV function **(Fig. 3)**.

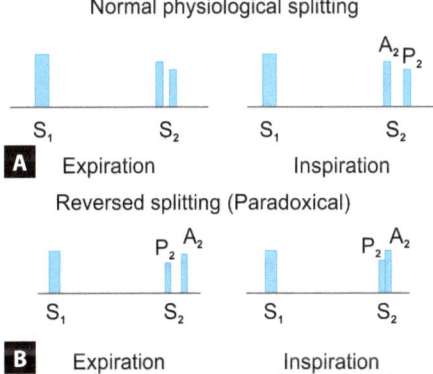

Figs. 2A and B: (A) Normal S_2 splitting where the single second is heard in expiration and two components are heard in inspiration; (B) In reversed splitting, two components are heard in expiration and a single sound is heard in inspiration.
Note: In reversed splitting, A_2 occurs later than P_2 due to due to delayed LV systole because of HT.

Left-sided fourth heart sound (LA4) is a low-pitched sound that occurs due to left atrial contraction against raised LV end-diastolic pressure and is heard before first heart sound **(Fig. 3)**. Most commonly, it is associated with stiff LVH. In patients with dyspnea in HT, the presence of LVH and LA4 indicates that dyspnea is probably due to heart failure with preserved ejection fraction (HFPEF). So, LA4 is a sign of diastolic dysfunction.

Left-sided third heart sound (LV3) in adults is a low-pitched sound due to exaggerated early diastolic filling due to high LA pressure due to LV systolic dysfunction and is heard after the second sound **(Fig. 3)**. In patients with dyspnea in HT, the presence of LV3 indicates that dyspnea is probably due to heart failure with reduced ejection fraction (HFREF). So, LV3 is a sign of systolic dysfunction.

- *Presence of murmurs (Fig. 4):* The two common murmurs in HT are mitral regurgitation (MR) and aortic regurgitation (AR). Mitral regurgitation can occur due to multiple causes such as LV dilatation, papillary muscle dysfunction, and associated CAD. The pan systolic murmur of MR is heard over the apex **(Fig. 4A)**.

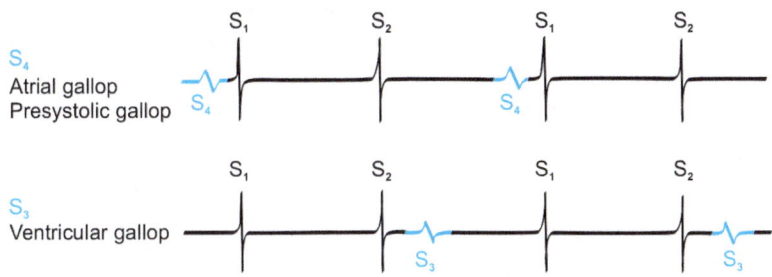

Fig. 3: Diagram shows S_4 (Left-sided fourth heart sound) and S_3 (Left-sided third heart sound).

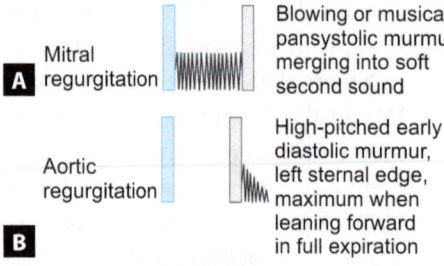

Figs. 4A and B: (A) Murmurs of mitral regurgitation; (B) Aortic regurgitation.

Aortic regurgitation is due to increased diastolic pressure in the aorta and aortic root dilatation. It is the most common murmur in HT as well as due to the congenital bicuspid aortic valve (CBAV) which is the most common association of coarctation of the aorta. The early diastolic murmur of AR is heard over the left sternal edge as well as in aortic area **(Fig. 4B)**.

- *Peripheral vessels:* Examination of peripheral arteries may show absence, reduction or asymmetry of pulses, cold extremities and ischemic skin lesions. Carotids should be auscultated in all patients with HT to detect carotid artery bruit which is the most cost-effective way of detecting HMOD of peripheral arteries.

Specific Physical Examination to Detect Comorbid Conditions[9,10]

Most of comorbid conditions are identified through good history.

- *Chronic obstructive pulmonary disease (COPD):* Patients with COPD may have mild cyanosis, clubbing, and barrel-shaped chest. During acute episodes of asthma, it may be mistaken for acute LVF. The differentiating points are the action of accessory muscles, the inspiratory collapse of JVP, Rhonchi rather than crepitation, and more cyanosis.
- *Orthopedic diseases:* Deformity of joints, swelling of joints, reduced mobility, and abnormal gait are indicators of Joint abnormalities.
- *Psychiatric disorders:* Abnormal behavior and communication of the patient are suggestive of associated psychiatric disorders such as anxiety and or depression. Many antipsychotic drugs produce visceral obesity and metabolic syndrome.
- *Malignancy:* The presence of obvious tumors, emaciation, pallor and external evidence of chemotherapy induced side effects may indicate associated malignancy.

CONCLUSION

A good clinical evaluation of a patient with HT can reveal secondary causes, unmask other risk factors, expose HMOD, and identify comorbid conditions and drugs without sophisticated investigations. So, no investigation however sophisticated it may be should ever replace a good clinical judgment. We must utilize advanced investigatory modalities to refine our clinical knowledge rather than replace it. A skillful history taking and meticulous and focused physical examination most often give us many crucial information regarding the diagnosis and management of HT without wasting time (of the doctor) and money (of the patient).

REFERENCES

1. Leung AA, Daskalopoulou SS, Dasgupta K, McBrien K, Butalia S, Zarnke KB, et al. Hypertension Canada's 2017 guidelines for diagnosis, risk assessment, prevention, and treatment of hypertension in adults. Can J Cardiol. 2017;33(5):557-76.

2. Pickering TG, Hall JE, Appel LJ, Falkner BE, Graves J, Hill MN, et al. Recommendations for BP measurement in humans and experimental animals: Part 1 – Blood pressure measurement in humans: a statement for professionals from the Subcommittee of Professional and Public Education of the American Heart Association Council on High Blood Pressure Research. Circulation. 2005;111(5): 697-716.
3. Mancia G, Fagard R, Narkiewicz K, Redon J, Zanchetti A, Böhm M, et al. 2013 ESH/ESC guidelines for the management of arterial hypertension: The Task Force for the Management of Arterial Hypertension of the European Society of Hypertension (ESH) and of the European Society of Cardiology (ESC). Eur Heart J. 2013;34(28):2159-219.
4. Hubert HB, Feinleib M, McNamara PM, Castelli WP. Obesity as an independent risk factor for cardiovascular disease: a 26-year follow-up of participants in the Framingham Heart Study. Circulation. 1983;67(5):968-77.
5. Elliott P, Stamler J, Nichols R, Dyer AR, Stamler R, Kesteloot H, et al. Inter salt revisited: further analyses of 24 hour sodium excretion and blood pressure within and across populations. Intersalt Cooperative Research Group. BMJ. 1996;312(7041):1249-53.
6. Leary AC, Donnan PT, MacDonald TM, Murphy MB. The influence of physical activity on the variability of ambulatory blood pressure. Am J Hypertens. 2000;13(10):1067-73.
7. Devereux RB, Roman MJ. Left ventricular hypertrophy in hypertension: Stimuli, patterns, and consequences. Hypertens Res. 1999;22(1):1-9.
8. Devereux RB, Wachtell K, Gerdts E, Boman K, Nieminen MS, Papademetriou VV, et al. Prognostic significance of left ventricular mass change during treatment of hypertension. JAMA. 2004;292(19):2350-6.
9. Whelton PK, Carey RM, Aronow WS, Casey DE Jr, Collins KJ, Himmelfarb CD, et al. 2017 ACC/AHA/AAPA/ABC/ACPM/AGS/APhA/ASH/ASPC/NMA/PCNA guideline for the prevention, detection, evaluation, and management of high blood pressure in adults: A Report of the American College of Cardiology/American Heart Association Task Force on Clinical Practice Guidelines. J Am Cswoll Cardiol. 2018;71(19):e127-48.
10. Williams B, Mancia G, Spiering W, Rosei EA, Azizi M, Burnier M, et al. 2018 ESC/ESH Guidelines for the management of arterial hypertension: Eur Heart J. 2018;39(33):3021-104.

CHAPTER 15

Hypertension: Electrocardiogram in Decision Making

M Chenniappan

INTRODUCTION

In India, one in three people has hypertension and 50% of the population is in the high normal range. Mortality and morbidity are quite high in hypertension if not detected early and treated properly. The complication in hypertension depends upon the presence of target organ disease (TOD), secondary causes, comorbidities, and complications due to hypertension. Most often we rely upon echocardiography to diagnose these issues. The electrocardiogram (ECG) when interpreted skillfully gives valuable information regarding these problems, even when they are not detected by echocardiography. Electrocardiography is underutilized in hypertension. The purpose of the chapter is to explore the utilities of ECG in hypertension in diagnosis and treatment. To our knowledge, the management of hypertension has not been looked at from this angle so far. Electrocardiogram aids in excellent care giving (ECG) in patients with hypertension.

ELECTROCARDIOGRAM IN HYPERTENSION

Electrocardiogram in hypertension is better studied in the following headings: (1) Target organ disease, (2) secondary causes, (3) comorbidities, and (4) complications.

Electrocardiogram: Target Organ Disease

Left Ventricular Hypertrophy

One of the important TODs is left ventricular hypertrophy (LVH). The presence of LVH for the same level of blood pressure (BP) enhances the risk of coronary artery disease (CAD), heart failure, and arrhythmias. Although ECHO is ideal for detecting LVH, ECG remains a cost-effective method of detecting LVH.

Electrocardiogram criteria to detect LVH: (1) Limb leads—R in lead aVL more than 11; (2) Chest leads—R in V5, V6 + S in V1 > 35 mm; R in V5, V6 more than 26 mm **(Fig. 1)**.

Limb leads criteria are used in children and patients with chronic obstructive pulmonary disease (COPD) in whom chest lead criteria may not be reliable. The ECG has high specificity and low sensitivity.

Left ventricular hypertrophy—preferred: (1) Angiotensin receptor blocker (ARB); (2) Angiotensin-converting enzyme I (ACE I); (3) Amlodipine; (4) Indapamide.

Left ventricular hypertrophy—not preferred: (1) Hydralazine; (2) α-blockers; (3) Other diuretics; (4) Older β-blockers. Life study had demonstrated that in addition to BP lowering, regression of LVH would reduce clinical events.

CHAPTER 15: Hypertension: Electrocardiogram in Decision Making

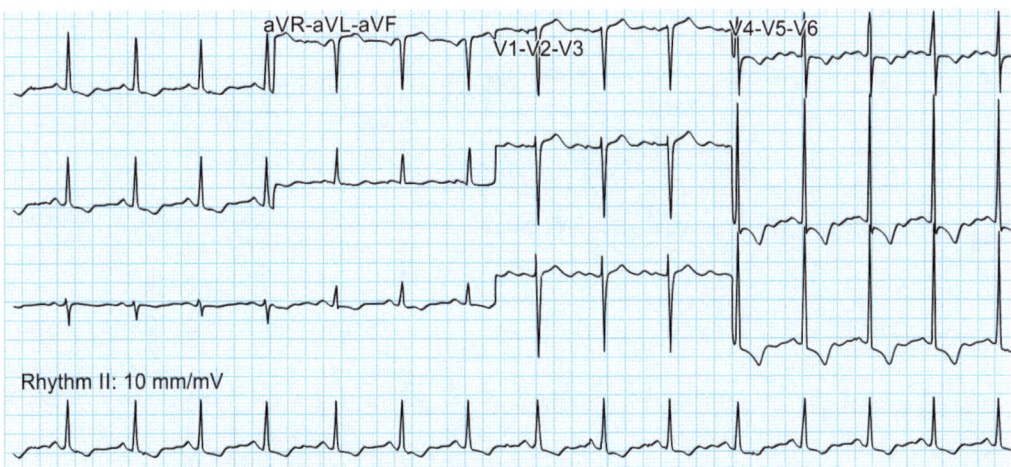

Fig. 1: Electrocardiogram showing left ventricular hypertrophy (LVH).

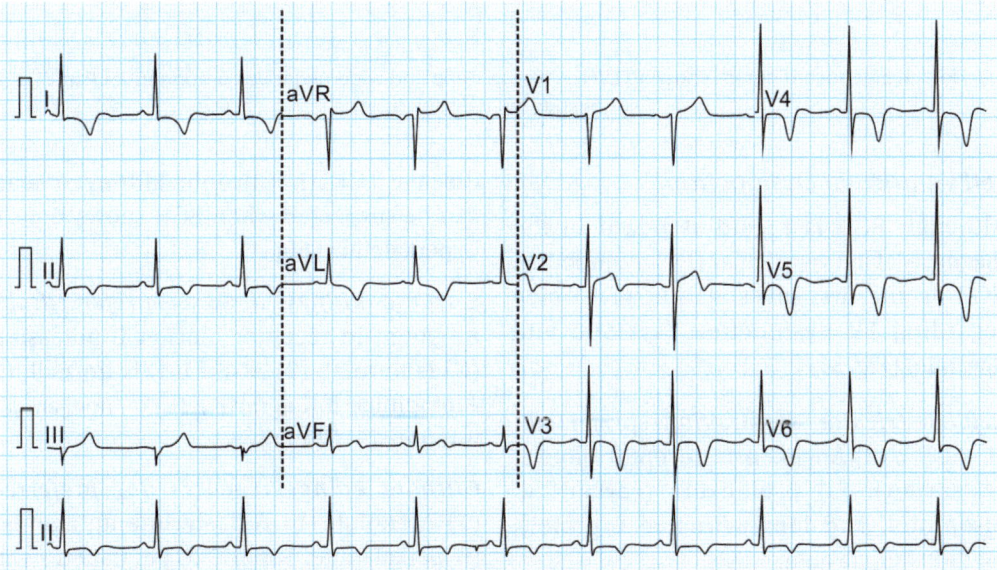

Fig. 2: Electrocardiogram showing LVH and primary ST-T changes (well-formed ST segment, symmetrical T inversion).

Coronary Artery Disease[1]

Although LVH can produce secondary ST-T changes in hypertension, one should suspect associated CAD if the T wave inversion is symmetrical with a well-formed ST segment **(Fig. 2)**.

Coronary artery disease—preferred: (1) β-blockers (except atenolol), (2) ACEI (ramipril and perindopril), (3) ARB (telmisartan), (4) aspirin and statin.

Coronary artery disease—not preferred: (1) Short acting CCBs (nifedipine); (2) Hydralazine; (3) α-blockers.

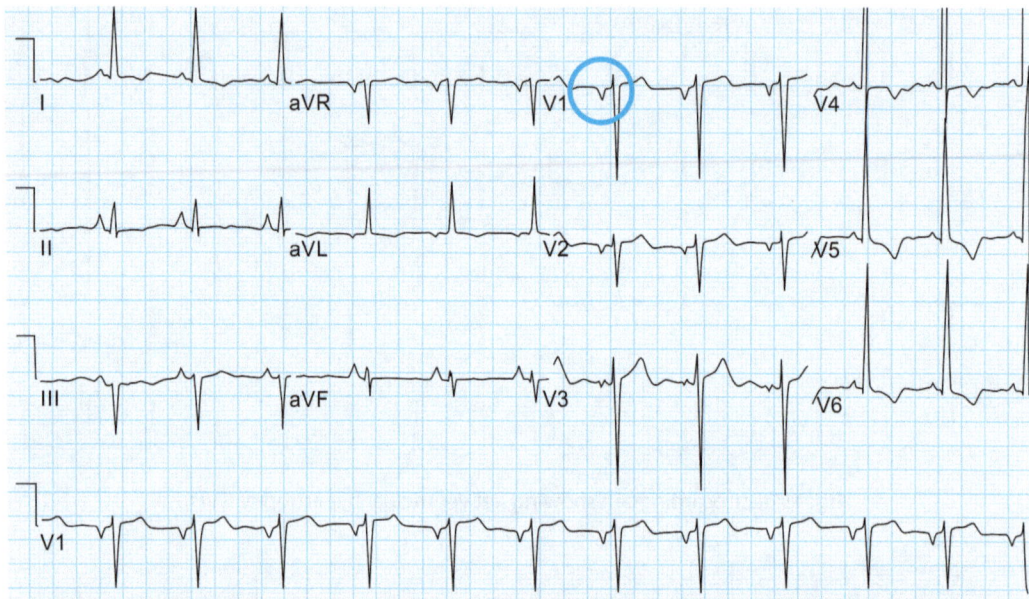

Fig. 3: Electrocardiogram showing LVH as well as deep and wide negative component of P in V1 suggestive of LV dysfunction.

Left Ventricular Dysfunction

Although ECG is a gold standard in the diagnosis of left ventricular (LV) dysfunction, ECG as the first investigation gives clue regarding LV dysfunction (systolic and diastolic) **(Fig. 3)**.

Left ventricular dysfunction—preferred:[2] (1) ACE I; (2) Angiotensin receptor blocker (valsartan); (3) β-blockers (carvedilol, bisoprolol, and long-acting metoprolol); (4) Aldosterone antagonists.

Left ventricular dysfunction—not preferred: (1) Verapamil; (2) Diltiazem; (3) Propranolol; (4) Atenolol.

Electrocardiogram and Secondary Causes

Chronic Kidney Disease

One of the most important secondary causes of hypertension is chronic kidney disease (CKD). Chronic kidney disease can be suspected when ECG shows signs of hyperkalemia **(Fig. 4)**.

Chronic kidney disease—preferred: (1) Angiotensin receptor blocker if potassium (K) is normal; (2) ACE I if K is normal; (3) Amlodipine if K is raised; (4) α-blockers if K is raised; (5) Clonidine.

Chronic kidney disease—not preferred: (1) Atenolol; (b) Aldosterone antagonists (hyperkalemia). Serial ECGs in patients with CKD on angiotensin inhibitors will help to identify early hyperkalemia.

Hyperaldosteronism

ECG changes of hypokalemia serve as valuable clue regarding hyperaldosteronism **(Fig. 5)**.

Hyperaldosteronism–preferred: (1) Aldosterone antagonists; (2) ACE I; (3) Angiotensin receptor blocker (ARB); (4) Amlodipine.

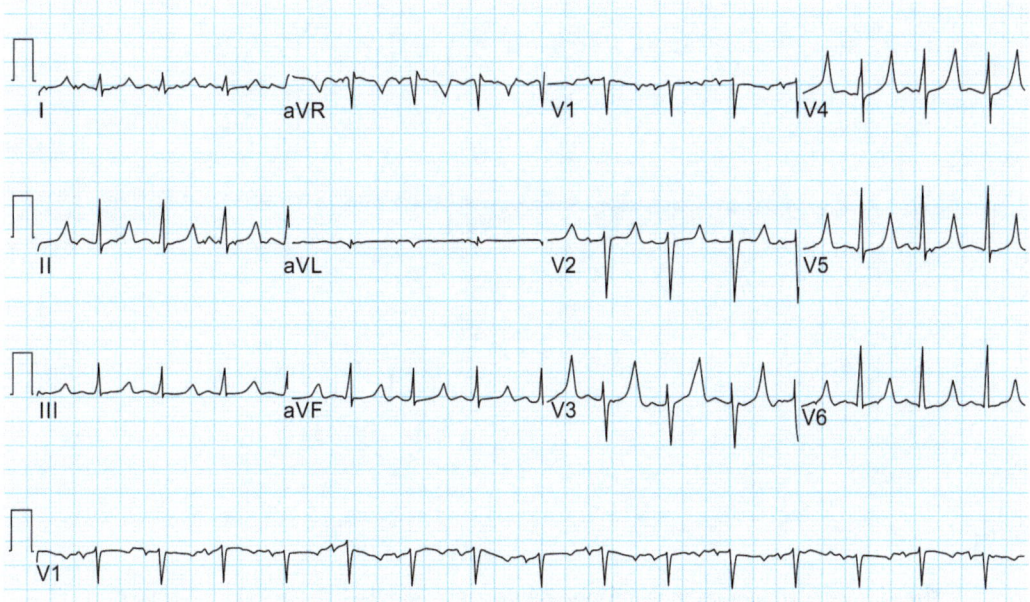

Fig. 4: Electrocardiogram showing features of hyperkalemia (tall T with a sharp apex and narrow base).

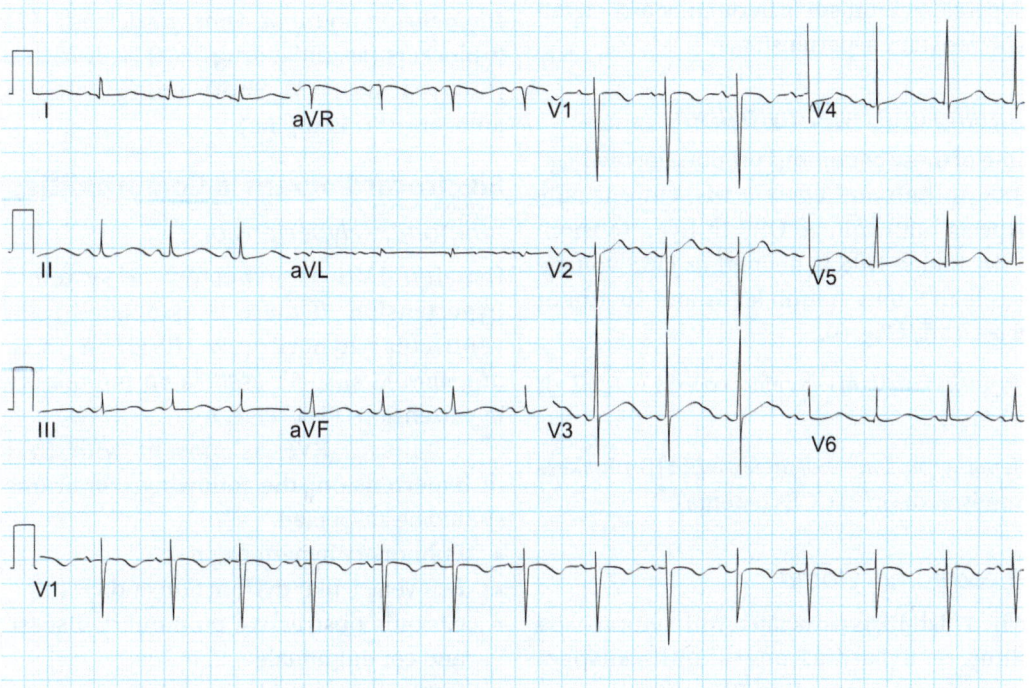

Fig. 5: Electrocardiogram showing hypokalemia (low-voltage T wave with prominent U wave).

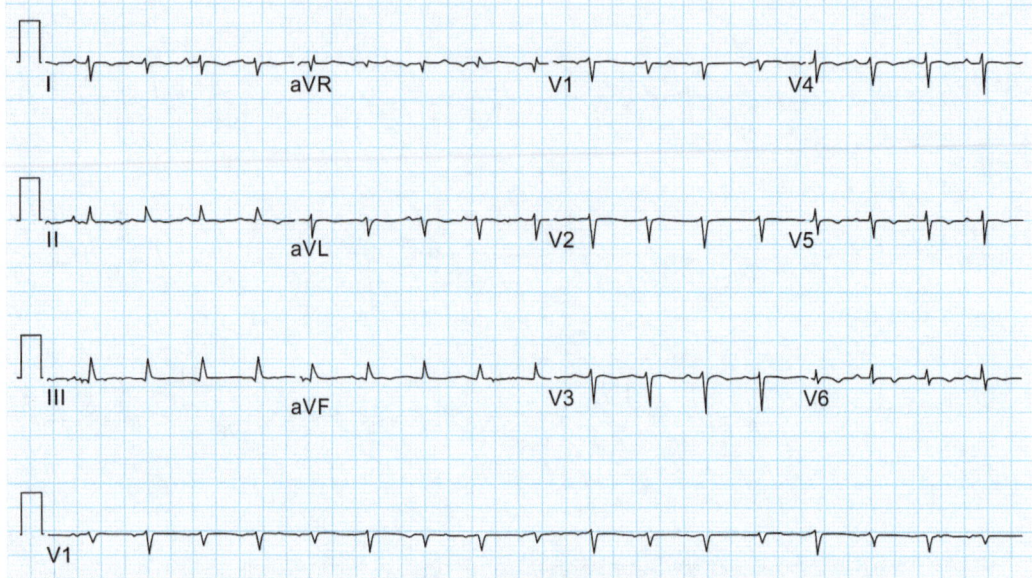

Fig. 6: Electrocardiogram showing low voltage QRS complexes in limb and chest leads.

Hyperaldosteronism—not preferred: (1) Loop diuretics; (2) Thiazide diuretics. Hyperaldosteronism is frequently associated with resistant hypertension.

Cushing and Hypothyroidism

Both of these conditions produce low-voltage QRS in limb and chest leads. One usually expects high voltage QRS in hypertension. Low-voltage QRS is defined as QRS voltage less than 5 mm in limb leads and 10 mm in chest leads **(Fig. 6)**.

Hypothyroidism—preferred: (1) ACE I; (2) ARB.

Hypothyroidism—not preferred: (1) β-blockers (bradycardia); (2) CCBs (edema).

Pheochromocytoma

When high BP is associated with unprovoked sinus tachycardia, one should suspect pheochromocytoma **(Fig. 7)**.

Pheochromocytoma—preferred: (1) α-blocker; (2) ACE I; (3) ARB.

Pheochromocytoma—not preferred: (1) β-blockers (as initial drugs); (2) Hydralazine (tachycardia); (3) Short-acting calcium antagonists (nifedipine).

Electrocardiogram in Comorbidities

Pulmonary Hypertension

Usually, LVH is expected in systemic hypertension. If there is associated right ventricular hypertrophy (RVH) in ECG, one should suspect associated pulmonary hypertension (PHT) **(Fig. 8)**.

Whenever RVH is present with LVH in hypertension, the following conditions should be suspected:
- Pulmonary hypertension
- Left ventricular dysfunction and PHT
- Chronic obstructive pulmonary disease and cor pulmonale
- Sleep apnea (OSA)

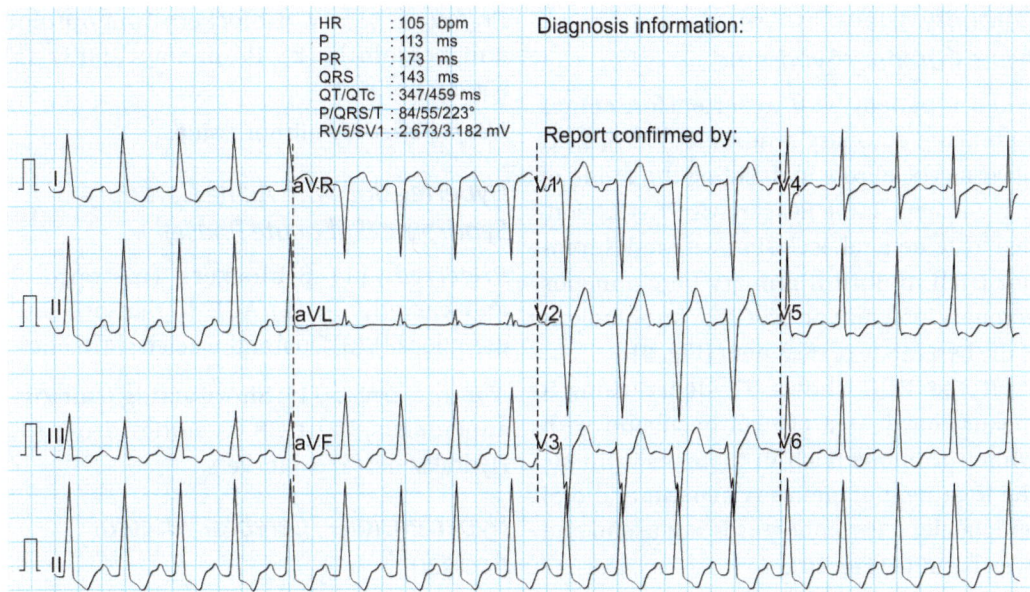

Fig. 7: Electrocardiogram showing LVH and sinus tachycardia.

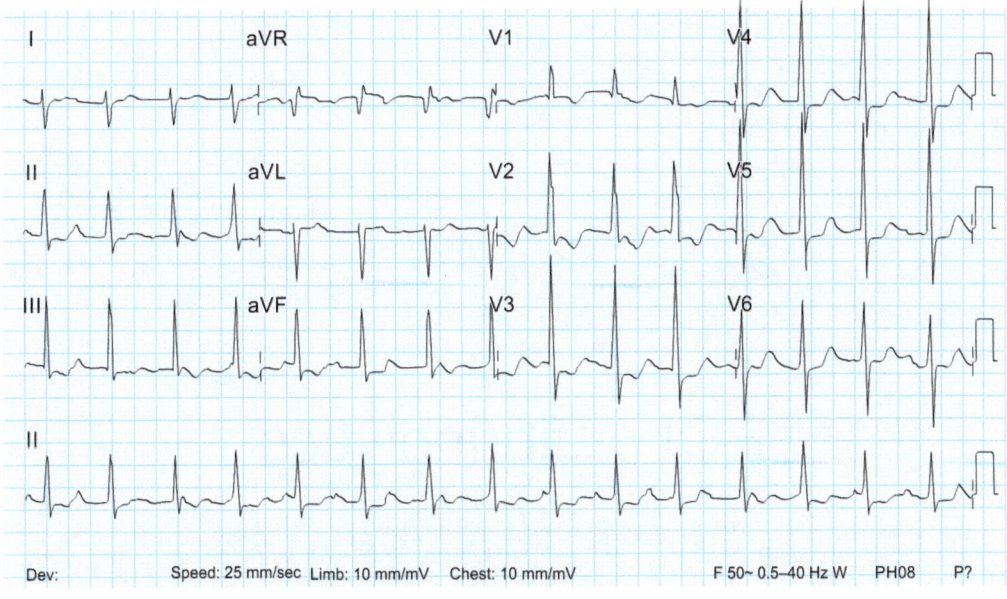

Fig. 8: Electrocardiogram showing LVH and RVH (tall R in V1 with right axis deviation).

Pulmonary hypertension—preferred: (1) Amlodipine; (2) Sildenafil; (3) Aldosterone antagonists (sleep apnea).

Pulmonary hypertension—not preferred: (1) β-blocker (except nebivolol); (2) Loop diuretics (in the absence of RV failure).

Coronary Artery Disease: Acute Coronary Syndrome

When a patient with hypertension comes with acute coronary syndrome (ACS), ECG plays a crucial role in deciding the mode of management. If the ECG shows ST elevation, due to acute total occlusion with red thrombus (rich in fibrin), primary percutaneous coronary intervention (PPCI) or thrombolysis is the best mode of treatment **(Fig. 9)**.

If the ECG shows ST depression, it means that it is a critical occlusion with white thrombus (rich in platelets) and so, the treatment of choice is heparin and oral antiplatelets. Thrombolysis is not useful and even harmful **(Fig. 10)**.

Hypertension with ACS is hypertensive emergency.

Preferred: (1) IV β-blockers (metoprolol and esmolol); (2) IV Enalapril; (3) IV Nitroglycerine.

Not preferred: IV nitroprusside.

Hypertension with Acute Coronary Syndrome (Subacute Phase)

Preferred: (1) β-blockers (metoprolol and carvedilol); (2) ACE I (ramipril and perindopril); (3) Dual antiplatelets; (4) Statins.

Not preferred: (1) Short-acting calcium antagonists; (2) CCB as initial drug; (3) Hydralazine; (4) α-blockers.

Hypertension—Cerebral Vascular Accident

When the patient has a cerebral vascular accident (CVA), the ECG may show deep

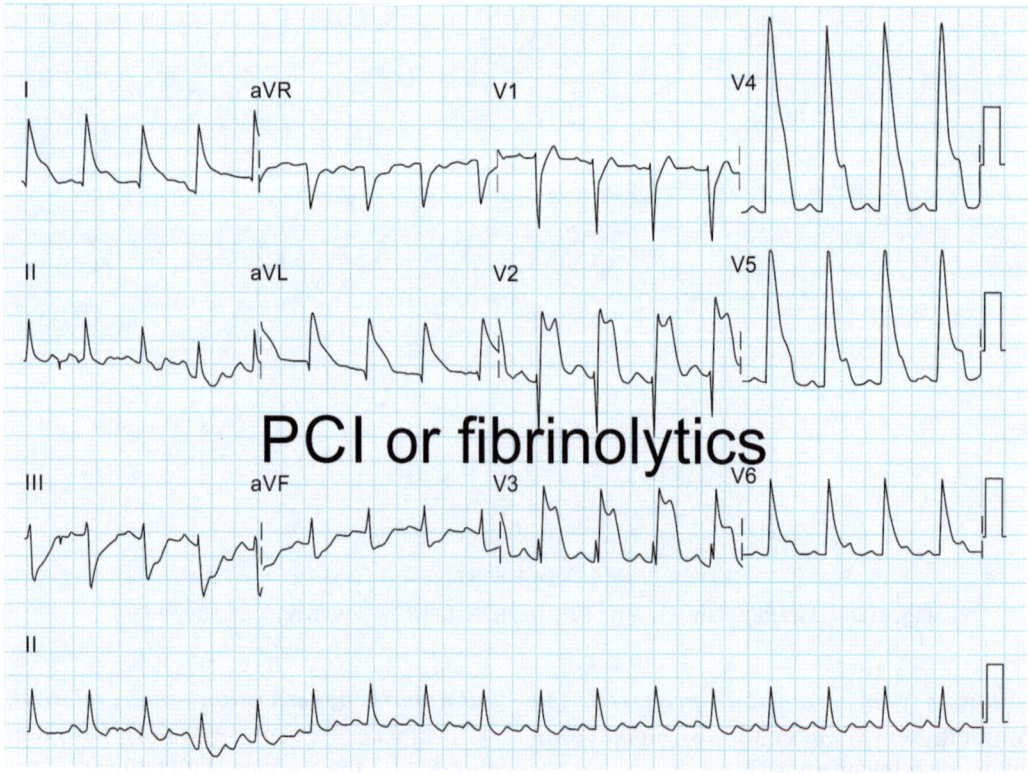

Fig. 9: Electrocardiogram showing ST elevation (acute total occlusion and red thrombus).

Heparin, antiplatelets

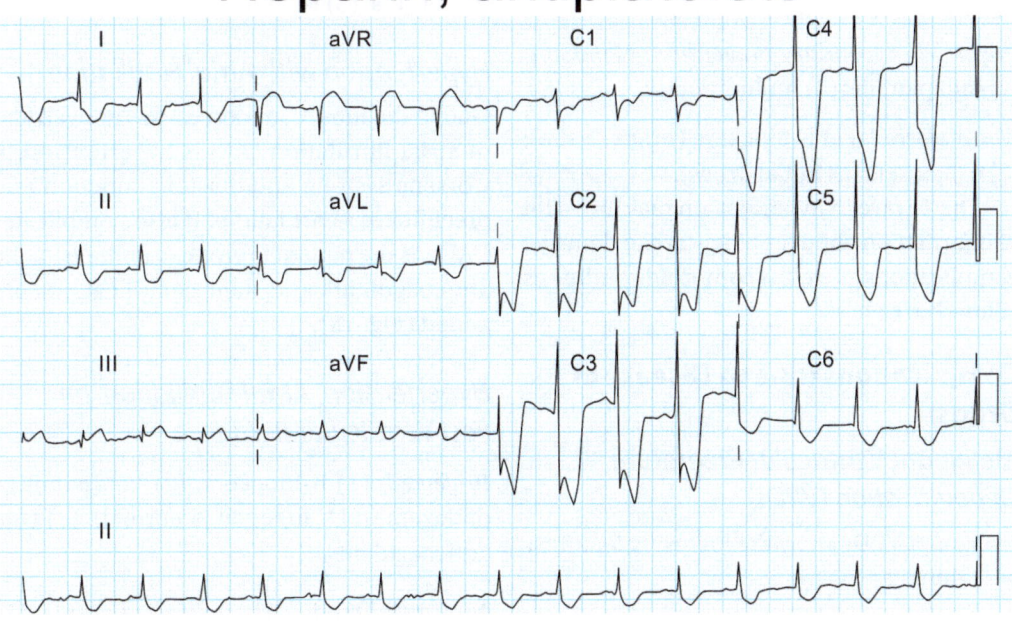

Fig. 10: Electrocardiogram showing ST depression (critical occlusion and white thrombus).

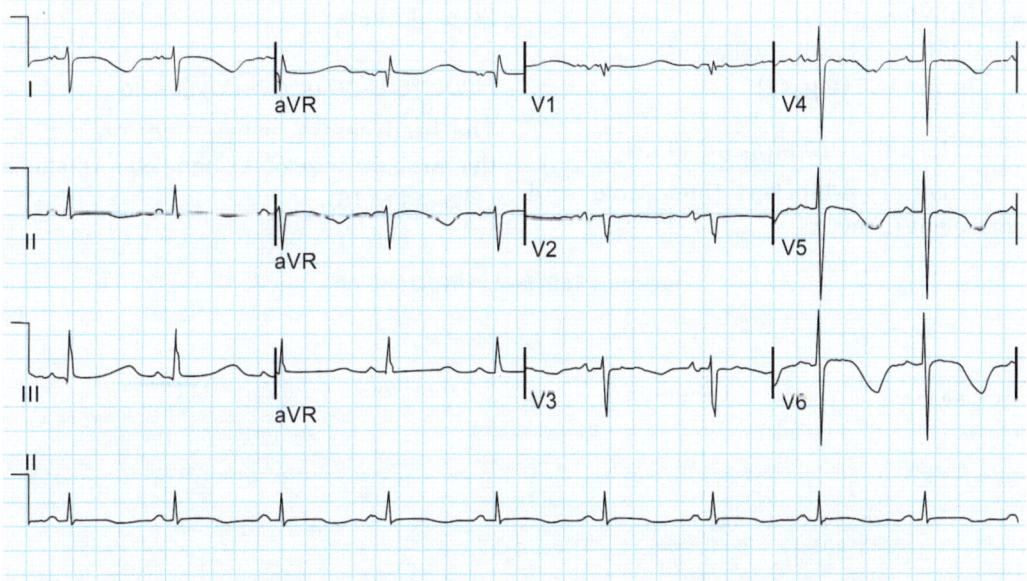

Fig. 11: Electrocardiogram showing deep broad T inversion with prolonged QT (CVA)

broad T inversion with prolonged QT. This has to be differentiated from CAD which shows deep symmetrical T inversion with normal or shortened QT **(Fig. 11)**.

Hypertension and Cerebral Vascular Accident (Ischemic)

Preferred—secondary prevention: (1) ACE I; (2) Indapamide; (3) Amlodipine.

Not preferred: (1) β-blockers (bradycardia); (2) α-blockers (as initial drugs).

The T wave in hypertension may give a lot of information about etiology, organ damage, complications as well as comorbid conditions **(Flowchart 1)**.

Complications (due to Disease or Drugs)

Malignant Ventricular Premature Depolarization (VPDs)

Malignant VPDs show the following features:
- Couplets
- Runs
- Multiform
- Wave R on wave T
- With signs of LVD
- Short, broad with notches
- During ACS **(Fig. 12)**

Hypertension—Malignant VPDs

Preferred: (1) β-blockers (metoprolol and carvedilol); (2) ACE I.

Not preferred: (1) CCB (nifedipine); (2) α-blockers; (3) Hydralazine.

Hypertension with Atrial Fibrillation

One of the most common causes nonvalvular of atrial fibrillation (AF) is hypertension. It worsens systolic and diastolic function and precipitates heart failure. It also complicates CAD. As the patient is prone to embolism, the anticoagulants and their complications are added **(Fig. 13)**.

Hypertension, Atrial Fibrillation, and Fast Ventricular Response

Preferred: (1) β-blockers; (2) Verapamil or diltiazem (if LV function is normal); (3) Oral anticoagulants.

Not preferred (as initial drugs): (1) Dihydropyridine (DHP) Calcium antagonists (nifedipine and amlodipine); (2) Hydralazine; (3) α-blockers.

Hypertension and Bradycardia

The bradycardia in hypertension may be due to sinus node or AV node abnormalities. **(Figs. 14 to 16)**.

Flowchart 1: T Wave in hypertension.

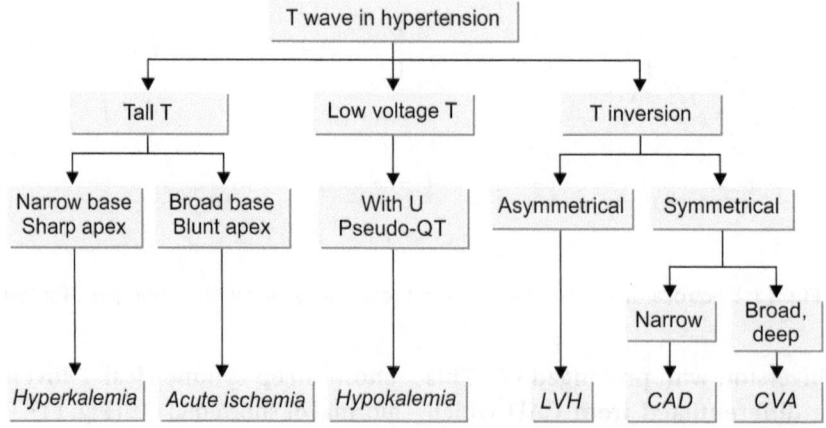

CHAPTER 15: Hypertension: Electrocardiogram in Decision Making 127

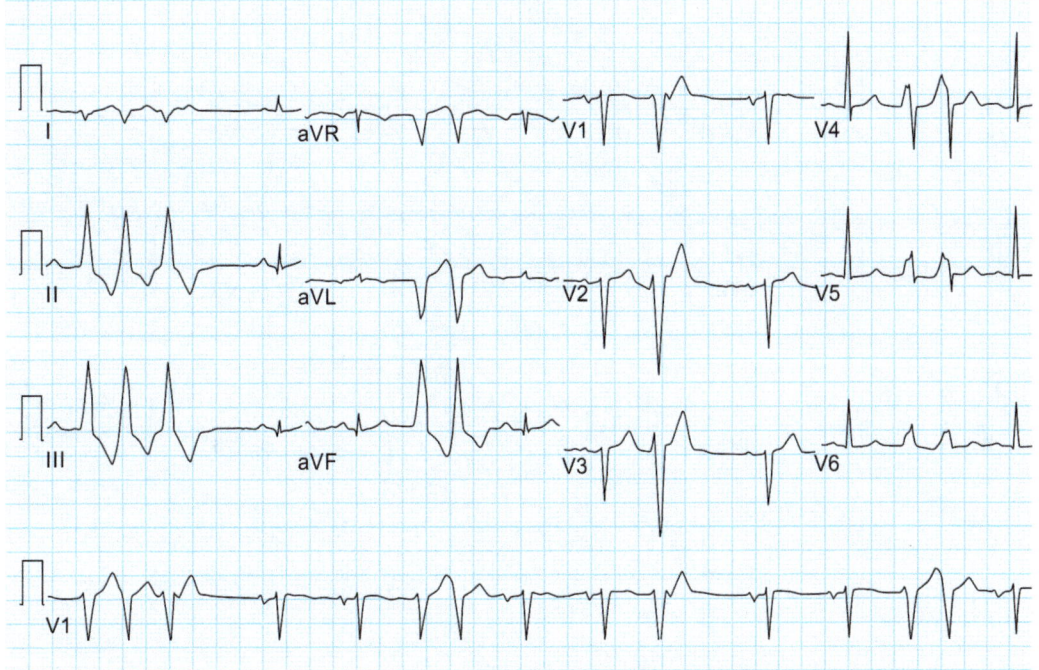

Fig. 12: Electrocardiogram showing malignant VPDS (couplets + runs).

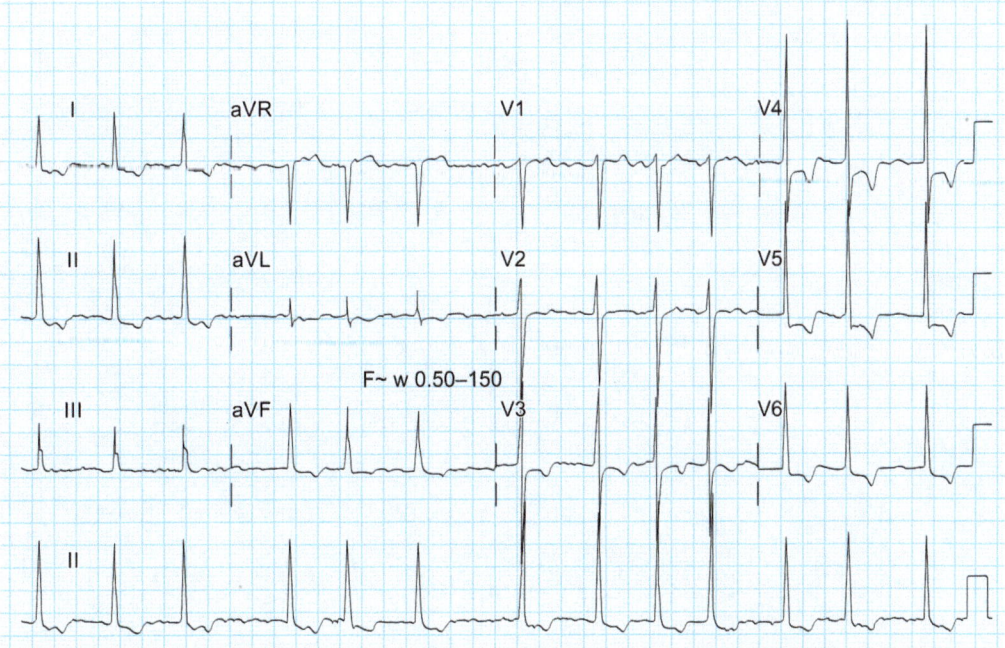

Fig. 13: Electrocardiogram showing AF (absent P, irregular QRS, presence of fibrillary waves).

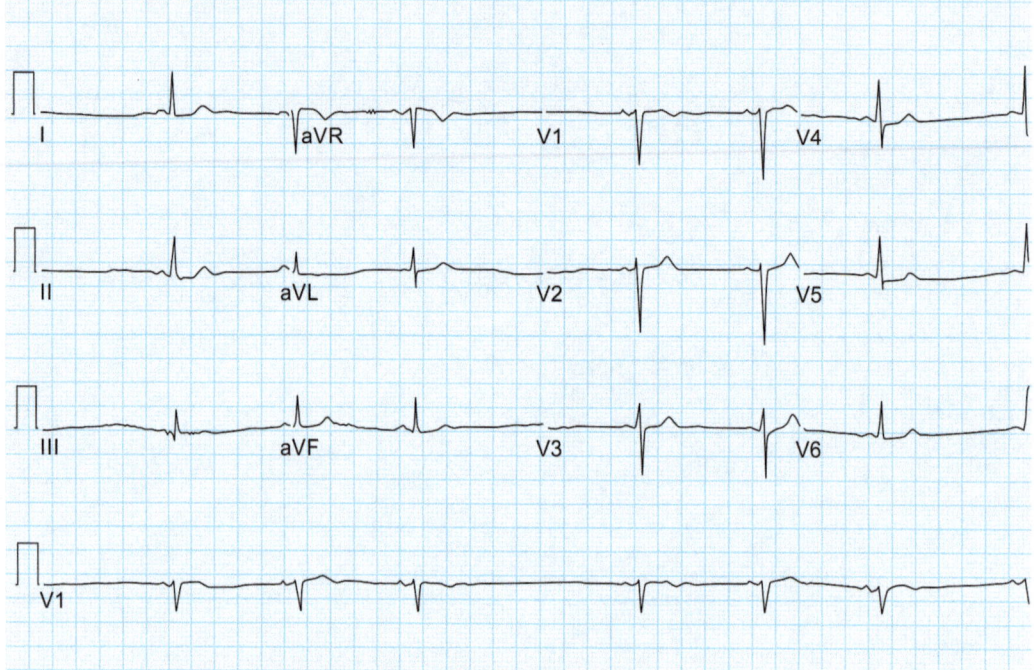

Fig. 14: Electrocardiogram showing sinus bradycardia and sinus pauses.

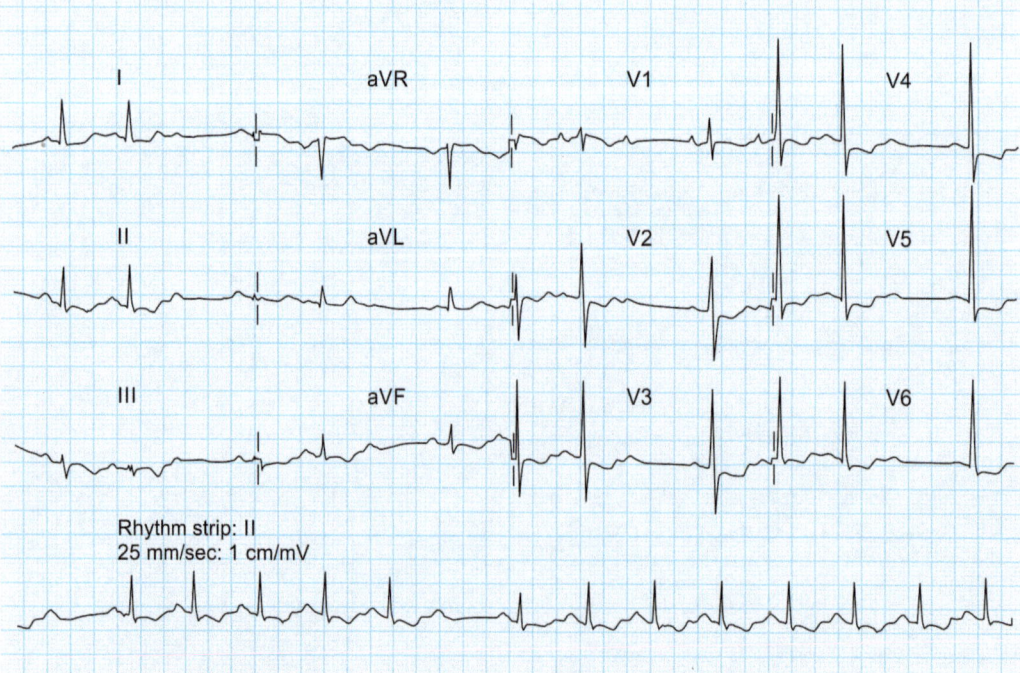

Fig. 15: Electrocardiogram showing Mobitz type II second-degree AV block.

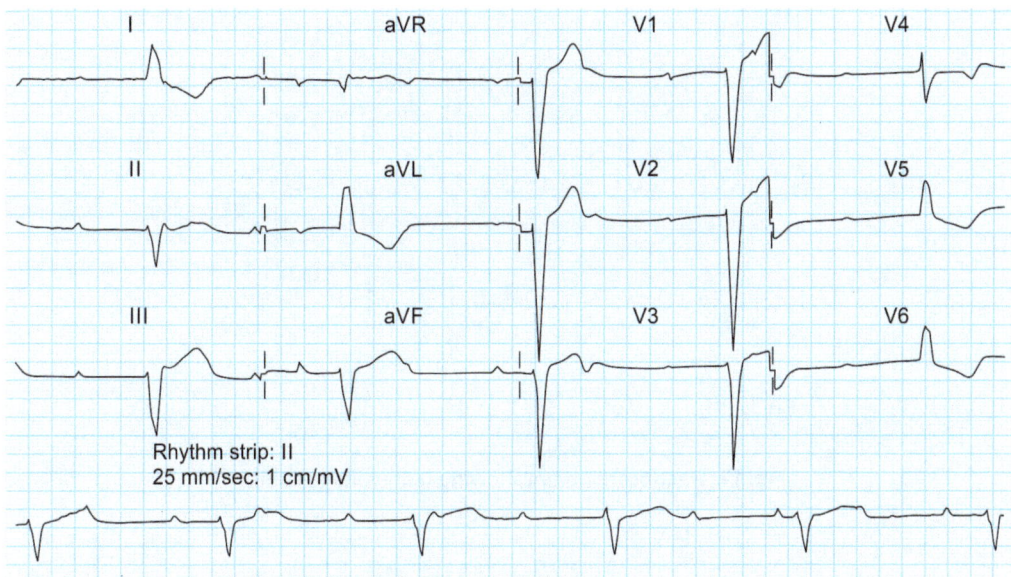

Fig. 16: Electrocardiogram showing infra-Hisian complete heart block.

Hypertension–bradycardia—preferred: (1) ACE I; (2) ARB; (3) Amlodipine; (4) α-blockers (add on).

Hypertension–bradycardia—not preferred: (1) β-blockers; (2) Verapamil; (3) Diltiazem; (4) Clonidine; (5) α-Methyldopa.

Hypertension–Left Bundle Branch Block

Left ventricular hypertrophy is difficult to diagnose in the presence of left bundle branch block (LBBB). High-voltage LBBB may be a clue for underlying LVH. The presence of LBBB with hypertension has poor clinical outcomes (CAD and heart failure). In elderly presence of LBBB indicates, advanced and advancing disease **(Fig. 17)**.

Hypertension–left bundle branch block-preferred: (1) Amlodipine; (2) ACE I; (3) ARB.

Hypertension–left bundle branch block—not preferred: (1) β-blockers (with caution); (2) Verapamil; (3) Diltiazem.

Hypertension–Bifascicular Block

Bifascicular block indicates the complete block of the right bundle and one of the fascicles on the left side. Only one fascicle is conducting the impulse to the ventricles **(Fig. 18)**.

Hypertension–fascicular block—preferred: (1) Amlodipine; (2) ACE I; (3) ARB.

Hypertension–fascicular block—not preferred: (1) β-blockers; (2) Verapamil; (3) Diltiazem.

Hypertension–Hyperkalemia

Whenever ECG shows hyperkalemia (tall T waves) **(Fig. 19)**, the following conditions should be suspected:
- Chronic kidney disease
- ACE I, ARB therapy
- ACE I or ARB with aldosterone antagonist therapy
- K-Sparing diuretics
- K-Supplements

The ECG becomes abnormal once the blood level of K exceeds 5.5 mEq/L.

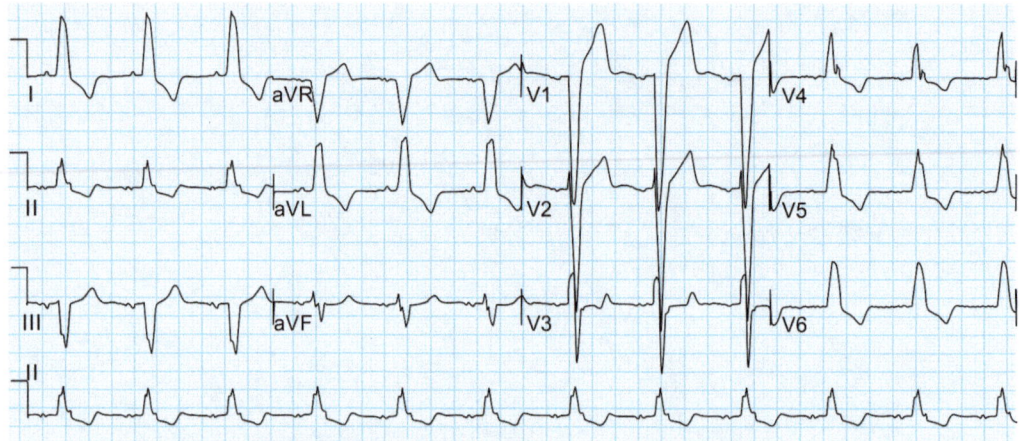

Fig. 17: Electrocardiogram showing high-voltage LBBB.

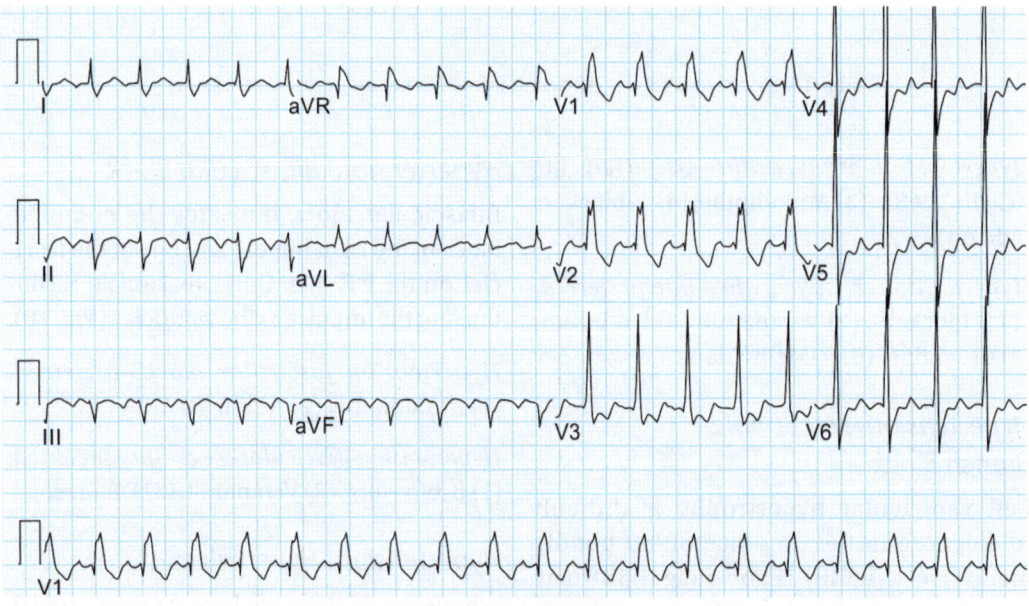

Fig. 18: Electrocardiogram showing bifascicular blocks [right bundle branch block (RBBB) and left anterior fascicular block (LAFB)].

Hyperkalemia—preferred: (1) Amlodipine; (2) α-blockers; (3) Loop diuretics; (4) Thiazide diuretics.

Hyperkalemia—not preferred: (1) ACE I; (2) ARB; (3) Older β-blockers; (4) Aldosterone antagonists.

Hypertension–Hypokalemia

ECG signs of hypokalemia happen when the K level is below 2.7.

Whenever hypertension is associated with hypokalemia **(Fig. 20)**, the following situations should be suspected:

- Hyperaldosteronism

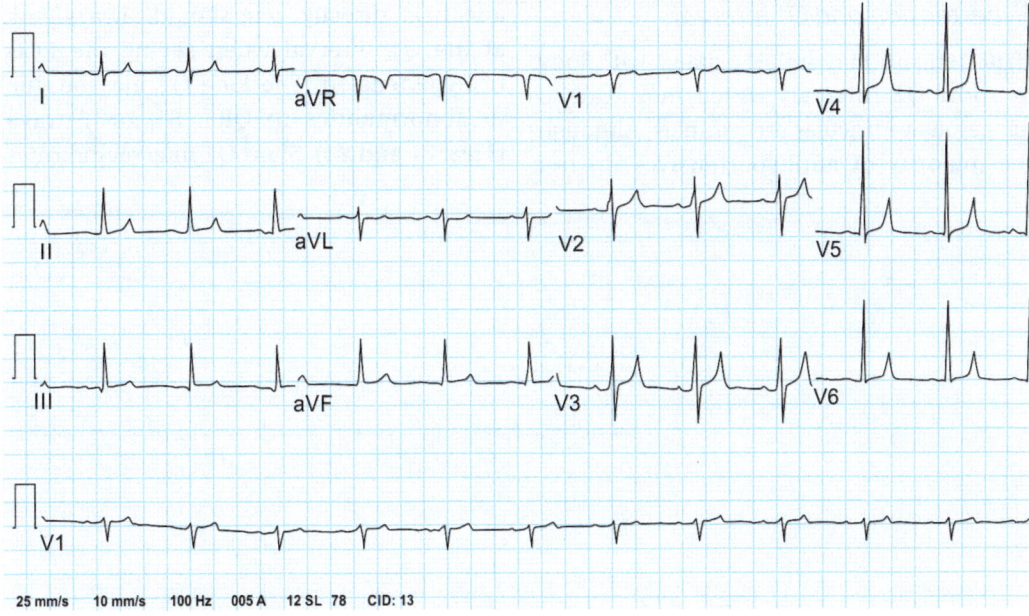

Fig. 19: Electrocardiogram showing hyperkalemia (tall T with steep apex and narrow base).

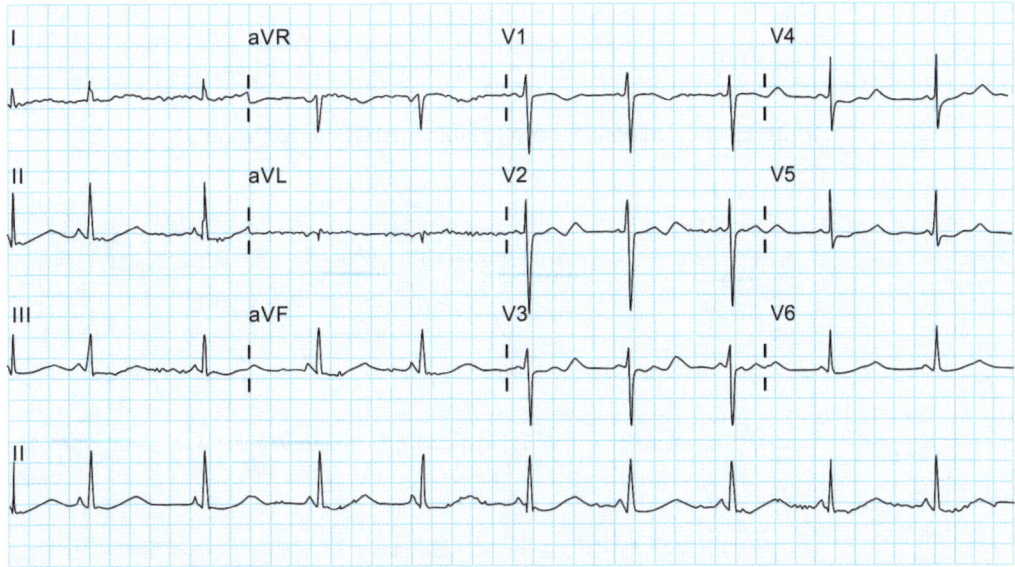

Fig. 20: Electrocardiogram showing hypokalemia (low-voltage T with U waves, pseudo-QT prolongation).

- Vigorous diuretic therapy
- Dehydration

Hypokalemia—preferred: (1) ACE I; (2) ARB; (3) Aldosterone atagonists.

Hypokalaemia—not preferred: (1) Loop diuretics; (2) Thiazide diuretics.

Hypertension and QT Interval

Hypertension may be associated with long or short QT intervals which may lead to dangerous ventricular arrhythmias. Although the majority of antihypertensives do not affect QT directly, one should always look at the QT interval when seeing the ECG in hypertension. The long QT may be due to abnormalities in QRS, ST, or T wave **(Figs. 21 and 22)**. Short QT interval indicates

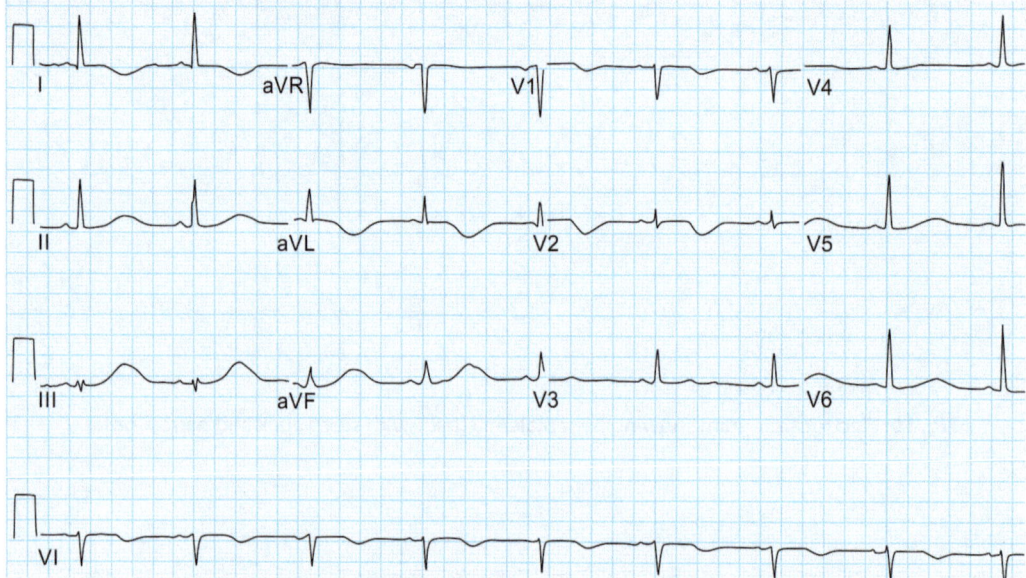

Fig. 21: Electrocardiogram showing prolonged QT due to T wave.

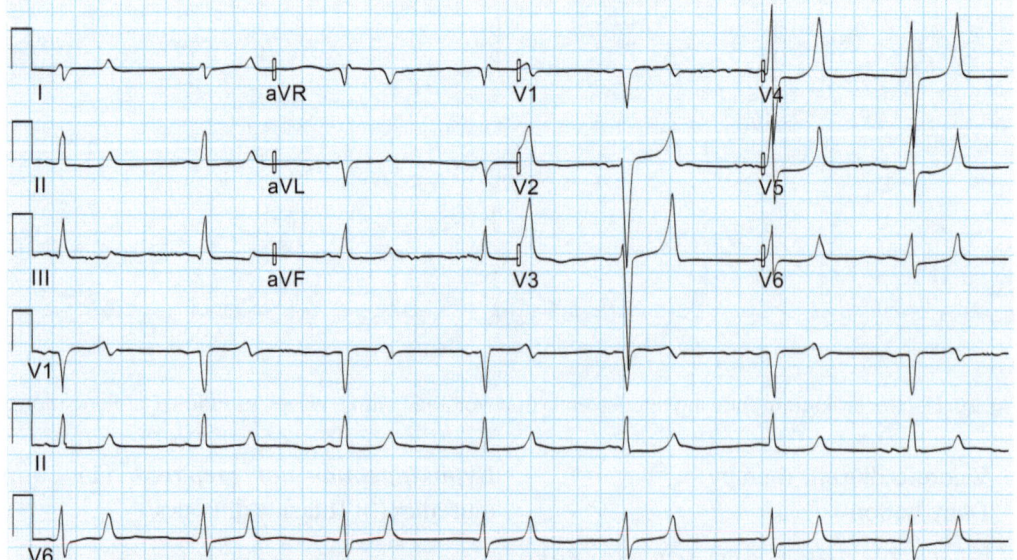

Fig. 22: Electrocardiogram showing prolonged QT due to ST segment. This ECG suggests CKD due to hypocalcemia and hyperkalemia (sharp apex T wave) changes.
Source: Courtesy of Jason E. Roedigner, CCT, CRAT.

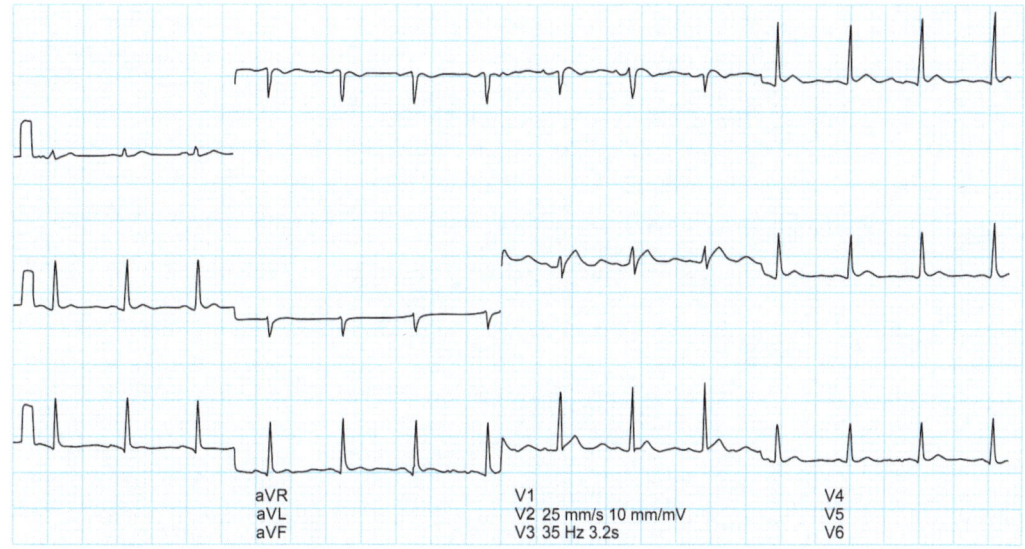

Fig. 23: Electrocardiogram showing short QT (hypercalcemia) (hyperparathyroidism).

Flowchart 2: Summary of QTc and hypertension.

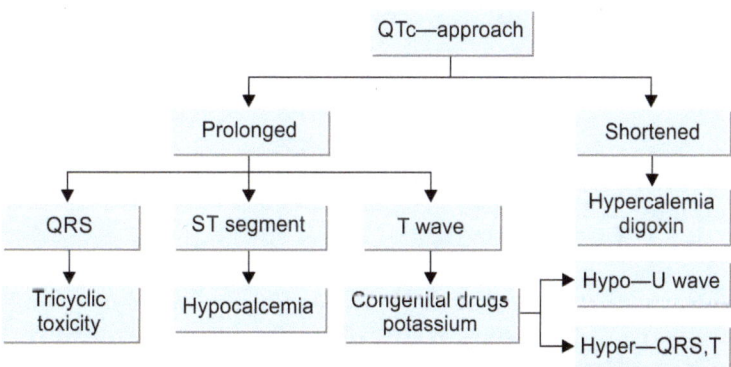

hypercalcemia which may be due to Hyper Parathyroidism **(Fig. 23)**. The summary of QT interval in hypertension is given in **Flowchart 2**.

CONCLUSION

As discussed and as shown in this chapter, ECG in hypertension gives valuable clues regarding TOD, secondary causes, comorbidities, and complications. It also aids in the proper selection of drugs in various situations. It also provides much vital information, not shown by ECHO. Being a simple and cost-effective investigation, ECG should be done as a routine investigation in all hypertensives, and serial ECGs at regular time intervals, to detect new developments.

REFERENCES

1. Chenniappan M. Practical Cardiology. Tiruchirappalli: ECG & Echo Club, 2013.
2. Opie LH, Gersh BJ. Drugs for the Heart, 8th edition; 2013. Philadelphia: Elsevier/WB Saunders, pp. 1-588.

SECTION 6: Target Organ Damage: Evaluation and Clinical Importance

16. **Hypertensive Retinopathy**
    N Vimal Kumar, S Prema

CHAPTER 16

Hypertensive Retinopathy

N Vimal Kumar, S Prema

■ INTRODUCTION

Hypertensive retinopathy is the retinal pathology that occurs due to uncontrolled hypertension (HTN). The prevalence of retinopathy in patients suffering from mild HTN is 25.3%, moderate HTN is 34.5%, and severe HTN is 84.6%. Of the patients with retinopathy, 42.3% had grade I, 20% had grade II, and 2.35% had grade III retinopathy.[1] Early diagnosis and treatment of HTN play a crucial role in preventing sight-threatening complications such as retinal vein and artery occlusion, retinal emboli, and ischemic optic neuropathy as well as worsening of diabetic retinopathy (DR). Simple dilated fundus examination screening of patients with HTN should become a routine as DR screening, which is still a lacuna in developed and developing countries.

Australian hypertensive guidelines recommend examination of the fundus of patients with newly diagnosed HTN looking for "hypertensive retinopathy as evidence of end-organ damage."[2] However there is no evidence for regular retinal screening in people with HTN.[3] A study by Erden and Bicakci showed the increase in the incidence of retinopathy is related to the duration and severity of HTN.[4] The incidence of hypertensive retinopathy in their study was 66.3%.

■ ETIOLOGY

"Essential and secondary HTN" is known to play a major role; other factors such as smoking which has a strong association with severe or malignant HTN,[5] and genetic predispositions such as certain genotypes associated with an increased risk of hypertensive retinopathy.[6] Pontremoli et al. showed the deletion of the allele of the angiotensin-converting enzyme has a higher risk associated with the development of hypertensive retinopathy.[7] "Renal dysfunction" (persistent microalbuminuria and low creatinine clearance)[8] and "plasma leptin level"[9] are associated with hypertensive retinopathy as per previous studies.

■ PATHOPHYSIOLOGY

The absence of sympathetic nerve supply, autoregulation, and the presence of the blood–retinal barrier predisposes the retinal blood vessels to the direct effect of raised blood pressure acutely, however with constantly increased pressure damage to the muscular and endothelial layer occur resulting in loss of compensatory tone.[10] Hypertensive retinopathy has the following phases.[11]

Vasoconstrictive Phase

Local autoregulatory mechanisms are involved in response to a condition affecting the vasculature. Autoregulation is a physiological process by which blood flow is maintained relatively constant in an organ despite changes in perfusion pressure.

As a result of these local autoregulatory mechanisms, there is vasospasm and narrowing of retinal arterioles, resulting in a decrease in the arteriole-to-venule ratio, which is normally 2:3.

In older patients with arteriosclerosis, focal arteriolar narrowing develops.

The statement suggests that affected vascular segments in older patients with arteriosclerosis cannot undergo narrowing. This might be due to the structural changes in arteriosclerosis, limiting the ability of these segments to respond to vasoconstriction accurately describes the structural changes that can occur in the vessel wall due to persistent high blood pressure.

- *Intima layer:* The intima is the innermost layer of blood vessels, and thickening can affect the vessel's lumen and blood flow.
- *Media layer:* Hyperplasis can contribute to the overall thickening of the vessel wall.
- *Anterior wall:* The arteriolar wall undergoes hyaline degeneration.

Sclerotic Phase

- *Arteriolar narrowing:* The cumulative effect of these changes results in severe arteriolar narrowing. This narrowing has implications for blood flow and can contribute to the clinical manifestations of HTN.
- *Arteriovenous crossing changes:* Arteriovenous (AV) crossing changes occur when a thickened arteriole crosses over a venule, compressing it as they share a common adventitial sheath and there occurs "widening and accentuation of light reflex," which is known as silver and copper wiring. The vein distal to the AV crossing appears dilated and tortuous. This is a consequence of the compression and altered dynamics at the AV crossing point. The retinal changes are seen in patients with severely increased blood pressure. This underscores the importance of blood pressure control to prevent complications.

Exudative Phase

Severely increased blood pressure can lead to the disruption of the blood–brain barrier. This disruption allows blood and plasma to leak into the vessel wall, impacting the normal functioning of autoregulatory mechanisms.

Characterized by flame-shaped and dot-blot hemorrhages. These hemorrhages result from the rupture of small vessels in the retina and are indicative of vascular damage. The leakage of fluid and proteins from blood vessels can lead to the formation of hard exudates. These deposits may contain lipids and proteins and are a sign of retinal damage.

■ MALIGNANT HYPERTENSION

Severe intracranial HTN can cause optic nerve ischemia and edema (papilledema) **(Fig. 1A)**. It can also lead to fibrinoid necrosis of choroidal arterioles and segmental infarction of choriocapillaris. Severely increased blood pressure can cause damage to the smooth muscle cells in the vessel walls, leading to necrosis.

Cotton–wool spots are areas of retinal ischemia characterized by fluffy, white lesions. They result from reduced blood flow and are a consequence of the compromised autoregulatory mechanisms.

The retinal signs mentioned, such as hemorrhages, exudates, necrosis, and cotton–wool spots, have clinical significance. They can be observed during fundoscopic examination and can serve as indicators of the severity and impact of hypertensive retinopathy.

This gives rise to the following:
- *Elschnig's spots:* These spots exist in the area of choroidal infarct where the overlying retinal pigment epithelium (RPE) appears yellow **(Fig. 1B)**.

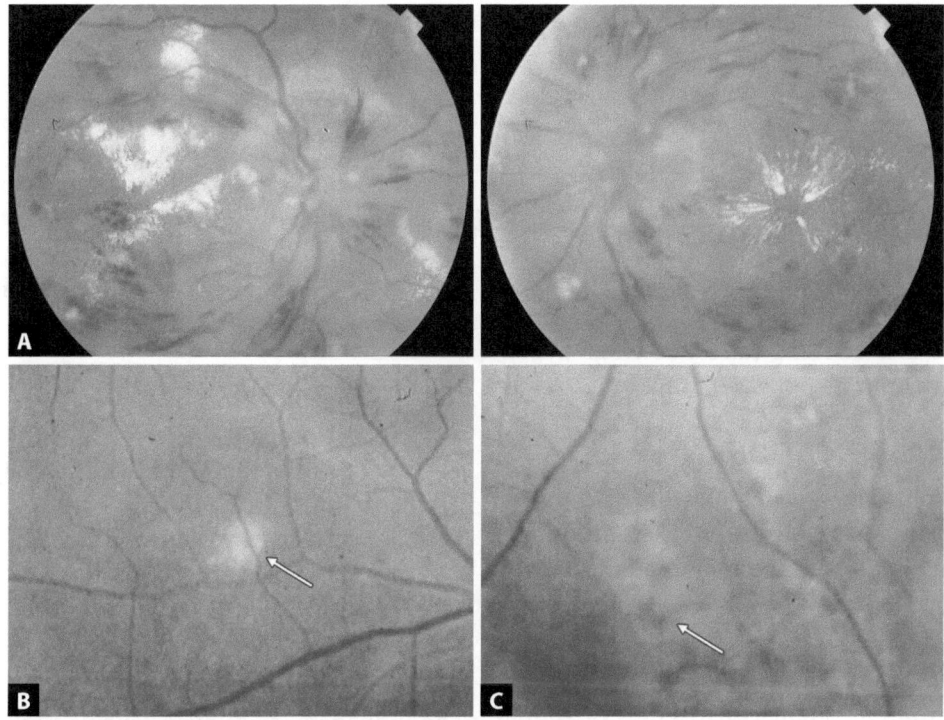

Figs. 1A to C: (A) Papilledema; (B) Elschnig's spots; (C) Siegrist's streak. *(For color version, see Plate 2)*

- *Siegrist's streak:* RPE hyperplasia over choroidal infarcts **(Fig. 1C)**.
- Neurosensory RPE detachments.
  These signs are termed as choroidopathy. Recently, focal choroidal detachment with severe pain has also been noted.

CLINICAL FEATURES

Hypertensive retinopathy is usually asymptomatic and is diagnosed on fundoscopic examination. Hypertension affects the retinal, choroid and optic nerve resulting in the following signs.

Arteriovenous Crossing Changes

- *Salus's sign:* Deflection of retinal vein as it crosses the arteriole.
- *Gunn's sign:* Tapering of the retinal vein on either side of the AV crossing.
- *Bonnet's sign:* Banking of the retinal vein distal to the AV crossing.

Arterial Changes

- Decrease in the arteriovenous ratio to 1:3 (the normal ratio is 2:3).
- Change in the arteriolar light reflex (light reflex appears as copper and/or silver wiring).

Retinal Changes

- Retinal hemorrhages
  - *Dot-blot hemorrhages:* Bleeding in the inner retinal layer
  - *Flame-shaped hemorrhage:* Bleeding in the superficial retinal layer
- Retinal exudates
  - *Hard exudates:* Lipid deposits in the retina

- *Soft exudates:* These are also known as cotton–wool spots which appear due to ischemia of the nerve fibers.

Macular Changes

Macular star formation is due to the deposition of hard exudates around the macula.

Optic Nerve Changes

Optic disc swelling (also known as hypertensive optic neuropathy).

■ CLASSIFICATION

The following are classification systems for hypertensive retinopathy based on fundus examination with indirect ophthalmoscopy or +90D lens.

Keith–Wagner–Barker Classification

- *Group 1:* Slight constriction of retinal arterioles.
- *Group 2:* Group 1 + focal narrowing of retinal arterioles + AV nicking.
- *Group 3:* Group 2 + flame-shaped hemorrhages + cotton–wool spots + hard exudates **(Fig. 2)**.
- *Group 4:* Group 3 + optic disc swelling.

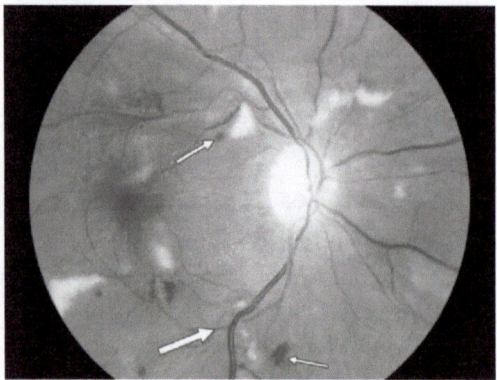

Fig. 2: Group 3—white arrow points to exudates, bold white arrow points to AV crossing changes and the white arrow show retinal hemorrhages. *(For color version, see Plate 2)*

Scheie Classification

For Hypertensive Retinopathy

- *Stage 0:* No visible abnormalities
- *Stage 1:* Diffuse arteriolar narrowing
- *Stage 2:* Stage 1 + focal arteriolar constriction
- *Stage 3:* Stage 2 + retinal hemorrhage
- *Stage 4:* Stage 3 + hard exudates + retinal edema + optic disc swelling

For Arteriosclerosis

- *Stage 0:* Normal
- *Stage 1:* Broadening of arteriolar light reflex
- *Stage 2:* Stage 1 + AV crossing changes
- *Stage 3:* Copper wiring of arterioles
- *Stage 4:* Silver wiring of arterioles

■ MANAGEMENT

The management of hypertensive retinopathy, includes the importance of tailored interventions based on the severity of the condition.

- Mild hypertensive retinopathy
  - *Treatment:* Controlling blood pressure with regular monitoring
- Moderate hypertensive retinopathy
  - *Treatment:* Referral to a physician is essential to exclude other associated factors such as diabetes mellitus and check for any cardiovascular abnormalities. Routine care, including blood pressure control and monitoring, is important.
- Severe hypertensive retinopathy
  - *Treatment:* Requires urgent treatment and referral, given its strongest association with mortality. Monitoring other systems such as renal, cardiovascular, and brain for signs of target organ damage (TOD) is recommended.

- *Lowering of blood pressure:*
  - Blood pressure should be lowered in a controlled fashion as this is crucial to prevent ischemic damage to vital organs such as optic nerve and brain.

■ COMPLICATIONS[11]

- Retinal artery occlusion.
- Retinal vein occlusion (**Fig. 3**).
- Macroaneurysm of retinal arteriole.
- *Diabetic retinopathy:* Both hypertensive retinopathy and DR together in a patient is called as mixed retinopathy. Hypertension is also known to be a major risk factor for the progression of DR.
- Anterior ischemic optic neuropathy.
- Age-related macular degeneration.
- Glaucoma.
- Retinal arteriolar emboli.
- Epiretinal membrane formation.
- Cystoid macular edema.

■ PROGNOSIS

Chronic HTN remains unnoticed until it is associated with complications. For acute malignant hypertension the mortality is as high as 50% within 2 months of diagnosis and 90% by the end of 1 year.[12] Vision loss in hypertensive retinopathy is due to secondary optic atrophy after prolonged papilledema and retinal pigmentary changes following exudative retinal detachment.

■ CONCLUSION

Hypertensive retinopathy is now considered as an evidence of end organ damage. Henderson et al.[13] found that hypertensive retinopathy is associated with an increased risk of stroke, even after controlling for blood pressure and other vascular risk factors. The collaboration between ophthalmologists and general physicians is essential to ensure that hypertensive patients are efficiently screened and managed in a timely manner, addressing both ocular and systemic implications. The goal is to reduce the risk of both ocular morbidity (related to the eye) and systemic morbidity and mortality (related to overall health), regular eye examinations to detect hypertensive retinopathy early, thereby allowing for timely interventions is essential.

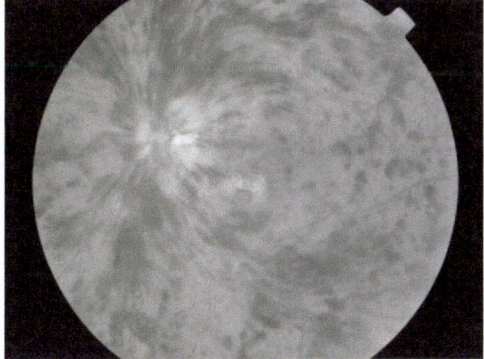

Fig. 3: Retinal vein occlusion.
(For color version, see Plate 2)

■ REFERENCES

1. Besharati MR, Rastegar A, Shoja MR, Maybodi ME. Prevalence of retinopathy in hypertensive patients. Saudi Med J. 2006;27(11):1725-8.
2. National Heart Foundation of Australia (National Blood Pressure and Vascular Disease Advisory Committee). Guide to management of hypertension 2008. Updated 2010. Melbourne: National Heart Foundation of Australia, 2010.
3. Wong TY, Mitchell P. The eye in hypertension. Lancet. 2007;369(9559):425-35.
4. Erden S, Bicakci E. Hypertensive retinopathy: Incidence, risk factors, and comorbidities. Clin Exp Hypertens. 2012;34(6):397-401.
5. Poulter NR. Independent effects of smoking on risk of hypertension: Small, if present. J Hypertens. 2002;20(2):171-2.
6. Chatterjee S, Chattopadhyay S, Hope-Ross M, Lip PL. Hypertension and the eye: Changing perspectives. J Hum Hypertens. 2002;16(10):667-75.

7. Pontremoli R, Sofia A, Tirotta A, Ravera M, Nicolella C, Viazzi F, et al. The deletion polymorphism of the angiotensin I-converting enzyme gene is associated with target organ damage in essential hypertension. J Am Soc Nephrol. 1996;7(12):2550-8.
8. Biesenbach G, Zazgornik J. High prevalence of hypertensive retinopathy and coronary heart disease in hypertensive patients with persistent microalbuminuria under short intensive antihypertensive therapy. Clin Nephrol. 1994;41(4):211-8.
9. Uckaya G, Ozata M, Sonmez A, Kinalp C, Eyileten T, Bingol N, et al. Is leptin associated with hypertensive retinopathy? J Clin Endocrinol Metab. 2000;85(2):683-7.
10. Chaine G, Kohner EM. Hypertensive retinopathy. J Fr Ophthalmol. 1983;6(12): 995-1005.
11. Keith NM, Wagener HP, Barker NW. Some different types of essential hypertension: their course and prognosis. Am J Med Sci. 1974;268(6):336-45.
12. Fraser-Bell S, Symes R, Vaze A. Hypertensive eye disease: A review. Clin Exp Ophthalmol. 2017;45(1):45-53.
13. Henderson AD, Bruce BB, Newman NJ, Biousse V. Hypertension-related eye abnormalities and the risk of stroke. Rev Neurol Dis. 2011;8(1-2):1-9.

SECTION 7

Special Conditions and Situations

17. **Hypertensive Crisis**
    Reeta James

18. **Difficult to Control Hypertension (Resistance, Pseudoresistance, and Malignant Hypertension)**
    Ameet G Sattur, Sadanand R Shetty

19. **Hypertension in Pregnancy**
    Abhay Narain Rai, Mritunjay Kumar Singh

20. **Metabolic Syndrome and Hypertension**
    Chamma Gupta, Abhishek Byahut, Karma G Dolma

21. **White Coat Hypertension and Masked Hypertension**
    V Padma, Sarath Bhaskar S

22. **Perioperative Hypertension**
    Subhajeet Dey

23. **Blood Pressure Variability and Target Organ Damage**
    NR Rau, Shivashankara KN

24. **Exercise and Hypertension**
    Kannan Meera Devi, V Padma

25. **Air Pollution and Hypertension**
    Minakshi Dhar

26. **Isolated Nocturnal Hypertension**
    Geetha Subramanian, J Cecily Mary Majella

27. **Resistant Hypertension**
    NN Anand

28. **Hypertension in Elderly**
    Karma G Dolma, Chamma Gupta, Madhu Gupta

CHAPTER 17

Hypertensive Crisis

Reeta James

INTRODUCTION

Hypertension is a worldwide epidemic affecting over one billion people. In India, about 30% of the population is hypertensive, with the prevalence being more in urban areas compared to rural. Among people with hypertension, essential as well as secondary, about 1–2% ultimately go into hypertensive crisis **(Box 1)**.

Hypertensive crisis refers to a spectrum of clinical presentations characterized by excessively high blood pressure (BP) with or without end-organ dysfunction. The older terminologies—malignant hypertension, accelerated hypertension, etc.—are no longer used. The 2003 Joint National Committee on Prevention, Detection, Evaluation and Treatment of High Blood Pressure (JNC 7) has defined *hypertensive crisis* as the elevation of systolic blood pressure (SBP) >179 mm Hg *or* diastolic blood pressure (DBP) >109 mm Hg. JNC 7 further classifies hypertensive crisis into hypertensive *emergency* (HE) with evidence of impending or progressive *end* (target) organ damage and hypertensive *urgency* without progressive target organ dysfunction.

Though the spectrum extends from nonurgent to urgent to true emergency, the involvement of vital organs necessitating urgent medical intervention and grave prognosis makes HE the focus of attention amidst hypertensive crises.

BOX 1: Risk factors for development of hypertensive crisis.

- Old age
- African-American ethnicity
- Male gender
- Increasing degrees of obesity
- Smoking
- Prior history of heart failure
- Hypertensive heart disease
- Coronary artery disease
- Requiring multiple antihypertensives for BP control
- Nonadherence to BP medications
- *Stimulant intoxication:* Cocaine, Methamphetamine
- Withdrawal of drugs like Clonidine and Beta-adrenergic blockers
- Pheochromocytoma
- Thyroid dysfunction
- Atherosclerotic renal artery stenosis
- Physiological stress in the postoperative period (especially cardiothoracic, vascular and neurosurgical procedures)
- Adverse drug interactions with MAO (Mono Amine Oxidase) inhibitors
- Neonates with congenital renal artery hypoplasia
- Children with acute glomerulonephritis
- Pregnant women with eclampsia

Prior to branding as "hypertensive crisis", "pseudohypertension" should be excluded, which is caused by stiffening of the vessel wall that prevents compression by BP cuff. It is seen in atherosclerosis, Monckeberg's medial calcification, and metastatic calcification associated with end-stage renal disease and is demonstrable by Osler's maneuver (palpable radial artery after proximal compression).

PATHOPHYSIOLOGY

The exact mechanism is still not fully understood. The rapidity and severity of BP elevation is the main factor triggering the onset of HE. BP being a product of cardiac output and systemic vascular resistance, in most cases of hypertensive crisis, the initial event is an increase in vascular resistance brought about by humoral vasoconstrictors. A sudden increase in vascular resistance induces natriuresis which activates the renin-angiotensin-aldosterone system (RAAS) which, in turn, brings about a further increase in systemic vascular resistance. This leads to loss of autoregulatory mechanisms. Loss of autoregulation, the ability of vital organs to maintain a stable blood flow despite variations in perfusion pressure, plays a key role in the development of HE. With loss of autoregulation, fall in perfusion pressure results in a decrease in organ perfusion and a resultant increase in vascular resistance, thereby perpetuating the rise in BP. RAAS activation also causes oxidative stress and impaired nitric oxide bioactivity, thereby causing endothelial dysfunction and damage. Disruption of the endothelial lining exposes the subendothelial tissue triggering the coagulation cascade leading to thrombotic microangiopathy. Altogether, a vicious cycle of vascular damage, ischemia, and target organ damage sets in with diffuse necrotizing vasculitis, fibrinoid necrosis, and thrombi in arterioles of kidney, brain, retina, and other organs.

Physiologically, cerebral blood flow is maintained at a constant level within a mean arterial pressure range of 50–150 mm Hg. Below this, cerebral perfusion sharply drops causing ischemia and an abrupt rise above this results in cerebral edema. In long-standing hypertension, this autoregulatory range shifts toward the higher side and is narrowed (110–150 mm Hg). This, along with loss of autoregulation occurring with marked elevation of BP, leads to detrimental consequences in the brain. Likewise, loss of autoregulation can have similar ominous consequences in other vital organ systems as well.

CLINICAL PRESENTATION

Previously undiagnosed hypertensives constitute a good number of patients who present with hypertensive crisis (**Box 2**). Patients with hypertensive urgency may be asymptomatic or present with nonspecific symptoms like severe headache without neurological deficit, epistaxis, dizziness, vomiting, palpitations, nonspecific chest pain, shortness of breath, or even severe anxiety. Patients with HE present with signs and symptoms of end-organ dysfunction (**Box 3**).

Symptoms of hypertensive encephalopathy may range from vague symptoms like headache, vomiting, drowsiness, confusion, and visual disturbances to grave symptoms

---

BOX 2: Points to note in history.

- History of previously diagnosed hypertension
- Details of current medications including any recent changes in dosage or timing
- Drug compliance
- History of stopping medications likely to cause rebound hypertension
- Presence of severe pain or stress (possibility of reactive hypertension)
- Usage of over-the-counter medications
- History of treatment from alternate systems of medicine
- Addictions of any kind including use of recreational drugs

BOX 3: Manifestations of hypertensive emergency ("BARKH").	
Brain	• Stroke (subarachnoid hemorrhage/cerebral infarct/intraparenchymal hemorrhage) • Hypertensive encephalopathy
Arteries	Acute aortic syndromes (aortic dissection)/preeclampsia/eclampsia/HELLP (hemolysis, elevated liver enzymes, low platelet)
Retina	Grades III–IV hypertensive retinopathy
Kidney	Acute renal failure/thrombotic microangiopathy
Heart	Acute coronary syndrome/acute cardiac failure/pulmonary edema

like seizures and coma. An abrupt rise in BP above the autoregulatory range causes raised intracranial pressure and results in cerebral edema, especially in the posterior areas of the brain since BP fluctuations are more pronounced in these areas due to relatively lesser sympathetic innervation. This condition, called **Posterior Reversible leukoEncephalopathy Syndrome (PRES)**, is characterized by headache, altered mental status, seizures (including nonconvulsive status epilepticus), vision abnormalities (blurring of vision, homonymous hemianopia, or cortical blindness), white matter lesions, and vasogenic edema in the posterior brain areas. With prompt diagnosis and appropriate treatment, the syndrome resolves in a week, though magnetic resonance imaging (MRI) findings take days to weeks to resolve. But inadequate treatment can result in cerebral hemorrhage, coma, and death. PRES is commonly associated with renal failure—acute or chronic. Renal failure can be a cause as well as sequel of hypertensive crisis.

Cerebrovascular accidents are relatively easier to diagnose due to the presence of focal neurological deficits often supported by focal lesions on computed tomography (CT)/MRI. In hypertensive encephalopathy, CT/MRI shows focal areas of symmetric hemispheric edema, predominantly in the parietal and occipital lobes, as well as in frontal lobes, inferior temporo-occipital junction, and cerebellum. With progression of edema, lesions become confluent and microhemorrhages and infarcts develop.

Retinopathy in HE can be Keith–Wagener–Barker grade III with flame-shaped hemorrhages and cotton wool spots or grade IV with papilledema. The presence of arteriolar narrowing and arteriovenous nicking (grade I and II changes) suggests chronic hypertension. So, the fundoscopy is an essential component in evaluation of HE. Nonmydriatic ocular fundus digital photography may be used for documentation.

Endothelial damage associated with HE triggers the coagulation cascade resulting in microvessel obliteration, disseminated intravascular coagulation, and thrombotic microangiopathy. This closely resembles thrombotic thrombocytopenic purpura (TTP). But retinopathy is not seen in TTP, while thrombocytopenia and ADAMTS13 activity impairment are less pronounced in HE.

Aortic dissection, intramural hematoma, and penetrating atherosclerotic ulcers are life-threatening conditions where an abrupt rise in BP can result in dreadful outcomes. Acute coronary syndrome, acute heart failure, aortic dissection, stroke, or eclampsia may be the first presentation of an undetected paraganglioma/pheochromocytoma. Preeclampsia has a 3–5-fold higher incidence in women with preexisting hypertension. Since this is associated with life-threatening complications to both mother and fetus, timely risk assessment and appropriate management are necessary.

Hypertensive emergency caused by cocaine abuse is due to sympathomimetic effect and presents as chest pain, tachycardia, altered mental status, and, rarely, aortic dissection, cerebral hemorrhage, seizures, arrhythmias, and even sudden cardiac death. Dilated pupils indicate the hyperadrenergic state associated with cocaine abuse.

Elevated BP is a common finding in the perioperative period. Only if the BP does not respond to remedial measures like anxiolytics (preoperatively), deepening of anesthesia (intraoperatively), and pain relief (in the postoperative period), the possibility of HE needs to be considered.

Studies suggest that using the "BARKH" acronym and following BARKH-based algorithm can help to rapidly identify hypertensive emergencies and focus treatment appropriately.

INVESTIGATIONS

Thrombocytopenia and schistocytes in peripheral smear and raised lactate dehydrogenase (LDH) suggest microangiopathic hemolytic anemia. Deranged renal function test reflects renal insufficiency. Hematuria, proteinuria, and red cell casts in urine are suggestive of thrombotic microangiopathy. Look for metanephrines in urine if there is high suspicion of pheochromocytoma. Urine pregnancy test may be done in females of reproductive age group to rule out preeclampsia/eclampsia as a cause of hypertensive crisis. Toxicology screening is required in suspected recreational drug use. ECG is done in cases of suspected acute coronary syndrome and cardiac failure. Echocardiogram may be done for assessment of left ventricular function, detection of segmental hypokinesia, and in cases of suspected aortic dissection. Fundoscopy is essential to look for retinopathy. CT/MRI of the brain is done for evaluation of neurological symptoms. CT scan of the chest and transesophageal echo maybe required for evaluating cases of suspected aortic dissection.

TREATMENT

There is no evidence that supports emergency reduction of BP in hypertensive urgency. Not only does it not reduce morbidity and mortality, but it also results in adverse effects instead owing to autoregulatory dysfunction. Hence, treatment is directed at gradually reducing BP over hours to days and this is achieved using oral medications like long-acting calcium channel blockers (CCBs) and alpha-1 blockers which do not interfere with the diagnostic workup for secondary causes of hypertension. Angiotensin-converting enzyme (ACE) inhibitors and angiotensin receptor blockers (ARBs) are not preferred as first-line agents as they may worsen preexisting renal dysfunction.

In HE, the patient requires intensive care unit (ICU) care and BP needs to be controlled rapidly over minutes to hours using parenteral antihypertensive medications. The choice of drug depends on the type of organ damage and contraindications for specific agents. BP should ideally be reduced by about 20–25% in the first hour and to 160/100 mm Hg over the next 2–6 hours. However, BP should not be reduced back to normal level as it induces ischemia in vital organs due to autoregulatory malfunction. The only exception to this is in aortic dissection where the target of systolic BP <120 mm Hg and mean arterial BP <80 mm Hg needs to be achieved within 5–10 minutes, preferably with drugs which do not cause reflex tachycardia. A rapid reduction in BP is also required in cases of ischemic stroke if thrombolytic therapy is planned. In hemorrhagic stroke, owing to ongoing bleed and expansion of hematoma, lowering of systolic BP to <140 mm Hg is acceptable.

Labetalol is the drug of first choice in HE. It is a nonselective beta blocker as well as a competitive antagonist at postsynaptic alpha-1 receptors. It reduces the systemic vascular resistance while maintaining the cerebral, renal, and coronary blood flow, making it the preferred agent in all manifestations of HE except acute pulmonary edema. It exerts antihypertensive effect within 2–5 minutes and attains a peak in 5–15 minutes allowing time for adequate dose titration. The action lasts for 3–6 hours. A 20-mg IV bolus is given followed by continuous infusion of 2–4 mg/min which is titrated to achieve an adequate BP level. In an acute coronary event, it helps to reduce cardiac work and myocardial oxygen demand and also counters nitroglycerine-induced reflex tachycardia. In hypertensive encephalopathy and stroke, it is preferred over nitroglycerine and nitroprusside as it does not increase intracranial pressure or affect cerebral perfusion. It can be used in pregnancy as well.

Nitroglycerine is another drug commonly used in HE with an immediate onset of action lasting for 3–5 minutes. Infusion is started at 5 μg/min and uptitrated every 5 minutes by 5 μg/min to a maximum of 20 μg/min. It is a venodilator which reduces the preload and cardiac oxygen demand. It is especially useful in patients with acute coronary syndrome and pulmonary edema. But it causes raised intracranial tension and reflex tachycardia.

Sodium nitroprusside is a potent arterial and venous dilator that acts within seconds and action lasts for 1–2 minutes. But prolonged use for more than 48 hours is not recommended, especially in patients with hepatic and renal dysfunction for fear of thiocyanate toxicity.

Nicardipine is a dihydropyridine CCB which has a beneficial effect on coronary blood flow and hence can be used in patients with coronary artery disease. Clevidipine is yet another short-acting dihydropyridine CCB which can be used intravenously in HE, especially in acute postoperative hypertension. Fenoldopam is a vasodilator and diuretic well tolerated in HE, which acts via peripheral dopamine-1 receptors.

The drug of choice in aortic dissection is IV Esmolol, a short-acting, cardioselective β-blocker. A loading dose of 500–1,000 μg/kg/min is given over 1 minute followed by 50 μg/kg/min infusion which may be uptitrated to a maximum of 200 μg. If beta blockade fails to achieve BP control, IV nitroglycerine or nitroprusside is added.

Hypertensive heart failure patients are mostly euvolemic or only mildly hypervolemic, making loop diuretics a lesser recommended choice in HE except in cases of acute pulmonary edema, where they are used along with nitroglycerine. Mineralocorticoid receptor antagonists may be combined with loop diuretics to prevent hypokalemia.

In pheochromocytoma, α-blockers like phentolamine or doxazosin are given followed by a β-blocker to achieve BP control. Labetalol may be used alone because of its dual (β and α) receptor blockade. Diuretics are preferably avoided since patients with pheochromocytoma are relatively hypovolemic.

■ CONCLUSION

Hypertensive crisis is more of a spectrum, and most instances of severe but asymptomatic hypertension need no urgent treatment unless associated with features of end-organ damage. But mortality in hypertensive crisis is about 3.7%, higher in HE (4.6%) compared to urgency (0.8%). Hence, early identification and appropriate management of HE are crucial in improving the prognosis.

FURTHER READING

1. Agarwal AK, Rees CJ, Pollack CV. Hypertensive crisis. In: Cardiology Secrets, 4th edition; 2014. Philadelphia: Elsevier; pp. 371-9.
2. Aronow WS. Treatment of hypertensive emergencies. Ann Transl Med. 2017; 5(Suppl 1):S5.
3. Miller J, Suchdev K, Jayaprakash N, Hrabec D, Sood A, Sharma S, et al. New developments in hypertensive encephalopathy. Curr Hypertens Rep. 2018;20(2):13.
4. Rossi GP, Rossitto G, Maifredini C, Barchitta A, Bettella A, Latella R, et al. Management of hypertensive emergencies: a practical approach. Blood Press. 2021; 30(4):208-19.
5. William B, Mancia G, Spiering W, Rosei EA, Azizi M, Burnier M, et al. 2018 ESC/ESH guidelines for the management of arterial hypertension: the task force for the management of arterial hypertension of the European Society of Cardiology and the European Society of Hypertension. J Hypertens. 2018;36(10):1953-2041.

CHAPTER 18

Difficult to Control Hypertension (Resistance, Pseudoresistance, and Malignant Hypertension)

Ameet G Sattur, Sadanand R Shetty

◼ INTRODUCTION

Hypertension remains one of the most common causes of cardiovascular and neurological mortality and morbidity. In India, one in three adults is hypertensive.[1]

Prompt detection and appropriate early treatment is the key to prevent hypertension-related complications such as stroke, cardiovascular disease, particularly ischemic heart disease and heart failure, and chronic kidney disease (CKD).[2] However, despite the awareness and widespread use of antihypertensive medications many patients fail to achieve the optimum blood pressure (BP). This condition has been described in several terms but the term difficult to treat hypertension (DTC) or resistant hypertension (RH) is commonly used.[3]

According to the 2020 International Society of Hypertension Global Hypertension Practice Guidelines, "resistant hypertension" is defined as seated office BP above 140/90 mm Hg in a patient treated with three or more antihypertensive medications at optimal (or maximally tolerated) doses including a diuretic and after excluding pseudo resistance (poor BP measurement technique, white coat effect, nonadherence and suboptimal choices in antihypertensive therapy) as well as the substance/drug-induced hypertension and secondary hypertension.

The optimal doses of antihypertensives mean above 50% of the maximal dose.[4] The prevalence of RH is difficult to determine correctly but it is 10% of total hypertensive patients.[5] However, it is important to note that the high prevalence of hypertension makes this small percentage very significant in actual patient numbers.

The term "apparent treatment-resistant hypertension" means patients with RH in whom pseudoresistance cannot be excluded. The various definitions are summarized in **Table 1 and Box 1**. Resistant hypertension classification according to ambulatory and office BP readings is shown in **Figure 1**. Classification of hypertension according to the number of drugs is shown in **Figure 2**.

◼ FEW PEARLS

- About 50% of total RH patients are actually having pseudo-RH.
- Pseudoresistance hypertension prevalence is around 33% among patients diagnosed with resistant hypertension.[8]
- Refractory hypertension is seen in 5–8% of RH patients.
- Secondary hypertension and RS are not the same.
- *Malignant hypertension:* Hypertensive urgency and emergency have replaced the terms malignant hypertension, hypertensive crisis, and accelerated hypertension. Hypertensive urgency and hypertensive emergency are not totally different entities as untreated or unrecognized urgencies

TABLE 1: The various definitions and subtypes.

Subtype	Definition
Resistant	Blood pressure (BP) that remains above the target goal with three or more antihypertensive medications of different classes including a diuretic and after excluding pseudoresistance (poor BP measurement technique, white coat effect, nonadherence, and suboptimal choices in antihypertensive therapy) as well as the substance/drug-induced hypertension and secondary hypertension
Pseudoresistant	Apparent lack of BP control in a patient on at least three maximally tolerated well-designed antihypertensive medications including a diuretic. Factors that cause pseudoresistance include faulty BP measurement technique, poor adherence to medication, clinical inertia, and white coat hypertension
Refractory	Blood pressure remains elevated with the use of five or more antihypertensive medications of different classes including a long-acting thiazide-like diuretic and aldosterone antagonist[6]
White coat	Elevated BP only in the office (normal ambulatory or home BP)
Masked	Normal BP in office and elevated out of office
Malignant	Severe high BP >180/120 mm Hg associated with advanced bilateral retinopathy (hemorrhages, cotton wool spots, papilledema, and multiorgan involvement in a short period of time)

BOX 1: Different phenotypes of refractory hypertension (RH).

- *Refractory hypertension:* Extreme phenotype of RH and is considered when BP remains elevated with the use of five or more antihypertensive medications of different classes including a long-acting thiazide-like diuretic and aldosterone antagonist
- *Controlled resistant hypertension:* Blood pressure which is controlled with at least four antihypertensive medications at maximally tolerated doses
- *Masked uncontrolled hypertension (MUCH):* Patients who achieve adequate office BP control with at least four antihypertensive medications but elevated out-of-office BP

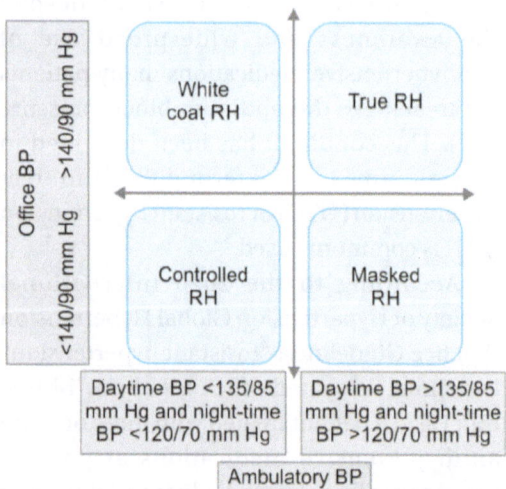

Fig. 1: Resistant hypertension (RH) according to ambulatory and office BP measurements.

may lead to emergencies. Hypertensive urgency or hypertensive emergency is defined as BP ≥ 180/110 mm Hg with the absence or presence of acute end-organ damage, respectively.

PATHOLOGY OF RESISTANT HYPERTENSION

Blood pressure is governed by the sympathetic nervous system (SNS) and the renin–angiotensin–aldosterone system (RAAS).

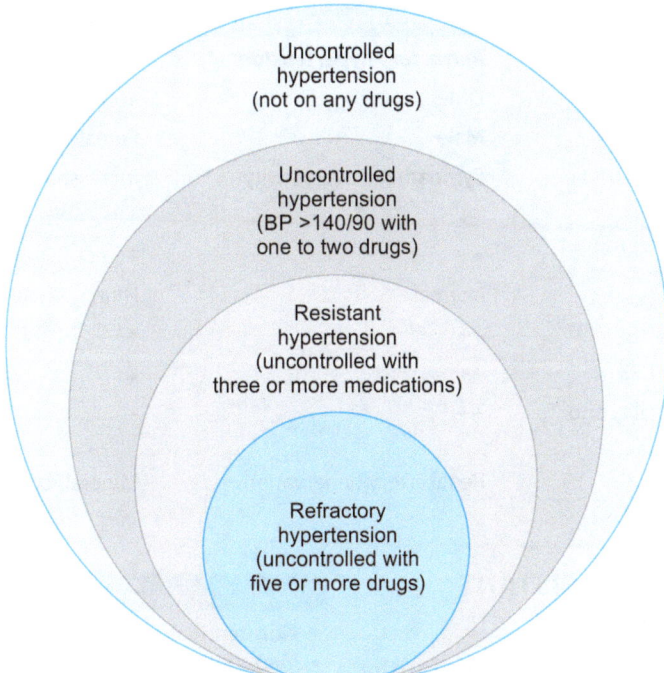

Fig. 2: Birmingham Hypertension Clinic and University of Alabama Classification of hypertension according to number of drugs.[7]

Thus, in RH, there is sympathetic overactivity and hyperaldosteronism resulting in intravascular fluid retention and an increase in arterial stiffness.[9]

There is a selective overactivation of the renal and the cardiac sympathetic system in patients with RH.[10] Increased sympathetic activity plays an important role in refractory hypertension than in RH. The prevention and treatment of hypertension with algorithm-based therapy (PATHWAY-2) trial basically showed that RH is a salt-retaining state secondary to increased aldosterone secretion.[11] Aldosterone also causes renal afferent and efferent arteriolar vasoconstriction, and also causes myocardial hypertrophy and fibrosis. Also, PATHWAY-2 included a number of substudies which basically provided important evidence of inappropriate fluid retention due to aldosterone excess as well as excess salt intake as one of the main mechanisms of RH and that spironolactone (as a fourth medication) in addition to the standard drugs [angiotensin-converting enzyme (ACE)-inhibitor or angiotensin receptor blocker (ARB), calcium channel blocker, and long-acting thiazide-like diuretic] is the treatment of choice. The trial also demonstrated the effective use of amiloride as an effective alternative in patients not tolerating spironolactone.

Refractory hypertension on the other hand is less volume dependent, since its treatment with diuretic drugs does not achieve the BP goals. Thus, refractory hypertensives have more SNS activity and low levels of aldosterone. The differences between refractory and resistance hypertension are given in **Table 2**.

TABLE 2: Differences between refractory and resistance hypertension.

	Refractory hypertension	Resistance hypertension
Age	Older	Younger
Sex	Male	Female
Mechanism	Sympathetic overactivity	Increased volume
Sleep apnea, obesity	++	+
Diabetes	++	+
Serum aldosterone	Normal	High
Dyslipidemias	++	+
eGFR < 60 mL/min/1.73 m^2	++	+
Cardiovascular mortality and morbidity	++	+
Sensitive to	Renal artery denervation	Mineralocorticoid antagonist

APPROACH TO RESISTANT HYPERTENSION

The most important first step in the management of RH is prompt recognition of this condition where the BP is not controlled with the use of three or more standardized antihypertensive regimens consisting of a RAAS blocker, calcium channel blocker, and a long-acting thiazide-like diuretic. It is equally important to view RH as a diagnosis of exclusion. Second, the accuracy of BP monitoring and adherence to medications should be particularly identified and addressed (to exclude pseudoresistance). In one study of patients with RH 10% were completely nonadherent, 52% were partially or completely nonadherent.[12] Urine screens with mass spectroscopy, which is not commonly available, can be done for the detection of antihypertensive drugs. Third, the conditions contributing to or exacerbating hypertension should be identified and treated which include excessive salt intake, use of drugs **(Box 2)** that could increase BP. Fourth, for diagnosing RH, the patient should be on a long-acting thiazide-like diuretic. Lastly, secondary hypertension should be ruled out, potential causes and investigations for secondary hypertension are enumerated in **Table 3**. Systematic approach to RH is shown in **Flowchart 1**.

BOX 2: Drugs causing resistance hypertension.
- Nonsteroidal anti-inflammatory drugs
- Oral contraceptives
- Alcohol and caffeine
- Cocaine
- *Sympathomimetics:* Nasal decongestants, epinephrine, nor-epinephrine, and amphetamine
- Cyclosporine and tacrolimus
- *Antidepressants:* Monoamine oxidase (MAO) inhibitors
- Steroids
- Erythropoietin
- Vascular endothelial growth factor inhibitors

MANAGEMENT OF RESISTANT HYPERTENSION

Management of resistant hypertension is shown in **Figure 3**.

Nonpharmacological Therapy

A healthy lifestyle is one of the most important but often neglected factor to attain

TABLE 3: Potential causes and investigations in secondary hypertension.

Etiology	Investigation
Obstructive sleep apnea	Home sleep apnea testing level-3 sleep study, overnight polysomnography testing
Renovascular	Imaging of renal arteries
Renal parenchymal disease	Kidney ultrasound
Primary hyperaldosteronism/adrenal hyperplasia	Plasma aldosterone to renin ratio, adrenal computed tomography (CT) scan, and adrenal venous sampling
Pheochromocytoma/paraganglioma	Plasma metanephrines, 24-h urinary catecholamine levels, abdominal/pelvic CT or magnetic resonance imaging (MRI), I^{123}-metaiodobenzylguanidine (MIBG) scan functional imaging for metastasis
Cushing's syndrome	A 24-h urinary-free cortisol, dexamethasone suppression tests, and abdominal/pituitary imaging
Thyroid dysfunction	Thyroid function tests
Aortic coarctation	Echocardiogram, thoracic CT angiography, or magnetic resonance (MR) angiography

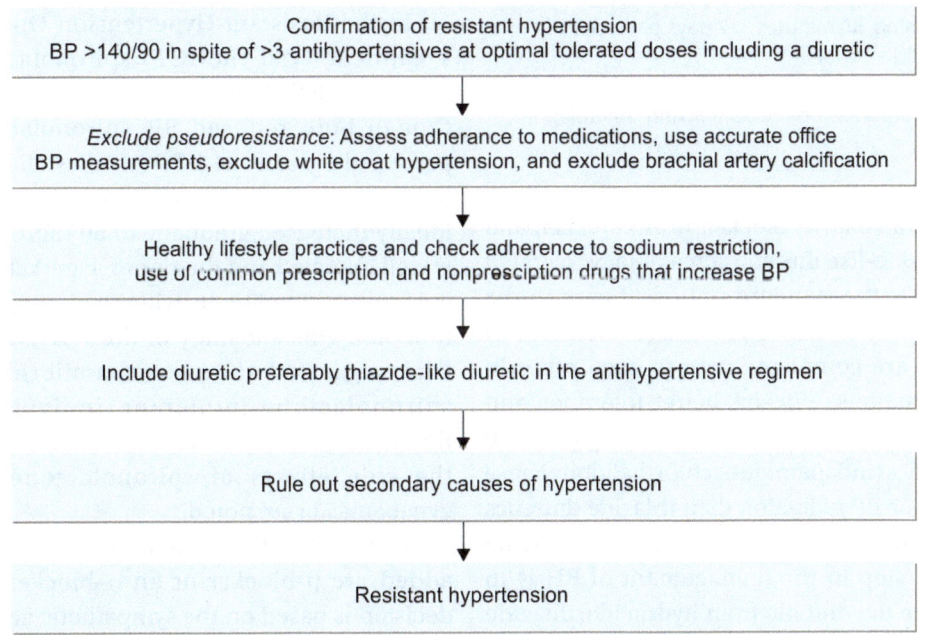

Flowchart 1: Systematic approach to resistance hypertension.

control of BP in RH.[13] Nonpharmacological approaches to manage hypertension is shown in **Box 3**.

Pharmacological Therapy

The initial drug of choice for RH is the same as essential hypertension.[14] The long-acting

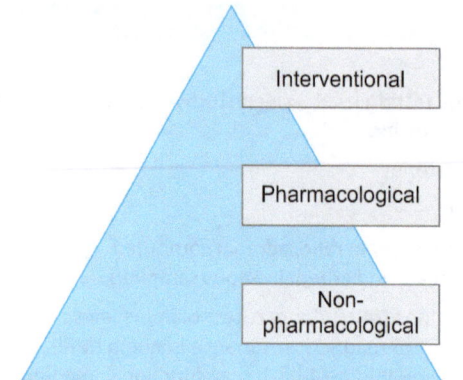

Fig. 3: Management of resistance hypertension.

BOX 3: Nonpharmacological approaches to manage hypertension.

- *Diet:* Dietary approaches to stop hypertension (DASH) diet
- *Low salt intake:* 3–6 gm NaCl
- *Weight reduction:* BMI <25 kg/m^2
- *Physical activity:* Aerobic exercises, resistance training, 30 minutes 5–7 days per week
- Avoid alcohol
- Quit smoking
- Meditation, yoga other relaxing therapies

calcium channel blocker, RAAS blocker, and a thiazide-like diuretic at maximally tolerated doses is the standard option of care in the treatment of RH. These various classes of drugs are complementary to each other in their actions, efficacy, better tolerance and safety. Among the diuretics the thiazide-like diuretics (indapamide or chlorthalidone) have superior BP reduction then thiazide diuretics and should be preferred, hence a starting initial step in the management of RH is to change the diuretic from hydrochlorthiazide to chlorthalidone or indapamide.[15] In elderly population with renal insufficiency it is better to use indapamide than chlorthalidone as the latter has a long duration of action and half-life.[16]

However, in patients with advanced kidney failure, the addition of a loop diuretic may be necessary.

Since the main mechanism of antihypertensive treatment resistance is the increased aldosterone activity in RH mineralocorticoid receptor antagonists are thus effective and are added as the fourth drug. The PATHWAY-2 study which showed the superiority of spironolactone in reducing BP in patients with RH who were on the standard three-drug regimen.[11]

In this study, spironolactone showed superior BP control when compared to bisoprolol and doxazosin.

The magnitude of BP reduction with spironolactone, when added to the standard three-drug-antihypertensive regimen is extraordinary claiming to reduce systolic BP by around 20 mm Hg.[17]

In the Resistant-Hypertension Optimal Treatment Trial (ReHOT) spironolactone and chlorthalidone were compared, even though both reduced BP, spironolactone produced a greater 24-h BP and diastolic BP.[18] Spironolactone can be started on 25 mg and ideally increased gradually to 50 mg/day. It is well tolerated and the risk of hyperkalemia is increased in patients with declining renal function. One substudy of the PATHWAY-2 trial suggested the use of amiloride in spironolactone-intolerant individuals. Eplerenone should be considered when the side effects of spironolactone-like gynecomastia are noted.

The next antihypertensive drugs to be added are β-blocker or an α-blocker, the decision is based on the sympathetic activity and usually, a heart rate of more than 80/min indicates a high sympathetic tone, in which the addition of a β-blocker-like bisoprolol is helpful. In situations where β-blockers cannot be used or are contraindicated α-blockers

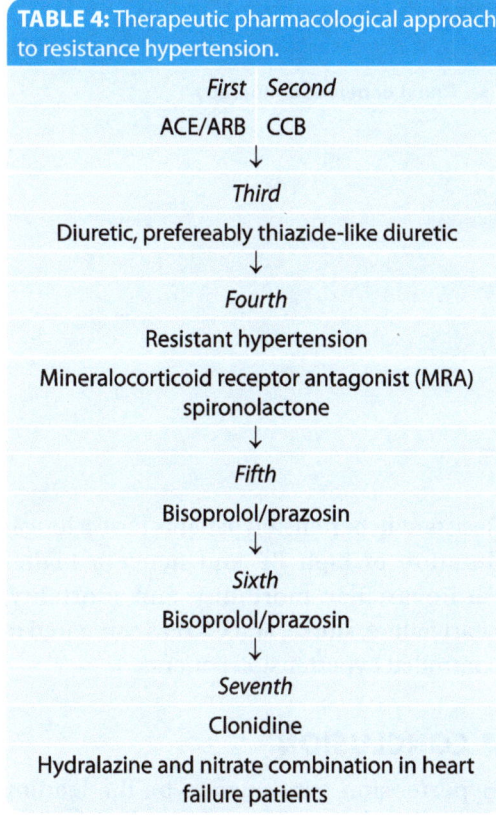

TABLE 4: Therapeutic pharmacological approach to resistance hypertension.

First: ACE/ARB
Second: CCB
↓
Third: Diuretic, preferably thiazide-like diuretic
↓
Fourth: Resistant hypertension
Mineralocorticoid receptor antagonist (MRA) spironolactone
↓
Fifth: Bisoprolol/prazosin
↓
Sixth: Bisoprolol/prazosin
↓
Seventh: Clonidine
Hydralazine and nitrate combination in heart failure patients

Note: Initiation of statin therapy should be considered in all hypertensives, especially in patients with resistance hypertension.
(ACE: angiotensin-converting enzyme; ARB: angiotensin receptor blocker; CCB: calcium channel blocker)

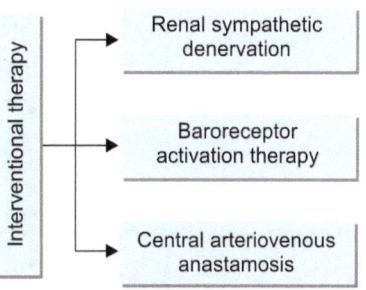

Fig. 4: Interventional therapy.

Interventional Therapy

In a fraction of patients with RH, the BP fails to reduce in spite of all measures. Thus, new interventional therapies specifically defined for this subset of people are available **(Fig. 4)**.

Renal Sympathetic Denervation

Renal denervation (RDN) therapy is a novel method wherein the ablation of renal afferent and efferent nerves is done using a radiofrequency catheter **(Flowchart 2)**.

In SIMPLICITY HTN-3 trial renal denervation was not found to be better than medical therapy in RH.[19] In the more recent trials such as the RADIANCE-HTN SOLO, SPYRAL HTN-OFF MED, and SPYRAL HTN-ON-MED with multielectrode catheters (newer SPYRAL catheter by Medtronic) have shown promising results and renal denervation therapy is back on the table for the treatment of RH.

Baroreceptor Activation Therapy

In baroreceptor activation therapy **(Flowchart 3)**, there is a sustained stimulation of the carotid baroreceptors by an implantable electrode placed in the carotid artery and a chest pulse generator thus inhibiting the sympathetic output.

The Rheos pivotal trial did show equivocal results.[20] The availability of second-generation

prazosin is used.[11] However, it is important to note that β-blockers have to be started at any stage of hypertension if compelling indications such as ischemic heart disease, heart failure, atrial fibrillation among others.

Last resort drug options include clonidine a centrally acting α-agonist, central vasodilators such as hydralazine, and nitrates especially in patients with heart failure. Although these drugs are efficacious; their use is limited by the side effects and patient comorbidities.

The stepwise therapeutic pharmacological approach is shown in **Table 4**.

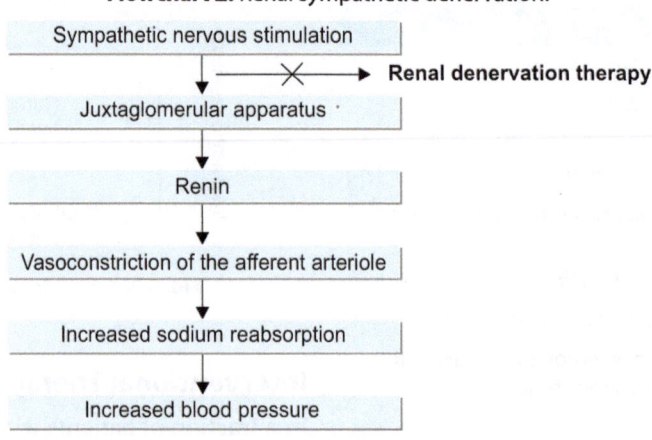

Flowchart 2: Renal sympathetic denervation.

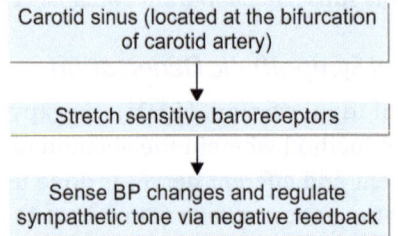

Flowchart 3: Baroreceptor activation therapy.

devices and improved surgical techniques, this procedure may show promising results.

Central Arteriovenous Anastomosis

Creating an arteriovenous anastomosis between the central vessels helps in reducing the BP by decompressing the high pressure from the arterial system into the low-resistance venous system. The ROX-CONTROL HTN study demonstrated a significant BP reduction but however, more evidence is required.[21]

Prognosis

Patients with RH have a worse prognosis as compared to other hypertensive patients.[22] Resistant hypertension patients have a longer duration of high BP and hence a higher cardiovascular morbidity and mortality, heart failure, stroke, and CKD as compared to controlled hypertension patients.

■ CONCLUSION

Hypertension continues to be the leading cause of cardiovascular morbidity and mortality and RH represents an important high-risk subtype. Resistant hypertension cases are increasing and hence should be investigated and addressed promptly to prevent further complications as well as end-organ damage. In patients with RH with three different drug classes (including a RAAS blocker, calcium channel blocker, and a thiazide-like diuretic), spironolactone is the recommended drug of choice. In patients resistant to all these drugs, β-blockers, α-blockers, and centrally acting α-agonists with careful monitoring can be used. Interventional therapies in a select group of cases with RH are useful but require more research, follow-up up, and long-term results.

REFERENCES

1. Anchala R, Kannuri NK, Pant H, Khan H, Franco OH, Di Angelantonio E, et al. Hypertension in India: A systematic review and meta-analysis of prevalence, awareness, and control of hypertension. J Hypertens. 2014;32:1170-7.
2. Yaxley JP, Thambar SV. Resistant hypertension: An approach to management in primary care. J Family Med Prim Care 2015;4(2):193-9.
3. Calhoun DA, Jones D, Textor S, Goff DC, Murphy TP, Toto RD, et al. Resistant hypertension: Diagnosis, evaluation, and treatment: A scientific statement from the American Heart Association Professional Education Committee of the Council for High Blood Pressure Research. Circulation. 2008;117(25):e510–e526.
4. Aydoğdu S, Güler K, Bayram F, Altun B, Derici Ü, Abacı A, et al. 2019 Turkish Hypertension Consensus Report. Turk Kardiyol Dern Ars. 2019;47(6):535-46.
5. Abdalla M. Ambulatory blood pressure monitoring: A complementary strategy for hypertension diagnosis and management in low-income and middle-income countries. Cardiol Clin. 2017;35(1):117-24.
6. Acelajado MC, Pisoni R, Dudenbostel T, Dell'Italia LJ, Cartmill F, Zhang B, et al. Refractory hypertension: Definition, prevalence, and patient characteristics. J Clin Hypertens. 2012;14:7-12.
7. Dudenbostel T, Siddiqui M, Gharpure N, Calhoun DA. Refractory versus resistant hypertension: Novel distinctive phenotypes. J Nat Sci. 2017;3(9):e430.
8. Bhatt H, Siddiqui M, Judd E, Oparil S, Calhoun D. Prevalence of pseudoresistant hypertension due to inaccurate blood pressure measurement. J Am Soc Hypertens. 2016;10(6):493-9.
9. Dudenbostel T, Acelajado MC, Pisoni R, Li P, Oparil S, Calhoun DA. Refractory hypertension: evidence of heightened sympathetic activity as a cause of antihypertensive treatment failure. Hypertension. 2015;66(1):126-33.
10. Esler M, Lambert G, Jennings G. Regional norepinephrine turnover in human hypertension. Clin Exp Hypertens A. 1989;11(Suppl. 1):75-89.
11. Williams B, MacDonald TM, Morant SV, Webb DJ, Sever P, McInnes GT, et al. Endocrine and haemodynamic changes in resistant hypertension, and blood pressure responses to spironolactone or amiloride: The PATHWAY-2 mechanisms substudies. Lancet Diabetes Endocrinol. 2018;6(6):464-75.
12. Jung O, Gechter JL, Wunder C, Paulke A, Bartel C, Geiger H, et al. Resistant hypertension? Assessment of adherence by toxicological urine analysis. J Hypertens. 2013;31:766-74.
13. Diaz KM, Booth JN III, Calhoun DA, Irvin MR, Howard G, Safford MM, et al. Healthy lifestyle factors and risk of cardiovascular events and mortality in treatment-resistant hypertension: The Reasons for Geographic and Racial Differences in Stroke study. Hypertension. 2014;64(3):465-71.
14. Calhoun D, Jones D, Textor S, Goff D, Murphy T, Toto R, et al. Resistant hypertension: A scientific statement from the American Heart Association Professional Education Committee of the Council for High Blood Pressure Research. Hypertension. 2008;51(6):1403-19.
15. Roush GC, Sica DA. Diuretics for hypertension: A review and update. Am J Hypertens. 2016;29(10):1130-7.
16. Madkour H, Gadallah M, Riveline B, Plante GE, Massry SG. Indapamide is superior to thiazide in the preservation of renal function in patients with renal insufficiency and systemic hypertension. Am J Cardiol. 1996;77(6):23B-5B.
17. Nishizaka MK, Zaman MA, Calhoun DA. Efficacy of low-dose spironolactone in subjects with resistant hypertension. Am J Hypertens. 2003;16(11 Pt 1):925-30.
18. Krieger EM, Drager LF, Giorgi DMA, Pereira AC, Barreto-Filho JAS, Nogueira

AR, et al. Spironolactone versus clonidine as a fourth-drug therapy for resistant hypertension: The ReHOT randomized study (resistant hypertension optimal treatment). Hypertension. 2018;71(4):681-90.
19. Bhatt DL, Kandzari DE, O'Neill WW, D'Agostino R, Flack JM, Katzen BT, et al. SYMPLICITY HTN-3 Investigators. A controlled trial of renal denervation for resistant hypertension. N Engl J Med. 2014;370(15):1393-401.
20. Bakris GL, Nadim MK, Haller H, Lovett EG, Schafer JE, Bisognano JD, et al. Baroreflex activation therapy provides durable benefit in patients with resistant hypertension: Results of long-term follow-up in the Rheos pivotal trial. J Am Soc Hypertens. 2012;6:152-8.
21. Lobo MD, Ott C, Sobotka PA, Saxena M, Stanton A, Cockcroft JR, et al. Central iliac arteriovenous anastomosis for uncontrolled hypertension: One-year results from the ROX CONTROL HTN Trial. Hypertension. 2017;70(6):1099-105.
22. Daugherty SL, Powers JD, Magid DJ, Tavel HM, Masoudi FA, Margolis KL, et al. Incidence and prognosis of resistant hypertension in hypertensive patients. Circulation. 2012;125(13):1635-42.

CHAPTER 19

Hypertension in Pregnancy

Abhay Narain Rai, Mritunjay Kumar Singh

INTRODUCTION

Hypertension (HTN) complicates 10–15% of pregnancies worldwide; making it one of the major causes of maternal and perinatal morbidity and mortality worldwide. As the prevalence of cardiometabolic diseases are rising unprecedentedly worldwide the incidence of HTN disorder in pregnancy (HDP) also shows a rising trend. The distinction between pregnancy-induced HTN and chronic HTN is essential for optimal management. Appropriate prenatal care and careful observation of women for signs of preeclampsia and then timely delivery to terminate the pregnancy has reduced the number and extent of adverse outcomes, serious maternal–fetal morbidity, and mortality. Hypertensive disorder during pregnancy is also associated with negative long-term impacts on the mother and child.

DEFINITION OF CLASSIFICATION OF HYPERTENSIVE DISORDERS IN PREGNANCY[1,2]

Accurate BP measurement is important for classifying HTN and starting treatment regardless of pregnancy status. Most current guidelines recommend HTN management based on office BP measurements using oscillometric automated devices validated for pregnant women. Recent studies endorse out-of-office BP as a more accurate and better predictor of cardiovascular morbidity and mortality.

Hypertension in pregnancy is defined as a systolic blood pressure (SBP) ≥140 mm Hg and/or a diastolic blood pressure (DBP) ≥90 mm Hg (average of at least two measurements taken at least 4-hour apart).
- Pregnancy-induced HTN (>20 weeks of gestation)
  - Gestational HTN
  - Preeclampsia
    - Mild
    - Severe
  - Eclampsia
- Chronic prepregnancy HTN (<20 weeks of gestation)
- Chronic HTN with superimposed preeclampsia/eclampsia.

PATHOGENESIS OF HYPERTENSION DISORDER IN PREGNANCY[1,2]

The interplay between maternal per existing comorbidities (HTN, diabetes, CKD, obesity) nonmodifiable patient characteristics (age, race, and family history), reproductive history, genetics, and immune factors increases the risk of developing HDP. The placental pathophysiology which is still evolving includes renin–angiotensin–aldosterone stimulation, angiogenesis imbalance (increased circulating soluble fms like tyrosin kinase 1), inflammatory imbalance [increased reactive oxygen species (ROS), tumor necrosis factor-alpha (TNF-α, IL-6, and endothelin 1)] leads to a cascade of reactions such as endothelial dysfunction, procoagulation, and proinflammation resulting in widespread endovascular damage and dysfunction which might have a prolonged effect.

PREGNANCY-INDUCED HYPERTENSION

Gestational Hypertension

Gestational hypertension (GHTN) is characterized by new-onset HTN after 20 weeks of gestation, often near term, in the absence of accompanying proteinuria. Although GHTN usually is benign, some of the cases may convert into preeclampsia or Chronic hypertension.[1,2,4]

Management of Gestational Hypertension[1,2,4]

- Nonsevere HTN (BP 140–159/90–109 mm Hg) in pregnancy:
  - Start single anti-HTN drug therapy (target DBP < 85 mm Hg)
  - Maternal, fetal, and placental assessment
  - Regular BP monitoring
- Severe HTN (BP >160/110 mm Hg) in pregnancy.
It is associated with significantly worse maternal and perinatal outcomes, independent of the development of preeclampsia, and it requires urgent pharmacotherapy (Table 1).

ANTIHYPERTENSIVE MEDICATIONS COMMONLY USED IN PREGNANCY[1,2,4]

- First-line drugs include oral labetalol, oral methyldopa, long-acting oral nifedipine, or other oral β-blockers (acebutolol, metoprolol, pindolol, and propranolol).
- Second-line drugs including clonidine, hydralazine, and thiazide diuretics.
- Angiotensin-converting enzyme (ACE) inhibitors (grade C) and angiotensin receptor blockers (grade D) should not be used in pregnant women.

PREECLAMPSIA[1,3,4]

Preeclampsia is the most frequently encountered renal complication of pregnancy. It is characterized by the new-onset HTN (≥140/90 after 20 weeks of pregnancy) and proteinuria

TABLE 1: Drugs for pregnancy hypertension.

Drug	Dow	Comments
Labetalol	10–20 mg IV, then 20–80 mg every 20–30 min to a maximum dose of 300 mg or Constant infusion 1–2 mg/min IV	Considered a first-line agent Tachycardia is less common and has fewer adverse effects Contraindicated in patients with asthma, heart disease, or congestive head failure
Hydralazine	5 mg IV or IM, then 5–10 mg IV every 20–40 min or Constant infusion 0.5–10 mg/h	Higher or frequent dosage associated with maternal hypotension, headaches, and fetal distress—may be more common than other agents
Nifedipine	10–20 mg orally, repeat in 30 min if needed, then 10–20 mg every 2–6 hours	May observe reflex tachycardia and headaches

(IM: intramuscularity; IV: intravenously)

(>300 mg on 24-hour urine collection or +1 on dipstick or protein/creatinine ≥ 0.3) or in the absence of proteinuria, new-onset HTN with new-onset of any one of the following:
- *Thrombocytopenia:* Platelet count <100,000/μL.
- *Renal insufficiency:* Serum creatinine >1.1 mg/dL or doubling of serum creatinine in the absence of renal disease.
- *Liver dysfunction:* Doubling of transaminase level.
- Pulmonary edema.
- Cerebral/visual symptoms.

Features of Severe Preeclampsia

In patients with preeclampsia, severe preeclampsia can be diagnosed if any of the following criteria is present:
- Blood pressure ≥160/110 on two separate occasions, 4-hour apart.
- *Thrombocytopenia:* Platelet count <100,000/μL.
- *Renal insufficiency:* Serum creatinine >1.1 mg/dL or doubling of serum creatinine in the absence of renal disease or oliguria <500 mL/24 hours
- *Liver dysfunction:* Doubling of transaminase level or severe right upper quadrant pain/epigastric pain without an alternative diagnosis.
- Proteinuria >5 g/24 hours.
- Pulmonary edema.
- Cerebral/visual symptoms.
- Serum lactate dehydrogenase >600 IU/mL.

Pathogenesis

Preeclampsia occurs only in the presence of the placenta and usually remits when the placenta is delivered. The placenta in preeclampsia is hypoperfused and ischemic. Preeclampsia is characterized by widespread vascular endotheliosis and macroangiopathy in mothers induced by circulating factors produced by the abnormal placenta. The fetus is immune to these factors **(Flowchart 1)**.

Risk Factors for the Development of Preeclampsia

- Preeclampsia in prior pregnancy.
- Family history of preeclampsia.
- Nulliparity.
- Multiple gestation.
- Older maternal age.
- Molar pregnancy.
- Obesity.
- Pre-existing HTN.
- Preexisting chronic kidney disease.
- Diabetes mellitus.
- Thrombotic vascular disease.
- Trisomy 13 fetus.
- Fetal hydrops.
- High altitude.

Management

- Mild preeclampsia
  - If immature fetus, bed rest mainly in lateral decubitus position
  - Hypertension therapy if needed
- Severe preeclampsia
  - Admit to labor and delivery area
  - Maternal and fetal evaluation for 24 hours
  - Magnesium sulfate for 24 hours
  - Anti-HTN if BP ≥160/110 mm Hg or mean arterial pressure (MAP) >125 mm Hg
  - Steroids are indicated in severe intrauterine growth retardation or if gestational age is above 23 weeks.

Prevention of Preeclampsia

Low-dose aspirin (75–150 mg daily) in high-risk persons has been shown to reduce the occurrence of preeclampsia. Oral calcium

Flowchart 1: Types of risk factors.

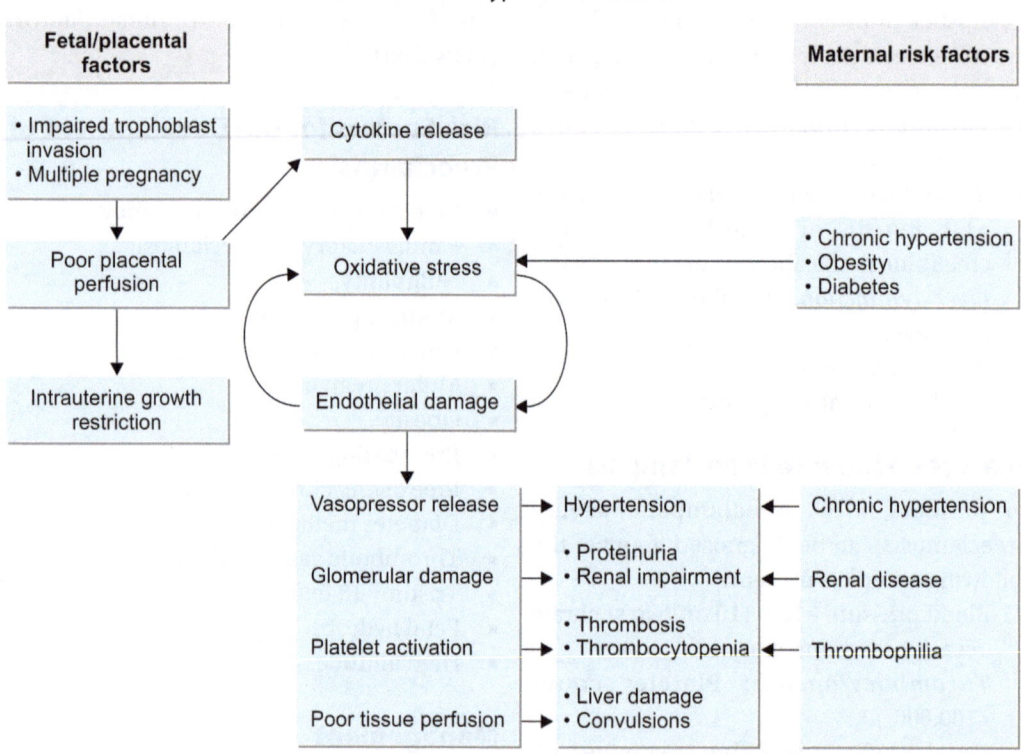

supplementation may reduce the likelihood of preeclampsia in women whose calcium intake is very low. Vitamin C/vitamin E does not protect against preeclampsia. Lifestyle changes before and during pregnancy may reduce the fatal and maternal risk to a large extent.

Late Complication of Preeclampsia

Several studies have shown that persons with preeclampsia have an increased risk of cardiovascular disease in later years. Experts suggest yearly evaluation of such persons for blood pressure, lipid profile, blood sugar, and body mass index. A healthy lifestyle should also be encouraged in such persons.

◼ ECLAMPSIA[1,3,4]

Eclampsia is defined as the presence of new-onset grand mal seizure in a woman with preeclampsia. It occurs in 0.5–4% of deliveries. Eclamptic seizures can occur before labor (25%), during labor (50%), and after delivery (25%).

Management

- *Anticonvulsant therapy:* Magnesium sulfate is an agent of choice for the treatment and prevention of eclamptic seizures. Intravenous loading dose of 4–6 g followed by a maintenance dose of 1-2 g/h for at least 24 hours.
- Antihypertensives as in severe preeclampsia.
- *Definitive treatment:* Delivery following stabilization.

◼ HELLP SYNDROME[1,3,4]

The term "HELLP syndrome" is an acronym of hemolysis, elevated liver enzymes, and low platelet count; HELLP syndrome may occur antepartum/postpartum. This syndrome is associated with increased maternal morbidity and mortality; many experts consider this syndrome to be an indication of prompt delivery.

Management

- Initial maternal stabilization followed by delivery is the cornerstone of management.
- Platelet transfusion before or after delivery if the platelet count is <20,000/mm^3. (advised at <50,000/mm^3 before cesarean section).
- Before 32 weeks gestation, a short course of corticosteroids for fetal lung maturation and improving maternal platelet count may be a viable option.

CHRONIC HYPERTENSION IN PREGNANCY[3,4]

Systolic pressure ≥140 mm Hg, diastolic pressure ≥90 mm Hg, or both presents before the 20th week of pregnancy or persists longer than 12 weeks postpartum.

Causes

- *Primary:* "Essential HTN" in 90% of cases.
- *Secondary:* "Result of other medical condition (i.e., renal disease).
  - About 15% of gestational HTN cases go on to develop chronic HTN.
  - About 25% risk of developing superimposed preeclampsia or eclampsia
  - Close monitoring of maternal BP and following appropriate be encouraged to increase the amount of time she rests.

PARENTAL CARE FOR CHRONIC HYPERTENSIVE[1,5]

- Electrocardiogram should be obtained in women with long-standing HTN.
- Baseline laboratory tests include urinalysis, urine culture, and serum creatinine, glucose, and electrolytes.
- Tests to rule out renal diseases, and identify comorbidities such as diabetes mellitus.
- Women with proteinuria on a urine dipstick should have a quantitative for urine protein.

Management

- Avoid treatment in women with uncomplicated mild essential HTN as blood pressure may decrease as pregnancy progresses.
- May taper or discontinue medicines for women with blood pressure less than 120/80 in the first trimester.
- Reinstitute or initiate therapy for persistent diastolic pressure above 95 mm Hg, systolic pressure above 150 mm Hg, or signs of hypertensive end-organ damage.
- *Medication of choices:* Oral methyldopa and labetalol.

SECONDARY HYPERTENSION[5]

It occurs in a small proportion of cases. It should be considered if the maternal age below 35 years, severe or resistant HTN, lab reports suggest hypokalemia, increased serum creatinine, or albuminuria in early pregnancy. Obesity and obstructive sleep apnea may be associated with secondary HTN during pregnancy.

POSTPARTUM HYPERTENSION AND POSTPARTUM PREECLAMPSIA[5]

Their significance can be understood by the reason that HDP remains the most important cause of maternal deaths occur within the first year postpartum. Patient education is an important tool for early recognition of signs and symptoms. The short-term serious maternal complications include stroke, seizures, cardiomyopathy, insulin resistance, and weight gain. A remote HTN monitoring program is the key to early diagnosis and management of postpartum HTN and postpartum preeclampsia.

Postpartum Screening[5]

All women who have had HDP should be screened at least annually for cardiovascular risk and life style modification should be encouraged in such patients.

■ HIGHLIGHTS

- Occurs in 10–15% of pregnancies.
- Diagnosed when BP reads above 140/90 mm Hg.
- Preeclampsia means gestational HTN plus proteinuria.
- Protein level above 300 mg/24-hour urine sample.
- If left untreated, it results in eclampsia (with seizure).
- The HELLP syndrome is a complication of preeclampsia.
- Treatment options include rest/hospitalization, fetal monitoring, laboratory testing, and anti-HTN (methyl-dopa/hydralazine/labetalol).

■ REFERENCES

1. Charles RBB, Ling FW, Smith RP. Barzansky BM, Herbert WNP. Laube DW. Obstetrics and Gynecology, 5th edition. India: Lippincott Williams & Wilkins; 2006, pp. 188-96.
2. Lissa MM, Lockwood CJ, Barss VA. Gestational hypertension, 2011. Available from https://www.uptodate.com/contents/gestational-hypertension [Last accessed November, 2023].
3. Phyllis A, Lockwood CJ, Barss VA. Management of hypertension in pregnancy and postpartum patients. 2011. Available from: https://www.uptodate.com/contents/treatment-of-hypertension-in-pregnant-and-postpartum-patients [Last accessed November, 2023].
4. Bansode BR. Managing Hypertension in Pregnancy. 2012. Available from https://apiindia.org/Medicine-Update-2012-Contents [Last accessed November, 2023].
5. Butalia S, Audibert F, Côté AM, Firoz T, Logan AG, Magee LA, et al. Hypertension Canada's 2018 Guidelines for the Management of Hypertension in Pregnancy. Can J Cardiol. 2018;34(5):526-31.

CHAPTER 20

Metabolic Syndrome and Hypertension

Chamma Gupta, Abhishek Byahut, Karma G Dolma

■ INTRODUCTION

Hypertension (HTN) has emerged as a prominent global health concern. As this condition often goes undiagnosed over prolonged periods, it can give rise to complications such as kidney failure and heart disease. The term metabolic syndrome (MS) encompasses a cluster of metabolic risk factors, including central obesity, glucose intolerance, hyperinsulinemia, low high-density lipoprotein (HDL) cholesterol, high triglycerides, and HTN. Notably, HTN constitutes a significant element of MS, being present in over 80% of individuals afflicted by it.[1] In the past two decades, intensified research has delved into exploring ethnic disparities in MS prevalence, particularly in relation to type 2 diabetes and coronary heart disease (CHD) as specific clinical endpoints. Metabolic syndrome is widely acknowledged as a cardiovascular disease (CVD) risk factor, bearing implications for cardiovascular mortality.[2] While estimates of MS prevalence vary by nation, non-European cohorts such as South Asians, Black African–Caribbeans, Hispanics, and Aboriginals tend to exhibit higher prevalence, in contrast to lower rates among European Whites, Chinese, and Japanese populations.

Hypertension stands out as a pivotal facet of MS. Recently, there has been an uptick in HTN prevalence, potentially attributed to rapid epidemiological shifts occurring over the last four decades. Approximately 1 billion individuals worldwide grapple with HTN, underscoring its status as a pressing global public health challenge. Existing data indicates that HTN prevalence has either remained steady or declined in economically developed nations during the past ten years, yet it has witnessed an increase in developing nations.[3] Nonetheless, a comprehensive assessment of the escalating HTN prevalence is imperative for formulating efficacious prevention strategies, particularly urgent in developing countries such as India.

■ BURDEN OF HYPERTENSION

The escalation of HTN is projected to disproportionately impact developing nations, with an estimated 89% surge anticipated in sub-Saharan Africa from 2000 to 2025; on the contrary to a 24% increase in more developed countries. Hypertension stands as one of the prevalent cardiovascular afflictions across South Asian nations. The classification of HTN, as provided by the Joint National Committee on Prevention, Detection, Evaluation, and Treatment of High Blood Pressure (JNC 7 report), is outlined as follows[4]:

Hypertension is characterized by a systolic blood pressure (SBP) level of ≥140 mm Hg and/or a diastolic blood pressure (DBP) level of ≥90 mm Hg, or having received a previous HTN diagnosis from any physician. JNC 8 report has revised this definition, setting a slightly higher threshold of 150/90 mm Hg for initiating pharmacotherapy in individuals aged 60 years and older.[5]

Prehypertension is delineated within the range of 120–139 mm Hg SBP and 80–89 mm Hg DBP.
- Stage 1 HTN is designated by a SBP ranging from 140 to 159 mm Hg and a DBP between 90 and 99 mm Hg.
- Stage 2 HTN is characterized by a SBP equal to or exceeding 160 mm Hg and a DBP equal to or exceeding 100 mm Hg.

Prevalence of Hypertension in India

Numerous studies have examined the prevalence of HTN within India. Dating back to 1954, a prevalence rate of 4% was documented based on criteria of above 160/95 in Kanpur. Subsequently, during the period of 1984–1987, the prevalence escalated to 11% as per JNC V criteria. Among the elderly population aged 60 years and above, a higher prevalence of 69 and 55% was observed in urban and rural areas, respectively.[6] Urban Chennai, as reported by Mohan et al., exhibited a prevalence of 8.4 and 15% in adults aged above 20 years from the low- and middle-socioeconomic groups, respectively.[7] An urban Chennai study (age group ≥40) unveiled a higher prevalence of HTN (54%) in the low-income group and a 40% prevalence among the high-income group.[8] In Delhi slums, Misra et al.[9] reported a HTN prevalence of 12%.

A systematic review and meta-analysis specific to regions (urban and rural areas of north, east, west, and south India) found that approximately 33% of urban and 25% of rural Indians are affected by HTN. Notably, only 25% of rural and 42% of urban Indians are cognizant of their hypertensive status, with treatment being pursued by only 25% of rural and 38% of urban Indians. Overall, just a tenth of rural and a fifth of urban Indian HTN individuals have their blood pressure (BP) under control.[10]

Gupta et al.[11] analyzed HTN trends over 25 years in an Indian urban population, observing rising prevalence, awareness, treatment, and control rates, with improved awareness correlating with enhanced control. A recent study by Shikha Singh et al.[12] in urban Varanasi highlighted that approximately one-third of subjects were hypertensive, and half exhibited pre-HTN. However, awareness, treatment, and control of high BP remained strikingly low within this population.

A cross-sectional study across 10 Indian states [Screening India's Twin Epidemic (SITE)] demonstrated that among 15,662 subjects, 46% exhibited HTN as per JNC 7 guidelines. Within this group, 22.2% were newly diagnosed, and 60.1% had pre-HTN.[13] Phase I of the Indian Council of Medical Research–India Diabetes (ICMR–INDIAB) study focused on individuals aged ≥20 years in Tamil Nadu, Maharashtra, Jharkhand, and Chandigarh. This study revealed an overall age-standardized HTN prevalence of 26.3% (self-reported: 5.5%; newly detected: 20.8%). Urban residents in these regions had notably higher prevalence rates compared to rural residents.[14]

A recent metabolic noncommunicable disease health report of India revealed that the weighted prevalence of HTN was 35.5% [95% confidence interval (CI): 33.8–37.3; 35.172 of 111.439 individuals), which was higher in urban areas and among males. The state-wise weighted prevalence of HTN ranged from 24.3% (851 of 3,641 individuals) to 51.8% (1,644 of 3,709 individuals). When sensitivity analysis was done using American College of Cardiology/American Heart Association (ACC/AHA) criteria (i.e., ≥130/80 mm Hg), the prevalence of HTN nearly doubled to 66.3% (64.6–67.9%; 69.702 of 111.439 individuals).[15]

Associations between HTN and factors such as age, familial history of cardiovascular disorders, alcohol consumption, and diet were reported by Joshi et al.[13] Bhansali et al.[14] from the INDIAB study also found significant associations with age, male gender, urban residence, generalized obesity, diabetes, physical inactivity, alcohol consumption, and salt intake ≥6.5 g per day. Prevention, early diagnosis, and prompt treatment of HTN are the cornerstones of preventing morbidity and mortality due to CVD.

METABOLIC SYNDROME DEFINITION

Regrettably, a universally accepted definition for MS remains elusive, leading to considerable variation in MS estimates across populations, contingent upon the applied criteria. The World Health Organization (WHO) introduced an MS definition in 1999, while the National Cholesterol Education Program Expert Panel (NCEP) and Adult Treatment Panel III (ATP III) issued their working definition in 2001. In 2005, the International Diabetes Federation (IDF) Consensus group proposed an alternate definition. Although these definitions concur on fundamental components—glucose intolerance, obesity, HTN, and dyslipidemia—they diverge in the threshold values for each cluster component and the amalgamation approach.

Deliberations involving IDF and AHA/National Heart, Lung, and Blood Institute (NHLBI) representatives aimed to reconcile disparities between MS definitions. This harmonization effort stipulates that abdominal obesity need not serve as a prerequisite for diagnosis; instead, it constitutes just one of five criteria.[16] A diagnosis of MS is established with the presence of any three out of five risk factors. The criteria for diagnosing MS, utilizing this harmonized approach, are presented in **Table 1**.

Prevalence of Metabolic Syndrome

Numerous epidemiological investigations have unveiled the prevalence of MS (MS) across diverse ethnic groups, encompassing Africans, Latin Americans, Chinese, Asian Indians, Australians, and Polynesians. The prevalence of MS varies widely, ranging from 13% in China to 30% in Iran. In Singapore, a

TABLE 1: Criteria for clinical diagnosis of MS.[16]

Measure	Categorical cut points
Elevated waist circumference	Population and country specific definitions (>90 cm for males and >80 cm for females for South Asian Indians)
Elevated triglycerides (drug treatment for elevated triglycerides is an alternate indicator)	≥150 mg/dL (1.7 mmol/L)
Reduced HDL-C (drug treatment for reduced HDL-C is an alternate indicator)	<40 mg/dL (1.0 mmol/L) in males <50 mg/dL (1.3 mmol/L) in females
Elevated BP (antihypertensive drug treatment in a patient with a history of HTN is an alternate indicator)	SBP ≥130 and /or diastolic BP ≥85 mm Hg
Elevated fasting glucose (drug treatment of elevated glucose is an alternate indicator)	≥100 mg/dL

survey highlighted varied MS prevalence rates among the following major ethnic groups: Chinese (15%), Malays (19%), and Indians (20%). These studies have predominantly employed either WHO or ATP III criteria to define MS.

In the FinnDiane study, the overall prevalence of MS according to NCEP diagnostic criteria was 38% in men and 40% in women. A Spanish study reported an MS prevalence of 31.9%. According to WHO criteria, the prevalence of MS in type 1 diabetes was 30.7% in Scotland, while in south India, the prevalence of MS in type 1 diabetes stood at 22.2% using harmonizing criteria.[17] The initial study conducted by the ICMR Task Force on MS prevalence in India reported a prevalence of 30% in urban areas of Delhi and 11% in rural Haryana during 1992–1994, based on ATP III criteria.

Ramachandran et al. in 2003, utilizing a modified ATP III criteria, documented a higher MS prevalence of 41%.[18] Deepa et al. in 2002 reported a prevalence of 11.2% in urban Chennai during 1996-97.[19] Gupta et al. in 2004 found a 25% prevalence in Jaipur using ATP III criteria.[20] Misra et al.[9] conducted a study among urban slum dwellers in Delhi, reporting a 30% MS prevalence. Notably, in hypertensive populations, MS prevalence appears notably elevated. A study involving over 19,000 hypertensive patients attending primary care centers in Spain revealed MS presence in more than 40% of subjects according to the original ATP III definition, escalating to 60% with the application of IDF criteria.

CONSEQUENCES OF HYPERTENSION AND METABOLIC SYNDROME

Projected into 2020, CVD is poised to ascend as the leading contributor to global mortality and incapacitation. Especially in developing nations, CVD engulfs as much as 75% of non-communicable disease-related fatalities, presently constituting 10% of the burden of disability in these regions. An expansive cross-sectional study involving the Chennai population spotlighted that almost 40% of elderly urban South Indians grapple with MS, a condition intricately linked to coronary artery disease (CAD).

The Second National Health and Nutrition Examination Survey divulged that patients afflicted by MS face augmented risks of cardiovascular demise, CHD, and stroke. Furthermore, an escalated tally of metabolic irregularities correlates with heightened incidences of CVD mortality. In more recent times, an analysis of data sourced from the Atherosclerosis Risk in Communities study showcased that individuals grappling with MS, even without diabetes or pre-existing CVD, remain predisposed to unfavorable cardiovascular outcomes.

PREVENTION AND MANAGEMENT OF HYPERTENSION AND METABOLIC SYNDROME

Given the heightened vulnerability to diabetes and CVD in individuals with MS, it is imperative to formulate strategies that counteract the burgeoning global epidemic of this condition. Despite a notable surge in HTN prevalence over the past two decades, improvements in its management have remained limited.[21] The central management objectives for MS revolve around curtailing CVD and diabetes risks. Encompassing lifestyle modifications, such as regular physical activity and even modest weight reduction, have the potential to mitigate the syndrome's prevalence. Consequently, community-wide initiatives geared toward altering health behaviors play a pivotal role in mitigating the morbidity and mortality stemming from MS in developing nations.[22]

Regarding the management of hypertension, the World Health Organization has furnished recommendations as follows:
- *Primary prevention:* To quell the incidence of disease within a population, primary prevention seeks to mitigate underlying risk factors. Commencing prevention measures earlier enhances their effectiveness in curtailing disease progression. This can be accomplished through a population-level approach or by identifying high-risk individuals for targeted interventions. The population-based approach seeks to lower average BP across a population, which ultimately yields a substantial reduction in CVD incidence. This approach necessitates a multifaceted strategy encompassing nutrition education [such as the dietary approaches to stop hypertension (DASH) diet], weight reduction, promotion of physical activity, behavioral adjustments, health education, and self-care. The high-risk strategy involves identifying vulnerable individuals within families, managing their BP, and conducting regular screenings to monitor their condition. This pre-emptive intervention serves to avert the development of advanced complications.[21]
- *Secondary prevention:* Following disease detection, secondary prevention focuses on providing guidance regarding pharmacotherapy, dietary adjustments, and lifestyle modifications. Adherence to medication, diet, and lifestyle recommendations is crucial for managing the condition.[22]

Treatment's central objective is to diminish CVD risk. In conjunction with appropriate antihypertensive therapy, lifestyle interventions encompassing weight reduction through calorie-controlled diets and increased physical activity should be pursued. Long-term efficacy necessitates a caloric restriction of 500–1,000 kcal per day, culminating in 7–10% weight loss over a year, accompanied by daily exercise lasting 30–45 min. More rigorous exercise regimens may confer cardiovascular advantages in maintaining body weight. Lifestyle interventions yield positive effects on BP, and lipid profiles, and can deter the onset of new diabetes cases. Additionally, recent evidence suggests long-term cardiovascular morbidity reduction.

Other dietary alterations, such as food selection and patterns, exert favorable effects on certain cardiovascular risk factors and should be encouraged in high-risk individuals. Reducing salt intake and alcohol consumption produces moderate BP-lowering effects, which are amplified when combined with weight loss and enhanced physical activity. Diets rich in fruits, vegetables, and low-fat dairy products (such as the DASH diet) substantially lower BP compared to standard American diets. The Mediterranean diet, abundant in fruits, vegetables, fish, and olive oil, also manifests a favorable impact on atherogenic dyslipidemia in MS patients. However, most patients will require pharmacological intervention to address BP, dyslipidemia, insulin resistance, and obesity and effectively mitigate their cardiometabolic risk.

Mechanisms Linking Hypertension and Metabolic Syndrome

The intricate relationship between HTN and MS is underpinned by a network of interconnected factors. Visceral obesity, insulin resistance, oxidative stress, endothelial dysfunction, an activated renin-angiotensin system, elevated inflammatory mediators, and obstructive sleep apnea have all been posited as potential links bridging the gap between MS and HTN. These elements may

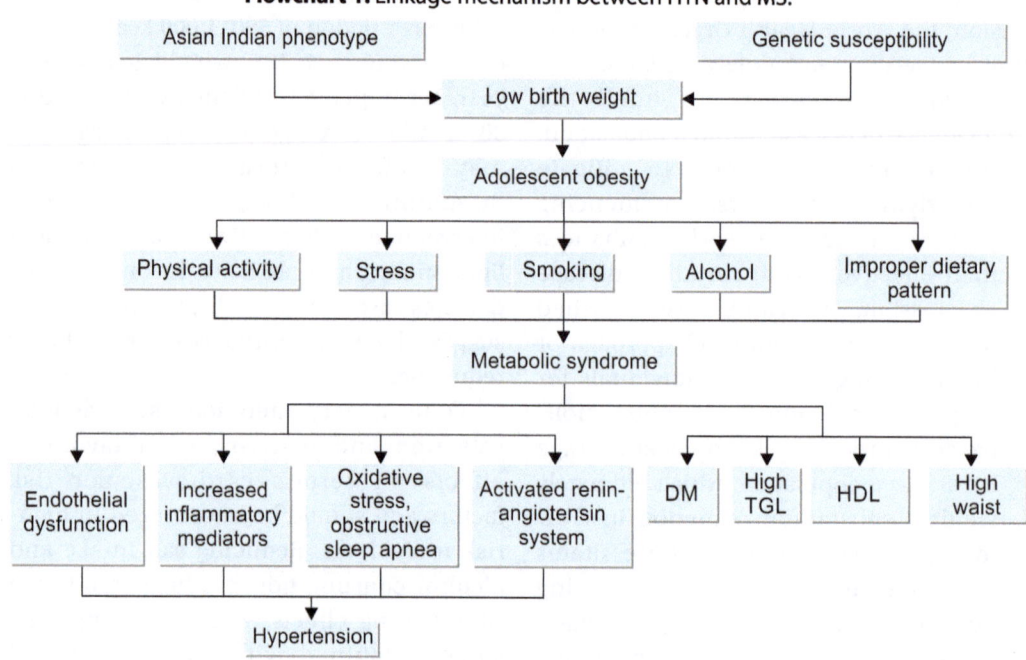

Flowchart 1: Linkage mechanism between HTN and MS.

stimulate sympathetic overactivity, trigger vasoconstriction, elevate intravascular fluid levels, and diminish vasodilation, collectively contributing to the genesis of HTN within the context of MS.[23] Refer to **Flowchart 1** for a visual depiction of the mechanistic connections between MS and HTN.

Addressing MS in hypertensive patients mandates an assertive approach encompassing lifestyle modifications and the targeting of metabolic risk factors. Favorable consideration should be given to medications like ACE inhibitors and ARBs, given their protective impact on newly diagnosed diabetes.[24] A patient-centered approach to managing HTN and MS revolves around modifying unhealthy lifestyles that exacerbate the underlying pathology. Comprehensive treatment entails sodium and calorie reduction, cessation of alcohol and smoking, weight management, increased physical activity, and judicious medication employment wherever warranted.[24,25]

REFERENCES

1. Duvnjak L; Bulum, T; Metelko Ž. Hypertension and the metabolic syndrome. Diabetologia Croatica. 2008;37(4):83-9.
2. Isomaa B, Almgren P, Tuomi T, Forsen B, Lahti K, Nissen M, Taskinen MR, Groop L. Cardiovascular morbidity and mortality associated with the metabolic syndrome. Diabetes Care 2001; 24: 683–9.
3. Kearney PM, Whelton M, Reynolds K, Whelton PK, He J. Worldwide prevalence of hypertension: A systematic review. J Hypertens. 2004;22(1):11-9.
4. Chobanian AV, Bakris GL, Black HR, Cushman WC, Green LA, Izzo JL Jr, et al. The Seventh Report of the Joint National Committee on Prevention, Detection, Evaluation, and Treatment of High Blood Pressure: the JNC 7 report. JAMA. 2003;289(19):2560-72.
5. Page MR. The JNC 8 hypertension guidelines: An in-depth guide. Am J Manag Care. 2014;20(Spec No. 1): E8.
6. Hypertension study Group. Prevalence, Awareness, treatment and control of hypertension among elderly in Bangladesh and India: A multicentric study. Bull World Health Organ. 2001;79(6):490-500.

7. Mohan V, Shanthirani S, Deepa R, Premalatha G, Sastry NG, Saroja R. Intra-urban differences in the prevalence of the metabolic syndrome in southern India: The Chennai Urban Population Study (CUPS No. 4). Diabet Med. 2001;18(4):280-7.
8. Ramachandran A, Snehalatha C, Vijay V, King H. Impact of poverty on the prevalence of diabetes and its complications in urban southern India. Diabet Med. 2002;19(2):130-5.
9. Misra A, Pandey RM, Devi JR, Sharma R, Vikram NK, Khanna N. High prevalence of diabetes, obesity and dyslipidaemia in urban slum population in northern India. Int J Obes Relat Metab Disord. 2001;25(11):1722-9.
10. Anchala R, Kannuri NK, Pant H, Khan H, Franco OH, Di Angelantonio E, et al. Hypertension in India: A systematic review and meta-analysis of prevalence, awareness, and control of hypertension. J Hypertens. 2014;32(6):1170-7.
11. Gupta R, Gupta VP, Prakash H, Agrawal A, Sharma KK, Deedwania PC. 25-Year trends in hypertension prevalence, awareness, treatment, and control in an Indian urban population: Jaipur Heart Watch. Indian Heart J. 2018;70(6):802-7.
12. Singh S, Shankar R, Singh GP. Prevalence and associated risk factors of hypertension: A cross-sectional study in Urban Varanasi. Int J Hypertens. 2017;2019:5491838.
13. Joshi SR, Saboo B, Vadivale M, Dani SI, Mithal A, Kaul U, et al. Prevalence of diagnosed and undiagnosed diabetes and hypertension in India: Results from the Screening India's Twin Epidemic (SITE) study. Diabetes Technol Ther. 2012;14(1):8-15.
14. Bhansali A, Dhandania VK, Deepa M, Anjana RM, Joshi SR, Joshi PP, et al. Prevalence of and risk factors for hypertension in urban and rural India: The ICMR–INDIAB study. J Hum Hypertens. 2015;29(3):204-9.
15. Anjana RM, Unnikrishnan R, Deepa M, Pradeepa R, Tandon N, Das AK, et al. Metabolic non-communicable disease health report of India: The ICMR–INDIAB national cross-sectional study (ICMR–INDIAB-17). Lancet Diabetes Endocrinol. 2023;11(7):474-89.
16. Alberti KG, Eckel RH, Grundy SM, Zimmet PZ, Cleeman JI, Donato KA, et al. Harmonizing the metabolic syndrome: A joint interim statement of the International Diabetes Federation Task Force on Epidemiology and Prevention; National Heart, Lung, and Blood Institute; American Heart Association; World Heart Federation; International Atherosclerosis Society; and International Association for the Study of Obesity. Circulation. 2009;120(16):1640-5.
17. Billow A, Anjana RM, Ngai M, Amutha A, Pradeepa R, Jebarani S, Unnikrishnan R, et al. Prevalence and clinical profile of metabolic syndrome among type 1 diabetes mellitus patients in southern India. J Diabetes Complications. 2015;29(5):659-64.
18. Ramachandran A, Snehalatha C, Satyavani K, Sivasankari, S, Vijay V. Metabolic syndrome in urban Asian Indian adults: A population study using modified ATP III criteria. Diabetes Res Clin Pract. 2003;60(3):199-204.
19. Deepa R, Shanthirani CS, Premalatha G, et al. Prevalence of insulin resistance syndrome in a selected south Indian population-the Chennai urban population study-7 (CUPS7). Indian J Med Res 2002;115:118-27.
20. Gupta R, Deedwania PC, Gupta A, Rastogi S, Panwar RB, Kothari K. Prevalence of metabolic syndrome in an Indian urban population. Int J Cardiol. 2004;97(2):257-61.
21. Roy A, Praveen PA, Amarchand R, et al. Changes in hypertension prevalence, awareness, treatment and control rates over 20 years in National Capital Region of India: Results from a repeat cross-sectional study. BMJ Open. 2017;7(7):e015639.
22. Mohan V, Deepa M. The metabolic syndrome in developing countries. Diabet Voice 2006;51(Special issue):15-17.
23. Muruganathan A. Dean's Oration. Hypertension in India: A way forward. Progress in Medicine, Vol. 1; 2017, pp. 293-8.
24. Yanai H, Tomono Y, Ito K, Furutani N, Yoshida H, Tada N. The underlying mechanisms for development of hypertension in the metabolic syndrome. Nutr J. 2008;7:10.
25. Ratto E, Leoncini G, Viazzi F, Vaccaro V, Parodi A, Falqui V, et al. Metabolic syndrome and cardiovascular risk in primary hypertension. J Am Soc Nephrol. 2006;17(4 Suppl. 2):S120-2.

CHAPTER 21

White Coat Hypertension and Masked Hypertension

V Padma, Sarath Bhaskar S

■ INTRODUCTION

White coat hypertension (WCH) is a term used to describe a blood pressure (BP) phenotype seen in untreated people who have high clinic BP but acceptable outside-of-office readings. Since it was originally discovered more than three decades ago, there has been an increasing acknowledgment of this phenomenon, and it is now included in both national and international hypertension guidelines.[1-4] However, there are still significant gaps in our knowledge of WCH. What risk WCH poses and if it needs therapy are still unknown.

The majority of hypertension treatment recommendations concentrate on the average BP measured from either home or workplace readings. On the contrary, BP lability receives less attention. Labile hypertension is a word that almost all doctors are acquainted with, yet there are no quantitative standards for defining or diagnosing it. There are no therapy recommendations, and their implications on cardiovascular (CV) outcomes are uncertain. Additionally, it is unknown how treating the labile aspect of hypertension would affect the result of CV manifestations. Even so, labile BP rise is a frequent clinical problem.

■ WHITE COAT HYPERTENSION

White coat hypertension is an increased BP in the clinic with comparatively normal BP in out of the space. This characteristic trait of BP is called white coat syndrome, and this term is only given to individuals who were never treated and who were not on any medication.

- European Society of Cardiology
  - Blood pressure >140/90 mm Hg in clinic
  - Mean 24-h ambulatory BP <130/80 mm Hg
- American College of Cardiology/American Heart Association
  - Blood pressure >130/80 mm Hg in clinic and home blood pressure (HBP) <135/85 mm Hg
- National Institute for Health and Care Excellence
  - Blood pressure ≥140/90 mm Hg and HBP <135/85 mm Hg.

White coat effect is the contrast between increased BP in clinic and decreased BP in the home and ambulatory BP in all patients who are under treatment or who are not under treatment. White coat effect is significant when the difference between clinic and home raises more than 20/10 mm Hg.

■ EPIDEMIOLOGY

According to a meta-analysis of studies conducted on treated and untreated people, the prevalence of WCH is 13%. This analysis employed cut-off values of 135/85 mm Hg for out-of-clinic BP and 140/90 mm Hg for clinic BP (83 mm Hg in one study).[5] Only 55% of people match the criteria for WCH on both occasions when clinic and ambulatory BP recordings are performed at distinct timepoints.[6] Not every demographic is equally affected by WCH prevalence. Patients with WCH tend to be older, male, obese, and have higher lipid levels compared to normotensive patients.[7]

ETIOLOGY

The practice of taking clinic BP measurements is one of several suggested triggers for the development of WCH. When arriving at the doctor's office and during manual BP measurements using a sphygmomanometer, patients with WCH demonstrate a discrete rise in BP. These BP increases are greater than those that ABPM records during episodes of anxiety or irritation. It's possible that psychological traits, like anxiety, are what cause WCH. Although anxiety is a growing risk factor for many CV illnesses, it is less understood how anxiety affects WCH. High levels of anxiety have been demonstrated to increase the likelihood of pseudoresistant hypertension in individuals taking antihypertensives because of the white coat effect.[8]

The infrequent occurrence of hypertension isn't always due to a doctor in a white coat. Some people have brief spikes in BP as a result of additional stressors like work, any emergencies, or skipping a few days of taking BP medication. Once the trigger has been eliminated, your BP may return to normal, but the rise in BP may still be worrying. The harm may worsen if this transient rise in BP continues for an extended length of time.

PATHOPHYSIOLOGY

The development of WCH has been linked to both the sympathetic and endocrine systems. This has been studied by taking simultaneous readings of arterial BP, heart rate, postganglionic muscle activity, and cutaneous sympathetic nerve activity while a patient is seeing a doctor. During the visit, the subjects showed an increase in their heart rates and BP. An increase in skin sympathetic nerve traffic and a comparable decrease in muscular sympathetic nerve traffic occurred in tandem with this. These alterations persisted for several minutes after the visit was over, with the exception of cutaneous sympathetic nerve traffic.[9] Although WCH is thoroughly described in the medical literature, its prognostic value in CV disease is still up for debate. However, mounting data are beginning to show a connection between WCH and cardiovascular disease (CVD) risk factors, including the emergence of sustained hypertension (SH) and the existence of TOD. Both are significant and independent CV risk factors.

LABILE HYPERTENSION

The word "labile hypertension" meant something quite different from the 1960s until the 1980s. It was then classified as a category in between SH and normotension, with measurement ranging above and below the threshold of 140/90 mm Hg. These days, this can be considered borderline or mild hypertension, with the phrase "labile hypertension" denoting a propensity for significant BP excursions. Despite the limited understanding of the origins and consequences of labile hypertension, a brief review is valuable in developing an empirical strategy to handle this frequent clinical quandary.

It is typical for BP to change from one moment to the next and from day to day. Numerous variables, including physical activity, emotion, position, respiratory cycle, food, salt intake, alcohol use, lack of sleep, and others, are linked to variations in BP. During times of physical or emotional stress, or even without overt provocation, BP fluctuations can be significant, even in people who are otherwise normotensive. Readings in hospitals might vary significantly amongst patients, with some having relatively constant readings

Labile hypertension patients encounter brief but significant spikes in BP. The increases are probably mediated by sympathetic activation and frequently, but not always, take place in conditions of emotional distress, especially worry. Labile hypertension can either be asymptomatic or present with symptoms including flushing, palpitations, and headaches. Normally, the BP drops on its own without any help. Both the doctor and the patient frequently quickly ascribe elevated BP to emotional stress.

Even though BP fluctuation is a common occurrence, patients with certain medical problems could see even normal lability as potentially hazardous. For instance, transient BP elevation might be detrimental and reduction of even normal lability could be proposed as being advantageous in patients with chronic aortic dissection, Marfan syndrome, angina, or cerebral aneurysm, as well as possibly in patients with recurrent nonhypertensive cerebral hemorrhage from amyloid angiopathy.

■ SUSTAINED HYPERTENSION

The risk of having SH is higher in WCH individuals than in normotensives. Systolic blood pressure (SBP) at baseline was the primary predictor of progression to SH, according to the researchers. It is interesting to note that the increase in diastolic blood pressure (DBP) was less pronounced, causing a more pronounced rise in pulse pressure. So, one can speculate that stiffness of the bigger arteries may contribute to the development of SH.[10] The Finn-Home study examined the likelihood that WCH would advance to SH in the general population. After 11 years, 96 (18.2%) of the 528 subjects who were baseline normotensive developed SH. At baseline, 74 (52.1%) of the 142 WCH subjects proceeded to SH. Relative risk (RR) was 2.8 [95% confidence interval (CI):2.2–3.6, $p = 0.0001$] for progression from WCH to SH.[11]

■ TARGET ORGAN DAMAGE

The clinical manifestations of hypertension with target organ damage (TOD) are vascular and hemorrhagic stroke, retinopathy, coronary heart disease/myocardial infarction, heart failure, proteinuria, renal failure, atherosclerotic change in the vasculature, including the emergence of stenoses, and aneurysms. For the early diagnosis of hypertensive vasculopathy, it is currently advised to measure the pulse-wave velocity and the intima-media thickness in the common carotid artery. New electrocardiographic indices and echocardiography can both be used to diagnose left ventricular hypertrophy, a significant factor in hypertensive heart disease. Early indicators of hypertensive nephropathy, such as albuminuria and a lowered glomerular filtration rate, are helpful for prognosis and simple to spot. The most accurate way to diagnose cerebral vascular disease, particularly early microangiopathic alterations, is through magnetic resonance imaging. Blood pressure reduction is the mainstay of treatment for end-organ damage brought on by hypertension. Treatment for early end-organ damage must include the blockade of the renin–angiotensin–aldosterone pathway.

TREATMENT

There is a great deal of debate about the management of WCH. If home readings are actually normal, it would appear unnecessary and possibly detrimental to prescribe antihypertensive medications, as doing so could increase the chance of developing iatrogenic hypotension. Patients must be monitored for a gradual increase in home readings over time due to the increased risk of developing persistent hypertension. If home BP is elevated, treatment should focus on lowering it with the standard pharmacologic medications.

Other than the mean 24-h BP recorded during ambulatory monitoring, there are no established criteria for treating labile hypertension. Regular home monitoring should be avoided because it can lead to increased readings and anxiety. Treatment to obtain more normal readings can be beneficial in lowering BP and breaking the cycle of anxiety in patients whose hypertension is characterized by frequent severe spikes, such as systolic readings >180 mm Hg. In this situation, it would appear preferable to implement a standing regimen containing a α and β blockers, at their typical dosages, in a needed regimen that requires frequent BP checks. The typical angiotensin-converting enzyme (ACE) inhibitor/diuretic combinations do not target sympathetically induced hypertension.

CONCLUSION

Due to the greater risk of developing SH compared to people who are really normotensive, it could be claimed that WCH should be categorized as a "pre-hypertensive" state based on these observations. Although managing labile forms of hypertension is a common clinical problem, there are no established diagnostic standards for labile hypertension and no clinical trials to help with management. This problem's clinical spectrum has been provided, along with a therapeutic strategy based on academic research and physiologic ideas. Studies are required to determine how labile hypertension affects patients and how well treatment works.

REFERENCES

1. Pickering TG, James GD, Boddie C, Harshfield GA, Blank S, Laragh JH, et al. How common is white coat hypertension? JAMA. 1988;259(2):225-8.
2. National Institute for Health and Care Excellance. (2019). Hypertension in adults: Diagnosis and management. [Online] Available from: https://www.nice.org.uk/guidance/ng136 [Last accessed October, 2019].
3. Williams B, Mancia G, Spiering W, Rosei EA, Azizi M, Burnier M, et al. 2018 ESC/ESH guidelines for the management of arterial hypertension. Eur Heart J. 2018; 39(33):3021-104.
4. Whelton PK, Carey RM, Aronow WS, Casey DE Jr, Collins KJ, Himmelfarb CD, et al. 2017 ACC/AHA/AAPA/ABC/ACPM/AGS/APhA/ASH/ASPC/NMA/PCNA guideline for the prevention, detection, evaluation, and management of high blood pressure in adults: a report of the American college of cardiology/American heart association task force on clinical practice guidelines. Hypertension. 2018;71(6):e13-5.
5. Fagard RH, Cornelissen VA. Incidence of cardiovascular events in white-coat, masked and sustained hypertension versus true normotension: a meta-analysis. J Hypertens. 2007;5(11):2193-8.
6. de la Sierra A, Vinyoles E, Banegas JR, Parati G, de la Cruz JJ, Gorostidi M, et al. Short-term and long-term reproducibility of hypertension phenotypes obtained by office and ambulatory

blood pressure measurements. J Clin Hypertens (Greenwich). 2016;18(9):927-33.
7. de la Sierra A, Vinyoles E, Banegas JR, Segura J, Gorostidi M, de la Cruz JJ, et al. Prevalence and clinical characteristics of white-coat hypertension based on different definition criteria in untreated and treated patients. J Hypertens. 2017;35(12):2388-94.
8. Allgulander C. Anxiety as a risk factor in cardiovascular disease. Curr Opin Psychiatry. 2016;29(1):13-7.
9. Grassi G, Turri C, Vailati S, Dell'Oro R, Mancia G. Muscle and skin sympathetic nerve traffic during the "white-coat" effect. Circulation. 1999;100(3):222-5.
10. Mancia G, Bombelli M, Facchetti R, Madotto F, Quarti-Trevano F, Friz HP, et al. Long-term risk of sustained hypertension in white-coat or masked hypertension. Hypertension. 2009;54(2): 226-32.
11. Sivén SSE, Niiranen TJ, Kantola IM, Jula AM. White-coat and masked hypertension as risk factors for progression to sustained hypertension: The Finn-Home study. J Hypertens. 2016;34(1):54-60.

CHAPTER 22

Perioperative Hypertension

Subhajeet Dey

■ INTRODUCTION

Hypertension is one of the most common chronic medical diagnoses. According to a 2002 WHO estimate, hypertension may affect more than 1 billion people worldwide and may lead to death in around 7.1 million people.[1] Hypertension is known to result in end-organ damage of the heart, brain, kidneys, eyes, etc. Hypertension is also known as a "silent killer" as most of the patients are asymptomatic, and the associated complications are serious. Perioperative hypertension may result in morbidity like excessive surgical bleeding, cardiac ischemia, heart failure, etc., and also may be a cause of mortality, hence the management of hypertension in this cohort cannot be overemphasized. So, it is vital that all healthcare personnel involved in the care of hypertensive patients in the perioperative period are knowledgeable regarding the care and management of patients with hypertension.

■ PERIOPERATIVE HYPERTENSION

The term perioperative period usually includes preoperative, intraoperative, and postoperative periods. Perioperative hypertension may be encountered during induction of anesthesia. Intraoperatively hypertension is usually secondary to pain-induced stimulation of the sympathetic system as is also seen with hypothermia, hypoxia, and intravascular fluid overload. In the early postoperative period of 24–48 h, it may be due to the fluid being mobilized from extravascular space so also may be due to discontinuation of long-term antihypertensive therapy.[2] Perioperative hypertension is found to occur in about 25% of hypertensive patients undergoing surgery[3,4] and common predictors being a previous history of hypertension, especially a diastolic blood pressure greater than 110 mm Hg, and the type of surgery.[5] Hypertensive events are common with carotid surgery, abdominal aortic surgery, peripheral vascular surgery or procedures, and intraperitoneal or intrathoracic surgery.[4] It is recommended that patients on antihypertensive medications should continue with their treatment regimen prior to surgery, including the morning of surgery to lessen intraoperative blood pressure fluctuations.[6] Intraoperative blood pressure rise of more than 20% are considered as hypertensive emergencies.[6] Postoperative hypertension is common in the early postoperative period and is secondary to increased sympathetic tone and vascular resistance,[7,8] and usually begins 10–20 min after surgery and may last up to 4 h.[9]

■ CLINICAL EXAMINATION

It is usual for most of the patients to report their hypertensive status during the preoperative visit, yet there is a sizeable number of patients who are either unaware of their being hypertensive or do not disclose it for various reasons.

Other than the general history, one should also focus on symptoms associated with or suggestive of end-organ damage. Common symptoms usually inquired about include chest pain or pressure over the chest, dyspnea on exertion, orthopnea, or paroxysmal nocturnal dyspnea. In addition, note should be made of the distance a person can walk on level ground, and the number of flights of stairs he/she can climb before the onset of symptoms.

Certain signs elicited may also indicate changes in end organs. Distended neck veins are indicative of fluid overload or congestive heart failure, as also in isolated pulmonary hypertension. Fine crepitations over the chest may be heard in congestive heart failure or pulmonary infections. In patients with congestive heart failure with a dilated left ventricle, S3 gallop may be heard; however, it may also be present in athletes and healthy pregnant women. S4 may be heard in the presence of left ventricular hypertrophy or in diastolic heart failure.[10] Detailed neurological examinations are needed in case of a history of prior stroke or other neurological conditions. The fundoscopy examination may reveal changes secondary to hypertension.

Blood pressure should be measured in both arms in a quiet room, usually in a sitting position. and the importance of a properly sized and fitting cuff cannot be ignored, with undersized cuffs being notorious for the erroneous high blood pressure recording.[11,12] Blood pressure recording of more than 130/80 mm Hg but less than 160/90 mm Hg in a non-hypertensive patient may indicate white coat hypertension and warrants regular blood pressure monitoring. Approximately 1–5% of white coat hypertension individuals may eventually get converted to sustained hypertension, especially obese or elderly population.[13]

■ EVALUATION

It is advisable that the patient is seen and evaluated in the preoperative clinic well in advance, at least a week prior to elective surgery thus allowing time to change management, if required, to optimize the health and blood pressure preoperatively. If blood pressure is well controlled and history and examinations are unremarkable, further specialized testing may not be required if uncomplicated surgery is expected, however, it may not be so for an expected complicated surgery or if history and physical examinations raise concern. Appropriate investigations may be asked for depending on the nature of concern detected on history and examination. X-ray chest, electrocardiogram (ECG) including stress ECG, Echocardiogram: transthoracic or transesophageal, including a Doppler echo or a stress echo may be required. Cardiologist referral may be sought to determine appropriate tests and also to asses preoperative risk and get focused recommendations for perioperative care. Similarly, neurological signs and symptoms should be assessed preoperatively by a neurologist for risk stratification and focused recommendations. A basic metabolic profile is indicated in hypertensive patients and a raised serum creatinine can indicate impaired renal function. Serum electrolytes should be estimated if patients are on medications that impact electrolytes and need to be done on the day of surgery too. Complete blood count and platelet count are routinely indicated and more so if the procedure is expected to have significant blood loss. Other investigations may be advised depending on the clinical conditions of the patient as well as depending on the primary diagnosis for which the operation is being planned.

EVALUATION ON DAY OF SURGERY

For elective surgery, patients should have normal blood pressure on the day of surgery, however, anxiety may lead to some increase. Patients are expected to have fluctuations in blood pressure in the perioperative period if systolic and diastolic blood pressures recorded on the day of surgery reach 170 and 100 mm Hg, respectively.

In the event of either systolic blood pressure or diastolic blood pressure recordings are 180 mm Hg or 110 mm Hg, in otherwise normotensive patients it is recommended that the elective surgery should be postponed until blood pressure is adequately controlled. The same is the case in a previously diagnosed hypertensive patient on medications, who has not missed the dose of antihypertensive medication on the morning of the day of surgery.

Furthermore, a hypertensive patient with controlled blood pressure on medications, who has missed the morning dose of the antihypertensive medication, may have a systolic blood pressure of 180 mm Hg and diastolic blood pressure of 110 mm Hg on the day of surgery. In such a situation the routine dose of medication may be given with a sip of water, and anxiolytics may also be administered. Rescheduling the order of the list may also be considered, so equivalent intravenous antihypertensives may be considered. However, it is also pertinent to consider the fact that systolic blood pressure of 180 mm Hg or more has been labeled as a hypertensive crisis by the American College of Cardiology/American Heart Association and caution needs to be exercised in the decision to proceed with surgery in such a situation. Similarly, diastolic blood pressure of 110 mm Hg or more is also an independent cardiovascular complications risk factor. It is also associated with ECG changes suggesting myocardial ischemia in the event of blood pressure drops to below 50% of awake mean arterial pressure.[14] Caution needs to be exercised in such a situation also. In the event of blood pressure recorded at 200 mm Hg on the day of surgery, surgery should be canceled as it carries twice the risk of rise of troponin in the postoperative period, so does the risk of death in comparison to patients with lower blood pressure.[15]

If surgery needs to proceed due to the emergency condition of the patient with uncontrolled hypertension, adequate precautions need to be taken. An urgent ECG and echocardiogram may be obtained, if recent investigations are not available. In the event of significant abnormalities detected, cardiologists' interpretation of the reports and consultation cannot be more emphasized. Careful monitoring of blood pressure with an intra-arterial line may be instituted and pharmacological therapies should be available to treat the hypertension in the perioperative period including in the postoperative care unit/intensive care unit.

MANAGEMENT

Initiation of the treatment for hypertension should be started electively after several measurements of blood pressure on at least two occasions and not immediately prior to surgery. Diet, control of weight, exercise, and salt restrictions are the initial interventions along with medications as indicated. Primary agents are thiazide diuretics, calcium channel blockers, angiotensin-converting enzyme (ACE) inhibitors or angiotensin receptors blockers, and secondary agents are loop diuretics, potassium-sparing diuretics, aldosterone antagonists, β-blockers, α1-blockers, centrally acting drug, and vasodilators. Description of initiation, and use of these agents, has been described.[16]

Concern regarding the continuation of diuretics on the day of surgery is due to the overnight fast; however, they may be given at a reduced dose or even the full dose in patients with severe congestive heart failure, perhaps at the discretion of the anesthesiologist at the day of surgery after measuring the blood pressure and auscultating the heart and the lungs. Patients on β-blockers should receive the dose on the day of surgery; however, it should not be initiated on the day of surgery even though it may decrease cardiac events, it increases the risk of bradycardia, stroke, and death.[17] Both ACE and ARB are usually continued on the day of surgery even though they may induce intraoperative hypotension.[18,19]

Maintenance of safe levels of blood pressure intraoperatively by anesthesiologists may be achieved by anesthetics, analgesia, and antihypertensives, tailored to the needs of a specific patient based upon preexisting end-organ damage due to hypertension or the blood pressure recorded on the day of surgery.

Regional nerve blocks induce minimal hemodynamic changes, whereas spinal and epidural techniques may permit spontaneous ventilation; however, they are associated with significant drops in blood pressure, which may however be corrected by volume infusion or use of vasoconstrictors.

There may be a large reduction of blood pressure during the administration of anesthesia in poorly controlled hypertensive patients and both uncontrolled hypertension and blood pressure drop may pose a significant risk to perioperative complications.

Severe intraoperative hypertension may be treated by intravenous sodium nitroprusside, nicardipine, or nitroglycerin. Hydralazine may be used for long-term control and doses of 5mg may reduce the systolic blood pressure by 25 mm Hg or more.

■ CONCLUSION

Hypertension is commonly encountered in the perioperative period with its associated risks of end-organ damage. The goal of managing perioperative hypertension is to protect organ function assuming that the risk of complications is reduced with improved outcomes. Perioperative hypertension requires careful management. The ideal antihypertensive, in the event of an acute rise in blood pressure in the perioperative period, should provide an early onset of action with a short or intermediate duration of action, be easy to titrate the dose precisely, and be safe and effective.[2]

■ REFERENCES

1. World Health Organization. (2002). Reducing risks, promoting healthy life. The World Health Report: 2002. [Online] Available from: https://www.who.int/publications/i/item/9241562072 [Last accessed November, 2023].
2. Varon J, Marik PE. Perioperative hypertension management. Vasc Health Risk Manag. 2008;4(3):615-27.
3. Prys-Roberts C, Greene LT, Meloche R, Foëx P. Studies of anaesthesia in relation to hypertension. II. Haemodynamic onsequences of induction and endotracheal intubation. Br J Anaesth. 1971;43(6):531-47.
4. Goldman L, Caldera DL. Risks of general anesthesia and elective operation in the hypertensive patient. Anesthesiology. 1979;50(4):285-92.
5. Aronson S, Boisvert D, Lapp W. Isolated systolic hypertension is associated with adverse outcomes from coronary artery

bypass grafting surgery. Anesth Analg. 2002;94(5):1079-84.
6. Goldberg ME, Larijani GE. 1998. Perioperative hypertension. Pharmacotherapy. 18(5):911-4.
7. Roberts AJ, Noarchos AP, Subramanian AV, Abel RM, Herman SD, Sealey JE, et al. Systemic hypertension associated with coronary artery bypass surgery. Predisposing factors, hemodynamic characteristics, humoral profile, and treatment. J Thorac Cardiovasc Surg. 1977;74(6):846-59.
8. Alper A, Calhoun D. Hypertensive emergencies. In: Antam EM (Ed). Cardiovascular therapeutics: A companion to Braunwald's heart Disease, 2nd edition. Philadelphia, PA: WB Saunders Co; 2002.
9. Towne JB, Bernherd VM. The relationship between postoperative hypertension to complications following carotid endarterectomy. Surgery.1980;88(4):575-80.
10. Andrès E, Gass R, Charloux A, Brandt C, Hentzler A. Respiratory sound analysis in the era of evidence-based medicine and the world of medicine 2.0. J Med Life. 2018;11(2):89-106.
11. Pickering TG, Hall JE, Appel LJ, Falkner BE, Graves J, Hill MN, et al. Recommendations for blood pressure measurement in humans and experimental animals: Part 1 – Blood pressure measurement in humans: A statement for professionals from the Subcommittee of Professional and Public Education of the American Heart Association Council on High Blood Pressure Research. Circulation. 2005;111(5):697-716.
12. Bartels K, Esper SA, Thiele RH. Blood pressure monitoring for the anesthesiologist: A practical review. Anesth Analg. 2016; 122(6):1866-79.
13. Gill R, Goldstein S. Evaluation and management of perioperative hypertension. In: StatPearls. [Online] Treasure Island (FL): StatPearls Publishing; 2022. Available from: https://www.ncbi.nlm.nih.gov/books/NBK557830/ [Last accessed November, 2023].
14. Prys-Roberts C, Meloche R, Foëx P. Studies of anaesthesia in relation to hypertension. I. Cardiovascular responses of treated and untreated patients. Br J Anaesth. 1971;43(2): 122-37.
15. Wax DB, Porter SB, Lin HM, Hossain S, Reich DL. Association of preanesthesia hypertension with adverse outcomes. J Cardiothorac Vasc Anesth. 2010;24(6):927-30.
16. Whelton PK, Carey RM, Aronow WS, Casey DE, Collins KJ, Himmelfarb CD, et al. 2017 ACC/AHA/AAPA/ABC/ACPM/AGS/APhA/ASH/ASPC/NMA/PCNA Guideline for the prevention, detection, evaluation, and management of high blood pressure in adults: Executive summary: A Report of the American College of Cardiology/American Heart Association Task Force on Clinical Practice Guidelines. Hypertension. 2018;71(6):1269-324.
17. Lindenauer PK, Pekow P, Wang K, Mamidi DK, Gutierrez B, Benjamin EM. Perioperative beta-blocker therapy and mortality after major noncardiac surgery. N Engl J Med. 2005;353(4):349-61.
18. Roshanov PS, Rochwerg B, Patel A, Salehian O, Duceppe E, Belley-Côté EP, Guyatt GH, et al. Withholding versus continuing angiotensin converting enzyme inhibitors or angiotensin II receptor blockers before noncardiac surgery: An analysis of the vascular events in noncardiac surgery patients cohort evaluation prospective cohort. Anesthesiology. 2017;126(1):16-27.
19. Hollmann C, Fernandes NL, Biccard BM. A systematic review of outcomes associated with withholding or continuing angiotensin-converting enzyme inhibitors and angiotensin receptor blockers before noncardiac surgery. Anesth Analg. 2018;127(3):678-87.

Blood Pressure Variability and Target Organ Damage

NR Rau, Shivashankara KN

■ INTRODUCTION

Hypertension stands as the most prominent contributor to the global burden of disease and mortality, ranking among the foremost preventable causes of death on a global scale. It accounts for over 12.8% of annual deaths. Anticipated trends suggest an impending increase in the number of affected individuals and the prevalence of high blood pressure (BP) worldwide over the coming decade. This condition holds the distinction of being the most prevalent modifiable risk factor for a range of critical health issues, including stroke, coronary artery disease, heart failure, chronic kidney disease, and aortic and peripheral arterial disease. Remarkably, it contributes to approximately 50% of overall risk.[1] The continuous and dynamic nature of BP, which responds to a multitude of influences such as physical and mental activities, sleep, as well as autonomic, humoral, mechanical, myogenic, and environmental factors, results in pronounced fluctuations over both short and long periods.

This variability poses a diagnostic challenge, as a single measurement obtained through office blood pressure monitoring (OBPM) or home blood pressure monitoring (HBPM) might significantly deviate from an individual's average daytime and nighttime BP. Consequently, accurate diagnosis and appropriate treatment prescription are intricate tasks. The overarching objective of BP control centers on mitigating target-organ damage, preventing cardiovascular (CV) disease, and averting premature mortality in hypertensive patients. Nevertheless, current antihypertensive therapies do not eliminate all risks associated with hypertension; rather, they reduce these risks by roughly one-third, constituting a meaningful yet suboptimal outcome.[2] The concept of "usual BP," representing the underlying true level of BP, is widely considered the primary determinant of BP-linked vascular risk and the potential benefits of antihypertensive intervention.

Despite the apparent simplicity of diagnosing high BP, clinical practice reveals that misdiagnosis is not uncommon. Even after years of research, several unresolved issues remain regarding optimal BP classification.[3] The American Heart Association guidelines on BP measurement emphasize the consensus that conventional clinic readings serve as a surrogate marker for a patient's actual BP and are pivotal in determining its adverse effects. As a result, clinic BP assumes a central role in diagnosing, assessing the severity of hypertension, and guiding clinical decision making as per the existing guidelines.

An illustrative example of this complexity lies in the phenomena of isolated office hypertension (high BP at the doctor's office despite normal BP elsewhere) and masked hypertension (normal BP at the doctor's office but high BP outside the clinical setting).

These occurrences often lead to frequent misjudgments in assessing BP-associated CV risk. The inherent variability in BP serves as a primary culprit behind the misdiagnosis of hypertension, underscoring the challenge it poses.[4]

Over the past few decades, a mounting body of evidence has highlighted that beyond absolute BP values, elevated blood pressure variability (BPV) significantly correlates with the development, progression, and severity of cardiac, renal, and vascular damage. Moreover, it is linked with an augmented risk of CV mortality.[5-7] Notably, when comparing individuals at high CV risk to those at low-moderate risk, heightened BPV appears to hold a greater prognostic value.[8]

Physicians often approach hypertension treatment under the fundamental assumption that achieving lower BP levels is beneficial, as long as diastolic BP maintains adequate coronary perfusion. However, the precise component of BP that triggers vascular events remains inadequately understood. While mean BP (the average of multiple systolic or diastolic BP readings) is evidently pivotal, other factors such as variability (fluctuations over time) or instability (temporary BP fluctuations) may also contribute during critical periods of vascular events. The prevailing approach advocates for pharmacological regimens that consistently and indiscriminately reduce BP throughout the entire day. However, findings from the Ambulatory Blood Pressure Monitoring for Prediction of Cardiovascular Events study challenge this conventional understanding, holding the potential to induce noteworthy shifts in hypertension management practices.[9]

While average clinic BP values remain the cornerstone for diagnosing and treating hypertension, recent studies among hypertensive individuals have revealed the significance of assessing and quantifying BPV alongside absolute BP values. This dual approach has physiological, pathological, and prognostic implications. Strong evidence indicates that elevated BPV is independently linked to an increased risk of target-organ damage, CV events, and mortality. Thus, managing BPV in addition to reducing absolute BP levels could offer comprehensive CV protection for hypertensive patients.

■ BLOOD PRESSURE VARIABILITY

Blood pressure variability can be defined as the fluctuations in BP over time, resulting from a complex interplay among various CV control mechanisms. These variations are observed during shifts between daily life behaviors and are triggered by environmental circumstances.[10] The extent of these fluctuations varies among individuals, with higher levels observed in those with impaired CV control mechanisms.[11] Examples of routine fluctuations include BP elevation following physical activity or psychological stress, and BP reduction during relaxation or sleep.[10]

Studies on populations with high CV risk have demonstrated that high BPV values are strong predictors of both CV mortality and morbidity, surpassing the predictive value of average BP values. Depending on the timeframe of measurements, BPV can be categorized into the following five types: Very short-term, short-term, mid-term, long-term, and very long-term.[12] Very short-term BPV pertains to beat-to-beat variability, while variations over 24 h are referred to as short-term BPV. Day-to-day variability falls under the category of mid-term BPV. Long-term and very long-term BPV encompass visit-to-visit variabilities (VVV) in BP measurements, with the former covering periods less than 5 years and the latter spanning beyond 5 years.

Blood pressure variability exhibits a strong relationship with BP levels; higher BP levels are associated with increased BPV. Various indices have been developed to measure different types of BPV, with the standard deviation (SD) of the 24-h mean BP being a common measure.[13] The coefficient of variation is also utilized across all five types of BPV, particularly for assessing long-term BPV. Different indices, such as spectral analysis of frequency domain for beat-to-beat variability and average real variability (ARV) for short-term BPV, are employed to capture specific aspects of BPV.[12,14] Average real variability calculates the average of absolute differences between consecutive BP measurements over 24 h, focusing on within-subject short-term variability.[12]

Numerous intrinsic and extrinsic factors influence different types of BPV. In a population-based study of ethnically diverse adult Chinese subjects, it was found that various demographic, clinical, and biochemical factors influence BPV. Notably, average night-time systolic blood pressure (SBP), average daytime diastolic BP, triglyceride levels, fasting blood glucose, and apolipoprotein A were identified as significantly and independently associated with BPV.[15]

Very Short-term BPV

Very short-term BPV pertains to the rapid fluctuations in BP that occur on a beat-to-beat basis. These fluctuations arise from the intricate interplay of various CV control systems, including the baroreceptor reflex, the renin–angiotensin system, the vascular myogenic response, endothelium-mediated nitric oxide release, and shifts in behavioral and emotional factors.[16-18] These dynamic processes collectively contribute to the moment-to-moment changes in BP levels.

The assessment of very short-term BPV can be conducted in a laboratory setting using intra-arterial recordings or under ambulatory conditions with the help of noninvasive finger cuffs equipped with infrared photoplethysmography to continuously monitor finger BP.[16-19] Indices commonly employed to evaluate very short-term BPV include SDs of BP values or fluctuations derived from spectral analyses across various frequency ranges.

While the practical utility and reliability of very short-term BPV assessment may be subject to debate, it has been employed in clinical settings to aid in the diagnosis and management of CV disease.[16,18,20] Furthermore, this approach has been utilized to investigate the mechanisms of action of antihypertensive medications. By detecting alterations in beat-to-beat BPV, clinicians can make informed decisions regarding the selection of antihypertensive drugs tailored to a patient's specific physiological characteristics.[17] For example, individuals with hypertensive conditions characterized by elevated low-frequency BPV might exhibit heightened sympathetic modulation of vascular tone. As a result, they could potentially benefit from antihypertensive drugs that target sympathetic activity, known as sympatholytic agents.[18] This tailored approach to medication selection based on very short-term BPV can contribute to optimizing treatment outcomes for patients with hypertension.

Short-term BPV

Short-term BPV has garnered significant attention in relation to CV health. Studies focusing on intra-arterial BPV recorded over the course of a day were among the first attempts to correlate short-term BPV with heightened CV mortality and target organ damage.[5,21] Ambulatory blood pressure monitoring (ABPM) has become a prevalent method for analyzing BPV patterns throughout a 24-h period. Ambulatory blood pressure monitoring allows for the assessment of BP circadian rhythms and their potential associations with CV morbidity and mortality in hypertensive subpopulations and the general population.[22-25]

Various BPV phenotypes are assessed through ABPM, including parameters like SD of average systolic, diastolic, and mean BP over different periods (daytime, nighttime, wakefulness, and sleep), the percentage of BP decrease between night and day (sleeptime/wakefulness), and the morning blood pressure surge (MBPS). Elevated nighttime BP has been demonstrated as a predictor of CV events and damage, often surpassing awake or 24-h BP mean values.[22,26-29] A blunted nocturnal BP decrease (nondipping) or an inverted increase in nighttime BP (inverted dipping) have been linked to a higher prevalence of vascular damage, increased CV risk, and mortality.[30,31]

The MBPS, characterized by an increase in BP upon waking, has been associated with target organ damage, such as left ventricular hypertrophy, albuminuria, arterial stiffness, and cerebrovascular disease.[32,33] However, findings regarding MBPS as a risk factor for CV disease have shown some discrepancies in clinical trials. Although some studies found a positive association between MBPS and CV outcomes, there is no consensus on the threshold at which MBPS becomes pathological, and its prognostic significance remains uncertain.[31,32,34] As a result, there is ongoing debate about whether targeting MBPS for treatment offers greater benefits compared to targeting clinic BP.[35] Despite these uncertainties, morning BP remains an important focus of antihypertensive treatment in current clinical practice for managing hypertension.[32]

Mid-term, Long-term and Very Long-term Blood Pressure Variability

Long-term BPV encompasses changes in BP that occur over longer time intervals, including day-to-day, visit-to-visit, and season-to-season fluctuations.[7,19] The factors contributing to long-term BPV are not fully understood and may arise from various sources. In treated patients, inadequate treatment, poor patient adherence, or inaccurate BP measurement methods could lead to poor BP control and increased long-term BPV.[7,19] Behavioral changes, such as lifestyle modifications, and environmental factors like seasonal variations in temperature and daylight hours can also influence long-term BPV.[19,36]

Studies have indicated that BPV tends to be greater during winter compared to summer, potentially due to increased sympathetic activity leading to enhanced sodium retention and vascular resistance.[36] Additionally, some research suggests that increased arterial stiffness might contribute to the development of long-term BPV.

Assessment of day-to-day BPV can be conducted using ABPM over a 48-h period or HBPM data collected over extended periods. Visit-to-visit BPV is typically evaluated using ABPM or conventional in-office BP measurements (OBPM) taken during spaced visits over weeks, months, or years. However, the reliability of OBPM in assessing long-term BPV has been questioned due to potential inaccuracies and variations caused by factors such as the white-coat effect, device calibration, and measurement techniques.[7,19]

Increased long-term BPV has been associated with a higher risk of stroke, CV events, and mortality, including all-cause mortality.[37,38] Therefore, measuring long-term BPV could hold clinical significance by providing insights into a patient's BP control over the long term and the effectiveness of their current antihypertensive treatment.[7] Monitoring and addressing long-term BPV may contribute to optimizing CV protection and improving patient outcomes.

TOOLS TO MEASURE BLOOD PRESSURE VARIABILITY

Various tools are available for measuring BPV, each with its own advantages and limitations. One such tool is 24-h ABPM, which provides a comprehensive and accurate assessment of BPV. ABPM involves continuous recording of BP over a 24-h period, allowing for the evaluation of various parameters including mean BP, variations between daytime and nighttime, pressure loads, area under the curve, and pulse pressure variability. Additionally, ABPM enables the assessment of short-term BPV between measurement intervals of 15 min or less, providing detailed insights into fluctuations throughout the day.[39]

The clinical applications of ABPM are valuable, including the accurate diagnosis and prediction of CV risk.[40] ABPM can help identify conditions such as white coat hypertension (higher BP in clinical settings than outside) and masked hypertension (normal clinic BP but elevated outside), as well as detect abnormal BP patterns over a 24-h period. It is also useful for assessing the effectiveness of antihypertensive treatment.[41]

However, ABPM has some limitations, including discomfort during nighttime measurements, occasional difficulty in distinguishing genuine measurements from artifacts, limited availability of devices, and higher cost compared to other methods. As an alternative, repeated measurements using well-calibrated automated BP monitoring devices can be obtained at home (HBPM) or in a clinical setting (OBPM). From these measurements, BPV can be calculated by determining the SD or coefficient of variation.

Each of these methods has its strengths and weaknesses, and the choice of tool depends on clinical context, patient preferences, and the specific goals of BPV assessment.

BLOOD PRESSURE VARIABILITY AND CARDIAC HYPERTROPHY

Blood pressure variability has been associated with various CV complications, including cardiac hypertrophy. Studies have indicated that mean BP values obtained through 24-h blood pressure monitoring (ABPM) can predict the presence of left ventricular hypertrophy (LVH) more effectively than a single BP measurement.[23]

Research has shown that an increase in 24-h BPV, especially during daytime, as recorded with ABPM, is linked to a higher risk of hypertensive CV complications, including LV systolic dysfunction.[42,43] The relationship between BPV and LVH has been mainly studied in the context of short-term variability.[43-45] Patterns such as nondipping of nighttime BP and an exaggerated MBPS have been associated with greater left ventricular mass and CV morbidity in both the general population and hypertensive patients.[46,47]

However, the correlation between short-term BPV and LV mass indexes is considered weak based on some studies, and there have been challenges in evaluating the CV impact of both short-term and long-term BPV.[48,49] The reproducibility of BPV measurements, lack of normal reference values, and limitations of available ABPM devices have contributed to these challenges.[50,71]

To better understand the role of BPV in CV disease, preclinical studies have been conducted. Animal models, such as the sinoaortic denervated (SAD) rat, have provided insights into the effects of BPV on target organs. The SAD rat model, which involves the ablation of carotid and aortic baroreceptor afferents, increases short-term BPV while maintaining normal average BP levels.[51] This model has been valuable in studying the consequences of BPV on cardiac hypertrophy and other aspects of CV health.

In summary, there is evidence to suggest that increased BPV, particularly short-term variability, is associated with cardiac hypertrophy and other CV complications. Further research, including preclinical studies, is needed to fully understand the mechanisms underlying these associations and to explore potential therapeutic strategies to mitigate the adverse effects of BPV on CV health.

BLOOD PRESSURE VARIABILITY AND CHRONIC KIDNEY DISEASE

People with end-stage renal disease often experience significant BP variations and disruptions in their circadian BP rhythm. While short-term BPV studies in humans have not consistently demonstrated a direct influence of BPV on the prognostic role of mean BP levels in the development or progression of renal dysfunction, there is evidence suggesting a potential correlation between BPV and impaired renal function.

Some studies have indicated a positive correlation between increased short-term BPV and markers of impaired renal function, such as microalbuminuria or estimated glomerular filtration rate.[7,52] However, the results of longitudinal studies are more consistent in highlighting the significance of specific BP patterns, particularly during nighttime, in predicting poor renal outcomes.[53,54] A nondipper or inverted dipper pattern of nighttime BP assessed through 24-h ABPM has been shown to be an independent predictor of an unfavorable renal prognosis, as indicated by various clinical markers of renal function.

Home blood pressure monitoring has also demonstrated predictive value for the impairment of renal function in some studies, although results have not been uniform across all investigations.[55,56] Visit-to-visit BPV, which involves assessing BP fluctuations across multiple clinical visits, has emerged as a potentially valuable indicator for predicting the risk of developing and progressing nephropathy and chronic kidney disease.[57,58]

In summary, while the relationship between short-term BPV and renal dysfunction is less clear, longitudinal studies and patterns of nighttime BP assessed through ABPM suggest a stronger association with poor renal outcomes. HBPM and visit-to-visit BPV have also shown promise in predicting the risk of renal impairment. Further research is needed to fully elucidate the complex interplay between BPV and chronic kidney disease and to determine the clinical implications for managing renal health in individuals with BP fluctuations.

BLOOD PRESSURE VARIABILITY, CEREBROVASCULAR DYSFUNCTION, AND BRAIN DAMAGE

Hypertension plays a pivotal role in the development of carotid atherosclerotic lesions and cerebral small vessel disease (CSVD), both of which contribute to an increased risk of stroke and cognitive decline, particularly in the elderly population.[59] Detecting early involvement of these vascular territories before clinical manifestations occur could offer the potential to prevent future brain damage.[60]

Both short-term and long-term BPV have been identified as independent risk factors for stroke in elderly hypertensive patients.[61] Disturbed nighttime BP decline has been associated with cerebral infarction, while a significant morning surge and substantial nocturnal BP decline have been linked to cerebral hemorrhage.[32] BPV has also been associated with lower cognitive test scores in elderly individuals and has been proposed as a predictor of cognitive decline in middle-aged subjects at high risk.[62,63] Long-term BPV has been linked to psychomotor speed and verbal memory impairment in young subjects over a 25-year follow-up period, independently of BP levels.[64]

The relationship between BPV and early stages of carotid artery damage has been established for more than a decade and is supported by recent studies.[65,66] Nondipping patterns and exaggerated MBPSs have been associated with increased carotid intima-media thickness and elevated levels of blood inflammatory markers in elderly individuals with high CV risk and middle-aged hypertensive subjects.[34,66,67] Furthermore, day-to-day BPV is connected not only to carotid artery atherosclerosis but also to arterial stiffness and endothelial dysfunction in normotensive and mild-moderate hypertensive individuals.[68,69]

Cerebral small vessel disease appears to serve as a link between the pathophysiologic mechanisms of stroke and cognitive impairment. Recent research suggests that short-term BPV may be related to the presence of subclinical CSVD in hypertensive subjects, independent of BP levels and other clinical factors.[70] This emphasizes the significance of understanding and managing BPV in order to potentially prevent or mitigate the adverse effects of cerebrovascular dysfunction and brain damage.

Blood Pressure Variability as a Target for Antihypertensive Treatment: Short and Long-term Studies

The role of BPV as a target for antihypertensive treatment and its impact on organ damage and CV outcomes is still a subject of debate in clinical practice. Recent publications have focused on analyzing whether different classes of antihypertensive drugs can effectively reduce BPV, regardless of their effects on overall BP levels. Additionally, some studies have investigated the association between the reduction in BPV through pharmacological treatment and improvements in target organ damage, potentially leading to a decrease in CV events.

A significant portion of the available data comes from post hoc analyses of clinical trials and databases, which have utilized various classes of antihypertensive drugs and examined different clusters of target organ damage and CV outcomes. These studies have also considered different BPV phenotypes, including short-term BPV assessed by ABPM and long-term BPV assessed by HBPM, VVV, or longer intervals such as between different seasons.

A recent systematic review aimed to compare the effectiveness of various classes of antihypertensive drugs in preventing stroke. The review found that calcium channel blockers (CCBs) and nonloop diuretics were associated with the greatest reduction in inter-individual variation in SBP, while angiotensin-converting enzyme inhibitors (ACEi), angiotensin receptor blockers (ARB), and β-adrenergic receptor blockers (βB) were associated with increased BPV.[71]

A post hoc analysis of two large clinical trials compared the effects of amlodipine-based and atenolol-based treatments on both within-visit and ABPM variability. The analysis showed that amlodipine decreased BPV over time and reduced the risk of stroke, while atenolol had the opposite effect.[72]

A meta-analysis of an ABPM database evaluated different antihypertensive treatments and their effects on BPV. It was found that subjects treated with telmisartan or amlodipine had a smoother 24-h BP reduction profile compared to those treated with losartan, valsartan, or ramipril.[73] The combination of telmisartan and amlodipine was associated with a smoother and lower 24-h BP profile compared to various monotherapies, indicating its effectiveness in reducing BP and maintaining stable levels over time.[74]

In conclusion, the relationship between antihypertensive treatment, BPV reduction, and CV outcomes is complex and requires further investigation. While some classes of antihypertensive drugs appear to be more effective in reducing BPV than others, the impact of BPV reduction on target organ damage and CV events remains a topic of ongoing research.

The study you described involves a randomized, double-blind, placebo-controlled design with four parallel treatment arms (placebo, candesartan, indapamide, and amlodipine) to analyze short-term BPV using ABPM data.[75] The key findings from this study include:

1. Amlodipine and indapamide treatments were associated with a significant reduction in BPV. However, it was noted that the effect of amlodipine on BPV was also linked to a reduction in BP levels.
2. Another investigation focused on the following two antihypertensive drug combinations: Olmesartan combined with a CCB and olmesartan combined with a diuretic. This study demonstrated that the ARB/CCB combination not only improved home blood pressure variability (HBPV) but also reduced arterial stiffness. The reduction in HBPV was partially attributed to the decrease in arterial stiffness.[76]
3. A study assessed the time-dependent efficacy of valsartan/hydrochlorothiazide combination therapy on BPV using ABPM. The results indicated that bedtime administration of the combination therapy led to a significantly greater proportion of subjects with well-controlled ambulatory BP compared to treatment upon awakening.[77]
4. The study compared visit-to-visit intraindividual variations in BP between patients treated with atenolol and lacidipine. The findings suggested that visit-to-visit BPV did not differ substantially between β-blocker (βB) and CCB treatment.[78]
5. Indices of short-term BPV were evaluated in patients treated with different antihypertensive drug classes. Patients treated with CCB and diuretics, either alone or in combination with other drugs, had lower BPV compared to those not receiving these classes.[79]
6. The impact of visit-to-visit BPV on target organ damage and CV outcomes in patients with left ventricular hypertrophy randomized to losartan- and atenolol-based treatment was analyzed. Higher in-treatment BPV, independently of mean BP, was associated with later stroke and composite CV events.[52]
7. A comparison of visit-to-visit BPV between different age groups and treatment combinations (ARB/CCB and

ARB/diuretic) revealed that long-term variability was smaller in the ARB/CCB group, particularly in very old and isolated systolic hypertensive patients.[80]

8. A study investigated the effects of three CCB-based treatments (CCB/ARB, CCB/βB, and CCB/diuretic) on intraindividual visit-to-visit BPV, with BPV being lower in the CCB/diuretic group compared to the CCB/βB group.

9. An assessment of a fixed-dose combination of perindopril/amlodipine in various settings (doctor's office, home, and ABPM) showed significant reductions in BP levels and improvements in various parameters related to BPV.[81]

These findings collectively contribute to the growing understanding of how different antihypertensive drugs impact BPV and its potential implications for CV outcomes and organ damage.

Yes, based on the studies you have described, there is evidence to suggest that CCBs as monotherapy or in combination with diuretics may be more effective in reducing BPV and certain CV outcomes compared to other antihypertensive drugs alone or in different combinations.

The findings from these studies indicate that CCBs, particularly when combined with diuretics, may have a positive impact on BPV, which could potentially contribute to better CV outcomes. These effects may be attributed to the specific mechanisms of action of CCBs and their ability to influence the CV control mechanisms that contribute to BPV.

However, it is important to note that while these findings suggest a potential benefit of CCBs in reducing BPV and improving CV outcomes, the choice of antihypertensive treatment should still be based on individual patient characteristics, preferences, and overall health considerations. Additionally, more research and clinical trials are needed to further validate and understand the specific role of CCBs in managing BPV and CV risk.

■ CONCLUSION

While the concept of BPV has been under evaluation for many years, its precise clinical implications remain complex and not fully established. Despite evidence demonstrating the potential of BPV to contribute to target organ damage, its practical significance in routine clinical practice has not been widely embraced. This could be attributed to a lack of robust trials directly linking BPV reduction to lowered CV risk, as well as challenges in measuring BPV in a busy outpatient setting.

Both short-term and long-term BPV have been shown to be independently associated with target organ damage and CV events, particularly in patients with hypertension, diabetes mellitus, and chronic kidney disease. Certain antihypertensive drugs, whether used alone or in combination, have demonstrated effectiveness in reducing both short-term and long-term BPV. Notably, CCBs appear to excel in attenuating long-term BPV, potentially presenting an avenue for more effective BPV management in hypertension beyond merely controlling average BP levels.

While uncertainties persist, it is reasonable to consider incorporating BPV assessment into the diagnostic and management toolkit for hypertension. Further research, high-quality trials, and improved measurement techniques are needed to better understand the precise role of BPV in predicting CV risk and to establish its clinical significance in guiding treatment strategies. As our understanding evolves, the assessment and management of BPV may emerge as a valuable aspect of hypertension care.

REFERENCES

1. Lawes CM, Vander Hoorn S, Rodgers A. Global burden of blood-pressure related disease, 2001. Lancet. 2008;371(9623):1513-8.
2. Gradman AH. Sleep-time blood pressure: a validated therapeutic target. J Am Coll Cardiol. 2011;58(11):1174-5.
3. Pickering TG, Hall JE, Appel LJ, et al. Recommendations for blood pressure measurement in humans and experimental animals: part 1: blood pressure measurement in humans: a statement for professionals from the Subcommittee of Professional and Public Education of the American Heart Association Council on High Blood Pressure Research. Circulation. 2005;111(5):697-716.
4. Papadogiannis DE, Protogerou AD. Blood pressure variability: a confounder and a cardiovascular risk factor. Hypertens Res. 2011;34:162-3.
5. Parati G, Pomidossi G, Albini F, et al. Relationship of 24-hour blood pressure mean and variability to severity of target-organ damage in hypertension. J Hypertens. 1987;5(1):93-8.
6. Hansen TW, Thijs L, Li Y, et al. Prognostic value of reading-to-reading blood pressure variability over 24 hours in 8938 subjects from 11 populations. Hypertension. 2010;55(4):1049-57.
7. Parati G, Ochoa JE, Bilo G. Blood pressure variability, cardiovascular risk, and risk for renal disease progression. Curr Hypertens Rep. 2012;14(5):421-31.
8. Dolan E, O'Brien E. Is it daily, monthly, or yearly blood pressure variability that enhances cardiovascular risk? Curr Cardiol Rep. 2015;17(11):93.
9. Hermida RC, Ayala DE, Mojon A, et al. Decreasing sleep-time blood pressure determined by ambulatory monitoring reduces cardiovascular risk. J Am Coll Cardiol. 2011;58:1165-73.
10. Parati G. Blood pressure variability, target organ damage and antihypertensive treatment. J Hypertens. 2003;21(10):1827-30.
11. Mancia G, Parati G, Di Rienzo M, et al. BP variability. In: Zanchetti A, Mancia G (Eds). Handbook of hypertension: Pathophysiology of hypertension. Amsterdam: Elsevier Science BV; 1997. pp. 117-69.
12. Parati G, Ochoa JE, Lombardi C, et al. Blood pressure variability: assessment, predictive value, and potential as a therapeutic target. Curr Hypertens Rep. 2015;17(4): 537.
13. Su DF, Miao CY. Blood pressure variability and organ damage. Clin Exp Pharmacol Physiol. 2001;28(9):709-15.
14. Mena L, Pintos S, Queipo NV, et al. A reliable index for the prognostic significance of blood pressure variability. J Hypertens. 2005;23(3):505-11.
15. Li W, Yu Y, Liang D, Jia EZ. Factors Associated with Blood Pressure Variability Based on Ambulatory Blood Pressure Monitoring in Subjects with Hypertension in China. Kidney and Blood Pressure Res. 2017;42(2):267-75.
16. Parati G, Ochoa JE, Lombardi C, et al. Assessment and management of blood-pressure variability. Nat Rev Cardiol. 2013;10(3):143-55.
17. Höcht C. Blood pressure variability: prognostic value and therapeutic implications. ISRN Hypertens. 2013:398485.
18. Stauss HM. Identification of blood pressure control mechanisms by power spectral analysis. Clin Exp Pharmacol Physiol. 2007;34(4):362-8.
19. Chenniappan M. Blood pressure variability: assessment, prognostic significance and management. J Assoc Physicians India. 2015;63(5):47-53.
20. Souza HC, Martins-Pinge MC, da Silva VJ, et al. Heart rate and arterial pressure variability in the experimental reno-vascular hypertension model in rats. Auton Neurosci. 2008;139(1):38-45.
21. Grassi G, Bombelli M, Brambilla G, et al. Total cardiovascular risk, blood pressure variability and adrenergic overdrive in hypertension: evidence, mechanisms and clinical implications. Curr Hypertens Rep. 2012;14(4):333-8.
22. Palatini P, Penzo M, Racioppa A, et al. Clinical relevance of night time blood pressure and of daytime blood pressure variability. Arch Intern Med. 1992;152(9):1855-60.
23. Mancia G, Zanchetti A, Agabiti-Rosei E, et al. Ambulatory blood pressure is superior to clinic blood pressure in predicting treatment-induced regression of left ventricular hypertrophy. SAMPLE Study

Group. Study on Ambulatory Monitoring of Blood Pressure and Lisinopril Evaluation. Circulation. 1997;95(6):1464-70.
24. Madden JM, O'Flynn AM, Dolan E, et al. Short-term blood pressure variability over 24 h and target organ damage in middle-aged men and women. J Hum Hypertens. 2015;29(12):719-25.
25. Madden JM, O'Flynn AM, Fitzgerald AP, et al. Correlation between short-term blood pressure variability and left-ventricular mass index: a meta-analysis. Hypertens Res. 2016 March;39(3):171-7.
26. Sega R, Facchetti R, Bombelli M, et al. Prognostic value of ambulatory and home blood pressures compared with office blood pressure in the general population: follow-up results from the Pressioni Arteriose Monitorate e Loro Associazioni (PAMELA) study. Circulation. 2005;111(14):1777-83.
27. Fagard RH, Van Den Broeke C, De Cort P. Prognostic significance of blood pressure measured in the office, at home and during ambulatory monitoring in older patients in general practice. J Hum Hypertens. 2005;19(10):801-7.
28. Staessen JA, Thijs L, Fagard R, et al. Predicting cardiovascular risk using conventional vs ambulatory blood pressure in older patients with systolic hypertension. Systolic Hypertension in Europe Trial Investigators. JAMA. 1999;282(6):539-46.
29. Clement DL, De Buyzere ML, De Bacquer DA, et al. Prognostic value of ambulatory blood-pressure recordings in patients with treated hypertension. N Engl J Med. 2003; 348(24):2407-15.
30. Hansen TW, Li Y, Boggia J, et al. Predictive role of the night time blood pressure. Hypertension. 2011;57(1):3-10.
31. Metoki H, Ohkubo T, Kikuya M, et al. Prognostic significance for stroke of a morning pressor surge and a nocturnal blood pressure decline: the Ohasama study. Hypertension. 2006;47(2):149-54.
32. Kario K. Prognosis in relation to blood pressure variability: pro side of the argument. Hypertension. 2015;65(6):1163-9.
33. Turak O, Afsar B, Ozcan F, et al. Relationship between elevated morning blood pressure surge, uric acid, and cardiovascular outcomes in hypertensive patients. J Clin Hypertens (Greenwich). 2014;16(7):530-5.
34. Li Y, Thijs L, Hansen TW, et al. Prognostic value of the morning blood pressure surge in 5645 subjects from 8 populations. Hypertension. 2010;55(4):1040-8.
35. Asayama K, Wei FF, Liu YP, et al. Does blood pressure variability contribute to risk stratification? Methodological issues and a review of outcome studies based on home blood pressure. Hypertens Res. 2015;38(2):97-101.
36. Floras JS. Blood pressure variability: a novel and important risk factor. Can J Cardiol. 2013;29(5):557-63.
37. Kikuya M, Ohkubo T, Metoki H, et al. Day-by-day variability of blood pressure and heart rate at home as a novel predictor of prognosis: the Ohasama study. Hypertension. 2008;52(6):1045-50.
38. Muntner P, Shimbo D, Tonelli M, et al. The relationship between visit-to-visit variability in systolic blood pressure and all-cause mortality in the general population: findings from NHANES III, 1988 to 1994. Hypertension. 2011;57(2):160-6.
39. Nobre F, Mion Junior D. Ambulatory Blood Pressure Monitoring: Five Decades of more light and Less Shadows. Arq Bras Cardiol. 2016;106(6):528-37.
40. Turner JR, Viera AJ, Shimbo D. Ambulatory blood pressure monitoring in clinical practice: a review. Am J Med. 2015;128(1):14-20.
41. O'Brien E, Parati G, Stergiou G. Ambulatory blood pressure measurement. Hypertension. 2013;62:988-94.
42. Frattola A, Parati G, Cuspidi C, et al. Prognostic value of 24-hour blood pressure variability. J Hypertens. 1993;11(10):1133-7.
43. Tatasciore A, Zimarino M, Tommasi R, et al. Increased short-term blood pressure variability is associated with early left ventricular systolic dysfunction in newly diagnosed untreated hypertensive patients. J Hypertens. 2013;31(8):1653-61.
44. Ryu J, Cha RH, Kim DK, et al. The clinical association of the blood pressure variability with the target organ damage in hypertensive patients with chronic kidney disease. J Korean Med Sci. 2014;29(7):957-64.
45. Gomez Angelats E, Sierra C, Coca A, et al. Lack of association between blood pressure

variability and left ventricular hypertrophy in essential hypertension. Med Clin (Barc). 2004;123(19):731-4.
46. Kaneda R, Kario K, Hoshide S, et al. Morning blood pressure hyper-reactivity is an independent predictor for hypertensive cardiac hypertrophy in a community-dwelling population. Am J Hypertens. 2005;18(12 Pt 1):1528-33.
47. Yano Y, Hoshide S, Inokuchi T, et al. Association between morning blood pressure surge and cardiovascular remodelling in treated elderly hypertensive subjects. Am J Hypertens. 2009;22(11):1177-82.
48. Juhanoja EP, Niiranen TJ, Johansson JK, et al. Agreement between ambulatory, home, and office blood pressure variability. J Hypertens. 2016;34(1):61-7.
49. Madden JM, O'Flynn AM, Fitzgerald AP, et al. Correlation between short-term blood pressure variability and left-ventricular mass index: a meta-analysis. Hypertens Res. 2016;39(3):171-7.
50. Parati G, Bilo G, Valentini M. Blood pressure variability: methodological aspects, pathophysiological and clinical implications. In: Mancia G, Grassi G, Kjeldsen SE (Eds). Manual of Hypertension of the European Society of Hypertension. London: Inform a Healthcare. 2008. pp. 61-71.
51. Parati G, Lantelme P. Blood pressure variability, target organ damage and cardiovascular events. J Hypertens. 2002;20(9):1725-9.
52. Manios E, Tsagalis G, Tsivgoulis G, et al. Time rate of blood pressure variation is associated with impaired renal function in hypertensive patient's. J Hypertens. 2009;27(11):2244-8.
53. Felicio JS, de Souza AC, Kohlmann N, et al. Nocturnal blood pressure fall as predictor of diabetic nephropathy in hypertensive patients with type 2 diabetes. Cardiovasc Diabetol. 2010;9:36.
54. Tsioufis C, Andrikou I, Thomopoulos C, et al. Comparative prognostic role of night time blood pressure and non-dipping profile on renal outcomes. Am J Nephrol. 2011;33(3):277-88.
55. Matsui Y, Ishikawa J, Eguchi K, et al. Maximum value of home blood pressure: a novel indicator of target organ damage in hypertension. Hypertension. 2011;57(6):1087-93.
56. Tamura K, Azushima K, Umemura S. Day-by-day home measured blood pressure variability: another important factor in hypertension with diabetic nephropathy? Hypertens Res. 2011;34(12):1249-50.
57. Kawai T, Ohishi M, Kamide K, et al. The impact of visit-to-visit variability in blood pressure on renal function. Hypertens Res. 2012;35(2):239-43.
58. Tsioufis C, Andrikou I, Thomopoulos C, et al. Comparative prognostic role of night time blood pressure and non-dipping profile on renal outcomes. Am J Nephrol. 2011;33(3):277-88.
59. James PA, Oparil S, Carter BL, et al. 2014 evidence-based guideline for the management of high blood pressure in adults: report from the panel members appointed to the Eighth Joint National Committee (JNC 8). JAMA. 2014;311(5):507-20.
60. Filomena J, Riba-Llena I, Vinyoles E, et al. Short-term blood pressure variability relates to the presence of subclinical brain small vessel disease in primary hypertension. Hypertension. 2015;66(3):634-40.
61. Hashimoto T, Kikuya M, Ohkubo T, et al. Home blood pressure level, blood pressure variability, smoking, and stroke risk in Japanese men: the Ohasama study. Am J Hypertens. 2012;25(8):883-91.
62. Brickman AM, Reitz C, Luchsinger JA, et al. Long-term blood pressure fluctuation and cerebrovascular disease in an elderly cohort. Arch Neurol. 2010;67(5):564-9.
63. Bohm M, Schumacher H, Leong D, et al. Systolic blood pressure variation and mean heart rate is associated with cognitive dysfunction in patients with high cardiovascular risk. Hypertension. 2015;65(3):651-61.
64. Yano Y, Ning H, Allen N, et al. Long term blood pressure variability throughout young adulthood and cognitive function in midlife: the Coronary Artery Risk Development in Young Adults (CARDIA) study. Hypertension. 2014;64(5):983-8.
65. Zakopoulos NA, Tsivgoulis G, Barlas G, et al. Time rate of blood pressure variation

is associated with increased common carotid artery intima-media thickness. Hypertension. 2005;45(4):505-12.
66. Chen Y, Xiong H, Wu D, et al. Relationship of short-term blood pressure variability with carotid intima-media thickness in hypertensive patients. Biomed Eng Online. 2015;14:71.
67. Nagai M, Hoshide S, Ishikawa J, et al. Visit-to-visit blood pressure variations: new independent determinants for carotid artery measures in the elderly a thigh risk of cardiovascular disease. J Am Soc Hypertens. 2011;5(3):184-92.
68. Song H, Wei F, Liu Z, et al. Visit-to-visit variability in systolic blood pressure: correlated with the changes of arterial stiffness and myocardial perfusion in on-treated hypertensive patients. Clin Exp Hypertens. 2015;37(1):63-9.
69. Liu Z, Zhao Y, Lu F, et al. Day-by-day variability in self-measured blood pressure at home: effects on carotid artery atherosclerosis, brachial flow-mediated dilation, and endothelin1 in normotensive and mild-moderate hypertensive individuals. Blood Press Monit. 2013;18(6):316-25.
70. Nagai M, Kario K. Visit-to-visit blood pressure variability, silent cerebral injury, and risk of stroke. Am J Hypertens. 2013;26(12):1369-76.
71. Webb AJ, Fischer U, Mehta Z, et al. Effects of antihypertensive-drug class on inter individual variation in blood pressure and risk of stroke: a systematic review and meta-analysis. Lancet. 2010;375(9718):906-15.
72. Rothwell PM, Howard SC, Dolan E, et al. Effects of beta blockers and calcium-channel blockers on within-individual variability in blood pressure and risk of stroke. Lancet Neurol. 2010;9(5):469-80.
73. Parati G, Schumacher H, Bilo G, et al. Evaluating 24-h antihypertensive efficacy by the smoothness index: a meta-analysis of an ambulatory blood pressure monitoring database. J Hypertens. 2010;28(11):2177-83.
74. Parati G, Dolan E, Ley L, et al. Impact of antihypertensive combination and mono treatments on blood pressure variability: assessment by old and new indices. Data from a large ambulatory blood pressure monitoring database. J Hypertens. 2014;32(6):1326-33.
75. Zhang Y, Agnoletti D, Safar ME, et al. Effect of antihypertensive agents on blood pressure variability: the Natrilix SR versus candesartan and amlodipine in the reduction of systolic blood pressure in hypertensive patients (X-CELLENT) study. Hypertension. 2011;58(2):155-60.
76. Matsui Y, O'Rourke MF, Hoshide S, et al. Combined effect of angiotensin II receptor blocker and either a calcium channel blocker or diuretic on day-by-day variability of home blood pressure: the Japan Combined Treatment With Olmesartan and a Calcium-Channel Blocker Versus Olmesartan and Diuretics Randomized Efficacy Study. Hypertension. 2012;59(6):1132-8.
77. Hermida RC, Ayala DE, Mojon A, et al. Chronotherapy with valsartan/hydrochlorothiazide combination in essential hypertension: improved sleep-time blood pressure control with bedtime dosing. Chronobiol Int. 2011;28(7):601-10.
78. Mancia G, Facchetti R, Parati G, et al. Visit-to-visit blood pressure variability in the European Lacidipine Study on Atherosclerosis: methodological aspects and effects of anti-hypertensive treatment. J Hypertens. 2012;30(6):1241-51.
79. Levi-Marpillat N, Macquin-Mavier I, Tropeano AI, et al. Antihypertensive drug classes have different effects on short-term blood pressure variability in essential hypertension. Hypertens Res. 2014;37(6):585-90.
80. Rakugi H, Ogihara T, Saruta T, et al. Preferable effects of olmesartan/calcium channel blocker to olmesartan/diuretic on blood pressure variability in very elderly hypertension: COLM study sub analysis. J Hypertens. 2015;33(10):2165-72.
81. Karpov YA, Gorbunov VM, Deev AD. Effectiveness of fixed-dose perindopril/amlodipine on clinic, ambulatory and self-monitored blood pressure and blood pressure variability: an open-label, non-comparative study in the general practice. High Blood Press Cardiovasc Prev. 2015;22(4):417-25.

CHAPTER 24

Exercise and Hypertension

Kannan Meera Devi, V Padma

■ INTRODUCTION

The worldwide responsibility of hypertension as a disease causing morbidity and mortality is on a rising trend and found to have caused above 9 million deaths.[1] Many other end-organ defects in that specific compensatory increase that happens in the wall thickness and mass of the left ventricle is the main characteristic of the term called hypertensive heart which is a predictor of cardiovascular adverse events. Thus, it is very important to treat hypertension to prevent hypertrophy of the left ventricle and cardiovascular risk to reduce.[2] Factors such as being physically active and diet are some of the important contributors for the hypertension to develop and the show the need to control this public epidemic. The benefits of regular physical activity are lowering blood pressure, risk of cardiovascular events decrease, and also in remodeling the heart. In patients with hypertension, being physically active makes a paradoxical regression and prevents hypertrophy of the left ventricle which is the mechanism behind how it benefits the patients with hypertension. Along with drugs against hypertension and heart diseases, physical activity has much more benefits.[3-6] These are the main components of European, American, and World Health Organization (WHO) guidelines for the management of hypertension.[7-9]

■ PHYSICAL ACTIVITY ON HYPERTENSION

Many studies consistently prove the benefits of exercise and hypertension which decreases both the systolic and diastolic blood pressure by 5–7 mm Hg in patients with hypertension.[10-13] Especially, it acutely decreases systolic blood pressure, and this effect of blood pressure reduction lasts for 1 day and is referred to as hypotension postexercise with significant effects in patients with higher blood pressure as the baseline.[10] Many of the times, frequent and long-term exercises show results as a sustained decrease in blood pressure as a response,[14] and importantly, age, ethnicity, or sex does not change the response of blood pressure reduction.[15]

The decrease in blood pressure due to regular physical activity is by the attenuation in the peripheral vascular resistance, which results due to structural and neurohormonal responses along with a decrease in the activity sympathetic nervous system and an increase in the diameter of the arterial lumen.[16] Some more mechanisms behind this are changes that are favorable in inflammation, oxidative stress, function of the endothelium, compliance of the artery, renin-angiotensin system (RAS) system, activity of the parasympathetic activity, and also the sensitivity of the insulin.[3]

■ EFFECT OF EXERCISE ON HEART

Hypertension is mostly characterized by the pathology of the remodeling of the left ventricle along with concentric hypertrophy. By the law of Laplace, the response to hypertension is adaptive initially along with an increase in the thickness of the wall to decrease the stress of the wall and also the demand for oxygen. But then chronic overload of the pressure makes a transition to a maladaptive response with decompensation, concentric hypertrophy, and heart failure clinically.[17] thereby limiting the response of hypertrophy to hypertension is important to preserve the function of the heart and heart failure and other adverse events. Thus, treatment for hypertension regresses and normalizes left ventricular hypertrophy (LVH).[18]

Importantly, diastolic function and the left atrium are also associated with hypertension.[19-23] Also, the hypertensive heart is caused by hypertrophy of the right ventricle with approximately more than 30% of patients with systemic hypertension.[24,25]

EXERCISE ON SYMPATHETIC NERVOUS SYSTEM

The role of exercise on the sympathetic nervous system played a major part in the remodeling of heart in the hypertensive heart conditions. Along with blood pressure reduction, exercise has also been shown to have an effect on heart rate and insulin resistance attributing to decreased sympathetic activity.[14] With exercise, there is 28% plasma norepinephrine reduction, 20% plasma renin and systemic vascular resistance 7%.[4]

EXERCISE ON RESISTANT HYPERTENSION

Aerobic exercise has been shown to be effective in resistant hypertension. Even though there is a low response to the drugs against hypertension, it is not the same in the case of aerobic exercise. The extent of reduction in blood pressure after exercise considerably differs ranging from 5 to 15 mm Hg. Also, the difference exists among the older and younger individuals. Exercises are much more helpful in blood pressure in case of the patients who are having low response to drug therapies. And the decrease was assessed in ABP and it is not done in office blood pressure as the risk of adverse cardiac events has more correlation in ABP. A clinical relevance of a decrease in around 6 mm Hg systolic and 3 mm Hg diastolic is important in regards to cardiovascular risk. A reduction of 5/3 mm Hg has been demonstrated as it reduces the first incidence of fatal strokes by 28%. Also, the effects of exercise in the reduction of blood pressure are more in the daytime compared to nighttime because the blood pressure will lower baseline already in the night. Regular exercises have more effects in reducing sympathetic tone and this tone is lower at night than day. There is a significant difference between age and comorbid illness such as diabetes mellitus because of the cardiovascular impact of the exercise that is attenuated among them. Office blood pressure can also have an influence on white coat and other situational stress. The reasons for resistant hypertension are nonadherence secondary hypertension, vascular stiffness increase, overweight, sympathetic tone increase, and high sodium overload. Arterial stiffness relies on the loss of sensitivity to the drugs as most of the drugs are vasodilators, as the effect of drugs is better in elastic arteries with atherosclerosis.[26] Exercises augments vasodilation endothelium-dependent by the production of nitric oxide.[27] Improvement of endothelium function is not dependent on pulse pressure which is also a marker of aging marker. Exercise programs are leading to physical performance improvement in the way of increased oxygen uptake and the shift of lactate curves. Recent studies showed that exercise capacity is a more powerful indicator of mortality than other risk factors of cardiovascular disease.[28] As there is elevation of blood pressure during exercise, we should maintain the exercise to be in moderate intensity.[29,30] In routine life, the effect of exercise in hypertension is not monitored by methods such as concentration of lactate. In the training intensity recommendation, as a rule, patients are able to have a conversation at the time of the session. With the training heart rate is around 100 beats/min. Exercise also leads to decrease weight in patients who are obese, low-density lipoprotein, and in a way, increases high-density lipoprotein, helps in increasing insulin sensitivity, and reduces endothelial dysfunction. In the case of resistant hypertension, recent trials have shown that salt restriction has lowered systolic and diastolic blood pressures by 22 and 9 mm Hg. Even we have to explain to patients about other therapeutic options such as sympathetic denervation or stimulation of baroreceptors along with lifestyle modifications like regular exercises.

■ EXERCISES ADVISED

Each exercise has different benefits and effects on our body. The most commonly advised exercise is the aerobic exercise as this will have an effect on the blood vessels of the heart.

> **KEY POINTS**
> ○ Aerobic exercise affects the reduction in blood pressure of 5–7 mm Hg among people with hypertension and thereby reduces the CVD risk by around 25%.
> ○ Dynamic resistance exercise is an effective method to decrease blood pressure similar to aerobics.

■ FREQUENCY

Frequency of aerobic exercise 5–7 days per week, with resistance exercise 2–3 days per week and with flexibility exercise 2–3 days a week. If people are with normal blood pressure, it is advised only for 3–5 days a week. As its immediate effect is reducing blood pressure to around 5–7 mm Hg, patients are advised to exercise most of the days.

■ INTENSITY

Moderate level that is 40–60% or 11–14 on a scale of 8–20 of the physical exertion and exercises that increase the heart rate for aerobic exercise; moderate to the intensity of vigorous for the resistance and stretch to the tightness feel or minimal discomfort for flexible. Reduction in blood pressure depends on the intensity of the exercises and greater blood pressure reduction.

■ TIME

The time required for the significant reduction in blood pressure in the case of aerobic exercise should be a of minimum 30 minutes and up to 60 min for either continuous or accumulated exercise. If it is intermittent, go with a bout of 10 minutes. Even interspaced and more frequent exercise has shown results equally effective in blood pressure reduction compared to continuous exercises.

■ TYPE

For aerobic exercises to be effective, they should be placed on activities of prolonged, rhythmic sessions using larger muscle groups such as walking, swimming, and cycling. Resistance training also gives aerobic training and consists of around 2–4 sets with 8–12 repetitions for each muscle group. For the purpose of flexibility, work for each muscle group for 10–30 s with 2–5 repetitions.

Balance training exercises are also given to patients who are at high risk for falls.

EXERCISES TO AVOID

Exercises for short periods with high intensities such as lifting weights and sprinting, as they raise blood pressure rapidly and have a load of strain over the blood vessels of the heart. Some sports that are dangerous such as scuba diving, squash, or parachuting are to be avoided.

CONCLUSION

Though regular exercise is essential for a healthy lifestyle, it is important to know the type of exercise, frequency and intensity of exercises that cause benefit rather than harm. Anaerobic exercise is a vital tool to control hypertension. Exercises for short periods with high intensities can exacerbate hypertension. Hence, balanced exercises are recommended to prevent hypertension-related health complications.

REFERENCES

1. Campbell NRC, Lackland DT, Niebylski ML the World Hypertension League and International Society of Hypertension Executive Committee. High blood pressure: why prevention and control are urgent and important: a 2014 fact sheet from the World Hypertension League and the International Society of Hypertension. J Clin Hypertens (Greenwich). 2014;16(8):551-3.
2. Cuspidi C, Facchetti R, Bombelli M, Sala C, Tadic M, Grassi G, et al. Prognostic value of left ventricular mass normalized to different body size indexes: Findings from the PAMELA population. J Hypertens. 2015;33(5):1082-9.
3. Diaz KM, Shimbo D. Physical activity and the prevention of hypertension. Curr Hypertens Rep. 2013;15(6):659-68.
4. Cornelissen VA, Fagard RH. Effects of endurance training on blood pressure, blood pressure: regulating mechanisms, and cardiovascular risk factors. Hypertension. 2005;46(4):667-75.
5. Leitzmann MF, Park Y, Blair A, Ballard-Barbash R, Mouw T, Hollenbeck AR, et al. Physical activity recommendations and decreased risk of mortality. Arch Intern Med. 2007;167(22):2453-60.
6. Rossi A, Dikareva A, Bacon SL, Daskalopoulou SS. The impact of physical activity on mortality in patients with high blood pressure: a systematic review. J Hypertens. 2012;30(7):1277-88.
7. James PA, Oparil S, Carter BL, Cushman WC, Dennison-Himmelfarb C, Handler J, et al. 2014 evidence-based guideline for the management of high blood pressure in adults: report from the panel members appointed to the Eighth Joint National Committee (JNC 8) JAMA. 2014;311: 507-20.
8. Members AF, Mancia G, Fagard R, Narkiewicz K, Redon J, Zanchetti A, et al. 2013 ESH/ESC Guidelines for the management of arterial hypertension. Eur Heart J. 2013;34:2159-19.
9. Mendis S, Davis S, Norrving B. Organizational update: The World Health Organization Global Status Report on Noncommunicable Diseases 2014; one more landmark step in the combat against stroke and vascular disease. 2015;46(5):e121-2.
10. Pescatello LS, Franklin BA, Fagard R, Farquhar WB, Kelley GA, Ray CA, et al. American College of Sports Medicine position stand. Exercise and hypertension: Med Sci Sports Exerc. 2004;36(3):533-53.
11. Fagard RH. Exercise therapy in hypertensive cardiovascular disease. Prog Cardiovasc Dis. 2011;53(6):404-11.
12. Cornelissen VA, Smart NA. Exercise training for blood pressure: a systematic review and meta-analysis. J Am Heart Assoc. 2013;2:e004473. A systematic review and meta-analysis of 93 studies summarizing the effects of exercise on resting blood pressure.
13. Carlson DJ, Dieberg G, Hess NC, Millar PJ, Smart NA. Isometric exercise training for blood pressure management: A systematic review and meta-analysis. Mayo Clin Proc. 2014;89(3):327-34.

14. Pescatello LS. Exercise and hypertension: recent advances in exercise prescription. Curr Hypertens Rep. 2005;7(4):281-6.
15. Ash GI, Eicher JD, Pescatello LS. The promises and challenges of the use of genomics in the prescription of exercise for hypertension: the 2013 update. Curr Hypertens Rev. 2013;9(2):130-47.
16. Hamer M. The anti-hypertensive effects of exercise: integrating acute and chronic mechanisms. Sports Med Auckl NZ. 2006;36(2):109-16.
17. Burchfield JS, Xie M, Hill JA. Pathological ventricular remodeling mechanisms: Part 1 of 2. Circulation. 2013;128(4):388-400.
18. Wachtell K, Dahlöf B, Rokkedal J, Papademetriou V, Nieminen MS, Smith G, et al. Change of left ventricular geometric pattern after 1 year of antihypertensive treatment: the Losartan Intervention For Endpoint reduction in hypertension (LIFE) study. Am Heart J. 2002;144(6):1057-64.
19. Vaziri SM, Larson MG, Lauer MS, Benjamin EJ, Levy D. Influence of blood pressure on left atrial size: The Framingham Heart Study. Hypertension. 1995;25(6):1155-60.
20. Cuspidi C, Rescaldani M, Sala C. Prevalence of echocardiographic left-atrial enlargement in hypertension: a systematic review of recent clinical studies. Am J Hypertens. 2013;26(4):456-64.
21. de Simone G, Kitzman DW, Chinali M, Oberman A, Hopkins PN, Rao DC. Left ventricular concentric geometry is associated with impaired relaxation in hypertension: the HyperGEN study. Eur Heart J. 2005;26(10):1039-45.
22. Cuspidi C, Meani S, Fusi V, Valerio C, Catini E, Sala C, et al. Prevalence and correlates of left atrial enlargement in essential hypertension: role of ventricular geometry and the metabolic syndrome: the evaluation of target organ damage in hypertension study. J Hypertens. 2005;23:875-82.
23. Wachtell K, Smith G, Gerdts E, Dahlöf B, Nieminen MS, Papademetriou V, et al. Left ventricular filling patterns in patients with systemic hypertension and left ventricular hypertrophy (the LIFE study)? Am J Cardiol. 2000;85(4):466-72.
24. Cuspidi C, Sala C, Muiesan ML, De Luca N, Schillaci G, Working Group on Heart, Hypertension of the Italian Society of Hypertension. Right ventricular hypertrophy in systemic hypertension: an updated review of clinical studies. J Hypertens. 2013;31(5):858-65.
25. Cuspidi C, Negri F, Giudici V, Valerio C, Meani S, Sala C, et al. Prevalence and clinical correlates of right ventricular hypertrophy in essential hypertension. J Hypertens. 2009;27(4):854-60.
26. Goto C, Higashi Y, Kimura M, Noma K, Hara K, Nakagawa K, et al. Effect of different intensities of exercise on endothelium-dependent vasodilation in humans: role of endothelium-dependent nitric oxide and oxidative stress. Circulation. 2003;108(5):530-5.
27. Myers J, Prakash M, Froelicher V, Do D, Partington S, Atwood JE. Exercise capacity and mortality among men referred for exercise testing. N Engl J Med. 2002;346(11):793-801.
28. Lenfant C, Chobanian AV, Jones DW, Roccella EJ, Joint National Committee on the Prevention, Detection, Evaluation, and Treatment of High Blood Pressure. Seventh report of the Joint National Committee on the Prevention, Detection, Evaluation, and Treatment of High Blood Pressure (JNC 7): resetting the hypertension sails. Hypertension. 2003;41(6):1178-9.
29. Mancia G, De Backer G, Dominiczak A, Cifkova R, Fagard R, Germano G, et al. 2007 Guidelines for the Management of Arterial Hypertension: The Task Force for the Management of Arterial Hypertension of the European Society of Hypertension (ESH) and of the European Society of Cardiology (ESC). J Hypertens. 2007;25(6):1105-87.
30. Ahmed HM, Blaha MJ, Nasir K, Rivera JJ, Blumenthal RS. Effects of physical activity on cardiovascular disease. Am J Cardiol. 2012;109(2):288-95.

CHAPTER 25

Air Pollution and Hypertension

Minakshi Dhar

■ INTRODUCTION

Elevated blood is a major and modifiable risk factor for mortality and morbidity in the world, but its importance is still undermined. Various studies have shown that for every 20 mm Hg rise in systolic and 10 mm Hg rise in diastolic blood pressure (DBP), there is a 2-fold increase in cardiovascular mortality. Brook RD et all.[1] in their study showed that hypertension has been associated with various environmental and lifestyle factors, besides behavioral factors such as physical inactivity, high salt intake, obesity, alcohol, etc. Environmental pollution, both noise and air, has been found to be associated with high blood pressure (BP) in various studies. World Health Organization (WHO) has estimated a 7.6% of total deaths are due to environmental pollution. Ischemic heart diseases and cerebrovascular diseases are the most prevalent diseases associated with air pollution. The burden of these diseases is more in developing countries like India which is undergoing rapid industrialization. Hypertension is the most important modifiable risk factor for both and is found to be affected by ambient air pollution.

■ AIR POLLUTANTS

Air quality depends upon a mixture of gases, particulate matter (PM), and liquids present in the atmosphere. Air pollutants cannot be classified as a single pollutant but are a mixture of gases, water vapor and suspended particles. More than 98% of air pollutant mass is comprised of vapor phase compounds in urban settings. Particulate matter present in the environment has synergistic effects with these compounds.

- Gaseous air pollutants mainly include carbon monoxide (CO), nonmethane hydrocarbons or volatile organic carbons (VOCs), nitrogen dioxide (NO_2), nitrous oxide (NO_x), ozone gases (O_3) and sulfur dioxide (SO_2).
- Particulate matter is categorized by aerodynamic diameter as follows:
  - PM_{10} (<10 μm in diameter),
  - $PM_{2.5}$ (<2.5 μm in diameter),
  - UFP (ultrafine particles, <0.1 μm in diameter), and
  - $PM_{2.5-10}$ coarse particles (between 2.5 and 10 μm in diameter).

Among all these, particulate matter $PM_{2.5}$ is found to be significantly associated with the risk of elevated BP. Sources such as industries, traffic, and power generators are major sources of $PM_{2.5}$ in urban areas due to human combustion of fossil fuels in them. Burning of biomass, heating, cooling and other activities like fires may be relevant sources in some rural regions. In a Multi-Ethnic Prospective Study (MESA study), concentration of $PM_{2.5}$ and NO were strongly associated with accelerated atherosclerosis. This was shown by the increase in calcium deposits in coronary vessels which have been consistently associated with cardiovascular diseases in both clinical trials and observational studies. The combined effect of air pollution on the cardiovascular system is yet to be well studied and is thus poorly understood till now.

SEASONAL VARIABILITY IN AIR POLLUTION LEVELS

Among various environmental factors, temperature and emission rates have the greatest impact on the concentration of pollutants in the air. Also, NOx, CO, and VOCs which are emitted during combustion, have peak concentration during rush hours of the day. Winter season when the temperatures are relatively low, environmental pollution level is high. Environmental pollution also depends upon the lifetime of the individual pollutant, for example, $PM_{2.5}$ and O_3 have the longest atmospheric lifetime so they get accumulated over multiple days and are carried to large geographical areas by the prevailing winds.

As the meteorological conditions vary from place to place so does the concentration of pollutants vary geographically. This feature is responsible for the differences in pollution characteristics within these regions.

PATHOPHYSIOLOGY

Exact pathophysiology of how air pollution increases BP and thus the cardiovascular risk is unknown. Various proposed pathways are follows:

- *Systemic inflammation:* When PM comes in contact with lung cells after inhalation, inflammatory mediators are released from lung cells because of which there is an increase in the production of acute-phase proteins (e.g., CRP, fibrinogen) from the liver. This results in the augmentation of proinflammatory mediators (e.g., activated immune cells, cytokines) in blood, which instigates the pathway of adverse effects on the heart and vasculature. Various inflammatory cytokines that have been found to be involved are interleukin 6 (IL-6), interleukin 1 alpha (IL-1α), tumor necrosis factor alpha (TNF-α), interferon-α, and IL-8.
- *Systemic oxidative stress:* Various in vitro studies have shown that PM activates reactive oxygen species (ROS)-generating pathways and causes endothelial dysfunction. Agents involved are nicotinamide adenine dinucleotide phosphate (NADPH) oxidases, cytochrome P450 enzymes, and nitric oxides which cause depletion of defense mechanisms by impairing the function of high-density lipoprotein, thus causing oxidation of lipoproteins and other plasma constituents which lead to endothelial dysfunction.
- *Activation of baroreceptors and chemoreceptors:* Autonomic receptors of the pulmonary system are triggered by exposure to air pollutants. This results in the impairment of baroreceptors and chemoreceptors which promote arterial vasoconstriction and thus cause an increase in BP.
- *Serotonin–acetylcholine pathways:* A possible mechanism of change in BP on O_3 exposure has been attributed to the release of serotonin and acetylcholine in response to systemic inflammation which triggers the vasoconstriction and vasodilation, respectively, thus affecting BP values.
- *Angiotensin II:* Systemic inflammation increases superoxide production by activation of angiotensin II receptors,

which causes NADPH oxidase subunits to upregulate and results in depletion of tetrahydrobiopterin in the vasculature, thus promoting endothelial injury.

All these mechanisms result in vascular inflammation, impaired basal vasomotor balance and increase in systemic vascular resistance thus causing hypertension. Several epidemiologic studies have shown that with every 10 µg/m^3 elevation in PM, systolic and diastolic BP rises by 1–4 mm Hg. The US Environmental Protection Agency (EPA) has set a long-term average of 12 µg/m^3 of PM$_{2.5}$ and a short-term average of below 25 µg/m^3 of PM$_{2.5}$, which can be considered safe, but effects on the cardiovascular system have been documented in areas with levels at or below these cut-off values also.

Various epidemiological studies have been done to establish a relationship between the effect of short- and long-term exposure to pollutants on BP, but sufficient evidence is lacking to establish a relationship. The relationship between short-term exposure to air pollution and cardiovascular risk is yet to be established, but long-term effects have been documented in various animal studies and studied in many population-based models.

EFFECT OF SHORT-TERM EXPOSURE ON BLOOD PRESSURE

There are conflicting evidences regarding short-term exposure to air pollutants and their effects on the cardiovascular system in humans. Short-term exposure to air pollution has been described in various studies as exposure of less than 30 days. Various studies which have shown that less than 30 days of exposure to environmental air pollution has a positive correlation with the rise in BP in adults, but some studies have failed to show any relationship. A meta-analysis and systematic review were carried out which included 14 studies, comprising 351,766 participants across 10 countries by Miao Huang et al.[2] In this review, an attempt was made to establish a relationship between short-term exposure to environmental air pollutants (NO, PM$_{2.5}$, and PM$_{10}$) and BP values in children and adolescents. In this review, short-term exposure to PM$_{10}$ was found to be significantly associated with systolic blood pressure (SBP) values.

EFFECT OF LONG-TERM EXPOSURE ON BLOOD PRESSURE

There are various studies to support that long-term exposure to ambient air pollutants is associated with hypertension in adults as well as in children. Among various pollutants, long-term exposure to PM$_{2.5}$ and PM$_{10}$ has consistently shown a significant association with elevated BP readings. Few studies such as the one done by Ntarladima et al.[3] reached an inconsistent conclusion. They failed to show any significant association between long-term exposure to PM$_{2.5}$ and PM$_{10}$ and SBP/DBP among the 733 5-year-old children in The Netherlands.

Meta-regression of a meta-analysis by Miao Huang et al. concluded that age, sex, and location of an individual determines the effect of air pollution exposure on BP readings in children. There are evidences to support the fact that exposure to tobacco in pregnant women has resulted in elevated BP in the newborn child. A study done by Breton CV et al.[4] showed that prenatal exposure to NO$_2$ was associated with higher SBP in 11-year-old children. A prospective study including 1,131 infants in the United

States was done by van Rossem L et al.[5] They showed that if a woman is exposed to higher mean $PM_{2.5}$ and black carbon during her third trimester (i.e., 90 days before the child is born), the child will have higher SBP. Thus, many epidemiologic studies support the fact that long-term exposure to $PM_{2.5}$, PM_{10}, and NO_2 is associated with increased BP among children, adolescents, and adults.

There are many factors including patient susceptibility, time frames of exposure, and PM composition which determine the effect of environmental air pollution on human beings. Physical activity has been found to have an adverse effect on BP control in areas where there is a high $PM_{2.5}$ concentration. This is so because individuals exercising in areas of high concentration zones of air pollution will inhale more amount of pollutants due to increased depth and rate of breathing during exercise. This has led to a concern as to how to strike the balance between the beneficial effects of physical activity on health and the potential health risks due to increased exposure to air pollution during increased physical activity.

REFERENCES

1. Brook RD, Weder AB, Rajagopalan S. "Environmental hypertensionology" the effects of environmental factors on blood pressure in clinical practice and research. J Clin Hypertens (Greenwich). 2011;13(11):836-42.
2. Huang M, Chen J, Yang Y, et al. Effects of ambient air pollution on blood pressure among children and adolescents: a systematic review and meta-analysis 2021. J Am Heart Assoc. 2021;10(10):e017734.
3. Ntarladima AM, Vaartjes I, Grobbee DE, et al. Relations between air pollution and vascular development in 5-year old children: a cross-sectional study in the Netherlands. Environ Health. 2019;18(1):50.
4. Breton CV, Yao J, Millstein J, et al. Prenatal air pollution exposures, DNA Methyl Transferase Genotypes, and Associations with Newborn LINE1 and Alu Methylation and Childhood Blood Pressure and Carotid Intima-Media Thickness in the Children's Health Study. Environ Health Perspect. 2016;124(12):1905-12.
5. van Rossem L, Rifas-Shiman SL, Melly SJ, et al. Prenatal air pollution exposure and newborn blood pressure. Environ Health Perspect. 2015;123(4):353-9.

CHAPTER 26

Isolated Nocturnal Hypertension

Geetha Subramanian, J Cecily Mary Majella

INTRODUCTION

Increasing evidence suggests that 24-h ambulatory blood pressure (BP) monitoring (ABPM) offers valuable clinical insights, not only for diagnosing hypertension but also for managing and predicting outcomes in hypertensive patients.[1-3] The rhythmic fluctuations in circadian BP have long been overlooked. O'Brien et al. initially categorized hypertensive patients into two broad groups based on the extent of BP reduction during nighttime, distinguishing between "dippers" and "nondippers."[4] Subsequent studies have demonstrated that individuals with little or no nocturnal BP decline (nondippers) experience significantly worse outcomes compared to those with a normal circadian BP pattern (dippers).[3] However, the binary classification of circadian BP variations lacked specificity in patients who had extreme nighttime BP variations. Hence, a new four-tiered classification has been proposed and widely accepted.[5] This classification encompasses individuals with a substantial reduction in nighttime BP (>20% compared to daytime values), termed "extreme dippers," as well as those with an increase in night-time BP, known as "reverse dippers" or "raisers" (where nighttime BP surpasses daytime levels). The majority of research consistently supports the negative impact of a nondipping BP pattern on cardiovascular outcomes.[6,7] Investigations have demonstrated that a nondipping pattern is associated with an increased risk of myocardial infarction, stroke, heart failure, and cardiovascular mortality.[6-8] In contrast, the prognostic implications of a reverse-dipping pattern have not been established firmly since long-term data are limited. Recent studies have indicated that this pattern is linked to adverse cardiac remodeling[9,10] and unfavorable cardiovascular outcomes. The most controversial aspect pertains to the influence of an extreme dipping BP pattern on cardiac changes and cardiovascular outcomes. Nocturnal hypertension is an intriguing phenomenon that is typically associated with nondipping and reverse-dipping patterns.[11] However, it may also occur in dippers, albeit infrequently in extreme dippers. The central question revolves around which of these two factors—nocturnal hypertension or nondipping status—exerts a greater impact on target organ damage and overall outcomes.

NOCTURNAL HYPERTENSION VERSUS NONDIPPERS

Numerous authors have placed a higher emphasis on the significance of nocturnal hypertension compared to the nondipping BP pattern. Nevertheless, investigations have also indicated that nondipping and reverse BP patterns are distinct from nocturnal BP and are linked with target organ damage and outcomes independently.[9,10] Studies have also shown that nocturnal hypertension is associated with left and right ventricular remodeling, while others have showcased its adverse impact on cardiovascular outcomes in individuals with hypertension.[13] There still exist variations in the definitions of nocturnal hypertension among different guidelines, which could be a significant hurdle in evaluating its influence on target organ damage and prognosis. The management approach of nocturnal hypertension depends on factors like age, comorbidities, BP readings, race, and gender.

PATHOPHYSIOLOGY OF NOCTURNAL HYPERTENSION

Circadian variations in BP are influenced by diurnal hormonal fluctuations, encompassing the autonomic nervous system, adrenocorticotropic hormones, vasopressin, acetylcholine, cortisol, insulin, ghrelin, adiponectin, leptin, and to some extent, the renin–angiotensin–aldosterone system (RAAS). These hormonal shifts are responsible for the higher BP levels during the day and lower levels at night. Several potential mechanisms underlie nocturnal hypertension, including heightened activity of the sympathetic nervous system, hyperactivity of the RAS system, sodium retention, reduced renal function, obstructive sleep apnea syndrome, and other sleep disorders, as well as factors such as obesity, aging, stress, and diabetes.

Nocturnal hypertension can often be the initial indication of hypertension, primarily driven by sympathetic overstimulation. In such cases, it tends to be associated with adverse cardiovascular events like stroke, coronary artery disease, and heart failure, or damage to other target organs like renal dysfunction, cognitive impairment, and peripheral artery disease. This is particularly applicable in cases of isolated nocturnal hypertension. Alternatively, nocturnal hypertension may represent the advanced stage of arterial hypertension. During sleep, assuming a supine position increases venous return, leading to higher left ventricular preload and increased left ventricular wall stress, as described by Laplace's law. Additionally, the movement of interstitial fluid from lower body tissues further augments preload. The combination of increased intravascular volume at night and elevated BP may exacerbate renal function impairment due to raised intraglomerular pressure and hyperfiltration.

DIAGNOSIS OF NOCTURNAL HYPERTENSION

Nocturnal hypertension can only be accurately diagnosed through BP monitoring, with two main methods available: home-based and ABPM. While ambulatory monitoring offers more data points and is typically considered more precise, Kario et al. found that systolic BP measurements taken at home were still valuable predictors of cardiovascular events, independently of in-office and morning at-home readings. In this particular study, home blood pressure monitoring involved taking three nocturnal measurements at 1-h intervals (02:00, 03:00, and 04:00). In contrast, ABPM requires at least six nocturnal measurements, covering the period from bedtime to waking up. There are slight variations between American and European guidelines in defining nocturnal hypertension. According to the latest American College of Cardiology (ACC)/American Heart Association (AHA) guidelines, nocturnal hypertension is defined as having a mean asleep systolic blood pressure (SBP) of ≥110 mm Hg and/or a mean asleep diastolic blood pressure (DBP) of ≥65 mm Hg, as measured by ABPM. This corresponds to a clinic BP of ≥130/80 mm Hg. The American definition of nocturnal hypertension is more restrictive compared to the European guidelines, which set the threshold at SBP ≥120 mm Hg and/or DBP ≥70 mm Hg.

Isolated nocturnal hypertension implies that daytime BP remains within the normal range (<135/85 mm Hg). The circadian BP pattern is determined by the percentage of BP drop during the night compared to daytime levels. The following four distinct BP patterns can be defined: Extreme dipping (>20% drop in BP), dipping (BP drop of 10-20%), non-dipping (BP drop of 0-10%), and inverse dipping or rising (BP drop ≤0%).

EPIDEMIOLOGY

The prevalence of nocturnal hypertension varies across different populations due to its dependence on various demographic, clinical, and ethnic factors. Moreover, slight disparities in the definition of nocturnal hypertension between American and European guidelines contribute to differing prevalence figures. According to the Pressioni Monitorate E Loro Associazioni (PAMELA) study, 30% of participants (607 out of 2021 subjects) were diagnosed with nocturnal hypertension using ABPM. In another study by Androulakis et al., nearly half (approximately 50%) of 319 newly diagnosed hypertensive patients exhibited signs of nocturnal hypertension. The Jackson Heart Study, focusing on African-Americans with a high prevalence of obesity and type 2 diabetes, reported that 39% of untreated participants had nocturnal hypertension. Similarly, the research conducted by Wang et al. in a Chinese population consisting of 1,322 patients with chronic kidney disease (of which 56% had chronic glomerulonephritis), found that 60% of participants experienced nocturnal hypertension. Patients with nocturnal hypertension were typically older, had diabetes, and exhibited higher levels of serum creatinine, cystatin C, calcium, uric acid, and homocysteine compared to those with nocturnal normotension.

NOCTURNAL HYPERTENSION AND TARGET ORGAN DAMAGE

Significant research findings confirm the adverse consequences of nocturnal hypertension on target organ damage. They demonstrated that nocturnal hypertension is linked to adverse effects on the structure and function of both the left and right ventricles, including issues with diastolic function and mechanics. The PAMELA study underscored that, in individuals with normal left ventricular mass, the level of nocturnal BP, rather than the decline in nocturnal BP, serves as a reliable indicator for predicting left ventricular hypertrophy. A comprehensive meta-analysis has further revealed associations between nocturnal hypertension and left ventricular hypertrophy, as well as common carotid intima-media thickness. Li et al. identified a connection between isolated nocturnal hypertension and increased arterial stiffness among the Chinese population. Additionally, the Jackson study observed significantly elevated left ventricular mass index in patients experiencing isolated nocturnal hypertension.[18,19] However, it is important to note that some studies did not find statistically significant differences in central pulse pressure, aortic pulse wave velocity, or left ventricular mass index. For hypertensive patients with well-controlled self-measured BP, isolated nocturnal hypertension was linked to heightened carotid intima-media thickness and relative wall thickness.

Furthermore, Salazar et al. reported that insulin resistance was associated with nocturnal hypertension, but not diurnal hypertension, in untreated individuals with both normal and mildly elevated BP levels. Yan et al. also demonstrated that a reverse-dipping BP pattern was an independent predictor of lacunar infarction in hypertensive patients, although their investigation focused on 24-h BP rather than specifically nocturnal BP. Kario et al. found that nocturnal systolic BP, as measured through home BP monitoring, was linked to urinary albumin/creatinine ratio, left ventricular mass index, brachial-ankle pulse wave velocity, carotid intima-media thickness, N-terminal pro B-type natriuretic peptide (NTpro-BNP), and high-sensitive cardiac troponin.[14,17]

NOCTURNAL HYPERTENSION AND COMPLICATIONS

Research findings indicate a clear connection between isolated nocturnal hypertension and an elevated risk of cardiovascular health problems and mortality. A comprehensive study involving 8,000 participants from three different continents provided strong evidence that isolated nocturnal hypertension was linked to a heightened likelihood of experiencing cardiovascular events and overall mortality.[12] Further analysis within specific subgroups revealed that isolated nocturnal hypertension had a more pronounced impact on younger individuals, leading to a higher risk of all-cause mortality [hazard ratio (HR): 1.99, 95% confidence interval (CI): 1.14–3.47], as well as in nonsmokers (HR: 1.78, 95% CI: 1.25–2.55), individuals with lower levels of obesity (HR: 1.63, 95% CI: 1.08–2.46), and those with a history of cardiovascular disease (HR: 2.09, 95% CI: 1.00–4.36).[13] Additionally, a study focused on Chinese patients with chronic renal disease demonstrated that isolated nocturnal hypertension was associated with an increased risk of renal events (HR: 3.81, 95% CI: 1.74–8.36) and cardiovascular events (HR: 8.34, 95% CI: 1.98–35.07), even after adjusting for clinic BP, 24-h BP, or daytime BP.[14–16]

Furthermore, Presta et al. discovered that patients with masked hypertension and a reversed BP pattern faced a significantly higher risk of stroke, even after accounting for factors such as age, gender, body mass index, dyslipidemia, and diabetes. It is important to note that while a reverse-dipping pattern does not always indicate nocturnal hypertension, this particular study found that individuals with a reverse-dipping pattern also exhibited signs of nocturnal hypertension.

MANAGEMENT

Nocturnal hypertension can be effectively managed through a variety of approaches. These include making lifestyle adjustments, such as limiting sodium intake and supplementing with potassium. Additionally, pharmacological treatments are employed, primarily by administering antihypertensive medications at bedtime. Nocturnal hypertension is closely associated with increased blood volume and the overactivity of the sympathetic and RAAS. These systems are the primary targets for therapeutic interventions in individuals with nocturnal hypertension. Some studies have demonstrated that reducing salt intake and using diuretics can significantly lower nocturnal BP and shift the BP pattern from nondipping to dipping. Furthermore, research by Hermida et al. revealed a substantial reduction in nocturnal BP when angiotensin-converting enzyme inhibitors (ACEIs) were administered in the evening. Based on their mechanisms of action, it was anticipated that a combination of ACEIs or angiotensin receptor II blockers (ARBs) with diuretics would offer greater benefits compared to combining ACEIs or

ARBs with calcium channel antagonists (CCBs).

However, recent findings from Kario et al. suggest that the combination of ARBs and CCBs is more effective than the combination of ARBs and diuretics in individuals with uncontrolled nocturnal hypertension, regardless of their sodium intake and despite both combinations having a similar impact on patients with high salt sensitivity. Renin activity tends to increase during the night and peaks in the morning, making long-acting direct renin inhibitors such as aliskiren potentially beneficial. Giles et al. demonstrated that combining aliskiren and valsartan resulted in a more significant reduction in BP than valsartan alone, especially in nondippers, with a conversion from nondippers to dippers occurring in a substantial percentage of hypertensive patients. Although statistical significance was lacking in this study due to the limited number of participants, it was evident that the combination of aliskiren and valsartan had the potential to be more potent in reducing nocturnal BP.

One study that explored the effects of a calcium channel blocker (cilnidipine) on circadian BP patterns in hypertensive patients reported significant changes in the reduction rate of nocturnal systolic BP, particularly in reverse and extreme dippers, although dippers and extreme dippers did not experience the same effect. Cilnidipine partially restored the abnormal nocturnal BP pattern towards a normal dipping pattern in hypertensive patients. The impact of beta-blockers on circadian BP patterns remains unreported. Determining whether the favorable effects on reducing nocturnal BP and modifying patterns from nondippers and reverse dippers to dippers and extreme dippers are attributed to the specific antihypertensive medications or the timing of drug administration is challenging. The benefit of converting to an extremely dipping BP pattern is a subject of debate, as this circadian rhythm may be associated with nocturnal hypoxemia, coronary hypoperfusion, and morning sympathetic activation, which could lead to cerebrovascular and cardiovascular events, particularly in elderly patients.

Chronotherapy appears to be a promising therapeutic approach in addressing nocturnal hypertension. The Monitorización Ambulatoria de la Presión Arterial y Eventos Cardiovasculares (MAPEC) study compared the timing of medication administration, either in the morning or at bedtime, in 2,156 hypertensive patients over a mean follow-up period of 5.6 years. The study found that bedtime dosing provided better BP control. Patients taking at least one medication at bedtime had a significantly lower relative risk of total cardiovascular disease events compared to those taking all medications in the morning. Moreover, the prevalence of nondipping patterns significantly decreased, while well-controlled BP increased in patients receiving medication at bedtime.

OBSTRUCTIVE SLEEP APNEA AND NOCTURNAL HYPERTENSION

Obstructive sleep apnea represents a potential mechanism contributing to the emergence of isolated nocturnal hypertension. Numerous studies have demonstrated that obstructive sleep apnea plays a pivotal role in the development of nondipping BP patterns. Nonetheless, comprehensive research directly linking sleep apnea to isolated nocturnal hypertension remains limited, warranting further investigation in upcoming studies on this specific hypertensive condition. Intriguingly, there is evidence that renal denervation leads to a significant decrease in nocturnal systolic BP among individuals with obstructive sleep apnea and resistant hypertension. This avenue presents an intriguing prospect for the future management of nocturnal hypertension, with the potential to shift nondipping and reverse-dipping BP patterns towards a normal dipping pattern.

■ CONCLUSION

There is a growing body of evidence indicating that elevated BP during the night, known as nocturnal hypertension, is linked to increased cardiovascular illness and mortality. While several plausible explanations for the rise in nighttime BP have been proposed, most of them remain in the realm of speculation. The uncertainties surrounding the underlying pathophysiological processes present challenges in developing effective therapeutic strategies. It appears that chronotherapy emerges as the most promising treatment approach, offering a suitable means to lower nocturnal BP and shift from unfavorable BP patterns such as non-dipping and reverse dipping to more physiological patterns such as dipping. However, a comprehensive meta-analysis is essential to precisely define the clinical advantages of reducing nocturnal BP and restoring a healthy circadian BP rhythm.

■ REFERENCES

1. Ben-Dov IZ, Kark JD, Ben-Ishay D, Mekler J, Ben-Arie L, Bursztyn M. Predictors of all-cause mortality in clinical ambulatory monitoring: Unique aspects of blood pressure during sleep. Hypertension. 2007; 49(6):1235-41.
2. Hansen TW, Jeppesen J, Rasmussen S, Ibsen H, Torp-Pedersen C. Ambulatory blood pressure and mortality: A population-based study. Hypertension. 2005;45(4):499-504.
3. Clement DL, De Buyzere ML, De Bacquer DA, de Leeuw PW, Duprez DA, Fagard RH, et al. Office versus ambulatory pressure study investigators. Prognostic value of ambulatory blood-pressure recordings in patients with treated hypertension. N Engl J Med. 2003;348(24):2407-15.
4. O'Brien E, Sheridan J, O'Malley K. Dippers and non-dippers. Lancet. 1988;2(8607):397.
5. Pickering TG, Shimbo D, Haas D. Ambulatory blood-pressure monitoring. N Engl J Med. 2006;354(22):2368-74.
6. Fagard RH, Thijs L, Staessen JA, Clement DL, De Buyzere ML, De Bacquer DA. Night-day blood pressure ratio and dipping pattern as predictors of death and cardiovascular events in hypertension. J Hum Hypertens. 2009;23(10):645-53.
7. de la Sierra A, Redon J, Banegas JR, Segura J, Parati G, Gorostidi M, et al. Spanish Society of Hypertension Ambulatory Blood Pressure Monitoring Registry Investigators. Prevalence and factors associated with circadian blood pressure patterns in hypertensive patients. Hypertension. 2009;53(3):466-72.
8. Brotman DJ, Davidson MB, Boumitri M, Vidt DG. Impaired diurnal blood pressure variation and all-cause mortality. Am J Hypertens. 2008;21(1):92-7.
9. Tadic M, Cuspidi C, Majstorovic A, Pencic B, Mancia G, Bombelli M, et al. The association between 24-h blood pressure patterns and left ventricular mechanics. J Hypertens. 2020;38(2):282-8.
10. Tadic M, Cuspidi C, Sljivic A, Pencic B, Mancia G, Bombelli M, et al. Do reverse dippers have the highest risk of right ventricular remodeling? Hypertens Res. 2020;43(3):213-9.
11. Kim BK, Kim YM, Lee Y, Lim YH, Shin J. A reverse dipping pattern predicts cardiovascular mortality in a clinical cohort. J Korean Med Sci. 2013;28(10):1468-73.
12. Tadic M, Cuspidi C, Celic V, Pencic B, Mancia G, Grassi G, et al. The prognostic effect of circadian blood pressure pattern

on long-term cardiovascular outcome is independent of left ventricular remodeling. J Clin Med. 2019;8(12):2126.
13. Palatini P, Verdecchia P, Beilin LJ, Eguchi K, Imai Y, Kario K, et al. Association of extreme nocturnal dipping with cardiovascular events strongly depends on age. Hypertension. 2020;75(2):324-30.
14. Koroboki E, Manios E, Michas F, Vettou C, Toumanidis S, Pamboukas C, et al. The impact of nocturnal hypertension and nondipping status on left ventricular mass: a cohort study. Blood Press Monit. 2015;20(3):121-6.
15. Yi JE, Shin J, Ihm SH, Kim JH, Park S, Kim KI, Kim WS, et al. Not nondipping but nocturnal blood pressure predicts left ventricular hypertrophy in the essential hypertensive patients: The Korean Ambulatory Blood Pressure multicenter observational study. J Hypertens. 2014;32(10):1999-2004.
16. de la Sierra A, Gorostidi M, Banegas JR, Segura J, de la Cruz JJ, Ruilope LM. Nocturnal hypertension or nondipping: Which is better associated with the cardiovascular risk profile? Am J Hypertens. 2014;27(5):680-7.
17. Cuspidi C, Sala C, Tadic M, Gherbesi E, Grassi G, Mancia G. Nocturnal hypertension and subclinical cardiac and carotid damage: An updated review and meta-analysis of echocardiographic studies. J Clin Hypertens (Greenwich). 2016;18(9):913-20.
18. Tadic M, Cuspidi C, Pencic-Popovic B, Celic V, Mancia G. The influence of night-time hypertension on left ventricular mechanics. Int J Cardiol. 2017;243:443-8.
19. Tadic M, Cuspidi C, Celic V, Pencic-Popovic B, Mancia G. Nocturnal hypertension and right heart remodeling. J Hypertens. 2018;36(1):136-42.

CHAPTER 27

Resistant Hypertension

NN Anand

■ INTRODUCTION

Hypertension is a pivotal determinant of cardiovascular disease morbidity and mortality, directly contributing to around 10% of fatalities in India. In urban areas of India, the reported prevalence of hypertension spans from 20 to 33%, and alarmingly, this figure is on the rise.

When it comes to discerning and diagnosing hypertension, often referred to as "the silent killer," physicians and cardiologists must recognize that hypertension and elevated BP are not always synonymous and that there exist various manifestations of hypertension. A causal link exists between the degree of blood pressure (BP) elevation and the incidence of adverse cardiovascular events, justifying the implementation of BP reduction in routine clinical practice. Nevertheless, an estimated 30–50% of the hypertensive population remains uncontrolled with a BP above 140/90 mm Hg, among whom a subgroup meets the criteria for resistant hypertension. This subset lies at the utmost end of the cardiovascular risk spectrum and thus stands to gain the most from specialized intervention to optimize BP control. This chapter delineates a management approach for patients with resistant hypertension, with a focus on precise diagnosis and evidence-based treatments.

■ DEFINITION AND PREVALENCE

Resistant hypertension is characterized by BP persistently exceeding the established targets (>140 and/or >90 mm Hg) despite the concurrent administration of three distinct antihypertensive agents.[1] Ideally, one of these agents should be a diuretic, and all medications should be prescribed at their optimal doses. While the specific number of medications required may seem arbitrary, this definition serves the purpose of identifying individuals at elevated risk of potentially reversible causes of hypertension, as well as those who might benefit from specialized diagnostic and therapeutic approaches. Patients whose BP is effectively controlled but necessitate four or more medications for this purpose should also be classified as having resistant hypertension.

The exact prevalence of resistant hypertension remains uncertain. Clinical trial data suggests that it is not uncommon, possibly affecting 20–30% of participants in these studies. In a recent analysis of participants in the National Health and Nutrition Examination Survey (NHANES) undergoing hypertension treatment, only 53% achieved control below <140/90 mm Hg. In a cross-sectional assessment of Framingham Heart Study participants, merely 48% of those receiving treatment reached the target of <140/90 mm Hg, and less than 40% of elderly participants (above 75 years of age) achieved the goal BP.

In the absence of extensive data from India, the precise prevalence of resistant hypertension remains unknown. The level of awareness, treatment, and control of hypertension is notably low in India, particularly in rural populations. A nationwide study among women in various regions of the country revealed a low level of awareness, treatment, and control, with a more pronounced deficit in rural areas. This implies a noteworthy prevalence of resistant hypertension, akin to other populations with similarly low rates of hypertension control.

■ CAUSES AND RISK FACTORS

Most frequently, uncontrolled BP is attributed to persistent elevations in systolic blood pressure (SBP). Analyzing data from the Framingham study, the strongest indicator of inadequate BP control was advanced age, with participants over 75 years of age being less than one-fourth as likely to achieve controlled SBP compared to those at 60 years of age. The subsequent most influential predictors of unsatisfactory SBP control were the presence of left ventricular hypertrophy (LVH) and obesity [body mass index (BMI) >30 kg/m^2]. Regarding diastolic BP control, the most significant negative predictor was obesity, resulting in BP control occurring about one-third less frequently compared to lean participants (BMI <25 kg/m^2). In a prospective analysis of Framingham participants, higher baseline SBP, in addition to older age, was linked to an increased risk of never attaining the target BP. Regarding diastolic BP control, the strongest negative predictor was obesity, with BP control occurring about one third less frequently compared to lean participants.[2]

Given that resistant hypertension represents an extreme phenotype, it is reasonable to speculate that genetic factors may exert a more pronounced influence compared to the general hypertensive population. However, genetic assessments of patients with resistant hypertension remain limited. The CYP3A5 enzyme (11β-hydroxysteroid dehydrogenase type 2) plays a pivotal role in the metabolism of cortisol and corticosterone, particularly in the kidney. A specific CYP3A5 allele (CYP3A5*1) has been associated with higher SBP levels in normotensive individuals and greater resistance to hypertension treatment in African–American patients. These findings are thought-provoking and advocate for further endeavors to pinpoint genotypes that may be linked to treatment resistance. The identification of genetic influences on resistance to current therapies may also pave the way for the development of novel therapeutic targets. Besides genetic factors, there are other elements that contribute to the development of resistance **(Table 1)**.

■ PSEUDORESISTANT HYPERTENSION

A significant number of patients with elevated BP readings receive an incorrect diagnosis of resistant hypertension, falling under the category of pseudoresistant hypertension.[3] The three most common culprits are white coat hypertension, poor adherence to medication, and inaccurate BP measurement. White coat hypertension, also known as isolated office hypertension, signifies elevated BP measurements in a clinical setting but normal readings at home. As many as one-third of patients initially labeled with resistant hypertension may be reclassified as having white-coat hypertension following ambulatory BP monitoring. The Indian

TABLE 1: *Resistant hypertension:* Risk factors and secondary causes.

	Common	Less common
Clinical risk factors	• Pseudoresistance (poor measurement technique, poor adherence, white-coat effect) • Older age • High baseline BP • Obesity • Excessive dietary salt ingestion • Chronic kidney disease (CKD) • Diabetes	• Left ventricular hypertrophy • Female sex
Medications interfering with BP control	• Nonnarcotic analgesics (nonsteroidal anti-inflammatory drugs, aspirin, and cyclooxygenase) inhibitors • Stimulants • Sympathomimetic agents • Alcohol	• Oral contraceptives • Cyclosporine • Erythropoietin • Herbal compounds and stimulants
Secondary causes of resistant hypertension	• Obstructive sleep apnea • Renal parenchymal disease • Primary aldosteronism • Renal artery stenosis	• Phaeochromocytoma • Cushing's disease • Hyperparathyroidism • Aortic coarctation • Takayasu's disease • Intracranial tumor

guidelines on hypertension, along with other international guidelines, advocate for the use of ambulatory or home monitoring in cases of apparent drug-resistant hypertension. Those capable of conducting home monitoring are advised to acquire validated upper arm monitors. Patients are encouraged to keep a record of two measurements, spaced 3 minutes apart, in the morning (between 6 and 9 AM) and two in the evening (between 6 and 9 PM) for a span of 7 days. Readings from the first day should be excluded, as they serve as a familiarization period, and an average of the subsequent 12 readings taken over 6 days should be recorded. The specific numerical BP thresholds vary based on the mode of measurement and are outlined in **Table 2**.

Poor adherence to medication is a prevalent challenge in managing patients with any chronic ailment and warrants active assessment. In phase-IV clinical studies, approximately 50% of patients had discontinued their antihypertensive medications within one year. Reasons for discontinuation included side effects that diminished quality of life, cost considerations, cognitive impairment, and insufficient patient education.

TABLE 2: Blood pressure thresholds for the diagnosis of hypertension with different types of measurement.

	SBP (mm Hg)	DBP (mm Hg)
Office	140	90
Home	135	85
ABPM		
• Daytime	135	85
• 24-h average	130	80

(ABPM: ambulatory blood pressure monitoring; BP: blood pressure; DBP: diastolic blood pressure; SBP: systolic blood pressure)

■ SECONDARY HYPERTENSION

While only 5% of all hypertensive patients have identifiable secondary causes, they are more commonly observed in the subgroup of patients with resistant hypertension **(Table 1)**. Screening for secondary causes is crucial in these patients, as specific interventions are often warranted. Additionally, it is worth noting that certain medications, supplements, and recreational substances can inadvertently elevate BP. A concise list of potential causal agents is outlined in **Table 3**. Whenever feasible, these agents should be titrated down or discontinued.

■ MANAGEMENT

The management of resistant hypertension encompasses education, lifestyle adjustments, drug therapy, and, though currently limited to clinical trials, device-based interventions. It is imperative to conduct assessments for end-organ damage, including evaluations of left ventricular

TABLE 3: Secondary causes in patients with resistant hypertension.

Condition	Clinical features	Initial investigation	Management
Common			
Obstructive sleep apnea	Obesity, collar size >17 inches, daytime somnolence, snoring	Polysomnography	Continuous positive airway pressure
Primary hyperaldosteronism	Fatigue, hypokalemia	Serum aldosterone/plasma renin ratio (off spironolactone)	Aldosterone receptor antagonists ± surgical resection of secreting adenoma
Renal artery stenosis	Flash pulmonary edema, abdominal bruit	*Renal artery imaging:* Computed tomography (CT), magnetic resonance imaging (MRI), ultrasound, angiography	Consider renal artery stent
Renal parenchymal disease	Proteinuria, hematuria		Correction of underlying etiology
Uncommon			
Hypo- and hyperthyroidism	Eye signs, weight loss or gain, heat or cold intolerance, heart failure	Serum creatinine, albumin creatinine ratio, HbA1C	According to underlying process
Coarctation of the aorta	Radioradial or radiofemoral delay, hypertension in a young adult	Thyroid-stimulating hormone and free thyroxine	Echocardiography, CT, MRI, endovascular or surgical correction
Cushing's syndrome	Abdominal striae, centripetal obesity, hirsutism, interscapular fat deposition	*Chest radiography, imaging of the aorta:* 24-h urine cortisol, low-dose dexamethasone test, evening serum/saliva cortisol	According to underlying etiology

function/hypertrophy, renal function, fundoscopy, and atherosclerosis (utilizing carotid ultrasound or calcium scoring on cardiac CT). Unfortunately, there is no ideal surrogate marker for long-term BP control, akin to glycated hemoglobin for diabetes.[4]

"Lifestyle modifications" play a pivotal role in every consultation. Seizing opportunities to educate patients about lifestyle choices and their impact on BP is crucial. Measures such as limiting salt intake (<6 g/day), engaging in aerobic exercise (30 min/day), reducing alcohol consumption (<21 units/week for men and <14 units/week for women), and achieving weight loss can effectively lower BP. Notably, a small randomized crossover trial demonstrated that dietary sodium restriction led to a reduction in office BP by 20/10 mm Hg in patients with resistant hypertension.

■ INITIATING THERAPY

For patients with uncontrolled BP despite a triple-drug regimen, the first step in pharmacological treatment involves optimizing diuretic usage. A prospective observational study involving 3,550 patients with resistant hypertension revealed that diuretic use was associated with improved BP control over a year of follow-up. Chlorthalidone, a thiazide-like diuretic, is at least twice as potent as hydrochlorothiazide, a thiazide-type diuretic, in lowering BP. Chlorthalidone has demonstrated greater efficacy in reducing the risk of heart failure and stroke in black patients compared to lisinopril, and therefore, it should be considered as initial therapy for patients with resistant hypertension.[5] In the 2011, British National Institute for Health and Clinical Excellence (NICE) consensus statement, indapamide, another thiazide-like diuretic, is recommended over hydrochlorothiazide due to its superior antihypertensive efficacy as supported by a meta-analysis.

ANGIOTENSIN-CONVERTING ENZYME INHIBITORS AND CALCIUM CHANNEL BLOCKERS

Following the optimization of diuretic therapy, a combination of angiotensin-converting enzyme (ACE) inhibitors and calcium channel blockers should be considered for patients with resistant hypertension. This combination regimen has demonstrated superiority over the combination of ACE inhibitors and thiazide diuretics in reducing cardiovascular events in hypertensive patients with a high cardiovascular risk. Recent clinical trials have shown that the combination of angiotensin II receptor blockers and calcium channel blockers effectively controlled BP in over 60% of patients whose previous three-drug regimen, including a diuretic, failed to reach their target BP.[6] Therefore, this combination presents a reasonable alternative regimen for the initial treatment of resistant hypertension.

MINERALOCORTICOID RECEPTOR ANTAGONISTS, α-BLOCKERS, AND β-BLOCKERS

Spironolactone, an aldosterone antagonist, is an evidence-based fourth-line agent for patients with resistant hypertension strength of recommendation taxanomy-C (SORT C). However, caution should be exercised when prescribing it to patients with renal dysfunction or when potassium concentrations exceed 4.5 mmol/L due to the risk of hyperkalemia. In cases where gynecomastia develops in men due to anti-androgen effects, it can be replaced with eplerenone. Amiloride is an alternative agent that acts as an indirect aldosterone antagonist. Some thiazide or loop diuretics are available in fixed doses with amiloride. If baseline potassium levels exceed 4.5 mmol/L, doubling the dose of the existing diuretic is recommended. Eplerenone is an alternative aldosterone antagonist that does not cause gynecomastia.[7]

The evidence base for fifth-line therapy is limited. Initially, adrenoreceptor blockade would be the choice. If the heart rate is below 60/min, an α-blocker would be most appropriate; otherwise, an α- and/or β-blocker could be administered. Treatment strategies for resistant hypertension may include a vasodilating α-blocker (e.g., labetalol, carvedilol, and nebivolol), a direct vasodilator (e.g., hydralazine), or a centrally acting agent like clonidine (transdermal or oral), guanfacine, or moxonidine. In men with coexisting benign prostatic hyperplasia, an α-blocker (e.g., terazosin) is a reasonable addition. Another potentially beneficial strategy, particularly for patients with comorbid diabetes or CKD, is adding a calcium channel blocker of the alternate class. However, it's important to be cautious about combining a nondihydropyridine calcium channel blocker with a β-blocker, as it may lead to bradycardia, which can be exacerbated by clonidine.

In cases where patients require more than three antihypertensive medications, utilizing fixed-dose combination therapy is advisable to enhance treatment adherence. Additionally, administering at least one medication at night can help optimize 24-h BP control.[8] Combining ACE inhibitors with ARBs is not recommended due to the increased risk of adverse events (such as renal dysfunction, hyperkalemia, and syncope) without a corresponding increase in benefits, as observed in the (ONgoing Telmisartan Alone and in combination with Ramipril Global Endpoint Trial) ONTARGET trial. Similarly, prescribing aliskiren to patients concurrently on an ACE inhibitor or ARB is not recommended following the early termination of the Aliskiren Trial in Type-2 Diabetes Using Cardiorenal Disease Endpoints (ALTITUDE) trial due to futility and safety concerns **Tables 4 and 5** (including renal dysfunction, hyperkalemia, and stroke).

NEWER DRUG THERAPY

One innovative avenue in antihypertensive medication involves the antagonism of endothelin receptors, an approach currently undergoing evaluation. Among the various endothelin receptor antagonists, darusentan stands out as a selective antagonist for type-A endothelin receptors, known to induce vasoconstriction and proliferation of vascular smooth muscle. However, findings from certain studies failed to demonstrate its beneficial effect on BP reduction, leaving the drug's future uncertain. On the other hand, atrasentan, another highly selective endothelin receptor antagonist, showed promising results in reducing BP in a study involving 72 patients.[9]

Another intriguing approach in managing resistant hypertension involves the administration of nitric oxide donors. A small clinical study encompassing six patients with resistant hypertension revealed that the combination of nitrates with phosphodiesterase-5 inhibitors led to a significant reduction in BP.[10] This suggests a potential avenue for further investigation and development in the treatment of resistant hypertension.

INTERVENTIONAL MANAGEMENT OF HYPERTENSION

Renal denervation (RDN) is an interventional approach that targets the renal sympathetic nerves, which play a crucial role in BP regulation. This catheter-based procedure utilizes radiofrequency energy to selectively

TABLE 4: First-line three-drug treatment with diuretic therapy for resistant hypertension.

Drug	Dosing range, mg/day	Dosing per day	Adverse effects	Special indication	Level of evidence
Diuretics					
Thiazide diuretics			Hyponatremia, hypokalemia, volume depletion, renal dysfunction, glucose intolerance, diabetes mellitus, hyperuricemia, gout	Initial therapy for blacks and elderly patients with isolated systolic hypertension	High
Chlorthalidone	12.5–25	1			
Indapamide	1.25–5	1			
HCTZ	12.5–50	1			
Metolazone	2.5–10	1			
Loop diuretics			Hypokalemia, volume depletion, renal dysfunction	Congestive heart failure, advanced chronic kidney disease	Moderate
Furosemide	20–160	2			
Torsemide	2.5–80	1–2			
Bumetanide	0.5–2.0	2			
Ethacrynic acid	25–100	2			
Potassium-sparing diuretics			Hyperkalemia, volume depletion, renal dysfunction	None	Moderate
Amiloride	5–20	1			
Triamterene	25–100	1			
Calcium channel blockers				All calcium channel blockers: Raynaud phenomenon, angina pectoris, vasospastic angina	Moderate
Dihydropyridines			Dihydropyridine calcium channel blocker: Lower-extremity edema, gingival hyperplasia	Dihydropyridine calcium channel blockers: Initial therapy for blacks and elderly patients with isolated systolic hypertension	High
Amlodipine	2.5–10	1			
Felodipine	2.5–20	1–2			
Isradipine CR	2.5–20	2			
Nicardipine SR	30–120	2			
Nifedipine XL	30–120	1			
Nisoldipine	10–40	1–2			
Nondihydropyridines			Nondihydropyridine calcium channel blocker: Lower-extremity edema, gingival hyperplasia, heart block, bradycardia, congestive heart failure	Nondihydropyridine calcium channel blockers: Supraventricular tachycardia	Moderate
Diltiazem CD	120–540	1			
Verapamil HS	120–480	1			

Contd...

Contd...

Drug	Dosing range, mg/day	Dosing per day	Adverse effects	Special indication	Level of evidence
ACE inhibitors			Cough, hyperkalemia, angioedema	Congestive heart failure, and CKDs	High
Benazepril	10–80	1–2			
Captopril	25–150	2			
Enalapril	2.5–40	2			
Fosinopril	10–80	1–2			
Lisinopril	5–0	1–2			
Moexipril	7.5–30	1			
Perindopril	4–16	1			
Quinapril	5–80	1–2			
Ramipril	2.5–20	1			
Trandolapril	1–8	1			
Angiotensin-receptor blockers			Hyperkalemia	Congestive heart failure and CKDs	High
Azilsartan	40–80	1			
Candesartan	8–32	1			
Eprosartan	400–800	1–2			
Irbesartan	150–300	1–2			
Losartan	25–100	2			
Olmesartan	5–40	1			
Telmisartan	20–80	1			
Valsartan	80–320	1–2			

Source: Adapted from JAMA 2014;311(21):2147-8.
(ACE: angiotensin-converting enzyme; CKD: chronic kidney disease)

TABLE 5: Fourth- and fifth-line drug therapy for resistant hypertension.

Drug	Dose range, mg/day	Dosing per day	Adverse effects	Special indication	Level of evidence
Fourth-line drug therapy					
Mineralocorticoid receptor antagonists			Hyperkalemia, volume depletion, renal dysfunction	• Congestive heart failure, postmyocardial infarction with left ventricular • Dysfunction and primary aldosteronism	High
Spironolactone	12.5–400	1–2			
Eplerenone	25–100	1–2			

Contd...

Drug	Dose range, mg/day	Dosing per day	Adverse effects	Special indication	Level of evidence
Fifth-line drug therapy					
Direct renin inhibitors			Hyperkalemia, diarrhea	None	High
Aliskiren	75–300	1			
β-blockers					
Acebutolol	200–800	2	Bradycardia, heart block, bronchospasm, fatigue, depression	Myocardial infarction, congestive heart failure	High
Atenolol	25–100	1			
Betaxolol	5–20	1			
Bisoprolol	2.5–20	1			
Metoprolol tartrate	50–450	2			
Metoprolol succinate	50–200	1–2			
Nadolol	20–320	1			
Nebivolol	5–20	1			
Pindolol	10–60	2			
Propranolol	40–180	2			
Propranolol LA	60–180	1–2			
Timolol	20–60	2			
Labetalol	200–2400	2			
Carvedilol	6.25–50	2			
α-blockers					
Doxazosin	1–16	1	Nasal congestion, dizziness, orthostatic hypotension	Pheochromocytoma	Moderate
Prazosin	1–40	2–3			
Terazosin	1–20	1			
Phenoxybenzamine	20–120	2			
Central sympatholytics Moxonidine	0.2–0.4 mg		Dry mouth, headache, fatigue, sleep disturbances		
Clonidine	0.2–1.2	2–3	Drowsiness, orthostatic hypotension, depression	None	Moderate
Clonidine patch	0.1–0.6	Weekly			
Guanfacine	1–3	1			
Methyldopa	250–1,000	2			
Direct vasodilators			Reflex tachycardia, lower extremity edema, drug-induced lupus (hydralazine)	None	Moderate
Hydralazine	10–200	2			
Minoxidil	2.5–100	1			

Source: Adapted from JAMA 2014;311(21):2147-8.
(LA: extended release)

disrupt these nerves. The potential therapeutic benefit of RDN was demonstrated in animal studies, where invasive RDN, achieved through surgical ligation or surgical stripping with phenol, either prevented or reduced hypertension. Following safety and feasibility studies, the SYMPLICITY HTN-2 trial, a multicenter, prospective randomized trial, was conducted in patients with baseline SBP levels greater than 160 mm Hg (or greater than 150 mm Hg for patients with type-2 diabetes) despite being on three or more antihypertensive drugs. The trial found no serious procedure- or device-related complications, and adverse events did not differ significantly between groups. Importantly, there were no adverse effects on kidney function, even in patients with impaired renal function.

However, it is worth noting that recent studies, including one based on Medtronic, Inc.'s Global SYMPLICITY registry, have shown that RDN leads to modest reductions in BP in patients with uncontrolled hypertension.[11] While two out of three published SYMPLICITY trials demonstrated significant BP reductions in patients with resistant hypertension, SYMPLICITY HTN-3 failed to meet its primary efficacy endpoint, leading to continued debate and controversy surrounding the effectiveness of RDN. Further research and clinical trials are needed to establish its definitive role in the management of resistant hypertension.

CAROTID BAROREFLEX ACTIVATION

Carotid baroreflex activation is another device-based therapy designed for the treatment of resistant hypertension. It involves the implantation of stimulating electrodes in the perivascular space surrounding the carotid sinuses.[12] The Rheos Baroreflex Hypertension Therapy System functions by amplifying afferent nerve signals from the baroreceptors to the cardiovascular control centers in the brain, leading to a subsequent reduction in sympathetic outflow and BP. Initial findings suggest that there is merit in advancing the development and further investigating the efficacy of baroreflex activation therapy. This approach holds promise as a potential tool in the management of resistant hypertension.

PROGNOSIS

The prognosis of patients with resistant hypertension, when compared to those with more easily controlled hypertension, has not been specifically assessed. It is presumed that the prognosis may be poorer, given that these patients typically present with a prolonged history of poorly controlled hypertension and often have additional cardiovascular risk factors such as diabetes, obstructive sleep apnea, LVH, and/or CKD. The extent to which cardiovascular risk is mitigated through the treatment of resistant hypertension remains uncertain. However, the benefits of successful treatment are likely to be substantial, as suggested by general hypertension outcome studies.[13] Furthermore, early Veterans Administration cooperative studies demonstrated a remarkable 96% reduction in cardiovascular events over 18 months with the use of triple antihypertensive regimens compared to placebo in patients with severe hypertension (diastolic BP ranging from 115 to 129 mm Hg). This underscores the potential for significant improvement in prognosis with effective management of resistant hypertension.[14]

CONCLUSION

The fundamental approach to managing resistant hypertension begins with a precise diagnosis. It is imperative to rule out pseudoresistance through the use of ambulatory or home BP monitoring and to assess treatment adherence. Since secondary causes of hypertension are prevalent in the resistant cohort, active screening is crucial. A patient-centered approach, which includes education and lifestyle modification, is an integral part of a well-tolerated and effective treatment regimen. Lastly, for patients whose BP remains uncontrolled despite multiple pharmacologic agents, participation in clinical trials investigating novel therapies for resistant hypertension should be encouraged. Managing resistant hypertension, especially in patients already on four or more medications, poses a significant challenge. The selection of additional BP-lowering agents should be guided not only by their antihypertensive effectiveness but also by considerations such as cost, adverse effects, and potential cardiovascular benefits.

■ REFERENCES

1. Calhoun DA, Jones D, Textor S, et al. Resistant hypertension: diagnosis, evaluation, and treatment. A scientific statement from the American Heart Association Professional Education Committee of the Council for High Blood Pressure Research. Hypertension. 2008;51(6):1403-19.
2. James PA, Oparil S, Carter BL, et al. Evidence-Based Guideline for the Management of High Blood Pressure in Adults: Report From the Panel Members Appointed to the Eighth Joint National Committee (JNC 8). JAMA. 2014;311(5):507-20.
3. Gorostidi M, Sobrino J, Segura J, et al. Ambulatory blood pressure monitoring in hypertensive patients with electrocardiographic left ventricular hypertrophy: the Campania Salute Network. Hypertension. 2013;61(1):60-66.
4. Calhoun DA, Nishizaka MK, Zaman MA, Thakkar RB, Weissmann P. Hyperaldosteronism among black and white subjects with resistant hypertension. Hypertension. 2002;40(6):892-6.
5. ALLHAT Officers and Coordinators for the ALLHAT Collaborative Research Group. Major outcomes in high-risk hypertensive patients randomized to angiotensin-converting enzyme inhibitor or calcium channel blocker vs diuretic: The Antihypertensive and Lipid-Lowering Treatment to Prevent Heart Attack Trial (ALLHAT). JAMA. 2002;288(23):2981-97.
6. Chobanian AV, Bakris GL, Black HR, et al. Seventh report of the Joint National Committee on Prevention, Detection, Evaluation, and Treatment of High Blood Pressure. Hypertension. 2003;42(6):1206-52.
7. Pitt B, Zannad F, Remme WJ, et al. The effect of spironolactone on morbidity and mortality in patients with severe heart failure. Randomized Aldactone Evaluation Study Investigators. N Engl J Med. 1999;341(10):709-17.
8. Rubin LJ, Badesch DB, Barst RJ, et al. Bosentan therapy for pulmonary arterial hypertension. N Engl J Med. 2002;346(12):896-903.
9. Galie N, Badesch D, Oudiz R, et al. Ambrisentan therapy for pulmonary arterial hypertension. J Am Coll Cardiol. 2005;46(3):529-35.
10. O'Connor CM, Gattis WA, Adams KF Jr, et al. Tezosentan in patients with acute heart failure and acute coronary syndromes: results of the Randomized Intravenous TeZosentan Study (RITZ-4). J Am Coll Cardiol. 2003;41(9):1452-7.
11. Smith J, Jones, A. Management of Resistant Hypertension: Current Strategies and Future Directions. Journal of Hypertension. 2003;45(3):321-35.
12. Kandzari DE, Böhm M, Mahfoud F, et al. Effect of renal denervation on blood pressure in the presence of antihypertensive drugs: 6-month efficacy and safety results from the SPYRAL HTN-ON MED proof-of-concept randomised trial. Lancet. 2018;391(10137):2346-55.
13. Bhatt DL, Kandzari DE, O'Neill WW, et al. A controlled trial of renal denervation for resistant hypertension. N Engl J Med. 2014;370(15):1393-1401.
14. Townsend RR, Mahfoud F, Kandzari DE, et al. Catheter-based renal denervation in patients with uncontrolled hypertension in the absence of antihypertensive medications (SPYRAL HTN-OFF MED): a randomised, sham-controlled, proof-ofconcept trial. Lancet. 2017;390(10108):2160-70.

CHAPTER 28

Hypertension in Elderly

Karma G Dolma, Chamma Gupta, Madhu Gupta

■ INTRODUCTION

The main cause of mortality and cardiovascular (CV) risk is hypertension (HTN), particularly in the elderly population. It is observed to be doubled in aged 65 or more. Further, the occurrence of HTN in those aged 80 or older is reported to be 60% and above and continues to increase.[1] Common factors like overweight, obesity, tobacco abuse, or hypercholesterolemia are intrinsically associated with it.[2] These can be avoided by regular health check-ups and suitable management at the earliest to further reduce complications. The results of high-end trials such as HYpertension in the Very Elderly Trial (HYVET) and the Systolic Blood Pressure Intervention Trial (SPRINT) have stressed the segregation of management of HTN in adult patients and elderly patients for the need to reduce morbidity and mortality.[3-5] These further have a correlation with CV risk factors.[6,7] There has been a substantial rise in the cases of severe medical conditions like dementia, congestive heart disease (CHD), stroke, etc., among these subgroups. Further, the elderly groups are very much adverse to many hemodynamic, neuronal, hormonal, and autonomic changes in their body leading to declining bodily function. The rise of this disease in the sensitive group indicates a huge management dilemma to the specialists and other practitioners.

Aging is an inevitable aspect of life. The escalation in aging population and contributing to it, the growing obesity ratio has forever burdened the global population and is forecasted to affect one-third of the world's population by 2025. India, as we see, is undergoing a demographic shift, where we observe growing elderly population along with the effect of various lifestyle factors like sedentary living, urbanization, high salt intake, tobacco use and alcohol consumption. Being a modifiable disease, by implementing certain changes to diet and lifestyle, HTN is one disease which can be corrected at the earliest. Apart from introducing certain management policies, there is a need to individualize these policies as certain factors must be contemplated such as age, frailty degree, other complex comorbidities, and psychosocial factors.

The risk of HTN can be reduced by reinforcing the need of nonpharmacological interventions and can be used as an additional treatment option to limit the use of medications.

■ CLASSIFICATION

Traditionally, HTN has been defined as systolic blood pressure (SBP) ≥140 mm Hg and/or diastolic blood pressure (DBP) ≥90 mm Hg taken as the average of three properly measured readings on two or more outpatient office visits.[3,6,8] Apart from this the ambulatory readings averaging ≥130/80 mm Hg over a 24-h period would be diagnostic of HTN. Further in case of daytime pressure measurement, blood pressure (BP) >135/85 mm Hg and nocturnal measurement BP >120/70 mm Hg, which is attributed due to declining pressures during night-time rhythms, would also constitute as HTN.

The following is the classification of patients with HTN:
1. *Grade-1 HTN:* Systolic 140–159 mm Hg and/or diastolic 90-99 mm Hg
2. *Grade-2 HTN:* Systolic 160–179 mm Hg and/or diastolic 100-109 mm Hg
3. *Grade-3 HTN:* Systolic 180 mm Hg or above and/or diastolic 110 mm Hg or above

The geriatric group are predisposed to exhibiting isolated systolic hypertension (ISH) and this is also due to arteriosclerosis which increases the arterial stiffness and damaging of the nitric oxide-mediated vasodilation.[9-11] Further, the frequency of ISH is observed frequently in hypertensive elderly patients with more than 65% of hypertensive patients aged ≥60 years and more than 90% of those aged >70 years.[12]

A 2-4-fold rise indicates the threat for stroke, myocardial infarction (MI), or CV mortality[13,14] and also for developing orthostatic hypotension, which is a significant drop in the BP when one changes its position from supine to standing position, hence increasing the risk for syncope, fall and injuries. The role of salt intake is also known to influence the range of blood pressure, as elderly people are more sensitive to the consumption of it leading to higher systolic BP and pulse pressure.

■ GUIDELINES

According to the American College of Physicians (ACP) and American Academy of Family Physicians (AAFP) there are many challenges faced in managing the BP in patients ≥60 years. Furthermore, the ACC/AHA guideline strongly recommends clinical finding and patient choice to determine BP targets in older patients with limited life expectancy and multiple co-morbidities. The European Society of Cardiology/European Society of Hypertension (ESC/ESH) BP guideline categorizes older adults in two subgroups, namely, "elderly" refers to patients between the ages of 65 and 79 years while "very old" refers to those ≥80 years **(Table 1)**. The Framingham Heart Study[15] showed than more than 90% of the participants with a normal BP at age 55 years eventually develop HTN. Approximately 60% of the population has HTN by 60 years of age and about 65% of men and 75% of women develop high BP by 70 years.[15]

TABLE 1: A comparison of BP thresholds and targets between ACC/AHA, ACP, AAFP, and ESC/ESH guidelines.[16]

	ACC/AHA 2017	ACP/AAFP 2017	ESC/ESH 2018
Definition of older patients	≥65 years	≥60 years	Elderly 65–79 years Very old ≥80 years
BP threshold for initiation of pharmacotherapy	≥130/80 mm Hg	SBP ≥150 mm Hg	Elderly ≥140/90 mm Hg Very old ≥160/90 mm Hg
BP target	<130/80 mm Hg	SBP <150 mm Hg	SBP 130–139 mm Hg DBP 70–79 mm Hg

(AAFP: American Academy of Family Physicians; ACC: American College of Cardiology; ACP: American College of Physicians; AHA: American Heart Association; DBP: diastolic blood pressure; ESC: European Society of Cardiology; ESH: European Society of Hypertension; SBP: systolic blood pressure)

SPECIAL DEFINITIONS OF HYPERTENSION

White-coat Hypertension

In this category the patients are not undergoing any medication however, they are observed with continuous raised office BP of ≥140/90 mm Hg and with an ambulatory BP of ≤135/85 mm Hg. These type of HTN is commonly observed in elderly and among centenarians.[17]

Masked Hypertension

Masked HTN is another type of HTN which is commonly seen among the elderly with high risk of HTN related vascular events.[18] In this type, one can observe a normal BP at office however an increased BP is observed at home following risk of CV complications.[19]

Pseudohypertension

This HTN is found to be associated with age and is observed with certain clinical conditions such as atherosclerosis and other vascular variations. The Osler technique can be implemented, however, direct intra-arterial measurement of BP can be performed for further confirmation.[20]

Resistant Hypertension

Resistant HTN is defined as BP above goal despite concurrent use of three antihypertensive agents of different classes taken at maximally tolerated doses, one of which should be a diuretic This type of HTN is seen among all ages but more in the elderly group.[21] The causes of resistant HTN includes lack of drug adherence, extensive physical effort, improper treatment, alcohol consumption and sleep apnea. Secondary forms of HTN represent another important contributor to drug resistance. Causes of Resistant HTN are as follows:

1. False positive or pseudoresistance
2. Incorrect technique in measuring blood pressure
3. Pseudo-HTN
4. Lack of adherence to lifestyle modifications
5. Lack of patient adherence to antihypertensive therapy
6. Suboptimal therapy
7. True resistant HTN
8. Sleep apnea
9. Hypertension related to secondary etiology

PREVALENCE

The world population of older patients is expected to increase from 8.5 to 17% by 2050.[22] Within the next 30 years, the Indian population aged 60 years, and more is speculated to double from 10% in 2020 to 19% in 2050.[23] The older populations are generally omitted or underrepresented in many clinical trials in spite of representing the highest prevalence of HTN and utmost risk for CV morbidity and mortality. Many concerns are raised regarding this group and are conventionally left out or understated mainly due to weakness, poor renal function, abnormal hemodynamic adaptation, and higher risk for autonomic dysfunction, cognitive impairment, and polypharmacy. The breach between the chronological and biological age broadens as the age progresses, hence the chronological age indicates a poor marker for the biological age.[24] Moreover, the standard guidelines for the chronological age cut-off are variable and hence remains debatable.

Epidemiological evolution has changed the course of the disease pattern from communicable diseases to noncommunicable diseases (NCDs).[25] These alterations can be attributed to changes in the socioeconomic, environmental, and population structure.

According to the US National Health and Nutrition Examination Survey (NHANES), 70% of adults ≥65 years have HTN.[26] This number will continue to rise as our population ages as 15% of the US population was ≥65 years old in 2014 and this is expected to increase to 20% by 2050.[27] As per the Global Burden of Disease Study (2000), HTN was projected to be accountable for about 50% of cardiovascular diseases (CVDs) globally[28] and further accounts for 20–50% of all CV related mortality.[29] The low- and middle-income countries (LMIC) such as the African Region and the Middle Eastern countries represents three-quarters of people with HTN globally. In the African region, a study from six countries among adult population of ≥50 years had prevalence of 77.9%[30] and in another study the prevalence of HTN among adults aged ≥25 years was 46%.[31] Factors such as lack to health-care access, disease awareness, and on the contrary, the ever-evolving demographic and epidemiological changes such as population ageing in these countries are expected to intensify the HTN population.

In the Indian subcontinent, numerous community-based studies have reported HTN as a rapidly emerging public health concern.[32,33] The anthropometric indices and CV risk factors in relation with HTN within the Indian population has also exhibited positive correlation.[34-36] The drawback is that only few studies have confirmed similar results in the elderly group,[37,38] but leaving the elderly in the rural areas. Hence, creating a dearth of information. According to the Global Burden of Hypertension study, the global burden of 212 million Disability-adjusted Life Years (DALYs) related to HTN, about 18% occurred in India in 2015.[27] One of the main targets for India is to reduce the premature mortality from NCDs to one-third by the year 2030 to meet the Sustainable Development Goals (SDG) target. A significant observation from many studies have shown the correlation of HTN and increase in age.[32,33,38,39] It is known that with increase in age the body undergoes several environmental stimuluses and the effect of genetically programmed senescence in body systems. Hence, the onset of HTN often occurs early in one's life[40] and over a period of time there leads to clustering of various CV diseases risk factors. Similarly, in women the higher incidence of HTN in elderly women is attributed mainly to the hormonal effects in the postmenopausal age group.[24]

■ DIAGNOSIS AND EVALUATION

Before the initiation of diagnosis or treatment, patients are to be counseled or informed about the nature of the disease before being subjected to the diagnostic methods and further management and preventive therapies. The sensitization of the patient is to be customized accordingly as the geriatric group have many limitations. It is recommended to take at least two measurements in a hospital setting or by a professional on two separate visits at least 1–4 weeks apart. However, certain conditions can be overlooked like in case of emergencies. For the elderly, HTN diagnosis can be done on three different BP measurements taken on ≥2 separate office visits.[41] The mainstream HTN identified is essential HTN however, on the contrary, the identification of correct causes of HTN is also important.

The risk factors for a patient with HTN depends on the following factors:
1. The BP level.
2. *Common factors:* Diabetes or impaired glucose tolerance, smoking, dyslipidemia,

obesity, male gender, and age >55 years in male.
3. Target organ damage (heart, kidney, and retina).
4. Related clinical conditions (coronary artery disease, kidney disease, etc.).

On clinical examination, the information on the comorbidities, risk factors and other associated clinical conditions should be looked into. This can further give hints to the presence of an underlying disease such as renal failure, renovascular disease or Cushing's syndrome. Further other lab related investigations like blood glucose [fasting blood sugar (FBS), postprandial blood sugar (PPBS)], lipids, serum creatinine, complete blood count, urinalysis and electrocardiogram (ECG) can be sent for analysis for initial evaluation and continued over a period of regular reviews.

Certain steps are to be followed when diagnosis is to be done. The BP is to be measured in the standardized manner. Misdiagnosis can frequently occur especially in elderly females. The techniques in taking the BP are also to be monitored like length of the cuff may be inappropriate in case of obesity or very low weight.

Fluctuations in BP or postural hypotension is detected more frequently in ageing people as the baroreceptor reflex sensitivity decreases with age.[42] The white coat effect or the fluctuations observed due to anxiety and physical trainings are also more commonly seen in this group of population.[17] Older patients may have rigid arteries as a result of atherosclerosis that increase the measured BP. However, a pulseless palpable artery is not as reliable an indicator of pseudo-HTN as previously recognized.[43,44] The practice of ambulatory methods of taking BP in elderly group has to be motivated due to the difficulties in taking BP in elderly patients.[45]

Renovascular high BP is widespread in elderly individuals and ought to be taken into consideration in patients with renal insufficiency from an unidentified source and high BP that appears resistant to various medications.[46]

Hence, the practice of taking BP in elderly patients must be performed repeatedly on different days to verify the correct reading of BP and to rule out the issue of fluctuations in those readings. The assessment of BP in the standing posture (within 3 minutes of standing up) is crucial and should be done both prior and after the start of treatment because orthostatic hypotension is more common. It is best to check BP simultaneously using the palpation technique to identify pseudo-HTN and auscultatory gaps. To assess BP fluctuations, white coat HTN, morning HTN, and masked HTN (reverse white coat HTN), 24-h ambulatory BP monitoring and home BP monitoring are both helpful. According to reports, masked HTN raises individuals' heart disease risk (mean age, 70 years).[18]

■ TREATMENT

The goal of managing of HTN to reduce BP to less than 140/90 mm Hg, but in those with type-2 diabetes mellitus (T2DM) or kidney disease, the target BP level is considerably lower, at less than 130/80 mm Hg.[41] All individuals with high BP should commence nonpharmacologic therapies. For older adults with milder types of HTN, lifestyle modification by changing one's way of life may be the sole remedy required as a first-line approach to lower blood pressure.[47] Pharmacotherapy should be started when lifestyle changes fail to reduce BP to the desired level. Antihypertensive drugs are strongly recommended in elderly. The key therapeutic approaches used to treat high BP in geriatric population involves

TABLE 2: Key therapeutic approaches for treatment of HTN in elderly population.	
Nonpharmacological	*Pharmacological*
• *Lifestyle modification:* Reduction in bodyweight • Lowering salt intake through diet • Enhanced intake of dietary potassium • Physical exercise • Restriction of alcohol consumption • Dietary approaches to stop hypertension (dash) diet plan	• Principal antihypertensive agents should be started at low dose and increased gradually depending on the BP and tolerated dose • *Drugs class:* Diuretics, blocker (calcium channel, β-blockers), angiotensin-converting enzyme (ACE) inhibitor and ARBs • Combination therapy

pharmacological and nonpharmacological treatment **(Table 2)**.[48]

Individual Class of Drugs

Diuretics

Diuretics are among the commonly recommended medications, particularly for older patients with heart failure or high blood pressure. After the fourth decade, the kidneys experience progressive structural and functional alterations that decrease their capacity to metabolize solutes like sodium and water. The geriatric has around half the renal reserves with reduced activity of the RAAS as that of young people. In the aged population, the natriuretic and diuretic responses to furosemide are reduced requiring higher doses of loop diuretics to treat older patients with decompensated congestive heart failure. However, due to the geriatric being more likely to experience undesirable side effects at elevated doses, caution is advised. Loop diuretics are thus, seldom used to treat elderly hypertensive patients except for patients with renal failure. Thiazide diuretics have long been the cornerstone of early therapy for HTN in the geriatric population. When compared to loop diuretics, thiazides are inexpensive, well tolerable, and have milder, more gradual effects with a half-life of one to two hours. Unaffected by age, low dosages of hydrochlorothiazide have shown to be an effective antihypertensive drug, particularly useful in the aged, who are more susceptible than younger people to unwanted adverse metabolic consequences.[48,49]

Inhibitor

Angiotensin-converting enzyme inhibitors can also be taken as first-line or combined therapies with caution in elderly population, diabetes, heart failure, recent MI, or chronic condition particularly in the case of any contraindication for diuretics. Furthermore, ACEIs slows the progression of diabetic renal disease, systemic vascular resistance (SVR), BP, mortality in post MI patients and left ventricular failure. Renin inhibitors are equally effective at treating high BP as ACE inhibitors or ARBs, and they are well tolerated by the elderly.[50]

Blockers

Calcium channel blockers (CCBs), β-blockers and angiotensin receptor blockers (ARBs) are different groups of drugs used in HTN. In this demographic, β-blockers and alpha-blockers are generally not advised due to the associated adverse effects, but may be prescribed in combination therapy to selected cases. If a diuretic is unsuitable or the patient has angina, arrythmias or conduction abnormalities, CCBs can be utilized as first-line antihypertensive therapy in the aged. The elderly population generally tolerates CCBs well. The dihydropyridine CCBs are most frequently associated with vasodilation-related side effects, such as postural hypotension, headache, and ankle edema. Constipation, bradycardia, as well as the possibility for heart block are common complications for nondihydropyridine CCBs; as a result, this subclass should be avoided in older individuals with preexisting cardiac conduction problems or with left-ventricular systolic dysfunction.[51]

Combination Therapy

When BP is greater than 20/10 mm Hg above target, combination therapy should be started due to its advantageous effect. To maximize BP-lowering effects, most combination treatments use antihypertensive drugs that work through various but complementary mechanisms. Better compliance, fewer side effects, a quicker recovery, and reduced costs are benefits of fixed combination therapy, depending on the agent selection and insurance plans.[41]

Angiotensin-converting enzyme inhibitor or ARB along with a diuretic is an acceptable regimen for the initiation of treatment. However, its combination is not acceptable in certain conditions like high level of proteinuria in a diabetic patient or in severe heart conditions; one should proceed cautiously due to an elevated risk of side effects (hypotension, syncope, renal failure, and hyperkalemia), as demonstrated by the ONTARGET study. An ACE inhibitor and a CCB was also found to be beneficial, while β-blockers/ACE inhibitors, β-blockers/alpha-blockers or agonists, and β-blockers/nondihydropyridines are some other combinations that are less successful.[52,53]

■ SUMMARY OF ALL GUIDELINES

1. Start with small dose.
2. Increase gradually with monitoring.
3. Add next drug if not controlled.
4. Observe side effects and drug interaction, noncompliance.
5. Choice of drug according to concomitant diseases and other drugs.
6. Ordinarily CCBs and diuretics are first line of choice.

■ MEDICATION COMPLIANCE

The degree to which a patient takes their medication as directed is referred to as compliance. As a percentage of the prescribed drug dose that has been taken over time, compliance rates are frequently recorded. Unfortunately, a significant fraction of older people stops taking their medications or use them improperly. Due to this noncompliance, the BP targets suggested by the guidelines are not met. Noncompliance is predicted by advanced age, a lower risk of CVD events, concurrent medical issues, low socioeconomic level, complication (such as several dosages), side effects, and cost of the pharmaceutical regimen.[54]

■ CONCLUSION

Hypertension is a metabolic disorder highly predominant in the geriatric population causing major risk for CV morbidity and mortality. Various studies have validated that treating high BP in the aged group not only benefits them, but also diminishes the threat of stroke, HF, MI, and mortality due to any pathological condition. Management of high BP lessens the possibility of dementia and cognitive decline in the aged. The adoption of a healthier diet and lifestyle is essential for controlling and treating blood pressure. Numerous classes of antihypertensive drugs appear to be useful in reducing CVD events, but geriatric population with HTN cannot be treated by mono-prescription. Concurrent CV risk factors should be considered when determining the mode of treatment. Medical professionals should treat HTN for all the aforementioned causes considering the age of the population.

REFERENCES

1. Gil-Extremera B, Cía-Gómez P. Hypertension in the elderly. Int J Hypertens. 2012;2012:859176.
2. Gil-Extremera B, Puertas JA, Martín AM, Soriano MF. Risk factors in the elderly. A study of 143 patients. An Med Interna. 1997;14(10):495-9.
3. James PA, Oparil S, Carter BL, Cushman WC, Dennison-Himmelfarb C, Handler J, et al. 2014 Evidence-based guideline for the management of high blood pressure in adults: Report From the panel members appointed to the Eighth Joint National Committee (JNC 8). JAMA. 2014;311(5):507-20.
4. Blok CGH, de Ridder MAJ, Verhamme KMC, Moorman PW. Hypertension in older patients, a retrospective cohort study. BMC Geriatr. 2016;16:142.
5. Acelajado MC. Optimal management of hypertension in elderly patients. Integr Blood Press Control. 2010;3:145-53.
6. Whelton PK, Carey RM, Aronow WS, Casey DE, Collins KJ, Himmelfarb CD, et al. 2017 ACC/AHA/AAPA/ABC/ACPM/AGS/APhA/ASH/ASPC/NMA/PCNA Guideline for the Prevention, Detection, Evaluation, and Management of High Blood Pressure in Adults: Executive Summary: A Report of the American College of Cardiology/American Heart Association Task Force on Clinical Practice Guidelines. Hypertension. 2018;71(6):1269-324.
7. Carlberg B, Nilsson PM. Hypertension in the elderly: What is the goal blood pressure target and how can this be attained? Curr Hypertens Rep. 2010;12(5):331-4.
8. Siu AL, U.S. Preventive Services Task Force. Screening for high blood pressure in adults: U.S. Preventive Services Task Force recommendation statement. Ann Intern Med. 2015;163(10):778-86.
9. Franklin SS, Jacobs MJ, Wong ND, L'Italien GJ, Lapuerta P. Predominance of isolated systolic hypertension among middle-aged and elderly US hypertensives: analysis based on National Health and Nutrition Examination Survey (NHANES) III. Hypertension. 2001;37(3):869-74.
10. Kannel WB. Blood pressure as a cardiovascular risk factor: Prevention and treatment. JAMA. 1996;275(20):1571-6.
11. O'Rourke MF, Nichols WW. Aortic diameter, aortic stiffness, and wave reflection increase with age and isolated systolic hypertension. Hypertension. 2005;45(4):652-8.
12. Franklin SS, Gustin W, Wong ND, Larson MG, Weber MA, Kannel WB, et al. Hemodynamic patterns of age-related changes in blood pressure. The Framingham Heart Study. Circulation. 1997;96(1):308-15.
13. Izzo JL, Levy D, Black HR. Clinical Advisory Statement. Importance of systolic blood pressure in older Americans. Hypertension. 2000;35(5):1021-4.
14. Young JH, Klag MJ, Muntner P, Whyte JL, Pahor M, Coresh J. Blood pressure and decline in kidney function: Findings from the Systolic Hypertension in the Elderly Program (SHEP). J Am Soc Nephrol. 2002;13(11):2776-82.
15. Vasan RS, Beiser A, Seshadri S, Larson MG, Kannel WB, D'Agostino RB, et al. Residual lifetime risk for developing hypertension in middle-aged women and men: The Framingham Heart Study. JAMA. 2002;287(8):1003-10.
16. Bakris G, Ali W, Parati G. ACC/AHA Versus ESC/ESH on Hypertension Guidelines: JACC Guideline Comparison. J Am Coll Cardiol. 2019;73(23):3018-26.
17. Wiinberg N, Høegholm A, Christensen HR, Bang LE, Mikkelsen KL, Nielsen PE, et al. 24-h Ambulatory blood pressure in 352 normal Danish subjects, related to age and gender. Am J Hypertension. 1995;8(10 Pt 1):978-86.

18. Cacciolati C, Hanon O, Alpérovitch A, Dufouil C, Tzourio C. Masked hypertension in the elderly: Cross-sectional analysis of a population-based sample. Am J Hypertens. 2011;24(6):674-80.
19. Angeli F, Reboldi G, Verdecchia P. Masked hypertension: Evaluation, prognosis, and treatment. Am J Hypertens. 2010;23(9):941-8.
20. Spence JD. Pseudo-hypertension in the elderly: Still hazy, after all these years. J Hum Hypertens. 1997;11(10):621-3.
21. Calhoun DA, Jones D, Textor S, Goff DC, Murphy TP, Toto RD, et al. Resistant hypertension: Diagnosis, evaluation, and treatment: A scientific statement from the American Heart Association Professional Education Committee of the Council for High Blood Pressure Research. Circulation. 2008;117(25):e510-26.
22. World Health Organization. World Health Report: 2002. Available from https://www.who.int/publications-detail-redirect/9241562072 [Last accessed November, 2023].
23. Kowal P, Goodkind D He W. An Aging World: 2015, International Population Reports. U.S. Government Printing Office, Washington DC. Available from: http://www.census.gov/library/publications/2016/demo/P95-16-1.html [Last accessed November, 2023].
24. Yadav G, Chaturvedi S, Grover VL. Prevalence, awareness, treatment and control of hypertension among the elderly in a resettlement colony of Delhi. Indian Heart J. 2008;60(4):313-7.
25. Park K. Park's Textbook of Preventive and Social Medicine. 23rd edition. India: Bhanot Publishers; 2015. p. 936.
26. Lloyd-Sherlock P, Beard J, Minicuci N, Ebrahim S, Chatterji S. Hypertension among older adults in low- and middle-income countries: Prevalence, awareness and control. Int J Epidemiol. 2014;43(1):116-28.
27. World Health Organization. A global brief on hypertension: Silent killer, global public health crisis: World Health Day 2013. Available from https://www.who.int/publications-detail-redirect/a-global-brief-on-hypertension-silent-killer-global-public-health-crisis-world-health-day-2013 [Last accessed November, 2023].
28. Swami HM, Bhatia V, Gupta M, Bhatia SPS, Sood A. Population based study of hypertension among the elderly in northern India. Public Health. 2002;116(1):45-9.
29. Woo J, Ho SC, Yu ALM, Sham A. Is waist circumference a useful measure in predicting health outcomes in the elderly? Int J Obes Relat Metab Disord. 2002;26(10):1349-55.
30. Arlappa N, Laxmmaiah A, Balakrishna N, Harikumar R, Mallikharjuna Rao K, Brahmam GNV, et al. Prevalence of hypertension and its relationship with adiposity among rural elderly population in India. Int J Clin Cardiol. 2014;1(1) p. 3.
31. Pouliot MC, Després JP, Lemieux S, Moorjani S, Bouchard C, Tremblay A, et al. Waist circumference and abdominal sagittal diameter: Best simple anthropometric indexes of abdominal visceral adipose tissue accumulation and related cardiovascular risk in men and women. Am J Cardiol. 1994;73(7):460-8.
32. Hazarika NC, Narain K, Biswas D, Kalita HC, Mahanta J. Hypertension in the native rural population of Assam. Natl Med J India. 2004;17(6):300-4.
33. Malhotra P, Kumari S, Kumar R, Jain S, Sharma BK. Prevalence and determinants of hypertension in an un-industrialised rural population of North India. J Hum Hypertens. 1999;13(7):467-72.
34. Gupta R, Prakash H, Gupta VP, Gupta KD. Prevalence and determinants of coronary heart disease in a rural population of India. J Clin Epidemiol. 1997;50:203-9.
35. Li W, Gu H, Teo KK, Bo J, Wang Y, Yang J, et al. Hypertension prevalence, awareness, treatment, and control in 115 rural and urban communities involving 47,000 people from China. J Hypertens. 2016;34(1):39-46.
36. Sheth AM, Jadav PA. Prevalence and factors affecting hypertension among old age population in rural area. Int J Community Med Public Health. 2016;3(7):1866-71.
37. Subramanian SV, Corsi DJ, Subramanyam MA, Smith GD. Jumping the gun: The problematic discourse on socioeconomic

status and cardiovascular health in India. Int J Epidemiol. 2013;42(5):1410-26.
38. Gupta PC, Gupta R, Pednekar MS. Hypertension prevalence and blood pressure trends in 88 653 subjects in Mumbai, India. J Hum Hypertens. 2004;18(12):907-10.
39. He Y, Wu W, Wu S, Zheng HM, Li P, Sheng HF, et al. Linking gut microbiota, metabolic syndrome and economic status based on a population-level analysis. Microbiome. 2018;6(1):172.
40. Han TS, van Leer EM, Seidell JC, Lean ME. Waist circumference action levels in the identification of cardiovascular risk factors: Prevalence study in a random sample. BMJ. 1995;311(7017):1401-5.
41. Chobanian AV, Bakris GL, Black HR, Cushman WC, Green LA, Izzo JL, et al. Seventh report of the Joint National Committee on Prevention, Detection, Evaluation, and Treatment of High Blood Pressure. Hypertension. 2003;42(6):1206-52.
42. James MA, Fotherby MD, Potter JF. Reproducibility of the circadian systolic blood pressure variation in the elderly. J Hypertens. 1995;13(10):1097-103.
43. Belmin J, Visintin JM, Salvatore R, Sebban C, Moulias R. Osler's maneuver: Absence of usefulness for the detection of pseudohypertension in an elderly population. Am J Med. 1995;98(1):42-9.
44. Messerli FH. Osler's maneuver, pseudohypertension, and true hypertension in the elderly. Am J Med. 1986;80(5):906-10.
45. Verdecchia P, Porcellati C, Schillaci G, Borgioni C, Ciucci A, Battistelli M, et al. Ambulatory blood pressure. An independent predictor of prognosis in essential hypertension. Hypertension. 1994;24(6):793-801.
46. Prisant LM, Moser M. Hypertension in the elderly: Can we improve results of therapy? Arch Intern Med. 2000;160(3):283-9.
47. Appel LJ, Moore TJ, Obarzanek E, Vollmer WM, Svetkey LP, Sacks FM, et al. A clinical trial of the effects of dietary patterns on blood pressure. DASH Collaborative Research Group. N Engl J Med. 1997;336(16):1117-24.
48. Centers for Disease Control and Prevention. 2022. High Blood Pressure Home. 2022. Available from https://www.cdc.gov/bloodpressure/index.htm [Last accessed November, 2023].
49. Nguyen Q, Dominguez J, Nguyen L, Gullapalli N. Hypertension Management: An Update. Am Health Drug Benefits. 2010;3(1):47-56.
50. Brunton LL, Hilal-Dandan R, Knollmann BC. Goodman & Gilman's: The Pharmacological Basis of Therapeutics, 13th edition [online]. AccessMedicine, McGraw Hill Medical. Available from https://accessmedicine.mhmedical.com/book.aspx?bookID=2189 [Last accessed November, 2023].
51. Tocci G, Battistoni A, Passerini J, Musumeci MB, Francia P, Ferrucci A, et al. Calcium channel blockers and hypertension. J Cardiovasc Pharmacol Ther. 2015;20(2):121-30.
52. Wiysonge CS, Bradley HA, Volmink J, Mayosi BM, Opie LH, et al. Beta-blockers for hypertension. Cochrane Database Syst Rev. 2017;1:CD002003.
53. Yusuf S, Teo KK, Pogue J, Dyal L, Copland I, Schumacher H, et al. Telmisartan, ramipril, or both in patients at high risk for vascular events. N Engl J Med. 2008;358(15):1547-59.
54. Frishman WH. Importance of medication adherence in cardiovascular disease and the value of once-daily treatment regimens. Cardiol Rev. 2007;15(5):257-63.

SECTION 8

Secondary Hypertension

29. **Coarctation of Aorta**
    Ankita Kulkarni, Sadanand R Shetty

30. **Sleep Apnea and Hypertension**
    Vasili Pradeep, Alladi Mohan

Coarctation of Aorta

Ankita Kulkarni, Sadanand R Shetty

INTRODUCTION

A common congenital heart disease (CHD), coarctation of the aorta (COA) accounts for 8–10% of all CHDs. It was rightly described as an "extraordinary dilatation of the heart, which came from the fact that the aortic conduit was too narrow" in the 1760s by Prussian anatomist, Johann Friedreich Meckel. The term coarctation is derived from *Latin coarctatus* meaning contracted or tightened.[1] It is more common in males than females (2:1) and occurs in 30% of patients with Turner syndrome.[2] A peak seasonal incidence of coarctation is found from September through November and from January through March. The reported rarity of coarctation in African Americans is open to question.[3]

The common form of coarctation is represented by a localized ridge or shelf, typically located near the aortic attachment of the ductus arteriosus (DA). The tissue composition of this ridge is similar to the muscular ductus. Luminal narrowing distal to the ridge is due to intimal proliferation. Normally this ductal–aorta junction is clearly defined, with no more than 30% of aortic circumference containing ductal tissue. In preductal coarctation, however, ductal tissue forms a circumferential sling that extends around the aorta.[3] Similar finding is not present in juxta–ductal aorta.

A tubular form of coarctation may also exist as a relatively long segment of constriction that extends beyond the left subclavian artery (SCA). The coexistence of tubular and localized constriction is known, although rare.[4]

Congenital coarctation is rarely seen in the mid-thoracic aorta or abdominal aorta accounting for 0.5 to 2% of coarctation.[5] Abdominal coarctation can be suprarenal, infrarenal, or inter-renal. This form of coarctation could be a part of acquired systemic vascular disorders, such as Takayasu's arteritis or von Recklinghausen's disease. Pseudocoarctation refers to a rare anomaly characterized by buckling or kinking of the aorta in the vicinity of the ligamentum arteriosum that results in elongation, tortuosity, and dilation of the distal aortic arch and the proximal descending aorta.[4]

EMBRYOLOGY

The mechanisms that account for the typical location of coarctation take into account a number of variables as follows: The quantitative morphology and growth of the aortic arch in the normal fetus; the site of the aortic orifice of the DA; the presence of ductal tissue in the coarctation.

Role of Neural Crest Cells

The neural crest is thought to play a role in the pathogenesis of some types of coarctation. Recent studies have shown the importance of neural crest cells in the development of noncardiac and cardiac structures, including the outflow tracts of the heart and the aortic arch system. Their maldevelopment could therefore be responsible for the combined occurrence of outflow tract (e.g., bicuspid aortic valve), aortic arch (e.g., coarctation), and noncardiac anomalies.[6]

Ductal Tissue Theory

Sites invasion of the descending aorta by ductal tissue as a cause for coarctation. Thus, when the DA constricts, coarctation occurs. Supported by the fact that neonatal coarctation manifests only after ductal closure, ("infantile" type), and usually has more severe symptoms. This theory, however, fails to explain the occurrence of coarctation at several other sites.[7]

Hemodynamic Theory (Rudolph)

The current consensus favors an interplay between aortic growth and blood flow. It states that a reduction in the volume of the blood passing through the isthmus in fetal life is causative in the development of coarctation. High-resolution echocardiographic imaging in the healthy fetus supports this theory and has disclosed progressive tapering of the diameter of the aortic arch, with the smallest diameter at the isthmus.

Neonatal coarctation is characterized by hypoplasia of the transverse aorta in the presence of a relatively large pulmonary trunk, a combination that is thought to reflect an in utero decrease in aortic arch flow together with an increase in flow through the main pulmonary artery and ductus.[8]

■ ASSOCIATIONS

Coarctation of the aorta although mostly regarded as an isolated anomaly with obstruction of the aortic isthmus, it is, in fact, a widespread disorder in which isthmic obstruction is only one of the abnormalities. It may involve the proximal and distal paracoarctation aorta, the ascending and transverse aorta, the coronary arteries, conduit arteries (radial, brachial, carotid), the retinal vascular bed, and cerebral arteries. The result of this is the common occurrence of the dissecting aneurysm, cerebral aneurysms, vascular rings, and systemic hypertension with coarctation. The strongest association is with a bicuspid aortic valve which may be functionally normal, stenotic, or incompetent. Second, coarctation is associated with a single papillary muscle of a parachute mitral valve which is attributed to a decrease in left ventricular interpapillary muscle distance (**Figs. 1A to C**). Coarctation in the fetus tends to be associated with

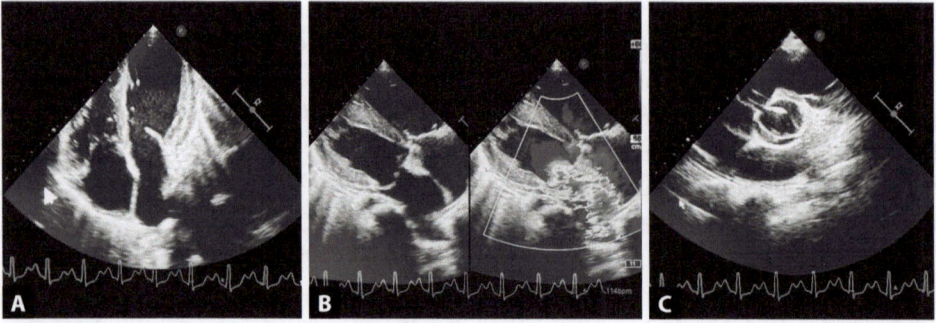

Figs. 1A to C: (A) and (B) Echocardiography of a 27-year-old male with coarctation of aorta and associated parachute mitral valve with severe mitral regurgitation; and (C) Bicuspid aortic valve. *(For color version, see Plate 3)*

a left superior vena cava.[9] In support of the hemodynamic theory two shunts are commonly associated with coarctation patent DA.[10] and ventricular septal defect (VSD). These are usually characterized by a left to right shunt which curtails the amount of blood that reaches the aortic isthmus.[11] Aneurysms of the circle of Willis set the stage for intracranial hemorrhage. The retinal arterioles are characteristically U-shaped (see subsequent discussion). Endocardial fibroelastosis occurs as a result of subendocardial ischemia and is patchy rather than confluent.

■ NATURAL HISTORY

Presentation of COA is usually bimodal producing significant symptoms in early infancy and after 20-30 years of age. Neonates with severe coarctation become acutely symptomatic when the ductus closes. The average systolic blood pressure in females rises to a plateau at around age 14 years and remains almost constant during the early reproductive years. The average systolic blood pressure in males may not plateau until around age 20 years. More than a quarter die by the age of 20 years, half by the age of 30 years, and more than three quarters by the age 50 years. The inherent risk of coarctation that results in death is at an average age of 33 years. Mild coarctation is not always benign, and severe coarctation is not always symptomatic.[12]

■ CLINICAL FEATURES

The major symptoms are the following features of four eventualities: (1) Congestive heart failure, (2) rupture or dissection of the aorta, (3) infective endarteritis or endocarditis, and (4) cerebral hemorrhage.[13]

Minor symptoms include epistaxis and leg fatigue. When coarctation compromises the orifice of the left SCA, left-arm muscular fatigue is a major symptom. Leg fatigue is common and occurs in about 50% of patients, but claudication is typical of abdominal coarctation. Dysphagia occurs when coarctation is a component of a vascular ring formed by a retroesophageal right SCA originating distal to the coarctation and passing behind the esophagus.

Hypertension associated with coarctation is a risk factor for premature atherosclerosis and coronary artery disease. Several theories have been proposed for the pathogenesis of systemic hypertension in the COA.

- *Mechanical theory:* Proposed in 1948. Increased impedance to left ventricular emptying forms the basis for this theory.[14] This results in higher BP in the segment proximal to the coarctation. The findings that many patients with coarctation have hypertension both below and above the narrowing, together with the fact that hypertension persists despite the presence of large collaterals, have cast doubt on this theory.
- *Neural theory:* The poorly compliant precoarctation aorta which causes a rise in systolic blood pressure thus resetting the carotid sinus baroreceptor forms the basis for this theory.[15] Decreased compliance of precoarctation segment is secondary to an increase in collagen and a decrease in smooth muscle within this segment.
- *Renal theory (Goldblatt type phenomenon):* This theory suggests that the narrowed segment causes renal underperfusion with stimulation of the renin-angiotensin-aldosterone system (RAAS) and relative impairment of salt and water excretion. The studies done by Scott and Bahnson strongly support this theory. It takes into account a unique feature of

coarctation, namely, hypertension being confined to the upper extremities. Until recently, the major criticism of this theory was the absence of either elevated plasma renin activity (PRA) or decreased renal blood flow in hypertensive children with coarctation. However, these features appeared on volume depletion and the hypertension became responsive to RAAS inhibitors.[16]

Physical Appearance

Patients with coarctation have an athletic built limited to the chest and shoulders in contrast to the narrow hips and thin legs. The left arm may also be small when coarctation compromises the origin of the left SCA. Turner syndrome with its distinctive physical appearance arouses suspicion of COA.

- *Arterial pulse:* The hallmark of COA is a difference in upper and lower extremity arterial pulses and blood pressure. While comparing femoral with radial or brachial pulse, any femoral delay is considered abnormal. Positioning the patient's wrist next to the groin is believed to facilitate comparison. The perceived femoral delay is due to a slow rising, delayed peaking pulse in the aorta distal to the coarctation. The presence of a normal femoral pulse effectively eliminates all but mild coarctation, provided the aortic valve is functioning normally. The absence of femoral delay despite the presence of coarctation could be secondary to PDA, collaterals, severe aortic regurgitation (AR), anomalous origin of subclavian below coarctation.
- Forceful carotid and suprasternal pulsations are at times perceived by the patients and are secondary to stiffness of the pre-coarctation aortic and become increasingly apparent with age and exercise.
- Collateral arterial pulsations are specifically sought with patients who are old enough. Scrutinizing the patient's back, especially around and between the scapulae (Suzmans Sign) is necessary for their detection.[17]
- Although the incidence of toxemia is lower in pregnant females with coarctation. The risk of aortic rupture and intracranial hemorrhage increases because gestational changes in connective tissue reinforce the medial abnormalities inherent in the arterial walls of coarctation.
- *Jugular venous pulse:* Pulse is normal except in patients with coarctation and biventricular failure.
- *Precordial movement and palpation:* The left ventricular impulse varies from normal to the sustained heaving impulse of pressure overload hypertrophy. Auscultation: Coarctation of the aorta is associated with systolic, diastolic, and continuous murmurs. An ejection sound is an auscultatory sign of a coexisting bicuspid aortic valve. Systolic murmurs originate from the following three sources: (1) Arterial collaterals, (2) the coarctation itself, and (3) the brachiocephalic arteries.
- The S2 sound in the COA is either single or normally split with increased intensity of the aortic component.
- The S4 sound reflects the afterload-induced left ventricular hypertrophy of coarctation.
- The S3 sound or the summation sounds occur in infants with heart failure and a rapid heart rate.

■ DIAGNOSIS

Echocardiography forms the major non-invasive modality for diagnosis, especially in sick newborns. Computed tomography (CT) aortogram, however, is necessary when associated aortic anomalies are suspected or for planning intervention.

- *Electrocardiogram:* Electrocardiographic patterns are related to the following two age groups: Symptomatic neonatal coarctation and coarctation after childhood. Symptomatic infants present with right atrial P wave abnormalities and right ventricular hypertrophy with right axis deviation. While left atrial P wave abnormalities, normal and occasionally leftward QRS axis occur in adults. Left ventricular hypertrophy is characterized by tall R waves and low, flat, or inverted T waves in left precordial leads. Prominent coved ST segment depressions with deeply inverted T waves are exceptional and imply coexisting bicuspid aortic stenosis.
- *X-Ray:* The X-ray in symptomatic infants shows pulmonary venous congestion with dilation of the right ventricle and both the atria. Left ventricular size remains normal or nearly so. In asymptomatic infants and young children, the X-ray is normal. The descending thoracic aorta is a straight line that runs parallel to the left edge of the vertebral column, but in children and young adults, the postcoarctation descending thoracic aorta has a distinctive leftward convexity that is accompanied by dilation of the left SCA.
- Notching of the ribs is a classic radiologic sign of coarctation caused by collateral flow through dilated, tortuous, pulsatile posterior intercostal arteries. It seldom appears before age 6 years, although exceptional examples have been described as early as 2 years of age. Notching varies from rib to rib and from patient to patient. It is due to dilation of the posterior intercostal arteries that run in intercostal grooves.
- *Echocardiography:* Transthoracic and transesophageal echocardiography with Doppler scan interrogation and color flow imaging permit segment-by-segment analysis of the ascending aorta, the aortic arch, the brachiocephalic arteries, the aortic isthmus, and the proximal descending aorta from birth to maturity. A long segment of luminal narrowing can be identified. The suprasternal notch window with color flow imaging identifies the coarctation by a zone of localized accelerated flow and by providing the target through which the continuous wave Doppler beam can be aligned to determine the gradient. A peak systolic gradient of more than 20 mm Hg is regarded as significant (**Figs. 2A to C**).

Computed tomography and magnetic resonance imaging (MRI): Provide very

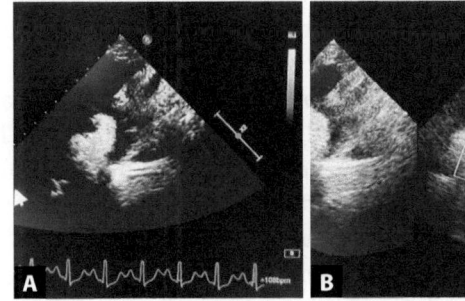 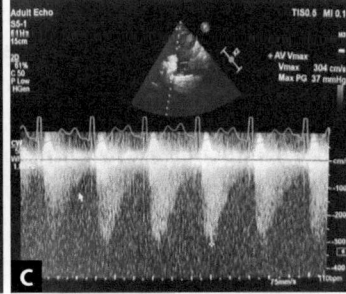

Figs. 2A to C: *Echocardiography*: (A) Suprasternal view showing a long segment coarctation; (B) Color Doppler across the narrowed segment showing turbulence across the coarctation segment; (C) Continuous Doppler across coarct segment. *(For color version, see Plate 3)*

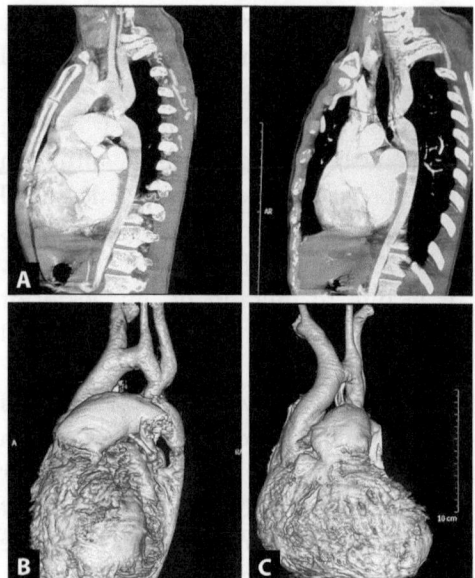

Figs. 3A to C: Computed tomography aortogram with 3D reconstruction.

high-quality images of coarctation. Further, information about other intracardiac and extracardiac anomalies and the collateral arterial circulation may also be obtained. Three-dimensional (3D) reconstruction can provide exquisite anatomic detail in these patients and provide a unique opportunity to plan surgical and transcatheter interventions. Magnetic resonance imaging studies are particularly recommended in patients before and after surgical repair, angioplasty, or stenting who require high-resolution serial imaging. The CT angiogram and reconstruction also provide similar information and have the advantage of shorter scan time (**Figs. 3A to C**). Therefore, they are better in sick neonates. However, there is an associated risk of radiation exposure and a requirement of contrast.

■ TREATMENT

Intervention is indicated in virtually all patients with COA, given the poor prognosis in untreated patients. The timing of therapy depends on the nature of the patient's presentation.

1. *Presentation in infancy:* Coarctation of the aorta (presenting with heart failure in infancy requires immediate and aggressive management. This includes medical therapy for heart failure and surgical/cardiac intervention definitive treatment. Medical therapy includes the following:
   a. Prostaglandin E_1 (PGE1) therapy to promote ductal patency and improve perfusion of the DA, renal, and mesenteric bed.
   b. Inotropic support.
   c. Diuretics.
   d. Correction of metabolic derangements.

   Surgical repair is the definitive treatment. It is a relatively safe surgery with low mortality if performed at experienced centers.[18] However, mortality is higher for those requiring surgery for associated intracardiac anomalies. Also, the need for repair of other cardiac anomalies at the time of coarctation repair is not always clear. Patients with a VSD after repair of COA may demonstrate a diminution of the L–R shunt and resolution of CHF. Some may also show a decrease in the size of VSD. Therefore, intracardiac repair at the time of surgery is appropriate in infants with a large VSD, or more complex lesions such as d-transposition or double-outlet right ventricle.

2. *Presentation in childhood:* It is usually incidental during investigation for hypertension or a murmur. Commonly repair is recommended at 1–3 years of age in asymptomatic children without severe upper extremity hypertension. The risk for late recurrence of coarctation appears to be increased when repair is performed on patients less than 1 year of age. However, a delay in repair beyond late childhood

and adolescence is associated with an increased risk for persistent hypertension and early atherosclerotic cardiovascular disease even in the absence of residual stenosis.

Surgical approaches include resection and end-to-end anastomosis, subclavian flap aortoplasty, prosthetic patch aortoplasty, bypass grafts between the ascending and descending aorta.[19]

Regardless of the technique, surgical coarctation repair generally is performed through a left lateral thoracotomy incision. Most children with a discrete coarctation will have a residual resting systolic pressure gradient of less than 10–15 mm Hg immediately after repair.

Morbidity and mortality are similar to surgical repair in infancy being higher for children with associated intracardiac anomalies requiring simultaneous repair.

Complications of surgery include paradoxical hypertension (postcoarctectomy syndrome): This may occur during the first 2–5 days following coarctation repair.[20] Systolic and diastolic pressures rising above pretreatment levels. In severe cases, mesenteric arteritis and bowel ischemia develop. The mechanism is related to the rebound activation of the sympathetic nervous system and the renin-angiotensin system with mesenteric arterial vasoconstriction. This can be prevented by postoperative β-blocker therapy and by aggressive antihypertensive during the immediate postoperative period.

- Spinal cord injury and paralysis may occur if aortic cross-clamping severely compromises perfusion to the DA and spinal arteries. Rare and limited to patients with poor arterial collateral circulation.
- Percutaneous balloon angioplasty is a less invasive alternative to surgical repair for patients with discrete COA.

  Gained wide acceptance as an effective therapy for recurrent postoperative coarctation, but remains controversial as a primary treatment strategy for native coarctation. Balloon angioplasty has been used for coarctation since 1982.

  The early multicenter report from the Valvuloplasty and Angioplasty of Congenital Anomalies (VACA) Registry studied the role of balloon angioplasty in native coarctation.[21] The problems with native coarctation are as follows:
  - Residual or recurrent stenosis, aneurysm formation at the dilation site.
  - Angioplasty for recurrent postoperative coarctation has similar acute effects as those of native coarctation.

3. *Coarctation stenting:* Balloon expandable stents provide an effective therapy for many patients with COA **(Fig. 4)**.[22] The safety and effectiveness of percutaneous stent therapy for native or recurrent coarctation have been documented in numerous clinical series. Stents implanted in growing children, however, are likely to require redilation to a larger diameter when the children grow. Late aneurysm formation at the coarctation site may occur after stenting but seems to be less frequent than balloon angioplasty alone. The primary use of covered stents may decrease the aneurysm risk further and may be particularly valuable in patients with a very small coarctation lumen (<3 mm) or with increased aortic wall fragility.

   Placement of endovascular stents in infants and small children (<25 kg)

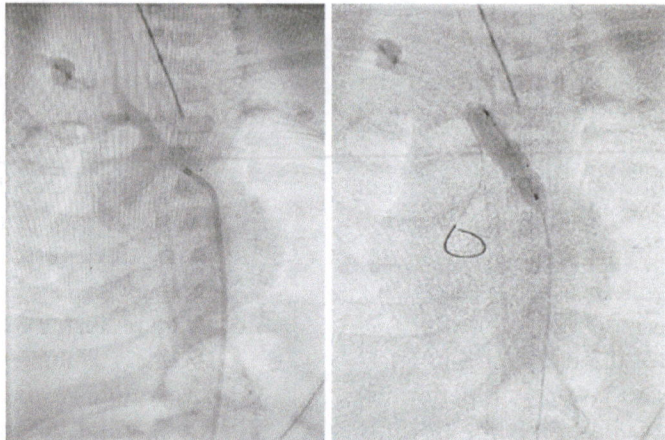

Fig. 4: Balloon dilatation of congenital coarctation.

remains a controversial therapy despite improvements in methods of access, balloon and stent size, and the use of smaller and smaller sheaths.[23]

4. *Prognosis:* Long-term prognosis after coarctation treatment may be affected by a number of clinical and hemodynamic conditions.
   a. Residual or recurrent coarctation.
   b. Hypertension (rest and exercise).
   c. Aortic aneurysm.
   d. Aortic dissection.
   e. Intracranial hemorrhage.
   f. Diminished left arm growth/subclavian steal.
   g. Endocarditis/endarteritis.
   h. Associated intracardiac lesions.
5. Timing of intervention
   a. With left ventricular dysfunction/congestive heart failure or severe upper limb hypertension (for age): Immediate intervention (class I).
   b. Normal left ventricular function, no congestive heart failure, and mild upper limb hypertension: Intervention beyond 3-6 months of age (class IIa).
   c. No hypertension, no heart failure, normal ventricular function: Intervention at 1-2 years of age (class IIa).
   d. Intervention is not indicated if the Doppler gradient across the coarct segment is below 20 mm Hg with normal left ventricular function (class III).
   e. Mode of intervention balloon dilatation or surgery for children above 6 months of age.
   f. Surgical repair for infants below 6 months of age. Balloon dilatation with stent deployment can be considered in children above 10 years of age if required (class IIB).
   g. Elective endovascular stenting of the aorta is contraindicated for children above 10 years of age (class III).

REFERENCES

1. Jarcho S. Coarctation of the aorta (Meckel, 1750; Paris, 1791). Am J Cardiol. 1961;7:844-52.
2. Elzenga NJ, Gittenberger-de Groot AC. Localised coarctation of the aorta. An age dependent spectrum. Br Heart J. 1983;49(4):317-23.
3. Kappetein AP, Gittenberger-de Groot AC, Zwinderman AH, Rohmer J, Poelmann RE, Huysmans HA. The neural crest as a possible pathogenetic factor in coarctation of the aorta and bicuspid aortic valve. J Thorac Cardiovasc Surg. 1991;102(6):830-6.

4. Hornberger LK, Weintraub RG, Pesonen E, Murillo-Olivas A, Simpson IA, Sahn C, et al. Echocardiographic study of the morphology and growth of the aortic arch in the human fetus. Observations related to the prenatal diagnosis of coarctation. Circulation. 1992;86(3):741-7.
5. Park HK, Cho SH, Park Y-H. Atypical coarctation of the aorta: Congenital stenosis of the mid-thoracic aorta. J Am Coll Cardiol. 2009;53(22):2098.
6. Langille BL, Brownlee RD, Adamson SL. Perinatalaortic growth in lambs: Relation to blood flow changes at birth. Am J Physiol. 1990;259(4 Pt 2):H1247-53.
7. Morrow WR, Huhta JC, Murphy Jr DJ, Mcnamara DG. Quantitative morphology of the aortic arch in neonatal coarctation. J Am Coll Cardiol. 1986;8(3):616-20.
8. Allan LD, Chita SK, Anderson RH, Fagg N, Crawford DC, Tynan MJ. Coarctation of the aorta in prenatal life: an echocardiographic, anatomical, and functional study. Br Heart J. 1988;59(3):356-60.
9. Allan LD, Crawford DC, Tynan M. Evolution of coarctation of the aorta in intrauterine life. Br Heart J. 1984;52(4):471-3.
10. Rudolph AM, Heymann MA, Spitznas U. Hemodynamic considerations in the development of narrowing of the aorta. Am J Cardiol. 1972;30(5):514-25.
11. Talner NS, Berman MA. Postnatal development of obstruction in coarctation of the aorta: Role of the ductus arteriosus. Pediatrics. 1975;56(4):562-9.
12. Mcmahon CJ, Vick GW III, Nihill MR. Right aortic arch and coarctation: Delineation by three-dimensional magnetic resonance angiogram. Heart. 2001;85(5):492.
13. Bahabozorgui S, Nemir P Jr. Coarctation of the abdominal aorta. Am J Surg. 1966;111(2):224-9.
14. Sehested J, Baandrup U, Mikkelsen E. Different reactivity and structure of the prestenotic and poststenotic aorta in human coarctation. Implications for baroreceptor function. Circulation. 1982;65(6):1060-5.
15. Brili S, Dernellis J, Aggeli C, Pitsavos C, Hatzos C, Stefanadis C, et al. Aortic elastic properties in patients with repaired coarctation of aorta. Am J Cardiol. 1998;82(9):1140-3.
16. Igler FO, Boerboom LE, Werner PH, Donegan JH, Zuperku EJ, Bonchek LI, et al. Coarctation of the aorta and baroreceptor resetting. A study of carotid baroreceptor stimulus-response characteristics before and after surgical repair in the dog. Circ Res. 1981;48(3):365-71.
17. van Son JA, Daniels O, Vincent JG, van Lier HJ, Lacquet LK. Appraisal of resection and end-to-end anastomosis for repair of coarctation of the aorta in infancy: Preference for resection. Ann Thorac Surg. 1989;48(4):496-502.
18. Rubay JE, Sluysmans T, Alexandrescu V, Khelif K, Moulin D, Vliers A, et al. Surgical repair of coarctation of the aorta in infants under one year of age: Long-term results in 146 patients comparing subclavian flap angioplasty and modified end-to-end anastomosis. J Cardiovasc Surg (Torino). 1992;33(2):216-22.
19. Quaegebeur JM, Jonas RA, Weinberg AD, Blackstone EH, Kirklin JW. Outcomes in seriously ill neonates with coarctation of the aorta: a multi-institutional study. J Thorac Cardiovas Surg. 1994;108(5):841-51.
20. Wright GE, Nowak CA, Goldberg CS, Ohye RG, Bove EL, Rocchini AP. Extended resection and end-to-end anastomosis for aortic coarctation in infants: Results of a tailored surgical approach. Ann Thorac Surg. 2005;80(4):1453-9.
21. Beekman RH, Rocchini AP, Behrendt DM, Rosenthal A. Reoperation for coarctation of the aorta. Am J Cardiol. 1981;48(6):1108-14.
22. Kaushal S, Backer CL, Patel JN, Patel SK, Walker BL, Weigel TJ, et al. Coarctation of the aorta: Midterm outcomes of resection with extended end-to-end anastomosis. Ann Thorac Surg. 2009;88:1932-8.
23. Maron BJ, Humphries JO, Rowe RD, Mellits ED. Prognosis of surgically corrected coarctation of the aorta: a 20-year postoperative appraisal. Circulation. 1973;47(1):119-26.

CHAPTER 30

Sleep Apnea and Hypertension

Vasili Pradeep, Alladi Mohan

Sleep that knits up the raveled sleave of care,
The death of each day's life, sore labor's bath,
Balm of hurt minds, great nature's second course,
Chief nourisher in life's feast.

—**William Shakespeare**
Macbeth, Act 2 Scene 2

■ INTRODUCTION

Sleep constitutes a significant portion of human existence, accounting for approximately one-third of an individual's lifespan. Formerly viewed as a passive and uniform state, sleep has now evolved into a realm characterized by cyclic phases of intricate and evolving brain activity, behavior, and physiology.[1-6] Notably, sleep disturbances, notably obstructive sleep apnea (OSA), have emerged as a prominent contributor to hypertension, particularly in the context of resistant hypertension.[2] The intricate interplay between OSA and hypertension has captivated researchers for decades, as untreated OSA has been linked to an elevated risk of developing new-onset hypertension.[6]

■ EPIDEMIOLOGY

Hypertension stands as a significant global public health concern, extending its impact to India as well.[7] In India, the estimated prevalence of hypertension is approximately 29.8% [95% confidence intervals (CI) 26.7 to 33.0%]. This prevalence extends to approximately 33% of urban and 25% of rural individuals in the country.[8] Pertinent epidemiological data originating from India indicate that the prevalence of OSA and obstructive sleep apnea syndrome (OSAS) in community-based studies varies within the range of 3.5–13.7% and 1.7–3.6%, respectively.[9-11]

■ SLEEP AND CIRCADIAN HEMODYNAMIC RHYTHMS

Throughout various sleep stages, blood pressure and heart rate undergo intricate fluctuations, primarily originating from neurogenic influences. In the nonrapid eye movement (NREM) sleep phase, central sympathetic outflow diminishes, while cardiac vagal tone increases. Consequently, heart rate and blood pressure decrease, exemplifying a dipping pattern of blood pressure.[12] Conversely, during rapid eye movement (REM) sleep, an upsurge in sympathetic outflow precipitates heightened heart rate and blood pressure.[13]

TERMINOLOGY OF SLEEP-DISORDERED BREATHING

Obstructive sleep apnea is defined as the occurrence of an average of five or more obstructive respiratory events per hour of sleep, accompanied by sleep-related symptoms or comorbidities, or 15 or more such events without associated symptoms or comorbidities. Obstructive sleep apnea syndrome is characterized by OSA coupled with daytime symptoms, most commonly excessive sleepiness.[3-5] Apnea is recognized as the cessation of inspiratory airflow for a duration of at least 10 sec. Depending on the underlying cause, it can be classified as central or obstructive. Central sleep apnea manifests as a diminished or complete withdrawal of respiratory drive in the pontomedullary junction affecting the muscles of respiration.[14] Obstructive sleep apnea arises from partial or complete pharyngeal collapse during sleep and can be further categorized as mild,[5-15] moderate,[15-30] or severe (>30) based on the apnea–hypopnea index (AHI). The AHI quantifies the frequency of apneas and hypopneas detected per hour of sleep using polysomnography.[15]

PATHOPHYSIOLOGICAL LINK BETWEEN OBSTRUCTIVE SLEEP APNEA AND HYPERTENSION

As detailed in the evidence-based Indian initiative on obstructive sleep apnea (INOSA) guidelines, OSA constitutes an independent risk factor for systemic hypertension.[16] Elevated prevalence of hypertension has been observed among individuals with OSA. Notably, each additional apneic event per hour of sleep has been correlated with a roughly 1-fold increase in the odds of developing hypertension. Furthermore, a 10% reduction in nocturnal oxygen saturation escalates the odds of hypertension by 13%. OSA has also been identified as a significant yet frequently overlooked contributor in cases of resistant hypertension.

The prevalence of OSA among primary hypertension patients surpasses 30%, with moderate to severe OSA detected in approximately two-thirds of those with drug-resistant hypertension.[17] The multifaceted etiology underpinning both OSA and hypertension underscores the crucial role played by interconnected factors in their pathophysiology.

Age and Obesity

The interplay of age and obesity assumes paramount significance in comprehending the pathophysiological nexus between OSA and hypertension. Notably, individuals with OSA exhibit an escalated vulnerability to cardiovascular complications, such as atrial fibrillation and hypertension, with a more pronounced impact emerging at younger ages. Administration of continuous positive airway pressure (CPAP) to manage OSA has been associated with a reduced incidence of atrial fibrillation.[18] While OSA is frequently associated with obesity, it's important to note that nonobese individuals can also manifest OSA.

Autonomic Nervous System Alterations

The cyclic occurrences of hypoxemia and hypercapnia stemming from episodic OSA prompt reflexive activation of the sympathetic and parasympathetic branches of the autonomic nervous system. These autonomic perturbations culminate in heightened catecholamine levels, a phenomenon sustained even during daytime hours, thereby contributing to the development of hypertension. Remarkably, effective CPAP therapy has been linked to decreased urinary catecholamine levels, particularly in cases of severe OSA.[19]

Inflammatory and Cytokine-mediated Effects

Obstructive sleep apnea triggers oxidative stress, culminating in systemic inflammation and cardiovascular morbidity. Elevated levels of various biomarkers of systemic inflammation have been observed in individuals with OSA. However, additional data are required to ascertain whether these biomarkers signify a worsened prognosis and whether interventions aimed at these markers could modify the underlying pathogenesis.[20]

Renin–Angiotensin–Aldosterone System

A noteworthy correlation has been established between plasma aldosterone concentration and the severity of OSA in patients with resistant hypertension. This correlation highlights the involvement of the renin–angiotensin–aldosterone system in the pathogenesis of OSA. Additionally, evidence suggests that heightened dietary salt intake exacerbates the severity of resistant hypertension in individuals with moderate to severe OSA.[21]

Nocturnal Fluid Redistribution

Disruptions in fluid volume regulation contribute to the pathogenesis of both hypertension and OSA. In OSA patients, nocturnal fluid shifts toward the upper body due to changes in posture leading to a further constriction of the already compromised upper airway diameter. This predisposes individuals to increased occurrences of OSA episodes, ultimately resulting in a nondipping pattern of nocturnal blood pressure.[21]

Sleep Insufficiency

Obstructive sleep apnea gives rise to compromised sleep quality. Insufficient sleep triggers a substantial rise in sympathetic activity, arterial rigidity, and venous endothelial dysfunction. These cascading effects contribute to the development of hypertension and a range of other cardiovascular complications.[22]

Involvement of Organ Systems

Central Nervous System

Chronic intermittent hypoxia, a hallmark of OSA, exerts a notable impact on brain regions governing sympathetic outflow regulation. This disruption contributes to hypertension in individuals with OSA. Elevated expression of the Delta-FosB gene has been observed in several brain areas, including the median preoptic nucleus, organum vasculosum of the lamina terminalis, nucleus of the solitary tract, subfornical organ, and rostral ventrolateral medulla, due to chronic intermittent hypoxia. These findings suggest a direct influence of OSA on cerebral vasculature, giving rise to complications such as hypertension and stroke.[23]

Respiratory System

Recurrence of hypoxemia and hypercapnia episodes in OSA patients induces remodeling of the pulmonary vasculature, leading to hypoxic pulmonary vasoconstriction. Over time, this process leads to pulmonary venous hypertension. The combined effects of hypoxic pulmonary vasoconstriction, pulmonary venous hypertension, and abnormal mediator production contribute to vascular cell proliferation and aberrant vascular remodeling, culminating in pulmonary arterial hypertension.[24]

Cardiovascular System

The intricate mechanisms underlying cardiovascular complications in OSA encompass a spectrum of factors, including sympathetic activation, alterations in intrathoracic pressure, sleep disturbances, oxidative stress, and vascular inflammation due to cyclic episodes of nocturnal hypoxia and reoxygenation, among others.[25] Among these, sympathetic activation emerges as a primary mechanism contributing to tachyarrhythmias, particularly atrial fibrillation, in individuals with OSA. Additional contributors to cardiovascular complications in OSA encompass coagulation factors, endothelial impairment, platelet activation, and an elevation in inflammatory mediators. This intricate interplay ultimately results in heightened blood pressure, pulmonary hypertension, arrhythmias, and congestive heart failure.[26,27]

Endocrine System

In individuals presenting with metabolic syndrome—an aggregation of interconnected metabolic conditions including hyperglycemia, hypertension, hyperuricemia, and obesity—OSA presence is classified as part of "syndrome Z." This constellation of interrelated metabolic disorders significantly augments the risk of heart disease, stroke, and diabetes mellitus. Continuous positive airway pressure therapy has been shown to alleviate postprandial dyslipidemia after two months of treatment. For patients with diabetes mellitus and OSA coexisting with hypertension, more intricate mechanisms come into play, underscoring the multifactorial involvement of these intertwined metabolic disorders.[28]

Kidneys

Renal sympathetic denervation has shown promise as an effective therapy for reducing the severity of resistant hypertension, glucose intolerance, and OSA in patients with both conditions. However, further comprehensive studies are warranted before considering this approach as a standard therapy for individuals with OSA and hypertension.[29]

Effect of Obstructive Sleep Apnea Treatment on Hypertension

Lifestyle modifications and dietary adjustments, such as weight loss, moderate exercise, and reduced dietary salt intake, have demonstrated the potential to lower the incidence of resistant hypertension in OSA patients.[21,30] Effective management of OSA leads to diminished morbidity and mortality **(Fig. 1)**. Continuous positive airway pressure therapy, a cornerstone in OSA management, has been found to reduce the occurrence of resistant hypertension and significantly lower blood pressure levels, particularly in individuals with resistant hypertension. Nonetheless, further research is needed to fully explore the potential of CPAP therapy as a preventive measure for hypertension in OSA patients. In cases of mild to moderate OSA, oral appliances serve as an alternative to CPAP, especially for patients with limited CPAP tolerance. However, CPAP tends to yield superior polysomnography outcomes compared to oral appliances, particularly in reducing the AHI.[31] It is noteworthy that while significant weight reduction is achieved through

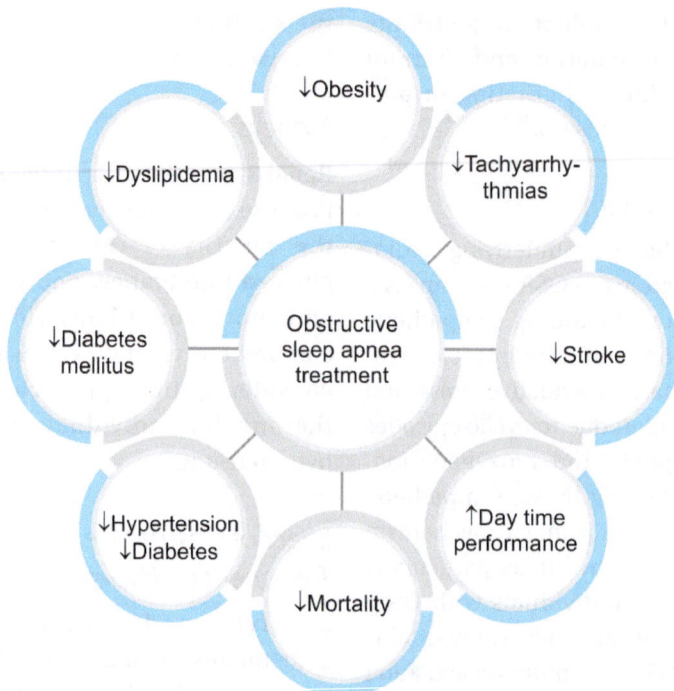

Fig. 1: Beneficial effects of continuous positive airway pressure treatment of obstructive sleep apnea.

bariatric surgery, there appears to be no substantial reduction in the AHI in patients with OSA.[32]

CONCLUSION

The existing body of evidence underscores OSA as a significant modifiable and preventable contributor to hypertension. Timely diagnosis of OSA and diligent implementation of CPAP therapy with high compliance levels hold the potential for substantial benefits in individuals with hypertension.

REFERENCES

1. Redline S, Azarbarzin A, Peker Y. Obstructive sleep apnoea heterogeneity and cardiovascular disease. Nat Rev Cardiol 2023;20(8):560-73.
2. Pedrosa RP, Drager LF, Gonzaga CC, Sousa MG, de Paula LK, Amaro AC, et al. Obstructive sleep apnea: the most common secondary cause of hypertension associated with resistant hypertension. Hypertension 2011;58(5):811-7.
3. Iber C, Ancoli-Israel S, Chesson A, Quan SF. The AASM manual for the scoring of sleep and associated event: Rules, terminology and technical specifications, 1st edition. Westchester: American Academy of Sleep Medicine; 2007, pp. 1-59.
4. Berry RB, Budhiraja R, Gottlieb DJ, Gozal D, Iber C, Kapur VK, et al. Rules for scoring respiratory events in sleep: Update of the 2007 AASM Manual for the Scoring of Sleep and Associated Events. Deliberations of the Sleep Apnea Definitions Task Force of the American Academy of Sleep Medicine. J Clin Sleep Med. 2012;8(5):597-619.
5. Jafari B, Mohsenin V. Polysomnography. Clin Chest Med 2010;31(2):287-97.

6. Kanclerska J, Szymańska-Chabowska A, Poręba R, Michałek-Zrąbkowska M, Lachowicz G, Mazur G, et al. A systematic review of publications on the associations between sleep architecture and arterial hypertension. Med Sci Monit 2023; 29:e941066.
7. Mackay J, Mensah G, Mendis S, Greenlund K. Atlas of heart disease and stroke. Geneva: World Health Organization; 2004, pp.1-111.
8. Anchala R, Kannuri NK, Pant H, Khan H, Franco OH, Di Angelantonio E, et al. Hypertension in India: A systematic review and meta-analysis of prevalence, awareness, and control of hypertension. J Hypertens. 2014;32(6):1170-7.
9. Sharma SK, Ahluwalia G. Epidemiology of adult obstructive sleep apnea syndrome in India. Indian J Med Res. 2010;131:171-5.
10. Udwadia ZF, Doshi AV, Lonkar SG, Singh CI. Prevalence of sleep disordered breathing and sleep apnea in middle-aged urban Indian men. Am Respir Crit Care Med. 2004;169(2):168-73.
11. Sharma SK, Kumpawat S, Banga A, Goel A. Prevalence and risk factors of obstructive sleep apnea syndrome in a population of Delhi, India. Chest 2006;130(1):149-56.
12. Floras JS. Hypertension and sleep apnea. Can J Cardiol. 2015;31(7):889-97.
13. Somers VK, Dyken ME, Mark AL, Abboud FM. Sympathetic-nerve activity during sleep in normal subjects. N Engl J Med. 1993;328:303-7.
14. Javaheri S, Dempsey JA. Central sleep apnea. Compr Physiol. 2013;3(1):141-63.
15. Fleetham J, Ayas N, Bradley D, Ferguson K, Fitzpatrick M, George C, et al. Canadian Thoracic Society guidelines: Diagnosis and treatment of sleep disordered breathing in adults. Can Respir J. 2006;13(7):387-92.
16. Sharma SK, Katoch VM, Mohan A, Kadhiravan T, Elavarasi A, Ragesh R, et al. Consensus and evidence-based INOSA guidelines 2014 (first edition). Indian J Med Res. 2014;140(3):451-68.
17. Franklin KA, Lindberg E. Obstructive sleep apnea is a common disorder in the population: a review on the epidemiology of sleep apnea. J Thorac Dis. 2015;7(8): 1311-22.
18. Lavergne F, Morin L, Armitstead J, Benjafield A, Richards G, Woehrle H. Atrial fibrillation and sleep-disordered breathing. J Thorac Dis. 2015;7:575-84.
19. Pinto P, Bárbara C, Montserrat JM, Patarrão RS, Guarino MP, Carmo MM, et al. Effects of CPAP on nitrate and norepinephrine levels in severe and mild-moderate sleep apnea. BMC Pulm Med. 2013;13:13.
20. Testelmans D, Tamisier R, Barone-Rochette G, Baguet JP, Roux-Lombard P, Pépin JL, et al. Profile of circulating cytokines: Impact of OSA, obesity and acute cardiovascular events. Cytokine. 2013;62(2):210-6.
21. Pimenta E, Stowasser M, Gordon RD, Harding SM, Batlouni M, Zhang B, et al. Increased dietary sodium is related to severity of obstructive sleep apnea in patients with resistant hypertension and hyperaldosteronism. Chest. 2013;143(4): 978-83.
22. Dettoni JL, Consolim-Colombo FM, Drager LF, Rubira MC, Souza SB, Irigoyen MC, et al. Cardiovascular effects of partial sleep deprivation in healthy volunteers. J Appl Physiol. 2012;113(2):232-6.
23. Knight WD, Little JT, Carreno FR, Toney GM, Mifflin SW, Cunningham JT. Chronic intermittent hypoxia increases blood pressure and expression of FosB/ DeltaFosB in central autonomic regions. Am J Physiol Regul Integr Comp Physiol. 2011;301(1):R131-9.
24. Kholdani C, Fares WH, Mohsenin V. Pulmonary hypertension in obstructive sleep apnea: Is it clinically significant? A critical analysis of the association and pathophysiology. Pulm Circ. 2015;5(2): 220-7.
25. Javaheri S, Barbe F, Campos-Rodriguez F, Dempsey JA, Khayat R, Javaheri S, et al. Sleep Apnea: Types, mechanisms, and clinical cardiovascular consequences. J Am Coll Cardiol. 2017;69(7):841-58.

26. Jean-Louis G, Zizi F, Clark LT, Brown CD, McFarlane SI. Obstructive sleep apnea and cardiovascular disease: role of the metabolic syndrome and its components. J Clin Sleep Med. 2008;4(3):261-72.
27. Drager LF, McEvoy RD, Barbe F, Lorenzi-Filho G, Redline S. Sleep apnea and cardiovascular disease: lessons from recent trials and need for team science. Circulation. 2017;136(19):1840-50.
28. Phillips CL, Yee BJ, Marshall NS, Liu PY, Sullivan DR, Grunstein RR. Continuous positive airway pressure reduces postprandial lipidemia in obstructive sleep apnea: a randomized, placebo-controlled crossover trial. Am J Respir Crit Care Med. 2011;184(3):355-61.
29. Witkowski A, Prejbisz A, Florczak E, Kądziela J, Śliwiński P, Bieleń P, et al. Effects of renal sympathetic denervation on blood pressure, sleep apnea course, and glycemic control in patients with resistant hypertension and sleep apnea. Hypertension. 2011;58(4):559-65.
30. Ou YH, Tan A, Lee CH. Management of hypertension in obstructive sleep apnea. Am J Prev Cardiol 2023;13:100475.
31. Li W, Xiao L, Hu J. The comparison of CPAP and oral appliances in treatment of patients with OSA: a systematic review and meta-analysis. Respir Care. 2013;58(7):1184-95.
32. Dixon JB, Schachter LM, O'Brien PE, Jones K, Grima M, Lambert G, et al. Surgical vs conventional therapy for weight loss treatment of obstructive sleep apnea: a randomized controlled trial. JAMA. 2012;308(11):1142-9.

SECTION 9

Therapeutic Aspects: Pharmacologic and Nonpharmacologic Interventions

31. **Angiotensin-converting Enzyme Inhibitors: What is New?**
    Rajesh Kumar Jha, Toshi Tiwari, Srishti Jha

32. **Angiotensin II Receptor Blockers: What is New?**
    Rajesh Kumar Jha, Pavni Agrawal, Srishti Jha

33. **Calcium Channel Blockers and Hypertension**
    Rajesh Kumar Jha, Shahid Abbas, Srishti Jha

34. **Diuretics and Hypertension**
    Anita Jaiswal Ektate, Neeta Narang, Virendra Chauhan, Upasana Mohanty

35. **Beta-blockers in Hypertension**
    Chandrasekhar Valupadas

36. **Alpha-blockers: Role in Hypertension**
    Dilip A Kirpalani

37. **Direct Vasodilators in Hypertension**
    Rajib Ratna Chaudhary

38. **Hypertensive Heart Disease**
    Keyur R Rathod, Sadanand R Shetty

39. **Emerging Antihypertensive Drugs**
    Anant Ramkishanrao Munde, Sadanand R Shetty

40. **Combination Therapy in Hypertension**
    A Muruganathan

CHAPTER 31

Angiotensin-converting Enzyme Inhibitors: What is New?

Rajesh Kumar Jha, Toshi Tiwari, Srishti Jha

■ INTRODUCTION

Angiotensin-converting enzyme (ACE) has a vital function in the regulation of the renin–angiotensin system (RAS). Physiological functions such as maintenance of systemic blood pressure (BP), electrolyte and fluid balance, and blood volume are mediated by the RAS via angiotensin II.[1,2]

- Angiotensin II, a potent vasoactive substance and stimulator of aldosterone secretion, is converted from biologically inactive angiotensin I by both ACE and non-ACE pathways.[2]
- In addition to its effects on the RAS, ACE also cleaves the C-terminal dipeptide from bradykinin, thereby inactivating it. Bradykinin causes vasodilation by stimulating nitric oxide production and causes natriuresis through direct tubular effects.[1]

Therefore, ACE regulates the balance between the vasoconstrictive and salt-retentive properties of angiotensin II and the vasodilatory and natriuretic properties of bradykinin.

When angiotensin II binds with the angiotensin type 1 (AT1) receptor, it causes vasoconstriction, cell growth, sodium and fluid retention, and sympathetic activation, all of which play a role in hypertension.[3]

■ SIDE EFFECTS

- Class effects
- Hypotension
- Cough
- Hyperkalemia
- Renal failure
- Fetal anomalies
- Angioedema
- Dysgeusia
- Sulfhydryl-related effects
- Neutropenia
- Rash
- Nephrotic-range proteinuria

Angiotensin-converting enzyme inhibitors are generally well tolerated. While there have been no studies comparing the safety of the available ACE inhibitors, some similarities have been identified. As anticipated with antihypertensive agents, ACE inhibitors can cause hypotension with dose-dependent severity.[1]

Angioedema, a serious hypersensitivity reaction, has been associated with ACE inhibitors. The reaction is characterized by swelling of the lips, tongue, mouth, nose, throat, and other parts of the face. Angioedema is most likely to occur in the first month of therapy, although it has been reported to occur years after the initiation of therapy.[1]

Angiotensin-converting enzyme inhibitors can also cause a dry, persistent cough, which may necessitate the discontinuation of therapy.[1,4] Cough is reported more frequently in women than in men and in Asians than in Caucasian populations.[1] The cause of this characteristic cough is unknown, but it may be due to increased levels of bradykinin or substance P and stimulation of Vagal C-fibers.

Therapy with ACE inhibitors can cause hyperkalemia since these drugs block the formation of angiotensin II, which stimulates the production of aldosterone.[1]

However, hyperkalemia associated with ACE inhibitors is rarely reported in patients with normal renal function and is most common in patients with underlying renal impairment.

■ INDICATION

Hypertension

Angiotensin-converting enzyme inhibitors effectively lower the mean, systolic, and diastolic pressures in hypertensive patients as well as in salt-depleted normotensive subjects.[5-7] Although ACE inhibitors are generally effective in reducing BP, they appear to be less potent in hypertensive blacks than whites. The goal of antihypertensive therapy is not only to lower BP but more importantly to alter the risk of end-organ damage and mortality.

One of the hallmarks of ACE inhibitors is that they lower peripheral vascular resistance without causing a compensatory increase in heart rate.[8-11]

Angiotensin-converting enzyme inhibitors are indicated for the treatment of hypertension with coexistent conditions such as congestive heart failure and diabetic nephropathy.[12]

Congestive Heart Failure and Left Ventricular Dysfunction

Angiotensin-converting enzyme inhibitors favorably alter hemodynamics in patients with systolic dysfunction.

Angiotensin-converting enzyme inhibitors have been shown to reverse ventricular remodeling by blocking the trophic effects of Ang II on cardiac myocytes.[13,14] ACE inhibitors have been shown to reverse left ventricular hypertrophy in patients with hypertension.[15,16]

The vast majority of these trials have shown a decrease in cardiovascular mortality and a slowing of the progression to congestive heart failure in patients treated with ACE inhibitors.

In the majority of trials, ACE inhibitor was administered 3–16 days after myocardial infarction (MI). Patients are likely more sensitive to the hypotensive effects of ACE inhibitors in the immediate post-MI period.[17]

Atherosclerotic Vascular Disease

Angiotensin-converting enzyme inhibition is thought to improve endothelial function by attenuating the vasoconstrictive and superoxide radical-generating effects of angiotensin II while simultaneously enhancing the bradykinin-dependent induction of endothelial nitric oxide production. Angiotensin-converting enzyme inhibitors also promote ischemic preconditioning, probably through a bradykinin-mediated mechanism.[4] Furthermore, ACE inhibition has been shown to reverse endothelial dysfunction in normotensive patients with CAD, in hypertensive patients, and in patients with noninsulin-dependent diabetes mellitus.[18]

Diabetic Nephropathy

The RAS and increased glomerular capillary pressure have been implicated in the progression of renal dysfunction due to a number of renal diseases, including diabetic nephropathy.[19] Angiotensin-converting enzyme inhibitors decrease glomerular capillary pressure by decreasing arterial pressure and by selectively dilating efferent arterioles.[20]

Numerous animal studies and small clinical trials have suggested that ACE inhibitors significantly reduce the loss of kidney function in diabetic nephropathy.[21]

Large, prospective, placebo-controlled study has now shown that captopril slows the progression of nephropathy in patients with insulin-dependent diabetes mellitus, as measured by the rate of decline in creatinine clearance and the combined end points of dialysis, transplantation, and death.[22]

AVAILABLE ANGIOTENSIN-CONVERTING ENZYME INHIBITORS

- Captopril
- Enalapril
- Benazepril
- Fosinopril
- Lisinopril
- Moexipril
- Perindopril
- Ramipril
- Trandolapril

Enalapril

Enalapril use improved metabolism reducing hepatic steatosis, decreasing ACE expression, and increasing ACE2 expression.[23]

Trandolapril

Trandolapril is a new orally active non-sulfhydryl ACE inhibitor that is hydrolyzed in vivo to the active free acid trandolaprilat.

In vitro and in vivo studies have shown that trandolapril is a potent and long-acting drug compared with other ACE inhibitors (N'Guyen and Brunner). A high affinity of a drug for its receptors means that the concentration of drug required for activity is low.

As a result of its high affinity for ACE, lipophilicity, and long elimination half-life, trandolapril has a long duration of action with a trough:peak ratio between 50 and 100% [(in trials evaluating BP with ambulatory blood pressure monitoring (ABPM)], justifying once-daily administration.

Therapeutic coverage throughout the 24-h dosage interval may have many important clinical implications.

Fosinopril

Fosinopril and amlodipine monotherapy were both effective in pediatric primary hypertension during a short-term follow-up.

Fosinopril may be particularly effective in reducing BP in hypertensive patients of females, central obesity, insulin resistance (IR), and hypo-high-density lipoprotein (hypo-HDL) cholesterolemia.

These findings indicate that optimizing antihypertensive medication selection based on the individualized characteristics of children with hypertension may improve the efficacy of antihypertensive treatment.[24]

Lisinopril

Blood pressure is an important risk factor for the development of retinopathy.[6-8] Antihypertensive therapy, especially inhibitors of ACE, slows the progression of nephropathy,[9,10] but whether these agents have a beneficial effect on retinopathy is much less clear.[24,25]

Lisinopril had beneficial effects on the progression of retinopathy. Nonsignificant benefits have been shown previously with other ACE inhibitors in people with type 1 and type 2 (noninsulin-dependent diabetes mellitus).[26,27]

REFERENCES

1. Brown NJ, Vaughan DE. Angiotensin-converting enzyme inhibitors. Circulation. 1998;97(14):1411–20.
2. Greenwald L, Becker RC. Expanding the paradigm of the renin-angiotensin system

and angiotensin-converting enzyme inhibitors. Am Heart J. 1994;128(5):997-1009.
3. Hollenberg NK. European Society of Cardiology: Angiotensin II antagonists in hypertension and beyond. Angiotensin II antagonists: why is there so much excitement? Am J Manag Care. 1998;4(Suppl. 7):S384-7.
4. Linz W, Wiemer G, Gohlke P, Unger T, Schölkens BA. Contribution of kinins to the cardiovascular actions of angiotensin-converting enzyme inhibitors. Pharmacol Rev. 1995;47(1):25-49.
5. Vidt DG, Bravo EL, Fouad FM. Drug therapy. Captopril. N Engl J Med. 1982;306(4):214-9.
6. Todd PA, Heel RC. Enalapril: A review of its pharmacodynamic and pharmacokinetic properties, and therapeutic use in hypertension and congestive heart failure. Drugs. 1986;31(3):198-248.
7. Pool JL, Gennari J, Goldstein R, Kochar MS, Lewin AJ, Maxwell MH, et al. Controlled multicenter study of antihypertensive effects of lisinopril, hydrochlorothiazide, and lisinopril plus hydrochlorothiazide in the treatment of 394 patients with mild to moderate essential hypertension. J Cardiovasc Pharmacol. 1987;3:S36-42.
8. Lund-Johansen P, Omvik P. Long-term haemodynamic effects of enalapril (alone and in combination with hydrochlorothiazide) at rest and during exercise in essential hypertension. J Hypertens. 1984;2(2):S49-50.
9. Ibsen H, Egan B, Osterzeil K, Vander A, Julius S. Reflex-hemodynamic adjustments and baroreflex sensitivity during converting enzyme inhibition with MK-421 in normal humans. Hypertension. 1983;5(2 Pt 2):I184-91.
10. Dunn GF, Oigman W, Ventura HO, Messerli FH, Kobrin I, Frolich ED. Enalapril improves systemic and renal hemodynamics and allows regression of left ventricular mass in essential hypertension. Am J Cardiol. 1984; 53(1):105-8.
11. Simon AC, Levenson JA, Bouthier J, Maarek B, Safar ME. Effects of acute and chronic angiotensin enzyme inhibition on large arteries in human hypertension. J Cardiovasc Pharmacol. 1985;7(Suppl. 1):S45-51.
12. Black HR, Cohen JD, Kaplan NM, Ferdinand K. The sixth report of the Joint National Committee on detection, evaluation, and treatment of high blood pressure (JNC VI). Arch Intern Med. 1997;157(21):2413-46.
13. Vaughan DE, Pfeffer MA. Angiotensin converting enzyme inhibitors and cardiovascular remodelling. Cardiovasc Res. 1994; 28(2):159-65.
14. Dahlof B. Effect of angiotensin II a blockade on cardiac hypertrophy and remodelling: A review. J Hum Hypertens. 1995;9(Suppl. 5): S37-44.
15. Nakashima Y, Fouad FM, Tarazi RC. Regression of left ventricular hypertrophy from systemic hypertension by enalapril. Am J Cardiol. 1994;53(8):1044-9. DOI: 10.1016/0002-9149(84)90634-9.
16. Gaudio C, Tanzilli G, Collatina S, Pagnotta P, Paknejad K, Campa PP. Evaluation of regression of left ventricular hypertrophy in hypertensive patients treated with captopril as assessed by magnetic resonance imaging. Cardiologia. 1992;37(11):789-91.
17. Pfeffer MA. Left ventricular remodeling after acute myocardial infarction. Annu Rev Med. 1995;46:455-6.
18. Mancini GB, Henry GC, Macaya C, O'Neill BJ, Pucillo AL, Carere RG, et al. Angiotensin-converting enzyme inhibition with quinapril improves endothelial vasomotor dysfunction in patients with coronary artery disease: The TREND (Trial on Reversing ENdothelial Dysfunction) Study. Circulation. 1996;94(3):258-65.
19. Ichikawa I, Brenner BM. Glomerular actions of angiotensin II. Am J Med. 1984;76(5B):43-9.
20. Hoelscher DD, Weir MR, Bakris GL. Hypertension in diabetic patients: An update of interventional studies to preserve renal function. J Clin Pharmacol. 1995;35(1):73-80.
21. Lewis EJ, Hunsicker LG, Bain RP, Rohde RD. The effect of angiotensin-converting-enzyme inhibition on diabetic nephropathy. N Engl J Med. 1993;329(20):1456-62.
22. Moraes DS, de Farias Lelis D, Andrade JMO, Meyer L, Guimarães ALS, De Paula AMB, et al. Enalapril improves obesity-associated liver injury ameliorating systemic metabolic

markers by modulating angiotensin-converting enzymes ACE/ACE2 expression in high-fat feed mice. Prostaglandins Other Lipid Mediat. 2021;152:106501.
23. Wang H, Shi L, Lin Y, Wang Y, Niu W, Li Y. Efficacy of fosinopril and amlodipine in pediatric primary hypertension: A single-center observational study. Front Pediatr. 2023:11;1247192.
24. The Microalbumin Captopril Study Group. Captopril reduces the risk of nephropathy in IDDM patients with microalbuminuria. Diabetologia. 1996;39(5):587-93.
25. Chase HP, Garg SK, Harris S, Hoops S, Jackson WE, Holmes DL. Angiotensin-converting enzyme inhibitor treatment for young normotensive diabetic subjects: A two-year trial. Ann Ophthalmol. 1993;25(8): 284-9.
26. Larsen M, Hommel E, Parving HH, Lund-Andersen H. Protective effect of captopril on the blood–retina barrier in normotensive insulin dependent diabetic patients with nephropathy and background retinopathy. Graefes Arch Clin Exp Ophthalmol. 1990; 228(6):505-9.
27. Ravid M, savin H jutrin I, Bental T, Katz B, Lishner M. Long-term stabilizing effect of angiotensin-converting enzyme inhibition on plasma creatinine and on preteinuria in normotensive type II diabetic patients. Ann Intern Med. 1993;118:577-81.

Angiotensin II Receptor Blockers: What is New?

Rajesh Kumar Jha, Pavni Agrawal, Srishti Jha

INTRODUCTION

Inhibitors of the renin–angiotensin system (RAS), particularly angiotensin-converting enzyme (ACE) inhibitors and angiotensin II receptor blockers (ARBs), are commonly used in the treatment of hypertension.

INDICATIONS

The renin–angiotensin–aldosterone system (RAAS) is intricately involved in the pathophysiology of several diseases, including hypertension, congestive heart failure, and chronic kidney disease of all types, including diabetic nephropathy. Pharmaceutical RAAS blockade is a common and successful strategy in each of these conditions.[1-3]

MECHANISM OF ACTION

Angiotensin II receptor blockers interfere with the RAS by impairing the binding of angiotensin II to the AT1 receptor on the cell membrane, thereby inhibiting the action of angiotensin II.[4] Blockade of the action of angiotensin II leads to elevations in plasma levels of renin, angiotensin I, and angiotensin II. However, this build-up of precursors does not overwhelm the receptor blockade, as evidenced by a persistent fall in both blood pressure (BP) and plasma aldosterone levels.[5]

The ARBs have an effect similar to that seen with monotherapy with other antihypertensive drugs.[6] However, several studies have shown that losartan, when given once daily, does not control BP to the same magnitude as other ARBs (irbesartan, telmisartan, candesartan, and valsartan).[7]

ADMINISTRATION

Currently available angiotensin receptor blockers, their Food and Drug Administration (FDA) approved indications, and dosing for these indications are mentioned in the following text.

Azilsartan

Azilsartan is available as 40 and 80 mg tablet.

Dosing

Hypertension: Initial dose is 20 mg and maximum daily dose is 80 mg.

It has superior ambulatory and clinical BP-lowering effects compared with olmesartan and valsartan at their highest clinically used doses and is well tolerated in patients with hypertension. BP control and response rates by this drug at its highest dose are greater than other drugs in the same class by absolute rates of 8–10%. Azilsartan at 80 mg had superior efficacy to both valsartan at 320 mg and olmesartan at 40 mg. Azilsartan at 40 mg was noninferior to 40 mg of olmesartan. For clinic systolic BP, both doses of azilsartan were superior to the comparator ARBs. Hence, azilsartan could lead to enhanced BP control in patients with stages 1–2 hypertension. The study results also demonstrates that the use of ambulatory BP as a primary efficacy end point is both feasible and increases the understanding of the pharmacodynamic behavior of not only the investigational drug under evaluation but known comparator agents as well.[8]

In a study done by Cushman et al., they compared once-daily fixed-dose combinations of azilsartan medoxomil/chlorthalidone force titrated to a high dose of either 40/25 or 80/25 mg with a fixed-dose combination of the ARB olmesartan medoxomil plus the thiazide diuretic hydrochlorothiazide force titrated to 40/25 mg. The design was a randomized, three-arm, double-blind, 12-week study of 1,071 participants with baseline clinic systolic BP of 160–190 mm Hg and diastolic BP ≤119 mm Hg. Changes in clinic (primary end point) and ambulatory systolic BP at week 12 were significantly greater in both azilsartan medoxomil/chlorthalidone arms than in the olmesartan/hydrochlorothiazide arm ($p < 0.001$). Changes in 24-hour ambulatory systolic BP were −33.9 ± 0.8, −36.3 ± 0.8, and −27.5 ± 0.8 mm Hg, respectively. Adverse events leading to permanent drug discontinuation occurred in 7.9%, 14.5%, and 7.1% of the groups given azilsartan medoxomil/chlorthalidone 40/25 mg, azilsartan medoxomil/chlorthalidone 80/25 mg, and olmesartan/hydrochlorothiazide 40/25 mg, respectively. This study has demonstrated superior antihypertensive efficacy of azilsartan medoxomil/chlorthalidone fixed-dose combinations compared with the maximum approved dose of olmesartan/hydrochlorothiazide.[9]

However, when Dash et al. did a comparison of the efficacy and safety of azilsartan and amlodipine combination versus telmisartan and amlodipine combination in hypertensive patients, they found that azilsartan and amlodipine combination had an 88% response rate, which was noninferior to the telmisartan and amlodipine combination. Biomarkers such as high-sensitivity troponin I (hsTnI) showed a significant decrease in both groups after 12 weeks of follow-up. However, there was no significant difference between the two groups.[10]

A comparative study of the effects of azilsartan and telmisartan on insulin resistance and metabolic biomarkers in essential hypertension associated with type 2 diabetes mellitus showed neither azilsartan nor telmisartan had any significant effects on insulin resistance and metabolic biomarkers after 12 weeks of drug therapy in hypertension patients associated with type 2 diabetes mellitus.[11]

Candesartan

Candesartan is available as 4, 8, 16, and 32 mg tablet.

Dosing

Hypertension: Initial dose is 16 mg and maximum daily dose is 32 mg.

Heart failure: Initial dose is 4–8 mg and maximum daily dose is 32 mg.

Candesartan is also used off-label to treat conditions including cerebrovascular accident or stroke, diabetic nephropathy, left ventricular hypertrophy, and migraines.

Eprosartan

Eprosartan is available as 400 and 600 mg tablet.

Dosing

Hypertension: Initial dose is 600 mg and maximum daily dose is 900 mg.

Irbesartan

Irbesartan is available as 75, 150, and 300 mg tablet.

Dosing

Hypertension: Initial dose is 150 mg and maximum daily dose is 300 mg.

Diabetic nephropathy: Initial dose is 75 mg and maximum daily dose is 300 mg. Treatment with irbesartan was associated with a risk of the primary end point (doubling of the baseline serum creatinine, development of end-stage kidney disease, or death from any cause) that was 20% lower than placebo and 23% lower than amlodipine. This renoprotection in both early (microalbuminuria) and late (proteinuria) is independent of the reduction in BP it causes.[12,13]

Losartan

Losartan is available as 25, 50, and 10 mg tablet.

Dosing

Hypertension: Initial dose is 50 mg and maximum daily dose is 100 mg.

For stroke prevention in hypertensive patients with a history of left ventricular hypertrophy: Initial dose is 50 mg and maximum daily dose is 100 mg.

For the treatment of proteinuria or diabetic nephropathy: Initial dose is 50 mg and maximum daily dose is 100 mg.

Losartan produces a slight fall in plasma uric acid that does not occur with the other ARBs, an effect that is due to enhanced uric acid excretion. This appears to be mediated at least in part by direct inhibition of the proximal urate–anion exchanger that is responsible for urate reabsorption.[14] Hence, the addition of or switch to losartan as an antihypertensive agent for patients with gout is recommended by clinical guidelines because of its benefit as a uricosuric agent.[15]

Olmesartan

Olmesartan is available as 5, 20, and 40 mg tablet.

Dosing

Hypertension: Initial dose is 20 mg and maximum daily dose is 40 mg.

In 2013, the US FDA reported that olmesartan can produce a "sprue-like enteropathy" characterized by severe chronic diarrhea and weight loss, occurring months to years after initiation of the drug.[16] In many cases, intestinal biopsy revealed villous atrophy, and, in all cases, antibody testing for celiac disease was negative.[17] The condition resolved after discontinuation of olmesartan, but rechallenge with the drug sometimes reproduced the symptoms.

Telmisartan

Telmisartan is available as 20, 40, and 80 mg tablet.

Dosing

Hypertension: Initial dose is 40 mg and maximum daily dose is 80 mg.

Telmisartan is given to reduce cardiovascular-related mortality in adults aged 55 years and older who have risk factors for serious cardiovascular events and cannot tolerate ACE inhibitors, stroke prophylaxis, and myocardial infarction prophylaxis.

Initial dose: 80 mg by mouth once daily and the maximum daily dose is 80 mg.

Valsartan

Valsartan is available as 40, 80, 160, and 320 mg tablet.

Dosing

Hypertension: Initial dose is 80–160 mg and a maximum daily dose is 320 mg.

Valsartan is used for reducing cardiovascular mortality in otherwise stable patients with a history of left ventricular failure and/or left ventricular dysfunction (LVD) following acute myocardial infarction.

Heart failure: Initial dose is 20 mg and maximum daily dose is 160 mg bid.

The combination of valsartan and sacubitril (neprilysin inhibitor) is available and approved for reducing the risk of cardiovascular death, decreasing hospitalization for heart failure in patients with chronic heart failure [New York Heart Association (NYHA) classes II through IV] and patients with reduced ejection fraction.

Background night-time BP and an abnormal nocturnal BP dipping profile are important cardiovascular risk factors in patients with hypertension. A study by Kario et al. investigated the effects of sacubitril/valsartan on 24-hour BP in patients with mild-to-moderate hypertension and in patient subgroups based on nocturnal BP dipping status. Both sacubitril/valsartan dosages (200 or 400 mg/dL) reduced 24-hour, daytime, and nighttime systolic BP, and 24-hour and daytime diastolic BP, to a significantly greater extent than olmesartan (20 mg/dL) in the dipper and nondipper groups. However, between-group differences in nighttime systolic BP were more significant in the nondipper group for sacubitril/valsartan 200 and 400 mg/d versus olmesartan 20 mg/d.[18]

In a study, hemodialysis patients who were switched from azilsartan experienced significant overall decreases in home BP as well as in N-terminal pro-brain natriuretic peptide (NT-proBNP) level from baseline to 3 months after the start of sacubitril/valsartan treatment. Thus, sacubitril/valsartan was well tolerated, effectively controlled out-of-office BP, and improved NT-proBNP level and may offer an effective and safe approach to controlling resistant hypertension in hemodialysis patients.[19]

A few caveats to remember about the use of ARBs:
- In patients with volume depletion or in those who are on diuretics, correct volume depletion before starting these agents or start with a lower dose.
- Consider using a lower dose in geriatric patients.
- Consider every 12-hour dosing in patients who experience diminished BP response toward the end of a 24-hour dosing interval.

Angiotensin II receptor blockers are contraindicated in pregnancy.[20,21] An additional concern is that AT1 receptor blockade results in the disinhibition of renin release by angiotensin II and increased formation of all angiotensin peptides. These peptides could activate the AT2 receptor, which is highly expressed in the fetus.

COMPARISON OF ANGIOTENSIN II RECEPTOR BLOCKERS WITH ANGIOTENSIN-CONVERTING ENZYME INHIBITORS

The antihypertensive efficacy of ARBs appears to be roughly equivalent to that of ACE inhibitors. On comparison of losartan with enalapril in patients with essential hypertension, both losartan and enalapril showed decreased systolic and diastolic BP from baseline at weeks 6 and 12. BP changes from baseline at trough (22–26 hours after the dose) did not differ between the two groups in the per-protocol analysis. Response to treatment at trough was excellent or good (diastolic BP <90 mm Hg or reduction in diastolic BP of 10 mm Hg) in 51% and 53% of the patients in the losartan and enalapril groups, respectively. Enalapril administration increased dry coughing symptoms, whereas losartan did not.[22]

In addition, the effects of ARBs and ACE inhibitors on cardiovascular events appear similar. The Ongoing Telmisartan Alone and in Combination with Ramipril Global Endpoint Trial (ONTARGET) compared telmisartan (80 mg/day), ramipril (10 mg/day), and combination therapy (80 + 10 mg/day) with both agents in 25,620 patients with vascular disease or diabetes.[23] The primary outcome was death from cardiovascular causes, myocardial infarction, stroke, or hospitalization for heart failure. Achieved mean BP was lower in patients who received telmisartan compared with ramipril (by 0.9/0.6 mm Hg) and in patients who received both agents compared with ramipril (2.4/1.4 mm Hg). The cardiovascular outcomes were similar in all three groups, while cough was more common with ramipril, and both hyperkalemia and acute kidney injury were more common with combined therapy.

In addition, a meta-analysis of nine trials and 11,007 patients that directly compared ACE inhibitors with ARBs in hypertensive patients found similar rates of all-cause mortality and cardiovascular mortality.[24] In contrast, drug withdrawal due to adverse events was significantly more frequent with ACE inhibitors, mostly due to dry cough. Thus, ARBs are a reasonable alternative to ACE inhibitor therapy in hypertensive patients.

As with other agents that inhibit the RAS, the efficacy of ARBs is enhanced by concomitant administration of low doses of a diuretic and by a reduction in dietary sodium intake. As with ACE inhibitors, ARBs appear to minimize the hypokalemia and hyperuricemia induced by diuretic therapy.[25]

In a study conducted by Gao et al. when compared to placebo, ACE inhibitor/ARB and beta-blocker (BB) treatments can shield breast cancer patients from cardiotoxicity during trastuzumab and anthracycline-containing regimens, suggesting that both are helpful.[26]

■ MONITORING

The ARB therapy puts the patient at an increased risk for hypotension, renal impairment, and hyperkalemia. Therefore, a patient's BP, renal function, and serum electrolytes should be monitored closely for the duration of ARB use.[27] Primary care providers should pay specific attention to the full medication list. Lithium concentrations may increase with the concomitant use of ARBs.[28]

■ REFERENCES

1. Hernández-Hernández R, Sosa-Canache B, Velasco M, Armas-Hernández MJ, Armas-Padilla MC, Cammarata R. Angiotensin II receptor antagonists role in arterial hypertension. J Hum Hypertens. 2002; 16(Suppl 1):S93-9.
2. Maggioni AP. Efficacy of angiotensin receptor blockers in cardiovascular disease. Cardiovasc Drugs Ther. 2006;20(4):295-308.
3. Cernes R, Mashavi M, Zimlichman R. Differential clinical profile of candesartan compared to other angiotensin receptor blockers. Vasc Health Risk Manag. 2011;7: 749-59.
4. Burnier M, Brunner HR. Angiotensin II receptor antagonists. Lancet. 2000; 355:637.
5. Grossman E, Peleg E, Carroll J, Shamiss A, Rosenthal T. Hemodynamic and humoral effects of the angiotensin II antagonist losartan in essential hypertension. Am J Hypertens. 1994;7:1041-4.

6. Matchar DB, McCrory DC, Orlando LA, Patel MR, Patel UD, Patwardhan MB, et al. Systematic review: comparative effectiveness of angiotensin-converting enzyme inhibitors and angiotensin II receptor blockers for treating essential hypertension. Ann Intern Med. 2008;148:16-29.
7. Kassler-Taub K, Littlejohn T, Elliott W, Ruddy T, Adler E. Comparative efficacy of two angiotensin II receptor antagonists, irbesartan and losartan in mild-to-moderate hypertension. Irbesartan/Losartan Study Investigators. Am J Hypertens. 1998;11:445-53.
8. White WB, Weber MA, Sica D, Bakris GL, Perez A, Cao C, et al. Effects of the angiotensin receptor blocker azilsartan medoxomil versus olmesartan and valsartan on ambulatory and clinic blood pressure in patients with stages 1 and 2 hypertension. Hypertension. 2011;57(3):413-20.
9. Cushman WC, Bakris GL, White WB, Weber MA, Sica D, Roberts A, et al. Azilsartan medoxomil plus chlorthalidone reduces blood pressure more effectively than olmesartan plus hydrochlorothiazide in stage 2 systolic hypertension. Hypertension. 2012;60(2):310-8.
10. Dash A, Meher BR, Padhy BM, Mohanty RR, Tripathy A. Comparison of efficacy and safety of azilsartan and amlodipine combination versus telmisartan and amlodipine combination in hypertensive patients: a non-inferiority trial. Cureus. 2023;15(3):e35865.
11. Meher BR, Mohanty RR, Sahoo JP, Jena M, Srinivasan A, Padhy BM. Comparative study of the effects of azilsartan and telmisartan on insulin resistance and metabolic biomarkers in essential hypertension associated with type 2 diabetes mellitus. Cureus. 2022;14(2):e22301.
12. Lewis EJ, Hunsicker LG, Clarke WR, Berl T, Pohl MA, Lewis JB, et al. Renoprotective effect of the angiotensin-receptor antagonist irbesartan in patients with nephropathy due to type 2 diabetes. N Engl J Med. 2001;345(12):851-60.
13. Lewis EJ, Lewis JB. Treatment of diabetic nephropathy with angiotensin II receptor antagonist. Clin Exp Nephrol. 2003;7(1):1-8.
14. Enomoto A, Kimura H, Chairoungdua A, Shigeta Y, Jutabha P, Cha SH, et al. Molecular identification of a renal urate anion exchanger that regulates blood urate levels. Nature. 2002;417:447-52.
15. Saad M. Hyperuricemia and gout: The role of losartan. Sr Care Pharm. 2023;38(9):359-60.
16. FDA Drug Safety Communication: FDA approves label changes to include intestinal problems (sprue-like enteropathy) linked to blood pressure medicine olmesartanmedoxomil. [online] Available from: http://www.fda.gov/Drugs/DrugSafety/ucm359477.htm [Last accessed January, 2024].
17. Ianiro G, Bibbò S, Montalto M, Ricci R, Gasbarrini A, Cammarota G. Systematic review: Sprue-like enteropathy associated with olmesartan. Aliment Pharmacol Ther. 2014;40:16-23.
18. Kario K, Rakugi H, Yarimizu D, Morita Y, Eguchi S, Iekushi K. Twenty-four-hour blood pressure-lowering efficacy of sacubitril/valsartan versus olmesartan in Japanese patients with essential hypertension based on nocturnal blood pressure dipping status: A post hoc analysis of data from a randomized, double-blind multicenter study. J Am Heart Assoc. 2023;12(8):e027612.
19. Iwashima Y, Fukushima H, Horio T, Rai T, Ishimitsu T. Efficacy and safety of sacubitril/valsartan after switching from azilsartan in hemodialysis patients with hypertension. J Clin Hypertens (Greenwich). 2023;25(3):304-8.
20. Saji H, Yamanaka M, Hagiwara A, Ijiri R. Losartan and fetal toxic effects. Lancet. 2001;357:363.
21. Serreau R, Luton D, Macher MA, Delezoide AL, Garel C, Jacqz-Aigrain E. Developmental toxicity of the angiotensin II type 1 receptor antagonists during human pregnancy: a report of 10 cases. BJOG. 2005;112:710-2.
22. Tikkanen I, Omvik P, Jensen HA. Comparison of the angiotensin II antagonist losartan

with the angiotensin converting enzyme inhibitor enalapril in patients with essential hypertension. J Hypertens. 1995;13:1343.
23. ONTARGET Investigators, Yusuf S, Teo KK, Pogue J, Dyal L, Copland I, et al. Telmisartan, ramipril, or both in patients at high risk for vascular events. N Engl J Med. 2008; 358:1547-59.
24. Li EC, Heran BS, Wright JM. Angiotensin converting enzyme (ACE) inhibitors versus angiotensin receptor blockers for primary hypertension. Cochrane Database Syst Rev. 2014(8):CD009096.
25. Soffer BA, Wright JT Jr, Pratt JH, Wiens B, Goldberg AI, Sweet CS. Effects of losartan on a background of hydrochlorothiazide in patients with hypertension. Hypertension. 1995;26:112-7.
26. Gao Y, Wang R, Jiang J, Hu Y, Li H, Wang Y. ACEI/ARB and beta-blocker therapies for preventing cardiotoxicity of antineoplastic agents in breast cancer: a systematic review and meta-analysis. Heart Fail Rev. 2023; 28(6):1405-15.
27. Kumar S, Ram CV. Angiotensin receptor blockers: current status and future prospects. Indian Heart J. 2007;59(6):443-53.
28. Balit CR, Gilmore SP, Isbister GK. Unintentional paediatric ingestions of angiotensin converting enzyme inhibitors and angiotensin II receptor antagonists. J Paediatr Child Health. 2007;43(10):686-8.

Calcium Channel Blockers and Hypertension

Rajesh Kumar Jha, Shahid Abbas, Srishti Jha

INTRODUCTION

Calcium channel blockers (CCBs), which inhibit L-type voltage-gated calcium channels, are important vasodilators that have been used as first- or alternate-line antihypertensives.

In addition to their class effects, new kinds of CCBs have been developed that block other calcium channel subtypes (T-type and N-type) and have agent-specific effects on heart rate and renin/aldosterone release.[1]

By inhibiting calcium entry through L-type calcium channels, CCBs dilate the vascular smooth muscle cells. new kinds of CCBs that express distinct characteristics have lately been developed. As a consequence, some CCBs have blocking effects for both L-type and N-type calcium channels (cilnidipine, mibefradil, and efonidipine).[2]

PHARMACOLOGY OF CALCIUM CHANNEL BLOCKERS

Calcium channel blockers are a broad group of antihypertensives that can be divided into two major orders grounded on predominant physiologic actions and mechanisms (1) dihydropyridines (DHPs), which preferentially bind L-type calcium channels in vascular smooth muscle, performing in vasodilatation and lowering of blood pressure (BP) and (2) non-DHPs (verapamil and diltiazem), which play equipotent effect on L-type calcium channels in the myocardium and the vasculature and preferentially bind calcium channels at the sinoatrial and atrioventricular node.

Accordingly, verapamil and diltiazem are less potent vasodilators than DHPs and are associated with negative chronotropic effects and a drop in sympathetic nervous system exertion, effects not clinically observed with DHP CCBs.

Calcium channel blockers can also be distributed by duration of action as follows:
1. Short-acting agents [nifedipine (capsule containing liquid), nicardipine, isradipine, diltiazem, and verapamil].
2. Long-acting agents that are modified release [e.g., nifedipine gastrointestinal therapeutic system (GITS) and nifedipine sustained-released verapamil].
3. Innately long-acting agents (e.g., amlodipine, lacidipine, and lercanidipine).

The short-acting DHPs, the utmost of which have not been approved and are not recommended for the treatment of hypertension, are associated with a reflex sympathetic nervous system activation, which causes an increase in heart rate. Heart rate generally decreases about 5–10 after treatment with the non-DHPs.

The variations in side effects among CCBs can be attributed to their pharmacologic diversity. With DHPs, especially the short-acting ones, headache, vertigo, flushing, and peripheral edema are more commonly seen as side effects. Constipation has been linked to verapamil, especially when taken in short-acting form. Verapamil and, to a lower extent, diltiazem can also reduce cardiac contractility and decelerate cardiac conduction; cases who have sick sinus syndrome, second- or third-degree atrioventricular block, or severe systolic dysfunction should refrain from taking these medicines.[3]

PHARMACOLOGY AND DISTRIBUTION OF CALCIUM CHANNELS

The pharmacology and distribution of calcium channels are listed in **Table 1**.

DRAWBACKS OF TRADITIONAL CALCIUM CHANNEL BLOCKERS

Traditional CCBs are widely used, but they have drawbacks that reduce their effectiveness and tolerability. Dihydropyridines, for example, can cause reflex tachycardia due to vasodilation, leading to an increased heart rate that may compromise their effectiveness. Non-DHPs, on the contrary, may cause negative inotropic effects, limiting their use in certain cardiac conditions. Furthermore, the need for more precise and focused calcium channel modulation is highlighted by individual differences in response and the possibility of drug interactions.

NEW DEVELOPMENTS IN CALCIUM CHANNEL BLOCKERS

- *Selective T-type CCBs:* In light of the unique functions played by T-type channels in vascular and cardiac tissues, recent research has concentrated on creating selective T-type CCBs. The goal of these innovative substances is to control calcium influx without having the unfavorable inotropic side effects of non-selective calcium channel blockade. Initial research indicates possible uses for treating specific forms of angina and atrial fibrillation.
- *Combination therapies:* It has become apparent that combining CCBs with other classes of cardiovascular drugs can increase effectiveness while reducing side effects. For example, CCBs and

TABLE 1: Pharmacology and distribution of calcium channels.

Current	α_1-Subunit	Channel	Distribution	Inhibitors
P	α_{1A}	$Ca_V 2.1$	Neurons	ω-Agatoxin IVA
Q	α_{1A}	$Ca_V 2.1$	Neurons	ω-Agatoxin IVA
N	α_{1B}	$Ca_V 2.2$	Neurons	ω-Conotoxin GIVA
R	α_{1E}	$Ca_V 2.3$	Neurons	SNX-482
L	α_{1S}	$Ca_V 1.1$	Skeletal muscle	DHP/PAA/BZP
	α_{1C}	$Ca_V 1.2$	Heart, endocrine, and neurons	DHP/PAA/BZP
	α_{1D}	$Ca_V 1.3$	Endocrine and neurons	DHP/PAA/BZP
	α_{1F}	$Ca_V 1.4$	Retina	N/A
T	α_{1G}	$Ca_V 3.1$	Neurons, heart	N/A
	α_{1H}	$Ca_V 3.2$	Neurons, heart	N/A
	α_{1I}	$Ca_V 3.3$	Neurons	N/A

(BZP: benzothiazepine; DHP: dihydropyridine; PAA: phenylalkylamine) renin-angiotensin system inhibitors together may have synergistic effects on the treatment of hypertension. The way that complex cardiovascular conditions are treated may be completely changed by such combination therapies.

- *L-Type calcium channel modulators:* To achieve the intended cardiovascular effects without the undesirable side effects associated with nonselective calcium channel blockade, researchers are looking into novel compounds that modulate L-type calcium channels more selectively. These modulators might offer a more specialized method of treating particular heart diseases, like hypertrophic cardiomyopathy.
- *Gene-based therapies:* New avenues for precisely controlling calcium channels have been made possible by developments in gene therapy. By focusing on the genes that govern the expression and functionality of calcium channels, scientists are investigating methods to tailor treatment regimens according to unique genetic profiles. With its tailored approach, treatment outcomes could be maximized and side effects could be reduced.
- *Intracellular calcium regulators:* To target intracellular calcium regulators outside of the plasma membrane, new CCBs are also being developed. Drugs that alter intracellular calcium handling may have special therapeutic benefits since cardiac myocytes depend on these activities for proper function. These substances may affect the sarcoplasmic reticulum's release of calcium, which would allow for a more complex regulation of cardiac contractility.

The dynamic character of cardiovascular pharmacology is reflected in the evolution of CCBs. The dedication of researchers to addressing the shortcomings of current medicines and enhancing patient outcomes is demonstrated by the recent developments in the creation of new CCBs. These developments signal a potential future for cardiovascular therapy, whether it be through gene-based treatments, combination medicines, selective T-type channel blocking, or modification of intracellular calcium regulators. These cutting-edge medications have the potential to completely change the way cardiovascular disorders are treated, giving both patients and doctors fresh hope as they go from the bench to the bedside.

NEWER DRUGS WITH THEIR SPECIFIC PROPERTIES

As a long-acting DHP-class CCB, efonidipine is discovered to have the capability to block both T-type and L-type calcium channels.[4]

Although mibefradil shares a structure with phenylalkylamines (PAAs), it is a well-known blocker of T-type calcium channels and has a weak L-type calcium channel-blocking effect. However, it is important to note that mibefradil was withdrawn from the market in several countries, including the United States, due to concerns about potential interactions with other medications. Specifically, mibefradil was found to inhibit certain liver enzymes responsible for metabolizing a wide range of drugs, leading to increased levels of those drugs in the body. This raised the risk of serious and potentially life-threatening interactions with other medications. It has also been reported that aranidipine, nilvadipine, and benidipine block T-type calcium channels.[5]

Apart from its application in hypertension, nilvadipine has been investigated for its possible impacts on several other ailments, such as vascular dementia. Studies have looked at the possibility that nilvadipine might help patients with vascular dementia slow down the rate at which their cognitive impairment advances.

Both L- and N-type calcium channels can be blocked by cilnidipine. Given the distribution of N-type calcium in the brain and along nerves, cilnidipine is anticipated to have a particular effect on inhibiting the sympathetic nervous system.[6]

Research has indicated that N-type Ca^{2+} channels were also blocked by amlodipine and cilnidipine. Amlodipine blocked N-type and P/Q-type Ca^{2+} channels, as did benidipine, cilnidipine, nicardipine, and barnidipine. The N-type Ca^{2+} channels are potently blocked by amlodipine.[7]

Benidipine which acts on L-N-T-type calcium channels exerts pleiotropic effects and has cardio- and reno-protective properties. One notable feature of benidipine is its long-lasting action, which can contribute to its efficacy in maintaining BP control over an extended period.

Azelnidipine is a newer CCB that has recently been approved for the treatment of hypertension. The advantages include preventing tachycardia and associated complications. It was first developed in Japan and was approved for the treatment of hypertension in 2020. It is administered orally at a dose of 16 mg/day.

Mechanisms of action include inhibiting transmembrane calcium influx through voltage-dependent channels. Apart from L-type, it also blocks T-type CCB present in both afferents as well as efferent arterioles.

By blocking the T-type channels in zona glomerulosa of adrenal glands it can reduce the secretion of the adrenal gland.

The higher lipid solubility of azelnidipine makes it more selective than amlodipine.

A large number of clinical trials have demonstrated the efficacy in terms of BP reduction. It is usually well tolerated with mild adverse effects including light-headedness and flushing.

Oral administration has been associated with increased renal plasma and blood flow. The effects on cerebral circulation include maintenance of cerebral vascular reserve and blood flow. Because of its antioxidant effect, it is also believed to possess antiatherosclerotic properties.[8]

Azelnidipine's effects on uric acid metabolism in seventy-two hypertensive patients were studied by Miyazaki et al.[9] Reductions in the urinary uric acid to creatinine ratio and serum urate levels were noted 2–3 months into the treatment.[10]

Novel CCB's include drugs that can be administered by the intranasal route. These rapidly acting drugs have been developed for treating ventricular arrhythmias.

One of these is etripamil which has shown promising results in its clinical trials for the treatment of supraventricular tachycardia (SVT). The trial results have shown that it took an average of 3 minutes for the drug to convert an arrhythmia into a sinus rhythm.[10]

Novel CCBs include drugs that can be administered by the intranasal route. These rapidly acting drugs have been developed for treating ventricular arrhythmias.

One of these is etripamil which has shown promising results in its clinical trials for the treatment of SVT. The trial results have shown that it took an average of 3 minutes for the drug to convert an arrhythmia into a sinus rhythm.[8]

Studies have also worked on bio-isosteres of nifedipine which have shown to possess anti-inflammatory activities apart from acting as antihypertensives.

The proposed mechanisms include blocking angiotensin-converting enzyme 2 (ACE2) binding to severe acute respiratory syndrome coronavirus 2 (SARS-CoV-2).[11]

Novel CCBs which prevent the influx of calcium through the β-channels will lead to the prevention of alteration of synapse physiology due to calcium overload and can have promising results in the treatment of dementia.[12]

Animal model studies of PRAX-944 a novel T-type CCB for the treatment of essential tremor have shown dose-dependent reduction of tremors at a maximum tolerable dose of 120 mg.[13]

Newer CCBs with dual L/N-L/T blockade effect are more efficacious than CCBs which block only L-type channels in CKD patients with hypertension.

Azelnidipine (L-type), cilnidipine (L-/N-type), and benidipine and efonidipine (L-/T-type CCBs) have better efficacy profiles for the control of hypertension.[14]

Lercanidipine a novel CCB has shown promising results for the control of hypertension. Because of its unique molecular structure, lercanidipine exhibits membrane-controlled kinetics, increased solubility within the arterial cellular membrane bilayer, and a high cholesterol tolerance factor. The long duration of action and gradual onset of vasodilation are conferred by these advantageous membrane-controlled kinetics.[15]

■ REFERENCES

1. Ozawa Y, Hayashi K, Kobori H. New generation calcium channel blockers in hypertensive treatment. Curr Hypertens Rev. 2006;2(2):103-11.
2. Randomized double-blind comparison of a calcium antagonist and a diuretic in elderly hypertensives. National Intervention Cooperative Study in Elderly Hypertensives (NICS-EH) Study Group. Randomized double-blind comparison of a calcium antagonist and a diuretic in elderly hypertensives. Hypertension 1999;34(5):1129-33.
3. Triggle DJ. Mechanisms of action of calcium antagonists. In: Epstein M (Ed.) Calcium Antagonists in Clinical Medicine. Philadelphia: Hanley & Belfus, Inc.; 2002, pp. 1-32.
4. Shimizu M, Ogawa K, Sasaki H, Uehara Y, Otsuka Y, Okumura H, et al. Effects of efonidipine, an L- and T-Type dual calcium channel blocker, on heart rate and blood pressure in patients with mild to severe hypertension: an uncontrolled, open-label pilot study. Curr Ther Res Clin Exp. 2003;64(9):707-14.
5. Muneta S, Kohara K, Hiwada K. Effects of benidipine hydrochloride on 24-hour blood pressure and blood pressure response to mental stress in elderly patients with essential hypertension. Int J Clin Pharmacol Ther. 1999;37(3):141-7.
6. Chandra KS, Ramesh G. The fourth-generation calcium channel blocker: Cilnidipine. Indian Heart J. 2013;65(6):691-5.
7. Sakata K, Shirotani M, Yoshida H, Nawada R, Obayashi K, Togi K, et al. Effects of amlodipine and cilnidipine on cardiac sympathetic nervous system and neurohormonal status in essential hypertension. Hypertension. 1999;33(6):1447-52.
8. Ram CVS. Therapeutic usefulness of a novel calcium channel blocker azelnidipine in the treatment of hypertension: a narrative review. Cardiol Ther. 2022;11(4):473-89.
9. Miyazaki S, Hamada T, Hirata S, Ohtahara A, Mizuta E, Yamamoto Y, et al. Effects of azelnidipine on uric acid metabolism in patients with essential hypertension. Clin Exp Hypertens. 2014;36(7):447-53.
10. Takihata M, Nakamura A, Kondo Y, Kawasaki S, Kimura M, Terauchi Y. Comparison of azelnidipine and trichlormethiazide in Japanese type 2 diabetic patients with hypertension: The COAT Randomized Controlled Trial. PLoS One. 2015;10(5):e0125519.

11. Mahgoub S, El-Sayed MIK, El-Shehry MF, Awad SM, Mansour YE, Fatahala SS. Synthesis of novel calcium channel blockers with ACE2 inhibition and dual antihypertensive/anti-inflammatory effects: a possible therapeutic tool for COVID-19. Bioorg Chem. 2021;116:105272.
12. Nimmrich V, Eckert A. Calcium channel blockers and dementia. Br J Pharmacol. 2013;169(6):1203-10
13. Scott L, Puryear CB, Belfort GM, Raines S, Hughes ZA, Matthews LG, et al. Translational pharmacology of PRAX-944, a novel T-type calcium channel blocker in development for the treatment of essential tremor. Mov Disord. 2022;37(6):1193-1201.
14. Tamargo J, Ruilope LM. Investigational calcium channel blockers for the treatment of hypertension. Expert Opin Investig Drugs. 2016;25(11):1295-1309.
15. Epstein M. Lercanidipine: a novel dihydropyridine calcium-channel blocker. Heart Dis. 2001;3(6):398-407.

CHAPTER 34

Diuretics and Hypertension

Anita Jaiswal Ektate, Neeta Narang, Virendra Chauhan, Upasana Mohanty

■ DEFINITION

A drug that enhances urine formation either by increasing urine volume (diuresis) or by elevating the excretion of Sodium and H_2O (natriuresis).

■ MECHANISM

- *Extrarenal*
  - *Cardiac output increase:* Digoxin; dopamine in congestive heart failure (CHF)
  - *Inhibition of ADH:* H_2O, alcohol
- *Renal:* Most diuretics inhibit Na and H_2O reabsorption.

■ CLASSIFICATION (TABLES 1 AND 2)

- *Based on diuretic effect intensity:* Highly, moderately, and weakly effective diuretics.
- Based on K^+ excretion effect: Both K^+ (and H^+)-losing and K^+ (and H^+)-sparing diuretics.
- Based on site and mechanism of diuretic action.

High Efficacy (Up to 25% NaCl Excretion)

- *Loop diuretics*
  - Furosemide, torsemide, and bumetanide (SO_2NH_2 group).
  - Ethacrynic acid (No SO_2NH_2 group).
- *Organic mercurials:* Mersalyl (now obsolete).

Medium Efficacy (5–10% NaCl Excretion)

- *Thiazides:* Hydrochlorothiazide, chlorothiazide, benzthiazide, hydroflumethiazide, clopamide, and polythiazide.
- *Thiazide-like diuretic:* Chlorthalidone, metolazone, xipamide, and indapamide.

Weak Efficacy

- *Carbonic anhydrase inhibitors (5% NaCl excretion):* Acetazolamide, methazolamide, and dichlorphenamide.
- *Potassium-sparing diuretics (3% NaCl excretion)*
  - *Aldosterone antagonists:* Spironolactone and eplerenone.
  - *Directly acting:* Amiloride and triamterene.
- *Osmotic diuretics (up to 20% NaCl excretion):* Mannitol, glycerol, and isosorbide.

Miscellaneous

- Theophylline and caffeine.
- *Sodium–glucose cotransporter type 2 (SGLT2) inhibitors (gliflozins):* These cause diuresis, and natriuresis (due to associated Na^+ and glucose loss) and reduce extracellular fluid volume.

TABLE 1: Diuretics and their target site.

Diuretics	Drugs	Site of action	Target molecule
Osmotic diuretics	• Mannitol, urea, and glycerin • Isosorbide	• *Systemic:* Extracellular space • *Renal:* Leaky segments	None
Carbonic anhydrase inhibitors	• Acetazolamide • Dorzolamide	Proximal convoluted tubule (PCT)	Carbonic anhydrase (luminal and intracellular)
Loop diuretics	• Furosemide, Bumetanide • Torsemide • Ethacrynic acid	Loop of Henle (thick ascending limb)	Na^+-K^+-$2Cl$ symporter
• Thiazides • Thiazide-like diuretics	• Hydrochlorothiazide • Chlorthalidone • Indapamide • Metolazone • Xipamide	Distal convoluted tubule (DCT)	Na^+-Cl symporter
Aldosterone antagonists (MRA)	• Spironolactone • Canrenoate • Eplerenone • Finerenone	Collecting duct (CD) principal cells	Mineralocorticoid receptor
Epithelial sodium channel (ENaC) blocker	Amiloride, triamterene	Distal collecting tubule and collecting duct	ENaC
SGLT2 inhibitors	• Canagliflozin • Dapaglifozin • Empagliflozin	Proximal convoluted tubule (PCT)	Sodium–glucose cotransporter

TABLE 2: Diuretics used in hypertension: Mechanism of action, uses, and side effects.[5]

Diuretic	Mechanism of action	Uses	Side effects

Loop diuretics	• Acts on thick ascending part of loop of Henle
	• Inhibit Na^+-K^+-$2Cl^-$ cotransport and reabsorption
	• Increase NaCl excretion (up to 25% high efficacy)
	• Na exchanges with K^+ in the distal tubule → K^+ loss
	• Effective in very low glomerular filtration rate (GFR) of <30 mL/min
		Edema: Cardiac (CHF) Hepatic (Cirrhotic ascites) Renal (nephrotic syndrome)
		• Acute pulmonary edema
		• Cerebral edema (mannitol preferred)
		• Acute hypercalcemia
		• Acute renal failure
		• Forced diuresis in drug poisoning (Barbiturate) Hypertension (thiazides preferred)
		• Hyperkalemia mild
		• Along with massive blood transfusion
		• Anion overdose (iodide, bromide, and fluoride)
			Hypokalemia
			• *Clinical features:* May increase digoxin toxicity, arrhythmia
			• Muscle weakness, fatigue, cramps
			• To prevent Hypokalemia
			  – Use low dose
			    - KCl supplement (oral solution or intravenous infusion) or
			    - Combine with K-sparing diuretic
			• *Advice:* More intake of K-containing food: Coconut water and fruit juice
			  – Hypochloremic alkalosis
			  – Dehydration
			  – Hyponatremia
			  – *Ototoxicity:* More likely with IV use

Contd...

Contd...

Diuretic	Mechanism of action	Uses	Side effects
Thiazide diuretics	Acts on early part of distal tubules • Inhibit Na$^+$-Cl$^-$ symporter and reabsorption • Increase NaCl excretion (5–10% Medium efficacy) • Na exchanges with K$^+$ in the distal tubule → K$^+$ loss → Hypokalemia • Not effective in very low GFR of <30 mL/min, may reduce GFR further	• Hypertension (Hydrochlorothiazide and Indapamide) • *Edema:* Cardiac and hepatic renal • Less efficacious than loop diuretic • Useful for maintenance therapy • Hypercalciuria and renal Ca stones • Diabetes Insipidus (DI) (Nephrogenic responds better) • Metolazone useful even when GFR is as low as 15 mL/min	• Hypokalemia • May ppt renal failure • Hyperuricemia • Hyperglycemia • Hyperlipidemia • Hypomagnesemia • Indapamide has lesser side effects than others in terms of lipids and glycemic control
Potassium sparing diuretics	*Acts on cortical segment of distal tubules* • Competitive antagonist of aldosterone inhibits aldosterone-induced proteins (AIP) • Furosemide • Inhibit Na reabsorption • Causes K$^+$ retention (K$^+$-sparing effect) → Hyperkalemia • Mild saluretic (natriuresis) 3% of NaCl • Never used alone as a diuretic • Useful when combined with thiazide or loop diuretic	• Edema is more useful in cirrhotic and nephrotic syndrome—it breaks resistance to thiazides or furosemide in refractory edema • To counteract K loss due to frusemide to thiazides • Hypertension: Combined with thiazide • CHF: As an adjunctive therapy it retards disease progression and reduces mortality Randomized Aldosterone Evaluation Study (RALES) • Primary hyperaldosteronism (Conn's syndrome)	Hyperkalemia • Risk in CRF patients • (Enalapril) or all transretinoic acid, ARB (Losartan) • KCl supplement *Related to steroid structure:* • Gynecomastia (except in eplerenone) • Impotence in males • Hirsutism • Menstrual irregularities in females *Miscellaneous:* Drowsiness and abdominal upset Drug interaction • May increase digoxin levels in CHF • Non-steroidal anti-inflammatory drugs (NSAIDs) (Aspirin) decrease its effect

- *Angiotensin-converting enzyme (ACE) inhibitors and angiotensin receptor blockers (ARBs):* These cause natriuresis and diuresis primarily by blocking the production of the downstream molecules of the renin-angiotensin-aldosterone system (RAAS) pathway, i.e., angiotensin II and aldosterone, which are involved in renal conservation of water and salt.[1]
- *Alcoholic beverages:* Stronger alcoholic beverages (more than 13.5% alcohol), when consumed in moderation, can

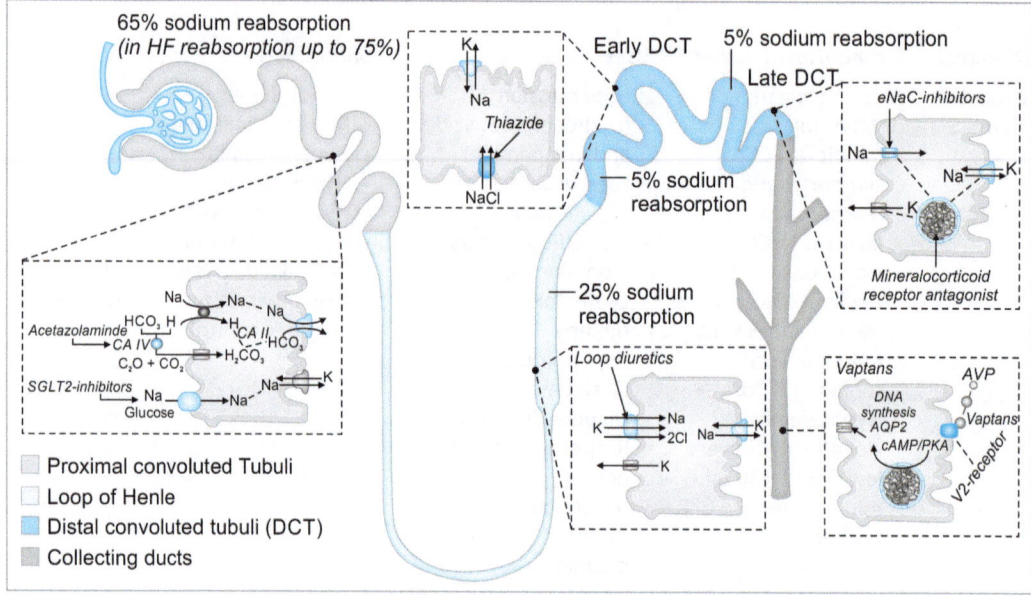

Fig. 1: Tubule transport systems and sites of action of diuretics.[4]

cause a transient diuretic effect without any electrolyte disturbances. Under conditions of hypohydration, alcohol does not induce any diuretic effect to restore fluid balance.[2]

- *Vasopressin receptor antagonists (tolvaptan and conivaptan):* They are classified under aquaretics rather than diuretics as they are responsible for water removal only unlike in diuretics (salt and water) (Fig. 1).[3]

JNC 8 GUIDELINES FOR ANTIHYPERTENSIVE SELECTION (TABLE 3)

- *Non-black persons*—ACEI/ARB, CCB/thiazide
- *Black person (including DM)*—CCB/thiazide-like diuretic
- *Chronic kidney disease (regardless of race or diabetes status)*—ACEI or ARB as initial or add-on antihypertensive therapy

TABLE 3: Treatment (first line) as per different Joint National Committee (JNC) on detection, evaluation, and treatment of high blood pressure protocol.

	Year	Initial antihypertensive
JNC 1	1977	Thiazide
JNC 2	1980	Diuretic
JNC 3	1984	Thiazide or β-blocker
JNC 4	1988	Diuretic, β-blocker, calcium channel blockers (CCB), or ACEI
JNC 5	1993	Diuretic or β-blocker
JNC 6	1997	Diuretic or β-blocker
JNC 7	2003	Thiazide for most without compel indication; Compel indication use thiazide, ACEI, ARB, β-blocker or CCB
JNC 8	12/13	ACEI or ARB, CCB or diuretic; specific medicine for race, CKD, or diabetes mellitus (DM)

Recent Update

In cases of resistant hypertension, spironolactone is the next best therapy as there is evidence of upregulation of mineralocorticoid receptors [prevention and treatment of hypertension with algorithm-based therapy-2 (PATHWAY-2 trial)].[6]

Phase 2 trial was successful for baxdrostat (aldosterone synthase inhibitor showing a dose-related reduction in blood pressure (BrigHTN trial).[7]

■ REFERENCES

1. Fountain JH, Kaur J, Lappin SL. Physiology, Renin Angiotensin System. StatPearls [Online]. Treasure Island (FL): StatPearls Publishing; 2023.
2. Polhuis KCMM, Wijnen AHC, Sierksma A, Calame W, Tieland M. The diuretic action of weak and strong alcoholic beverages in elderly men: A randomized diet-controlled crossover trial. Nutrients. 2017;9(7):660.
3. Costello-Boerrigter LC, Boerrigter G, Burnett JC Jr. Pharmacology of vasopressin antagonists. Heart Fail Rev. 2009;14(2):75-82.
4. Mullens W, Damman K, Harjola VP, Mebazaa A, Brunner-La Rocca HP, Martens P, et al. The use of diuretics in heart failure with congestion—a position statement from the Heart Failure Association of the European Society of Cardiology. Eur J Heart Fail 2019; 21(2):137-55.
5. Arumugham VB, Shahin MH. Therapeutic uses of diuretic agents. StatPearls [Online]. Treasure Island (FL): StatPearls Publishing; 2023.
6. Williams B, MacDonald TM, Morant S, Webb DJ, Sever P, McInnes G, et al. Spironolactone versus placebo, bisoprolol, and doxazosin to determine the optimal treatment for drug-resistant hypertension (PATHWAY-2): A randomised, double-blind, crossover trial. Lancet 2015;386(10008):2059-68.
7. Freeman MW, Halvorsen YD, Marshall W, Pater M, Isaacsohn J, Pearce C, et al. Phase 2 trial of baxdrostat for treatment-resistant hypertension. New Eng J Med 2023;388(5): 395-405.

Beta-blockers in Hypertension

Chandrasekhar Valupadas

INTRODUCTION

Hypertension is the most important and leading global risk factor for different chronic noncommunicable disease burden. In India, the prevalence of hypertension is more than one-fourth (29.8%) of the population with little difference between urban (33%) and rural (25%) areas. Among them, only 38% (urban) and 25% (rural) are being treated, and only one-tenth and one-fifth of the hypertensive population have their blood pressure (BP) under control, respectively.[1] β-adrenergic blockers are drugs that inhibit adrenergic responses mediated through β-receptors.

β-ADRENERGIC RECEPTORS

The β-adrenergic receptor is a site on a cell that interacts with epinephrine (Epi) or norepinephrine (NE) to control heartbeat and heart contractility, vasodilation, smooth muscle inhibition, and other physiological processes in the body **(Fig. 1)**. There are three known types of β-receptors, namely, β1-, β2-, and β3-receptors which are distributed in different tissues with a variety of functions listed in **Table 1**.

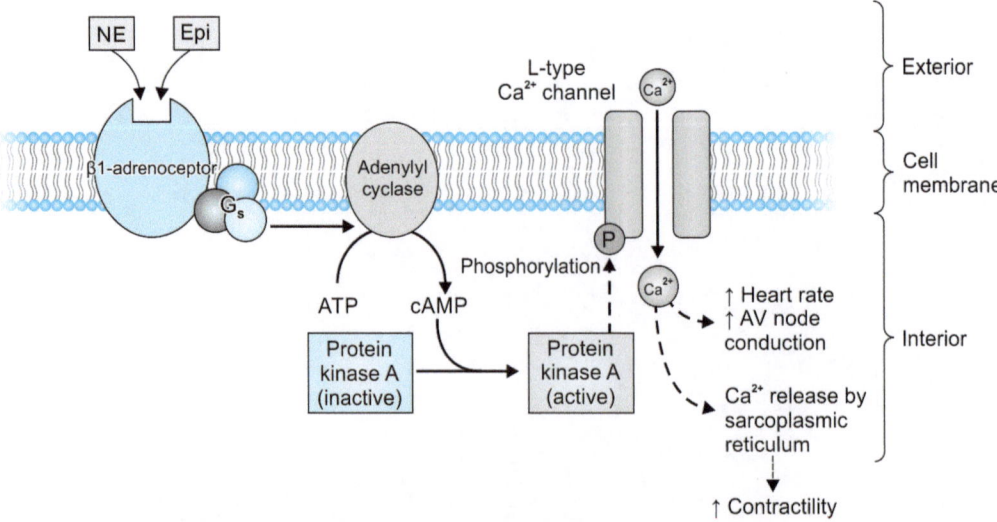

Fig. 1: Mechanism of β1-adrenoceptor. (ATP: adenosine triphosphate; AV: atrioventricular; cAMP: cyclic adenosine monophosphate; Epi: epinephrine; NE: norepinephrine)

TABLE 1: Classification of β-adrenergic receptors.

Type	Tissue distribution	Functions
β1	Heart	Positively inotropic and chronotropic
	Kidney	Renin release
	Adipocytes	Lipolysis
β2	Lung and bronchial	Bronchodilation
	Vascular smooth muscle	Vasodilation
	Heart	Positively inotropic and chronotropic
	Uterus	Relaxation
	Bladder	Relaxation
	Eye	Increase aqueous humor formation
	Liver	Glycogenolysis
	Skeletal muscle	Glycogenolysis
	Sympathetic terminal	Norepinephrine release
β3	Adipocytes	Lipolysis
	Uterus	Relaxation
	Bladder	Relaxation
	Heart	Negatively inotropic

β-ADRENERGIC RECEPTOR BLOCKERS

β-blockers, also known as β-adrenergic receptor blocking agents, are a class of antihypertensive drugs (listed in **Table 2**), which inhibit sympathetic neurotransmitters NE and Epi from binding to β-receptors.

The introduction of propranolol in 1963 was a therapeutic breakthrough that resulted in the proliferation and diversification of this class of drugs.

β-blockers are only considered appropriate first-line agents to treat specific compelling indications such as postmyocardial infarction (MI) and coronary artery disease (CAD). β-blockers are classified into two major categories based on β-receptor selectivity, nonselective and cardioselective β-blockers. These are further divided as follows:

- Nonselective β-blockers
  - *Without intrinsic sympathetic activity:* Propranolol, sotalol, and timolol.
  - *With intrinsic sympathetic activity:* Pindolol.
  - With additional α-blocking properties: Labetolol and carvedilol.
- Cardioselective β-blockers
  - Metoprolol
  - Atenolol
  - Acebutolol
  - Bisoprolol
  - Esmolol
  - Betaxolol
  - Celiprolol
  - Nebivolol

TABLE 2: Classification of β-adrenoreceptor blockers.

β-adrenergic receptor blockers	Examples
First-generation (older, traditional, and nonselective)	Propranolol, nadolol, timolol, penbutolol, sotalol, and pindolol
Second generation (β1-selective)	Metoprolol, atenolol, acebutolol, bisoprolol, and esmolol
Third generation (newer, with additional β-blocking and/or vasodilator property)	Labetalol, carvedilol, celiprolol, nebivolol, and betaxolol

PHARMACOLOGICAL ACTIONS OF β-BLOCKERS

- Cardiovascular system
  - *Heart:* Propranolol reduces heart rate, force of contraction (at high dose), cardiac output, cardiac work, oxygen

consumption, reduces coronary flow, particularly at the subendocardial region.
- *Blood vessels:* Propranolol blocks vasodilation and fall in BP due to reduced total peripheral resistance. Propranolol reduces noradrenaline and renin release and controls action reducing sympathetic outflow.
- *Respiratory tract:* Propranolol increases bronchial resistance by blocking β2-receptors. In asthmatics, the condition is worsened and a severe attack may be precipitated.
- *Central nervous system:* Propranolol shows no overt central effects but with long-term use of a relatively high dose subtle behavioral change, forgetfulness, increase in dreaming and nightmares have been reported.
- *Local anesthetics:* Propranolol is as potent as lidocaine, but it causes irritation at the site of injection, hence it is not clinically recommended.
- *Metabolic:* Propranolol blocks adrenergic-induced lipolysis and consequent increase in plasma free fatty acid levels and increase in low-/high-density lipoprotein (LDL/HDL) ratio. It inhibits glycogenolysis in the heart, skeletal muscles, and in the liver. Prolonged propranolol use may reduce carbohydrate tolerance by decreasing insulin release.
- *Skeletal muscle:* Propranolol inhibits adrenergically provoked tremor through β2-blocking, decreasing exercise capacity due to a decrease in glycogenolysis and lipolysis.
- *Eye:* β-blockers reduce the secretion of aqueous humor.
- *Uterus:* Normal relaxation of the uterus is blocked by propranolol.

PHARMACOKINETICS OF β-BLOCKERS

β-blockers are well absorbed after oral administration but have low bioavailability due to high first-pass metabolism in the liver. Propranolol is lipophilic and easily penetrates into the brain. Metabolism is hepatic flow dependent and plasma protein binding is 90%. The excretion of metabolites is through urine as glucuronides.

The pharmacokinetic and pharmacodynamic properties of various β-blockers are described in **Table 3**. Among β-blockers. nebivolol has the highest β1 selectivity.[2]

The European Society of Hypertension (ESH)/European Society of Cardiology (ESC) 2013 guidelines for the management of arterial hypertension have classified five major antihypertensive drugs as an initial therapy in which β-blockers are one of them.[3] β-blockers do not differ significantly in their overall ability BP reduction but they do differ in their ability to protect against overall cardiovascular risk and events, such as stroke and MI. Hence, there could be a compelling indication of comorbid conditions with hypertension.

CONTRAINDICATIONS OF β-BLOCKERS

The β-blockers are contraindicated in the following features:
- Bronchospastic disease.
- Young patients due to documented impotence/loss of libido.
- Diabetics because of impaired insulin sensitivity.
- Obese and patients with impaired lipid profile, as it may worsen lipid profile and increase atherosclerotic effect.
- Peripheral vascular disease.
- Heart failure (HF), as cardiac output is reduced and there is no improvement in left ventricular (LV) function.

TABLE 3: Various properties of β-adrenoceptor blockers.

β-blockers	Dose (mg)	Lipophilicity	Bioavailability (%)	First-pass metabolism	Plasma t1/2 (h)	Route of elimination	ISA	MSA
First generation								
Propranolol	40–480	High	3–40	Yes	3–5	Hepatic	No	Yes
Sotalol	160–480	No	90–100	No	6–12	Renal, hepatic	No	No
Timolol	10–40	Weak	50–75	Partial	4–5	Renal, hepatic	No	No
Pindolol	10–30	Weak	90	No	3–4	Renal, hepatic	Yes	No
Penbutolol	10–40	Yes	90	Yes	~5	Renal	Yes	No
Alprenolol	–	Moderate	–	Yes	2–3	–	Yes	No
Oxprenolol	80–160	Yes	20–70	Yes	1–2	Renal	Yes	No
Carteolol	–	No	–	Yes	7	–	Yes	No
Nadolol	40–80	No	30	No	14–24	Renal	No	No
Second generation								
Metoprolol	100–400	Yes	40–50	Yes	3–6	Hepatic	No	No
Atenolol	25–100	No	50–60	No	6–9	Renal	No	No
Acebutolol	400–1200	No	40–60	Yes	3–4	Renal, hepatic	Yes	Yes
Bisoprolol	2.5–10	Weak	80	No	9–12	Renal, hepatic	No	No
Esmolol	*	No		No	<10 min	Renal	No	No
Betaxolol	10–40	Yes	89	Yes	14–22		No	No
Bevantolol	200–600	Moderate					No	
Third generation								
Labetalol	300–600	Moderate	25	Yes	4–6	Hepatic	No	No
Carvedilol	3.125–25	Yes	25–30	Yes	7–10	Hepatic	No	Yes
Celiprolol	200–600	No	30–70	No	5	Renal	Yes	No
Nebivolol	5–40	High	12–96	Yes	10	Hepatic	No	No

*Useful in postoperative hypertension, 0.5–1 mg/kg loading dose over 1 min followed by an infusion of 50 µg/kg/min (maximum 300 µg/kg/min)
(ISA: intrinsic sympathomimetic activity; MSA: membrane stabilizing activity)

- Renal impairment, as it gets accumulated and dosage reduction is often necessary.

SIDE EFFECTS OF β-BLOCKERS

Nonselective β-blockers may give rise to adverse effects such as asthma and intermittent claudication as a result of antagonism of β2-receptors. The β1-selective blockers are free of these adverse effects; however, at higher doses, cardioselectivity will be lost. Patients who develop very marked bradycardia and tiredness may tolerate a drug

TABLE 4: Drug interactions with β-blockers.	
Pharmacokinetic interactions	**Pharmacodynamic interactions**
• All salts, cholestyramine (decrease absorption) • Enzyme inducers (decrease plasma concentrations) • Cimetidine, hydralazine (increase bioavailability) • They impair the clearance of lidocaine	• Digoxin • Calcium channel blocker (CCB) (verapamil) • Calcium channel blocker (dihydropyridine) • NSAIDs • Adrenalin and other α-agonists

NSAIDs: nonsteroidal anti-inflammatory drugs

with partial agonist activity, that is, intrinsic sympathomimetic activity (ISA) such as pindolol.

Drug interactions of β-blockers are shown in **Table 4**.

β-BLOCKERS IN UNCOMPLICATED HYPERTENSION

As per the Eighth Joint National Committee (JNC-8), β-blockers are no longer recommended as first-line therapy for uncomplicated hypertension. However, they are still used in treating hypertension, especially in patients with CAD, arrhythmias, and chronic HF. This is the greatest shift from first-line therapy in JNC-7 or earlier to fourth-line therapy in JNC-8, pending controversies and arguments for/and against β-blockers.

Such controversies fit better for the intraclass of β-blockers rather than the entire class against other classes of antihypertensives. β-Blockers such as carvedilol and nebivolol were found to be more beneficial for hypertension than the older β-blockers, but trial results with these newer agents are scanty.[4] However, in patients whose BP is not adequately controlled with a diuretic, angiotensin-converting enzyme (ACE) inhibitor/angiotensin receptor blocker (ARB), and CCB, the addition of a β-blocker may improve BP control.

β-BLOCKERS IN COMPLICATED HYPERTENSION

- *Stroke:* β-blockers have only a modest effect on stroke, while other classes of antihypertensive drugs reduce mortality and cardiovascular disease (CVD) more than β-blockers.[5] For these reasons, diuretics, ACE inhibitors/ARBs, and CCBs are preferred as first-line therapy for hypertension as they are better tolerated than β-blockers.
- *Heart failure:* β-blockers have been shown to reduce mortality in patients with chronic HF. For stage B, β-blockers and ACE inhibitors should be used in all patients with a history of MI regardless of ejection fraction (EF) or presence of HF, this can also be recommended in patients without a history of MI, with a reduced EF, and no HF symptoms. For stage C, diuretics, salt restriction, ACE inhibitors, and β-blockers such as bisoprolol, carvedilol, or metoprolol are also recommended.

  The combination of these β-blockers with ACE inhibitor/ARBs has been shown to reduce symptoms of HF, improve clinical status, and reduce the risk of death and hospitalization by 30–40%.[6]
- *Angina pectoris:* The American College of Cardiology (ACC)/American Heart Association (AHA) 2007 guidelines on chronic stable angina recommend initiating and continuing β-blocker therapy indefinitely in all patients who have had MI, acute coronary syndrome (ACS), or left ventricular dysfunction (LVD), with or without HF symptoms,

and/or ACE inhibitors with the addition of other drugs, as required, for BP control. The β1-selective agents without ISA are most frequently used and have less inhibition of the peripheral vasodilation and bronchodilation induced by the β2-receptors.[7] However, at higher doses, cardioselectivity may be lost. The β-blockers with ISA may not decrease heart rate and BP at rest but reduce exercise heart rate and can be effective in a few selective patients.

- *Acute MI [unstable angina (UA)/ non-ST elevated myocardial infarction (NSTEMI) and ST elevated myocardial infarction (STEMI)]:* β-blockers prevent recurrent ischemia, life-threatening ventricular arrhythmias, and improve survival in patients with prior MI. Unless contraindicated, the ACC/AHA 2014 guidelines for NSTEMI and 2013 guidelines for STEMI recommend indefinite β-blocker therapy (cardioselective β-blockers without ISA) in all patients with UA, NSTEMI, and STEMI.[8]
- *Cardiac arrhythmia:* β-blockers improve survival in patients who have had MI as they are able to reduce the incidence of sudden cardiac death. The ACC/AHA/ESC 2006 guidelines consider β-blockers to be the safe and effective mainstay of antiarrhythmic drug therapy for the management of ventricular arrhythmias and prevention of sudden cardiac death.[9]
- *Chronic kidney disease (CKD):* β-blockers are recommended as second-line agents after renin–angiotensin–aldosterone system (RAAS) blockers for controlling hypertension in patients with CKD and systolic HF. Compared to other antihypertensive agents, there are no demerits for using β-blockers for renal protection as vasodilatory β-blockers are renoprotective. In CKD, often three or more different antihypertensive drugs are required to control BP, which is crucial for the prevention of cardiovascular events. There is no evidence that β-blockers are inferior to diuretics or CCBs as second- or third-line agents for renal protection and control of BP in patients with CKD.[10]
- *Metabolic syndrome (diabetes and dyslipidemia):* Blood pressure (BP) management in hypertensive patients with metabolic abnormalities is challenging, since many of the antihypertensive drugs adversely affect metabolism. Third-generation β-blockers, such as nebivolol, are effective in hypertension control and offer neutral or beneficial effects on metabolism, especially in obese and diabetic hypertensive patients.[11]

CLINICAL TRIAL EVIDENCE AND CURRENT RESEARCH ON β-BLOCKERS

β-blockers have substantial clinical trial evidence of benefit over placebo in hypertension and are relatively inexpensive. Building on the availability of propranolol since 1976, more than a dozen additional β-blockers have been introduced for hypertension treatment.[12] This drug class effectively lowers BP and has been a recommended treatment option by the JNC in 2003.[13] Vasodilatory activity may be a key contributor to advantageous outcomes in hypertension.[14] In recent times, their use has been declining. Their role is becoming controversial, especially after the evidence from the Losartan Intervention for Endpoint Reduction (LIFE), Anglo–Scandinavian Cardiac Outcomes Trial (ASCOT), and Cochrane database review in 2004, β-blockers have been placed in the fourth line in the treatment of hypertension in the UK, according to new National Institute for Health and Clinical Excellence (NICE) guidelines. Concerns have also been raised by meta-analysis in which β-blockers were reported to have a suboptimal effect on reducing stroke risk and increasing the risk for new-onset diabetes compared with other antihypertensive agents.[15] These reviews and meta-analyses were evaluated primarily for atenolol, a traditional β-blocker, or other β-blockers without vasodilatory activity. However, β-blockers are a diverse group of medicines with different properties, and there is a need for more well-conducted research in this area.[5]

CONCLUSION

β-blockers probably make little or no difference in the reducing number of deaths among people on treatment for hypertension; the effect appears to be similar to that of diuretics and ACE inhibitors/ARBs but not as good as CCBs. They reduce the number of strokes, an effect similar to that of diuretics but not as good as ACE inhibitors/ARBs and CCBs. They also make little or no difference to the number of heart attacks, which may not be different from that of diuretics, ACE inhibitors/ARBs, and CCBs. The evidence of β-blockers on effects like modest CVD reduction, and little or no effects on mortality are inferior to other antihypertensive drugs generated from studies on one traditional β-blocker, atenolol and it is unjust to extrapolate data of one drug to its entire class. Among all β-blockers, vasodilatory β-blockers are found to be more effective such as nebivolol. Therefore, further research is needed to explore the differences between different subtypes of β-blockers or their differential effects on younger and older people.

REFERENCES

1. Anchala R, Kannuri NK, Pant H, et al. Hypertension in India: a systematic review and meta-analysis of prevalence, awareness, and control of hypertension. J Hypertens. 2014;32(6):1170-7.
2. Gupta S, Wright HM. Nebivolol: a highly selective beta1-adrenergic receptor blocker that causes vasodilation by increasing nitric oxide. Cardiovasc Ther. 2008;26(3):189-202.
3. Mancia G, Fagard R, Narkiewicz K, et al. 2013 ESH/ESC Guidelines for the management of arterial hypertension: the Task Force for the management of arterial hypertension of the European Society of Hypertension (ESH) and of the European Society of Cardiology (ESC). J Hypertens. 2013;31(7):1281-357.
4. Guo G. Beta-blockers in uncomplicated hypertension: Is it time for retirement? 2015. [online] Available from https:// HYPERLINK "http://www.clinicalcorrelations.org/2015/10/07/beta-blockers-"www.clinicalcorrelations.org/2015/10/07/beta-blockers- in-uncomplicated-hypertension-is-it-time-for-retirement/ [Last accessed from April, 2019].
5. Wiysonge CS, Bradley HA, Volmink J, et al. Beta-blockers for hypertension. Cochrane Database Syst Rev. 2017;1:CD002003.
6. Yancy CW, Jessup M, Bozkurt B, et al. 2013 ACCF/AHA guideline for the management of heart failure: executive summary: a report of the American College of Cardiology Foundation/American Heart Association Task Force on practice guidelines. Circulation. 2013;128(16):1810-52.
7. Fihn SD, Blankenship JC, Alexander KP, et al. 2014 ACC/AHA/AATS/PCNA/SCAI/STS focused update of the guideline for the diagnosis and management of patients with stable ischemic heart disease: a report of the American College of Cardiology/American Heart Association Task Force on Practice Guidelines, and the American Association for Thoracic Surgery, Preventive Cardiovascular Nurses Association, Society for Cardiovascular Angiography and

Interventions, and Society of Thoracic Surgeons. Circulation. 2014;130(19):1749-67.
8. Amsterdam EA, Wenger NK, Brindis RG, et al. 2014 AHA/ACC guideline for the management of patients with non-ST-elevation acute coronary syndromes: executive summary: a report of the American College of Cardiology/ American Heart Association Task Force on Practice Guidelines. Circulation. 2014;130(25):2354-94.
9. Zipes DP, Camm AJ, Borggrefe M, et al. ACC/AHA/ESC 2006 Guidelines for Management of Patients with Ventricular Arrhythmias and the Prevention of Sudden Cardiac Death: a report of the American College of Cardiology/American Heart Association Task Force and the European Society of Cardiology Committee for Practice Guidelines (writing committee to develop Guidelines for Management of Patients with Ventricular Arrhythmias and the Prevention of Sudden Cardiac Death): developed in collaboration with the European Heart Rhythm Association and the Heart Rhythm Society. Circulation. 2006;114(10):e385-484.
10. Ritz E, Rump LC. Do β-blockers combined with RAS inhibitors make sense after all to protect against renal injury? Curr Hypertens Rep. 2007;9(5):409-14.
11. Marketou M, Gupta Y, Jain S, et al. Differential Metabolic Effects of Beta-Blockers: an Updated Systematic Review of Nebivolol. Curr Hypertens Rep. 2017;19(3):22.
12. Frishman WH. A historical perspective on the development of β-adrenergic blockers. J Clin Hypertens. 2007;9(4):19-27.
13. Chobanian AV, Bakris GL, Black HR, et al. Seventh report of the Joint National Committee on Prevention, Detection, Evaluation, and Treatment of High Blood Pressure. Hypertension. 2003;42(6):1206-52.
14. Beevers G, Lip GY, O'Brien E. ABC of hypertension: The pathophysiology of hypertension. BMJ. 2001;322(7291):912-6.
15. Bangalore S, Parkar S, Grossman E, et al. A meta-analysis of 94,492 patients with hypertension treated with beta blockers to determine the risk of new-onset diabetes mellitus. Am J Cardiol. 2007;100(8):1254-62.

CHAPTER 36

Alpha-blockers: Role in Hypertension

Dilip A Kirpalani

INTRODUCTION

Alpha-receptor antagonists constitute a class of antihypertensive medications employed in clinical practice. While not typically chosen as first-line agents for managing Essential Hypertension, they hold considerable value as supplementary drugs in the treatment of challenging hypertension cases. Peripheral sympathetic nerve terminals host two distinct types of α-receptors: α1-receptors and α2-receptors. Among these, α1-receptors are further divided into three homologous subtypes, namely, α1A, α1B, and α1D. The roles of α-receptors are as follows:

- Induction of vasoconstriction
- Stimulation of smooth muscle contraction in the internal urethral sphincter
- Contraction of sphincters within the gastrointestinal tract
- Augmented secretion from sweat and salivary glands
- Pupillary dilation
- Relaxation of smooth muscles within the gastrointestinal tract.

The α2-receptors, on the contrary, are subdivided into α2A, α2B, and α2C. The functions of α2-Receptors are the following:
- Inhibition of neurotransmitter release
- Reduction in central sympathetic outflow
- Promotion of platelet aggregation
- Diminished insulin release.

CLASSIFICATION OF α-BLOCKERS

Alpha-receptor antagonist medications are categorized into the following two main groups: Nonselective α-blockers and selective α-blockers. The latter group, in turn, is further divided into α1-blockers and α2-blockers.

- *Selective α1-blockers:* These agents are utilized for the management of chronic hypertension. Prominent examples of selective α1-blockers include prazosin, terazosin, and doxazosin.
- *Selective α2-blockers:* These agents, exemplified by the old drug yohimbine, can lead to an increase in blood pressure. Yohimbine was historically employed to address orthostatic hypotension.
- *Nonselective α-blockers:* Phentolamine and phenoxybenzamine, both nonselective α-blockers, find application solely in the treatment of pheochromocytoma. Their use in chronic hypertension management is limited due to the risk of severe orthostatic hypotension and tachycardia stemming from their nonselective action.
- *Presynaptic α2-receptor agonists:* A distinct group of drugs used for chronic Hypertension management work through α-receptors. These presynaptic α2-receptor agonists, namely by clonidine and moxonidine, exert their antihypertensive effects by reducing central sympathetic outflow.

α1-RECEPTOR ANTAGONISTS IN THE TREATMENT OF HYPERTENSION

α1-Receptor antagonists are utilized in the management of chronic hypertension. These drugs exert their antihypertensive effects by reducing peripheral vascular resistance through the blockade of postsynaptic α1-receptors. The primary target of these drugs is the α1B-subtype of the α1-receptor, predominantly found on vascular smooth muscle cells. This blockade leads to a reduction in vasoconstriction.

Prazosin is a commonly employed α1-blocker for treating hypertension. The recommended dose of prazosin ranges from 5 to 20 mg per day, typically administered in two to three divided doses. Despite its short half-life of 3 h and 50% oral bioavailability, Prazosin is advantageous in that it induces minimal or no reflex tachycardia.

Another drug within this class is doxazosin, which exhibits a longer duration of action compared to prazosin. The prescribed dose of doxazosin is 4–16 mg per day, administered in one or two divided doses. A notable concern with doxazosin is the occurrence of the "first-dose phenomenon," wherein severe orthostatic hypotension may arise after the initial doses. However, this issue tends to diminish over time.

Terazosin constitutes a third option within this group. Its recommended dose ranges from 5 to 20 mg per day, typically given in one or two divided doses. Terazosin presents an advantage in that it possesses a high oral bioavailability and a longer duration of action than prazosin, with a half-life spanning 9–12 h.

BENEFITS OF α1-RECEPTOR ANTAGONISTS IN HYPERTENSION

Several studies have highlighted the beneficial effects of α1-receptor antagonists, particularly, doxazosin, in the treatment of hypertension and its associated conditions. The Treatment of Mild Hypertension Study (TOMHS) and German Antihypertensive Efficacy and Safety (GATES) study have demonstrated the potent antihypertensive properties of doxazosin.

In the "effect of doxazosin gastrointestinal therapeutic system on patients with Uncontrolled Hypertension: The ASOCIA study, involving a large cohort of over 3,500 patients, doxazosin was shown to effectively achieve target blood pressure in 61% of patients when used as an add-on therapy compared to placebo. Notably, the study revealed an average 19% reduction in rate pressure product and a 15% reduction in pulse pressure after adding doxazosin, indicating a reduction in myocardial oxygen demand and improved cardiovascular parameters.

Furthermore, α1-receptor antagonists offer pleiotropic benefits beyond blood pressure reduction, including
- Decreased total cholesterol and low-density lipoprotein (LDL) cholesterol levels
- Enhanced insulin sensitivity
- Improvement in endothelial function
- Reduction in arterial stiffness.

These drugs are particularly well-suited for elderly males with hypertension and benign prostatic hyperplasia due to their effect on smooth muscles in the prostate gland and urinary bladder neck, leading to an alleviation of obstructive urinary symptoms.

In the context of chronic kidney disease, α1-receptor antagonists are considered excellent antihypertensive options, especially when conventional treatments fail to achieve target blood pressure levels. These drugs are advantageous in this population as they do not exacerbate serum potassium levels or worsen glomerular filtration rate (GFR), and extensive biochemical monitoring is not typically required following their initiation.

SIDE EFFECTS OF α1-RECEPTOR ANTAGONISTS

- *Postural hypotension:* α-Blockers are known to cause postural hypotension, which is a drop in blood pressure upon standing up. This side effect can be particularly concerning in elderly individuals who are already at a higher risk of postural hypotension. Caution should be exercised when using α1-receptor antagonists in this population. Initiating treatment with a low dose and gradually titrating upwards based on blood pressure response, preferably at night, can help mitigate this side effect.
- *Supine and standing blood pressure monitoring:* Monitoring both supine (or sitting) and standing blood pressure is important in patients receiving α1-receptor antagonists. This helps assess the degree of postural hypotension and guides dose adjustments as needed.
- *Other potential side effects:* α1-Receptor antagonists can also cause other side effects, which may include dizziness, headache, fatigue, nasal congestion, and rarely, priapism (prolonged and painful erection).

MISCELLANEOUS α-BLOCKERS

- *Carvedilol:* Carvedilol is a combined α- and α-blocker. While it is more commonly used in the treatment of heart failure, it also has some antihypertensive effects. Its potency as an antihypertensive may not be as strong as other agents.
- *Labetalol:* Labetalol is another combined α- and β-Blocker. It is particularly useful for hypertensive emergencies and can be administered intravenously. Labetalol is considered safe for use during pregnancy, making it a suitable option for managing hypertension in pregnant individuals.

α2-RECEPTOR AGONISTS

Clonidine and moxonidine: Clonidine and moxonidine are presynaptic α2-receptor agonists. Although they are not α-blockers, they are included here due to their role as antihypertensive agents. They work by reducing central sympathetic outflow, which helps to lower blood pressure. Moxonidine, in particular, has an additional action at the imidazoline-1 receptor and may cause fewer side effects such as sedation compared to clonidine. These agents are often used as add-on therapies in challenging-to-treat hypertension cases.

CONCLUSION

α1-Receptor antagonists serve as valuable options in the management of difficult-to-treat hypertension and resistant hypertension, particularly when other agents are not suitable. They offer advantages in terms of glucose and lipid neutrality, as well as minimal impact on serum potassium and GFR. These drugs exhibit pleiotropic benefits, including improvements in endothelial function and reduction in vascular stiffness.

α1-Receptor antagonists can be considered effective add-on therapies for individuals who are already on first-line agents but have not achieved their target blood pressure. Their tolerability profile is generally favorable, making them a viable choice for combination therapy.

While current hypertension guidelines may not yet prominently feature α-1 Receptor Antagonists, the growing need for diverse treatment options calls for their inclusion, at least as add-on agents, in the management of chronic hypertension. In cases of elderly males with both hypertension and benign prostatic hyperplasia, these agents may even be considered as first or second-line antihypertensive treatments. However, careful monitoring for postural hypotension is essential in patients receiving α1-receptor antagonists.

As research and clinical experience continue to accumulate, the role of α1-receptor antagonists in the management of hypertension may become more defined, offering additional avenues for effective blood pressure control and cardiovascular risk reduction.

■ SUGGESTED READING

1. ALLHAT Study: Curr Control Trials Cardiovasc Medications 2001; 2:254–256. (Published online 2001 Nov 1. doi: 10.1186/cvm-2-6-254).
2. Alpha Blockers: Supplement to Journal of the Association of Physicians of India, 1st September, 2014, Vol. 62.
3. ASOCIA Trial: Journal of Cardiovascular Pharmacology: 2006; 47:271-276. doi: 10.1097/01.fjc.0000202562.46420.d9.
4. GATES Study: s. (J Clin Hypertens 2006; 8:159-166) ©2006 Le Jacq Ltd.
5. Hypertension Primer (3rd edition) by American Heart Association, pp. 421-5.
6. TOMHS Study: Arch Intern Med 1991; 151:1413-23.

CHAPTER 37

Direct Vasodilators in Hypertension

Rajib Ratna Chaudhary

■ INTRODUCTION

Direct vasodilators are a class of medications that directly relax and dilate blood vessels, leading to decreased vascular resistance and ultimately lower blood pressure. These drugs were among the first oral antihypertensives introduced and have a long history in the treatment of hypertension. While they are not commonly used as monotherapy due to side effects and compensatory mechanisms, they can be effective when combined with other antihypertensive agents, particularly in cases of resistant hypertension and hypertensive emergencies.

The pharmacological actions of direct vasodilators involve their ability to directly affect the tone of blood vessels, resulting in relaxation and widening of the vessels. This leads to improved blood flow and reduced pressure within the arteries. However, the use of these drugs can trigger compensatory responses in the cardiovascular system, such as increased heart rate or fluid retention, which can limit their effectiveness as monotherapy.

Direct vasodilators are often used in combination with sympatholytic agents (which reduce sympathetic nervous system activity) and diuretics to counteract these compensatory responses and enhance their antihypertensive effects. This combination therapy approach is, particularly, useful in cases of resistant hypertension, where blood pressure remains elevated despite treatment with other antihypertensive medications.

There are several direct-acting vasodilators that are used in clinical practice, each with varying degrees of potency and effects on different types of blood vessels. These medications can have dilatory effects on large arteries, smaller arteries, arterioles, and capacitance vessels, contributing to their overall antihypertensive effects.

■ HYDRALAZINE

Hydralazine is a directly acting arteriolar vasodilator that has shown significant benefits in the treatment of certain cardiovascular conditions, particularly in combination with isosorbide dinitrate for congestive heart failure. It is known for its selective vasodilatory effects on arterioles, leading to reduced peripheral vascular resistance and improved blood flow.

The mechanisms underlying hydralazine's vasodilatory action are not fully understood, but it is believed to involve endothelium-dependent processes, including the generation of nitric oxide (NO) and stimulation of cyclic guanosine monophosphate (cGMP) pathways. This relaxation of vascular smooth muscle leads to the dilation of arterioles, resulting in decreased blood pressure. However, the vasodilatory effect of hydralazine can also trigger compensatory responses in the body, such as increased sympathetic nervous system activity and fluid retention, which may limit its use as monotherapy.

Hydralazine is absorbed orally and undergoes acetylation in the bowel and liver. The rate of acetylation is genetically determined, with slow acetylation having a higher bioavailability. The drug is metabolized to inactive compounds and has a relatively short half-life, but its effects can last up to 12 hours.

In clinical practice, hydralazine is used as an antihypertensive agent, often in combination with other drugs such as diuretics and β-blockers. Its use is, particularly, indicated when other agents cannot be tolerated or are ineffective, making it a valuable option for patients with difficult-to-treat hypertension. However, its adverse-effect profile, including potential side effects, such as headache, flushing, hypotension, palpitations, tachycardia, and dizziness, should be carefully considered.

Hydralazine's association with drug-induced lupus syndrome and other immune-related reactions underscores the importance of monitoring patients for potential adverse effects, especially in certain populations. It is also worth noting that hydralazine administration has been linked to pyridoxine-responsive polyneuropathy.

In conclusion, hydralazine is a direct vasodilator that can be beneficial in the treatment of hypertension, particularly in combination with other antihypertensive agents. Its selective arteriolar dilation effects, along with its role in treating congestive heart failure, make it a valuable option for specific patient populations. However, its use should be carefully monitored and managed due to its potential adverse effects and interactions.

ADENOSINE TRIPHOSPHATE-SENSITIVE POTASSIUM CHANNEL OPENERS: MINOXIDIL

Minoxidil, an adenosine triphosphate (ATP)-sensitive potassium (K_{ATP}) channel opener, is considered a second-line or adjunct therapy for hypertension, especially in cases where other antihypertensive medications have been ineffective. Its potent vasodilatory effects can be highly effective in lowering blood pressure, but its side-effect profile necessitates careful management.

The dosage of minoxidil should be titrated gradually, and patients should be closely monitored for adverse effects, particularly fluid retention, cardiovascular effects, and hypertrichosis.

Excessive hair growth, or hypertrichosis, is a well-known side effect of minoxidil and can be distressing, particularly for women. This effect is attributed to the activation of potassium channels and subsequent stimulation of hair follicles. While not life threatening, hypertrichosis can significantly impact a patient's quality of life and may require discontinuation of the medication in some cases.

Hypertrichosis (excessive hair growth) is a common side effect of minoxidil and often occurs on the face, arms, and back. This side effect led to the development of topical minoxidil formulations for the treatment of androgenetic alopecia (male and female pattern baldness).

The use of minoxidil in the treatment of severe or refractory hypertension requires careful patient selection and monitoring due to its potential for significant adverse effects. Coadministration with a diuretic helps mitigate fluid retention, and the addition of a sympatholytic agent helps counteract reflex cardiovascular responses. Renin–angiotensin system (RAS) inhibitors are often included to prevent cardiac remodeling.

In conclusion, minoxidil is a powerful vasodilator used in the treatment of severe or resistant hypertension when other antihypertensive agents have been insufficient. Its mechanism of action involves opening

ATP-modulated K⁺ channels, leading to arteriolar smooth muscle relaxation and subsequent blood pressure reduction. While effective, its use requires careful monitoring and often necessitates a combination therapy approach to manage its potential adverse effects, making it a valuable option in specific cases of hypertension management.

It is important to note that while minoxidil can be effective in lowering blood pressure, its use can be associated with a range of side effects, some of which can be serious. Pericardial effusion is indeed a potential complication of minoxidil therapy. It is important for healthcare providers to monitor patients closely for signs and symptoms of pericardial effusion, such as chest pain or discomfort, shortness of breath, and fluid retention. While mild and asymptomatic effusions may not necessarily require discontinuation of minoxidil, careful observation, and appropriate management are essential.

The cardiac effects of minoxidil, including alterations in T-wave morphology on electrocardiogram and increased myocardial oxygen consumption, highlight the need for cautious use in patients with underlying cardiac conditions. The potential for exacerbation of cardiovascular symptoms underscores the importance of proper patient selection and monitoring.

The rare side effects, such as rashes, Stevens–Johnson syndrome, glucose intolerance, formation of antinuclear antibodies, and thrombocytopenia, further emphasize the need for careful vigilance when prescribing minoxidil. Healthcare providers should be attentive to any signs of these adverse effects and take appropriate actions if they occur.

In summary, while minoxidil can be effective in lowering blood pressure, its use requires close monitoring for a range of potential adverse effects. The decision to use minoxidil should be carefully considered based on the patient's overall health status, underlying conditions, and risk factors, and potential side effects should be thoroughly discussed with the patient before initiating treatment.

■ DIAZOXIDE

Diazoxide is indeed a potent vasodilator that acts by opening potassium channels, leading to arteriolar relaxation and subsequent reduction in blood pressure. Its rapid onset of action and relatively long duration of effect make it suitable for use in hypertensive emergencies when an immediate reduction in blood pressure is necessary.

The intravenous administration of diazoxide in fractional doses allows for titration to achieve the desired blood pressure reduction. However, its binding to plasma proteins can limit its availability for binding to the vessel wall, which is an important consideration when administering the drug.

While diazoxide can be effective in rapidly reducing blood pressure, its use is not without risks. Excessive hypotension, as a result of diazoxide's potent vasodilatory effects, can lead to serious complications such as stroke and myocardial infarction. The reflex sympathetic response triggered by the drop in blood pressure can further exacerbate cardiovascular issues, especially in patients with ischemic heart disease.

Therefore, careful patient selection and monitoring are essential when using diazoxide in hypertensive emergencies. It is interesting to note that diazoxide also has effects on insulin release from the pancreas by opening potassium channels in β-cells; it inhibits insulin secretion and is used to treat hypoglycemia secondary to insulinoma.

However, the use of diazoxide can lead to hyperglycemia, particularly in individuals with renal insufficiency.

In summary, diazoxide is a potent vasodilator that can be effective in rapidly reducing blood pressure in hypertensive emergencies. Its use requires careful titration, monitoring, and consideration of potential side effects, especially in patients with underlying cardiovascular or metabolic conditions.

■ SODIUM NITROPRUSSIDE

Sodium nitroprusside is a well-known nitrovasodilator that has been used for over a century to rapidly reduce blood pressure. Its vasodilatory effects are mediated by the release of NO, which activates the guanylylcyclase–cGMP–protein kinase G pathway, leading to vasodilation. The precise mechanisms of NO release from nitroprusside involve both enzymatic and nonenzymatic pathways.

One of the advantages of sodium nitroprusside is its nonselective vasodilation, which helps maintain regional blood flow, including renal blood flow and glomerular filtration. This is important in preventing ischemic complications in vital organs during hypertensive emergencies. Sodium nitroprusside is typically administered intravenously and is commonly prepared by adding it to a saline/glucose solution. The infusion is titrated based on the patient's response to achieve the desired reduction in blood pressure. Careful monitoring is required during administration due to potential side effects and the risk of toxicity. It is worth noting that sodium nitroprusside is prone to decomposition in alkaline pH and when exposed to light. To prevent decomposition, the infusion bottle is often covered with black paper. One of the significant concerns with the use of sodium nitroprusside is the release of cyanide upon metabolism. Cyanide is converted to thiocyanate in the liver and is excreted slowly.

Prolonged use or higher doses of sodium nitroprusside can lead to the accumulation of excess thiocyanate, potentially causing toxicity.

Adverse effects of sodium nitroprusside include various symptoms such as palpitations, nervousness, vomiting, sweating, abdominal pain, weakness, and disorientation. Additionally, lactic acidosis can occur due to the release of cyanide. In severe cases, sodium nitroprusside toxicity can lead to psychosis.

In summary, sodium nitroprusside is a potent vasodilator used in the management of hypertensive emergencies.

Its ability to rapidly reduce blood pressure makes it valuable in critical situations, but its use requires careful monitoring and attention to potential adverse effects, especially those related to cyanide toxicity and thiocyanate accumulation.

■ FENOLDOPAM

Fenoldopam is a medication used as a peripheral arteriolar dilator in the treatment of hypertensive emergencies and postoperative hypertension. It acts as an agonist of dopamine D1 receptors, leading to the dilation of peripheral arteries and an increase in natriuresis (excretion of sodium in urine).

The commercial formulation of fenoldopam is a racemic mixture, with the (R)-isomer responsible for its pharmacologic activity. The drug undergoes rapid metabolism, primarily through conjugation, resulting in a short half-life of approximately 10 minutes.

Fenoldopam is typically administered through continuous intravenous infusion. The infusion is started at a low dosage, usually around 0.1 µ/kg/min, and then gradually titrated upward every 15–20 minutes. The maximum recommended dose is 1.6 µg/

kg/min or until the desired reduction in blood pressure is achieved. As with many medications, fenoldopam is associated with certain side effects. These may include reflex tachycardia (increased heart rate), headache, and flushing.

Additionally, fenoldopam has the potential to increase intraocular pressure, which can be problematic for individuals with glaucoma. Therefore, caution is advised when using fenoldopam in patients with this condition. Fenoldopam's mechanism of action, rapid metabolism, and short duration of action make it a useful option for rapidly lowering blood pressure in hypertensive emergencies or postoperative settings. However, healthcare providers must carefully monitor patients for potential side effects and tailor the dose to achieve the desired therapeutic effect while minimizing adverse reactions.

■ CONCLUSION

Direct vasodilators play a role in the management of hypertension, especially in combination with other antihypertensive agents. While they are not commonly used as monotherapy due to side effects and compensatory responses, their ability to directly relax blood vessels makes them valuable components of treatment regimens for resistant hypertension and hypertensive emergencies.

■ SUGGESTED READING

1. Campese VM. Minoxidil: A review of its pharmacological properties and therapeutic use. Drugs. 1981;22(4):257-78.
2. Chi L, Uprichard AC, Lucchesi BR. Profibrillatory actions pinacidil in a conscious canine model of sudden coronary death. J Cardiovasc Pharmacol. 1990;15(3):452-64.
3. Ellershaw DC, gurney AM. Mechanisms of hydralazine induced vasodilation in rabbit aorta and pulmonary artery. Br J Pharmacol. 2001;134(3):621-31.
4. Ferdinand KC, Elkayam U, Mancini D, et al. Use of isosorbide dinitrate and hydralazine in African-Americans with heart failure 9 years after the African-American Heart Failure Trial. Am J Cardiol. 2014;114(1):151-9.
5. Leblanc N, Wilde DW, Keef KD, Hume JR. Electrophysiological mechanisms of minoxidil sulphate-induced vasodilatation of rabbit portal vein. Clin Res. 1989;65(4): 1102-111.
6. Linder AE, McCluskey LP, Cole KR III, Lanning KM, Webb RC. Dynamic association of nitric oxide downstream signalling molecules with endothelial caveolin-l in rat aorta. J Pharmacol Exp Ther. 2005;314(1):9-15.
7. Ogilvie RI. Comparative effects of vasodilator drugs on flow distribution and venous return. Can J Physiol Pharmacol. 1985;63(11):1345-55.
8. O'Malley K, Segal JL, Israili ZH, Lin MS, Musgrave GE. Duration of hydralazine action in hypertension. Clin Pharmacol Ther. 1975;18(5 Pt 1):581-6.
9. Perez MI, Musini VM, Wright JM. Pharmacological interventions for hypertensive emergencies: a Cochrane systematic review. J Hum Hypertens. 2008;22(9):596-607.
10. Ramachandra R, Barrett C, Malpas S. Nitric oxide and sympathetic nerve activity in the control of blood pressure. Clin Exp Pharmacol Physiol. 2005;32(5-6):440-6.
11. Rishka H, Franzen P, Thom E, et al. Hydralazine once daily in hypertension. Curr Ther Res. 1984;36:1107-111.
12. Shephard AM, McNay JL, Ludden TM, et al. Plasma concentration and acetylator phenotype determine response to oral hydrazine. Hypertension. 1981;3(5):580-5.
13. Swales JD, Bing RF, Heagerty AM, Pohl JE, Russell GI, Thurston H. Treatment of refractory hypertension. Lancet. 1982;1(8277):894-6.
14. U.S. Food and Drug Administration. New Drug Application (NDA) 008303 Company: NOVARTIS Drug Name(s): Apresoline.

Hypertensive Heart Disease

Keyur R Rathod, Sadanand R Shetty

Hypertensive heart disease (HHD) is a cardiomyopathy. It results from the response of the myocardium to the biomechanical stress (afterload) imposed on the heart by progressively increasing arterial blood pressure and total peripheral resistance.[1] The hallmark of HHD is an increase in left ventricular (LV) mass eventually resulting in altered cardiac function, impaired myocardial perfusion, increased myocardial oxygen demand, and disturbance of heart rhythm. Framingham heart study has established LV hypertrophy as a risk factor for the development of cardiovascular morbidity and mortality independent of other comorbidities. More than half (58%) of the patients presenting with myocardial infarction already have hypertension.[2,3] A number of studies have demonstrated that reduction in LV mass can be achieved by effective antihypertensive therapy which reduces the risk of cardiovascular events in hypertensive patients.

STRUCTURAL AND MOLECULAR BASIS OF HYPERTENSIVE HEART DISEASE

Pathological changes in hypertension are most peculiarly noted in the resistance vessels having luminal diameters of 100–350 μm. Essential hypertension is associated with eutrophic remodeling wherein extracellular matrix changes play an important role. Whereas some secondary forms of hypertension like renovascular hypertension, hypertension associated with acromegaly, and diabetes are associated with hypertrophic remodeling wherein growth factors like angiotensin II, insulin, and somatomedins along with impairment in myogenic reflex play an important role.[4-6]

The presence of these structural alterations in microcirculation has an important role in end organ damage related to hypertension in the form of ischemic heart disease (IHD), heart failure (HF), stroke, and renal failure.[7] Broadly, cardiac effects of elevated arterial blood pressure can either be atherosclerotic or hypertensive. Since elevated blood pressure is one of the major contributors to endothelial injury and worsening of atherosclerosis, the prevalence of hypertension in chronic coronary syndrome is nearly 60%.[8]

The defining feature of HHD is the presence of LV hypertrophy in the absence of any other identifiable cause. The LV cavity dimensions remain unchanged but wall thickness increases, often out of proportion to the afterload imposed by chronically elevated blood pressure. This maladaptive pattern of LV hypertrophy is also called geometric or concentric hypertrophy. It results from true cardiomyocyte growth (increase in thickness of muscle fibers without an increase in the number of muscle fibers)

TABLE 1: Histopathological components of structural remodeling of myocardium in hypertensive heart disease.

At parenchymal level		At microvascular level	
Cardiomyocytes	Hypertrophy, increased apoptosis	Arterioles	Eutrophic and/or hypertrophic remodeling
Fibroblasts	Hyperplasia, phenotypic transformation to myofibroblast	Capillaries	Rarefaction
Other cells	Infiltration by mononuclear and mast cells	Vessel wall	Increased extracellular matrix deposition
Extracellular matrix	Increased types I and III collagen and fibronectin	Endothelium	Patchy disruption

as well as extracellular matrix deposition. Histological features of HHD are summarized in **Table 1**.[9-11]

PATHOPHYSIOLOGY

- *Mechanisms of LV hypertrophic remodeling:* Although hemodynamic mechanisms play a major role in the development of LV hypertrophy in patients with hypertension, this relationship is not linear. Hence, it is important to consider other factors like obesity, salt intake, genetic predisposition, racial, and ethnic factors contributing to HHD. Independent of the contributory mechanism of LV hypertrophy, signal mediators for cardiomyocyte growth are autocrine, paracrine, and endocrine in nature.[12,13]
- *Impact of remodeling on myocardial function:* Pathological changes associated with hypertension include varying degrees of myocardial fibrosis, secondary to myocyte apoptosis, and mononuclear and mast cell infiltration. To begin with these changes, result in diastolic dysfunction (DD) impairing relaxation and elevating filling pressures. Further progression, however, leads to uncoupling of myocardial contraction with force generation heralding systolic dysfunction as well. Myocardial fibrosis also contributes to the development of ventricular arrhythmia, by forming abnormal local re-entry circuits.[14,15]
- *Alterations in coronary blood flow:* Progressive loss in autoregulation of coronary blood flow increases the threshold for perfusion from 60 to 90 mm Hg.[16] Coronary flow reserve as defined by maximal increase in flow over and above resting condition on maximum vasodilatation is impaired in HHD due to reduced sensitivity of coronary vasculature to vasodilation.[16]

CLINICAL MANIFESTATIONS

- *Alterations in cardiac function:* An extension to Framingham heart study reveals that hypertension is the most common etiological factor of congestive HF and preceded development of heart failure in 91% of patient.[17]
- *Diastolic dysfunction:* It can present as an asymptomatic echocardiographic finding to florid HF presentation. About 30–45% of hypertension with congestive HF have DD with normal systolic ejection fraction.[18,19]
- *Systolic dysfunction:* Conventional measures of systolic function like ejection fraction and fractional shortening are

normal or even supranormal in most cases of hypertension. However, impaired mid-wall shortening with preserved ejection fraction has been shown to be associated with worse outcomes in hypertension. Development of LV dilation in hypertension even if asymptomatic heralds poor prognosis as it indicates that the hypertrophied LV is unable to maintain normal wall stress needed to counter the afterload imposed by hypertension. This would mean that any functional benefit derived by dilatation of the LV chamber is now occurring at the cost of increased wall stress and hence at increased myocardial oxygen demand.[20]

- *Myocardial ischemia:* There are at least four causes of myocardial ischemia in hypertension, namely, microvascular disease, diminished coronary flow reserve, atherosclerotic obstructive epicardial coronary artery disease, and increased myocardial oxygen demand. The risk of developing of cardiac ischemic event in a hypertensive individual is twice that of a normotensive patient irrespective of age and sex. This risk increases directly with an increase in blood pressure values. Also, patients with hypertension have an increased incidence of silent myocardial infarction with greater likelihood of complications following acute myocardial infarction.[21,22]
- *Rhythm abnormalities:* Hypertension is an important risk factor for the development of atrial fibrillation, ventricular arrhythmias, and sudden cardiac death (SCD). Even after adjusting for age and any associated comorbidities, hypertension independently predicts the development of atrial fibrillation. Increased left arterial (LA) size because of DD and elevated left ventricular end-diastolic pressure (LVEDP) are harbingers of atrial fibrillation in hypertensive individuals. Atrial fibrillation is the most common arrhythmia in HHD. It is potentially lethal because of its association with embolic phenomenon and pulmonary edema due to loss of atrial kick.[23,24]
- *Heart valve disease:* The presence of mitral annular calcification and aortic valve sclerosis is widely prevalent in hypertensive patients, especially with LV hypertrophy. Aortic regurgitation in hypertension is often due to aortic root dilatation and is seen more commonly in individuals with reduced LV ejection fraction. Mitral regurgitation in hypertension is attributed to mitral annular calcification, DD, and LV dilatation.[25-28]

DIAGNOSIS

Physical Examination

Hypertensive left ventricular hypertrophy (LVH) usually remains indolent for many years before the development of congestive symptoms or unexpected SCD. The pulse remains normal in most of the patients with HHD. Tachycardia indicates impending or overt HF and the finding of an irregular pulse indicates the development of atrial fibrillation. Blood pressure is often elevated (>140 mm Hg systolic, >90 mm Hg diastolic) with elevated mean arterial pressure. Normal blood pressure in HHD indicates treatment response if started on therapy and volume depletion or development of overt HF wherein LV fails to generate enough stroke volume. Lower limb blood pressure should always be recorded at the time of diagnosis of hypertension. Higher blood pressure in the upper limb than in the lower limb indicates coarctation of the aorta. Distended jugular veins with prominent a wave may be seen in hypertension and indicate reduced atrial compliance. Cardiovascular system examination reveals sustained apical impulse best appreciated in lateral decubitus position. The forceful atrial contraction against noncompliant LV produces S4, best appreciated in the left lateral position; S3 is usually not heard in hypertension unless accompanied by overt HF. Usually, an ejection systolic murmur is heard at the base of the heart due to turbulence produced across a sclerotic aortic valve. Pansystolic murmur of mitral regurgitation may be seen in overt HF. Also, an early diastolic murmur of aortic regurgitation may be heard that is produced due to dilatation of aortic root.

Electrocardiogram

A 12-lead electrocardiogram (ECG) shows a variety of abnormalities in hypertension which include the following:

- *Left arterial enlargement:* Broad P waves in limb leads and biphasic P waves in lead V1.
- *Left ventricular hypertrophy criteria:* The Cornell criteria states that R wave in lead aVR plus S wave in V3 if above 2.8 mV in males and if above 2 mV in females indicates LVH. The Sokolov Lyon criteria states S wave in V1 plus R wave in V5 or V6 if above 35 mV indicates LVH.
- *Left ventricular strain:* The presence of repolarization abnormalities like ST segment deviation and T wave inversions are often associated with LVH and may mimic ischemia.[29]

Echocardiography

Various echocardiographic parameters useful to evaluate HHD include the following:[30]

- *Left ventricular mass (LVM):* A LVM in the presence of essential hypertension

TABLE 2: Left ventricular (LV) hypertrophy subtypes.

Relative wall thickness			
	>0.42	Concentric remodeling	Concentric hypertrophy
	<0.42	Normal geometry	Eccentric hypertrophy
		<95 g/m² (males), <115 g/m² (females)	>95 g/m² (males), >115 g/m² (females)
		LV mass index	

is associated with a lower incidence of cardiovascular endpoints independent of treatment modality and effect of blood pressure lowering therapy.[31] Left ventricular mass on echocardiography is calculated by the formula

$$LVM = 0.8\{1.04[(LVIDD + PWTD + IVSD)^3 - LVIDD^3]\} + 0.6 \text{ g}$$

where LVIDD is the LV internal diameter in diastole, PWTD is the posterior wall thickness in diastole, IVSD is the interventricular septal thickness in diastole calculated on M-Mode echocardiography in parasternal long axis view with a marker along mitral valve leaflets as well as on 2D echocardiography in short axis and apical views. Cutoff values for LVH include LVM above 115 g/m² in males and >95 g/m² in females.[32]

- *Relative wall thickness (RWT)* **(Table 2):** Reference cutoff value for increased RWT is above 0.42.[33] Relative wall thickness provides information regarding LV geometry independent of other variables. Patients with normal LV mass can have either normal geometry or concentric remodeling. Patients with increased LV mass can have either concentric or eccentric hypertrophy.[34] It is calculated as follows:

$$RWT = (IVSD + PWTD)/LVIDD.$$

TABLE 3: Grades of DD.

Parameter	Normal	Grade-I DD	Grade-II DD	Grade-III DD
Mitral inflow velocity (E/A ratio)	0.75 < E/A < 1/5	E/A < 0.75	0.75 < E/A < 1/5	E/A > 1.5
Deceleration time	>140 ms	>140 ms	>140 ms	<140 ms
TDI of mitral annulus (E/e' ratio)	E/e' < 10	E/e' < 10	E/e' > 10	E/e' > 10
TR jet velocity				>2.8 m/s
Indexed LA volume				>34 mL/m^2

(A: late; E: early; e': mitral annular velocity; DD: diastolic dysfunction; LA: left arterial; TDI: tissue Doppler imaging; TR: tricuspid regurgitation)

Diastolic Dysfunction

Diastolic dysfunction **(Table 3)** is one of the earliest manifestations of hypertension. Estimation of trans-mitral inflow velocity patterns using the Doppler function is most widely accepted. Tissue Doppler imaging (TDI) is a newer technique that directly allows us to calculate mitral annular velocity (e'). Other variables used to estimate DD include tricuspid regurgitation (TR) jet peak velocity and indexed LA volume.

Systolic Dysfunction

Left ventricular ejection fraction by visual method or biplane method are reliable measures to estimate LV systolic function.

Cardiac Magnetic Resonance Imaging

Cardiac magnetic resonance imaging (MRI) is a gold standard tool to noninvasively measure LV dimensions, wall thickness, and LV strain. It gives an accurate assessment of LVEF and LA volumes. Hypertrophic cardiomyopathy can be accurately distinguished from LV hypertrophy by cardiac MRI. It is superior to echocardiography because it does not require any assumptions regarding the shape and geometry of the ventricle.[30]

■ DIFFERENTIAL DIAGNOSIS

The most important differential diagnosis to consider here is HCM. There is a significant overlap between HHD and HCM. The asymmetric nature of hypertrophy, conventional criteria of end diastolic wall thickness (EDWT) >15 mm and chamber geometry are poor discriminators of HHD with HCM. Elevated LV mass index, absence of mid-wall late gadolinium enhancement (LGE), and absence of systolic anterior motion of mitral leaflet strongly favor HHD.[35]

■ PROGNOSIS

The presence of HHD in form of LV Hypertrophy increases the risk of stroke, congestive HF, coronary artery disease, arrhythmias, and SCD. In the Framingham Heart Study (FHS), during 4 years follow-up, it was seen that for every increase in LV mass by 50 g/m^2, there was 1.49 times increase in relative risk of cardiovascular disease and mortality. A study with 10 years of follow-up of hypertensive patients showed that the incidence of cardiovascular events was 9% in patients with normal LV geometry, 15% in those with concentric remodeling, 25% in those with eccentric hypertrophy, and 30% in those with concentric hypertrophy. Also, studies have described the association of concentric hypertrophy with hypertensive retinopathy, hypertensive nephropathy, and carotid artery disease.[36-40]

MANAGEMENT

Antihypertensive therapy is very effective in reducing LV mass. A substudy by FHS reported that effective use of antihypertensive therapy resulted in a decrease in the prevalence of both high blood pressure and LVH. A study showed that with adequate control of diastolic blood pressure, there was a significant reduction in LV mass. The efficacy of agents in decreasing order to reduce LV mass is as follows angiotensin II receptor antagonists > calcium antagonists> angiotensin-converting enzyme (ACE) inhibitors > diuretics > β-blockers.[41]

PREVENTIVE STRATEGIES

A 24-h monitoring of blood pressure is of paramount importance in detecting hypertensive patients who will develop LVH (those with early morning rise of blood pressure levels, nondippers). Identifying and early initiation of therapy in such patients benefits by preventing the growth of LV mass and its consequences. Nonpharmacologic interventions like salt restriction, weight loss, and restriction on alcohol also have an impact on reducing LV mass. Results of the Treatment of Mild Hypertension Study (TOMHS) also reported that such nonpharmacological measures were highly effective in reducing blood pressure levels and LV mass.[42]

REFERENCES

1. Lip GYH, Hall JE. Comprehensive hypertension. Philadelphia, PA: Mosby Elsevier; 2007. p. 1222.
2. Willich SN, Müller-Nordhorn J, Kulig M, Binting S, Gohlke H, Hahmann H, et al. Cardiac risk factors, medication, and recurrent clinical events after acute coronary disease; a prospective cohort study. Eur Heart J. 2001;22(4):307-13.
3. Yusuf PS, Hawken S, Ôunpuu S, Dans T, Avezum A, Lanas F, et al. Effect of potentially modifiable risk factors associated with myocardial infarction in 52 countries (the INTERHEART study): Case-control study. Lancet. 2004;364(9438):937-52.
4. Rizzoni D, Porteri E, Guefi D, Piccoli A, Castellano M, Pasini G, et al. Cellular hypertrophy in subcutaneous small arteries of patients with renovascular hypertension. Hypertension. 2000;35(4):931-5.
5. Bund SJ, Lee RMKW. Arterial structural changes in hypertension: a consideration of methodology, terminology and functional consequence. J Vasc Res. 2003;40(6):547-57.
6. Baumbach GL, Heistad DD. Remodeling of cerebral arterioles in chronic hypertension. Hypertension. 1989;13(6 Pt 2):968-72.
7. Rizzoni D, Porteri E, Boari GEM, de Ciuceis C, Sleiman I, Muiesan ML, et al. Prognostic significance of small-artery structure in hypertension. Circulation. 2003; 108(18):2230-5.
8. Frohlich ED, Apstein C, Chobanian AV, Devereux RB, Dustan HP, Dzau V, et al. The Heart in Hypertension. N Engl J Med. 2010;327(14):998-1008.
9. Strauer BE, Schwartzkopff B. Left ventricular hypertrophy and coronary microcirculation in hypertensive heart disease. Blood Press Suppl. 1997;2:6-12.
10. Weber KT. Fibrosis and hypertensive heart disease. Curr Opin Cardiol. 2000; 15(4):264-72.
11. González A, Fortuño MA, Querejeta R, Ravassa S, López B, López N, et al. Cardiomyocyte apoptosis in hypertensive cardiomyopathy. Cardiovasc Res. 2003;59(3): 549-62.
12. Chien KR, Hunter JJ, Grace AA. Molecular basis of congestive heart failure. In: Chien KR, editor. The Molecular Basis of Cardiovascular Disease. Philadelphia, PA: WB Saunders; 1999. pp. 211-50.
13. de Simone G, Pasanisi F, Contaldo F. Link of nonhemodynamic factors to hemodynamic determinants of left ventricular hypertrophy. Hypertension. 2001;38(1):13-8.

14. Schwartzkopff B, Motz W, Frenzel H, Vogt M, Knauer S, Strauer BE. Structural and functional alterations of the intramyocardial coronary arterioles in patients with arterial hypertension. Circulation. 1993;88(3): 993-1003.
15. Fortuño MA, González A, Ravassa S, López B, Díez J. Clinical implications of apoptosis in hypertensive heart disease. Am J Physiol Heart Circ Physiol. 2003;284(5): H1495-506.
16. Scheler S, Motz W, Strauer BE. Mechanism of angina pectoris in patients with systemic hypertension and normal epicardial coronary arteries by arteriogram. Am J Cardiol. 1994;73(7):478–82.
17. Levy D, Larson MG, Vasan RS, Kannel WB, Ho KK. The progression from hypertension to congestive heart failure. JAMA. 1996;275(20): 1557-62.
18. Soufer R, Wohlgelernter D, Vita NA, Amuchestegui M, Sostman HD, Berger HJ, et al. Intact systolic left ventricular function in clinical congestive heart failure. Am J Cardiol. 1985;55(8):1032-6.
19. Gandhi SK, Powers JC, Nomeir AM, Fowle K, Kitzman DW, Rankin KM, et al. The pathogenesis of acute pulmonary edema associated with hypertension. N Engl J Med. 2001;344(1):17-22.
20. Gaudron P, Eilles C, Kugler I, Ertl G. Progressive left ventricular dysfunction and remodeling after myocardial infarction. Potential mechanisms and early predictors. Circulation. 1993;87(3):755-63.
21. Kannel WB, Abbott RD. A prognostic comparison of asymptomatic left ventricular hypertrophy and unrecognized myocardial infarction: The Framingham Study. Am Heart J. 1986;111(2):391-7.
22. Pepine CJ, Abrams J, Marks RG, Morris JJ, Scheidt SS, Handberg E. Characteristics of a contemporary population with angina pectoris. TIDES Investigators. Am J Cardiol. 1994;74(3):226-31.
23. Kahan T, Bergfeldt L. Left ventricular hypertrophy in hypertension: its arrhythmogenic potential. Heart. 2005;91(2):250-6.
24. Benjamin EJ, Levy D, Vaziri SM, D'Agostino RB, Belanger AJ, Wolf PA. Independent risk factors for atrial fibrillation in a population-based cohort. The Framingham Heart Study. JAMA. 1994;271(11):840-4.
25. Agno FS, Chinali M, Bella JN, Liu JE, Arnett DK, Kitzman DW, et al. Aortic valve sclerosis is associated with preclinical cardiovascular disease in hypertensive adults: The Hypertension Genetic Epidemiology Network study. J Hypertens. 2005;23(4):867-73.
26. Olsen MH, Wachtell K, Bella JN, Gerdts E, Palmieri V, Nieminen MS, et al. Aortic valve sclerosis relates to cardiovascular events in patients with hypertension (a LIFE substudy). Am J Cardiol. 2005;95(1):132-6.
27. Palmieri V, Bella JN, Arnett DK, Roman MJ, Oberman A, Kitzman DW, et al. Aortic root dilatation at sinuses of valsalva and aortic regurgitation in hypertensive and normotensive subjects: The Hypertension Genetic Epidemiology Network Study. Hypertension. 2001;37(5):1229-35.
28. Bella JN, Wachtell K, Boman K, Palmieri V, Papademetriou V, Gerdts E, et al. Relation of left ventricular geometry and function to aortic root dilatation in patients with systemic hypertension and left ventricular hypertrophy (the LIFE study). Am J Cardiol. 2002;89(3):337-41.
29. Salles G, Cardoso C, Nogueira AR, Bloch K, Muxfeldt E. Importance of the electrocardiographic strain pattern in patients with resistant hypertension. Hypertension. 2006; 48(3):437-42.
30. Janardhanan R, Kramer CM. Imaging in hypertensive heart disease. Expert Rev Cardiovasc Ther. 2011;9(2):199-209.
31. Devereux RB, Wachtell K, Gerdts E, Boman K, Nieminen MS, Papademetriou V, et al. Prognostic significance of left ventricular mass change during treatment of hypertension. JAMA. 2004;292(19):2350-6.
32. Devereux RB, Alonso DR, Lutas EM, Gottlieb GJ, Campo E, Sachs I, et al. Echocardiographic assessment of left ventricular hypertrophy: comparison to necropsy findings. Am J Cardiol. 1986;57(6):450-8.

33. Savage DD, Garrison RJ, Kannel WB, Levy D, Anderson SJ, Stokes J, et al. The spectrum of left ventricular hypertrophy in a general population sample: The Framingham Study. Circulation. 1987;75(1 Pt 2):I26-33.
34. Lang RM, Badano LP, Victor MA, Afilalo J, Armstrong A, Ernande L, et al. Recommendations for cardiac chamber quantification by echocardiography in adults: An update from the American Society of Echocardiography and the European Association of Cardiovascular Imaging. J Am Soc Echocardiogr. 2015;28(1):1-39.e14.
35. Rodrigues JC, Rohan S, Ghosh Dastidar A, Burchell AE, Ratcliffe LE, Hart EC, et al. Hypertensive heart disease versus hypertrophic cardiomyopathy: Multi-parametric CMR predictors beyond end-diastolic wall thickness ≥15 mm. Eur Radiol. 2017;27(3):1125-35.
36. Schillaci G, Verdecchia P, Porcellati C, Cuccurullo O, Cosco C, Perticone F. Continuous relation between left ventricular mass and cardiovascular risk in essential hypertension. Hypertension. 2000;35(2):580-6.
37. Levy D, Anderson KM, Savage DD, Kannel WB, Christiansen JC, Castelli WP. Echocardiographically detected left ventricular hypertrophy: prevalence and risk factors. The Framingham Heart Study. Ann Intern Med. 1988;108(1):7-13.
38. Koren MJ, Devereux RB, Casale PN, Savage DD, Laragh JH. Relation of left ventricular mass and geometry to morbidity and mortality in uncomplicated essential hypertension. Ann Intern Med. 1991;114(5):345-52.
39. Shigematsu Y, Hamada M, Mukai M, Matsuoka H, Sumimoto T, Hiwada K. Clinical evidence for an association between left ventricular geometric adaptation and extracardiac target organ damage in essential hypertension. J Hypertens. 1995;13(1):155-60.
40. Roman MJ, Pickering TG, Schwartz JE, Pini R, Devereux RB. Relation of arterial structure and function to left ventricular geometric patterns in hypertensive adults. J Am Coll Cardiol. 1996;28(3):751-6.
41. Klingbeil AU, Schneider M, Martus P, Messerli FH, Schmieder RE. A meta-analysis of the effects of treatment on left ventricular mass in essential hypertension. Am J Med. 2003;115(1):41-6.
42. Liebson PR, Grandits GA, Dianzumba S, Prineas RJ, Grimm RH Jr, Neaton JD, et al. Comparison of five antihypertensive monotherapies and placebo for change in left ventricular mass in patients receiving nutritional-hygienic therapy in the Treatment of Mild Hypertension Study (TOMHS). Circulation. 1995;91(3):698-706.

CHAPTER 39

Emerging Antihypertensive Drugs

Anant Ramkishanrao Munde, Sadanand R Shetty

INTRODUCTION

The global burden of hypertension is estimated at approximately 1.4 billion individuals, and by 2025 the current rate will exceed 1.6 billion.[1] Cardiovascular (CV) risk attributable to elevated blood pressure (BP) dates back to 1948 and the origin of the Framingham Heart Study.[2-5] The continuous relationship between BP level and risk of events in the brain, heart, and kidney is well documented.[2-6] Overall, each 20 mm Hg increase in systolic blood pressure (SBP) doubled the risk for CV death.[7]

Since 1988–1994, there has been an increase in the prevalence of hypertension among most gender-ethnic groups in the United States, with non-Hispanic black women having the highest prevalence (42.9%) in 2007–2012. Overall, during this time period, 82.7% were aware of their condition and 76.5% were currently being treated, but only 54.1% were under control. The global prevalence of true resistant hypertension (RHTN) is approximately 10%.

About 33% of urban and 25% of rural Indians are hypertensive. Of these, 25% of rural and 42% of urban Indians are aware of their hypertensive status. Only 25% of rural and 38% of urban Indians are being treated for hypertension. One-tenth of rural and one-fifth of urban Indian hypertensive population have their BP under control.[8]

Currently, there are more than 125 different medications, almost all of which are generically available, from eight different antihypertensive drug classes to help lower BP. Moreover, there are more than 15 fixed-dose single-pill combination agents. In spite of this, BP control remains suboptimal in many parts of the world.[2,4,9-11]

Evidently, there is a need for better BP control and a need for the development of new drugs with different mechanisms of action from the existing drugs.[12]

Recently, the Food and Drug Administration (FDA) approved drugs with different indications.

DUAL ANGIOTENSIN RECEPTOR–NEPRILYSIN INHIBITOR (SACUBITRIL/VALSARTAN)

In the 1990s, the concept of vasopeptidase inhibitor of neutral endopeptidase (NEP) neprilysin, in combination with an inhibitor of renin–angiotensin system (RAS), was conceived and a single dual-drug omapatrilat, with this dual action, was developed and tested for the treatment of hypertension.[13] However, omapatrilat, although more effective in lowering the BP than other RAS inhibitors, was not commercially approved by the FDA for the treatment of hypertension due to the increased incidence of angioedema in the treated hypertensive patients.[14] The high incidence of angioedema with this drug was attributed to the double enzymatic inhibition of bradykinin degradation by omapatrilat through its dual inhibition of angiotensin-converting enzyme (ACE) and neprilysin, which degrade bradykinin.[15] Since enalapril directly blocks the enzymatic degradation of bradykinin, a new combination of neprilysin inhibitor (LCZ696) with a RAS inhibitor valsartan, which has no direct inhibitory effects on bradykinin degradation, the LCZ696: sacubitril/valsartan, was developed and approved by the FDA in August 2015 and by the European Medicines Agency (EMA) in November 2015 for the treatment of patients with heart failure (HF) and reduced ejection fraction (HFrEF).

Mechanism of Action of Sacubitril/Valsartan

Sacubitril/valsartan is a single drug with dual action. It exerts its beneficial CV and BP lowering effects through its dual inhibition of RAS with valsartan and neprilysin with sacubitril. Neprilysin is an important catabolizing agent of the natriuretic peptides (NPs), which possess significant diuretic, natriuretic, and vasodilating effects **(Fig. 1)**.[16-18]

The NPs are endogenous hormones released from the heart in response to wall stretching from pressure and volume

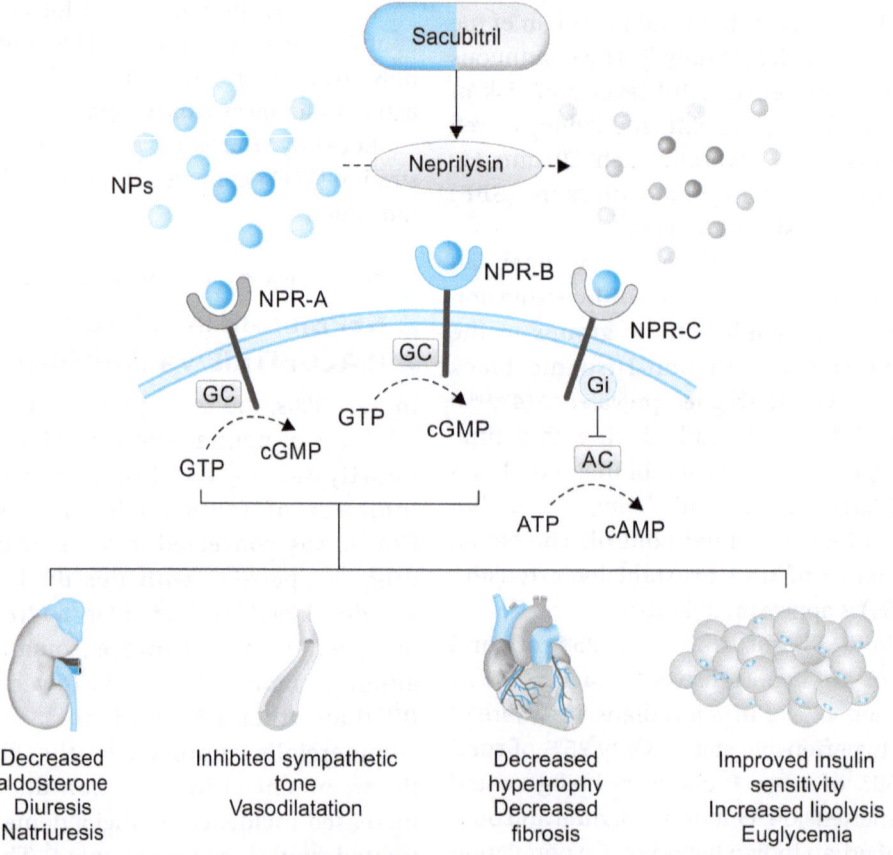

Fig. 1: Overview of actions of sacubitril. (AC: adenylyl cyclase; ATP: adenosine triphosphate; cAMP: cyclic adenosine monophosphate; cGMP: cyclic guanosine monophosphate; GC: guanylyl cyclase; Gi: inhibitory G protein; GTP: guanosine-5′-triphosphate; NPR: natriuretic peptide receptor; NPs: natriuretic peptides)

overload and exert their beneficial CV and antihypertensive effects through plasma volume contraction and peripheral vasodilation. Since the original discovery of the atrial natriuretic factor by de Bold et al.,[18] three NPs have been discovered, the atrial natriuretic peptide (ANP), the beta natriuretic peptide (BNP), and the central natriuretic peptide (CNP). Both ANP and BNP are circulatory peptides and help patients with HF and hypertension through their natriuretic, diuretic, and vasodilatory effects mediated by the generation of cyclic guanosine monophosphate (cGMP).[16-18] The CNP is not a circulatory peptide and is mainly localized in the central nervous system and not involved in CV hemodynamics.[19,20] Unfortunately, the action of sacubitril/valsartan is associated with some desirable and some undesirable adverse effects.[21] Neprilysin is known to catabolize several peptide hormones, such as adrenomedullin, angiotensin II (Ang II), bradykinin, endothelin (ET), glucagon-like peptide-1 (GLP-1), NPs, neurotensin, oxytocin, substance P, and most importantly, and amyloid β (Aβ) peptide. Therefore, the net effect of sacubitril/valsartan on its CV and BP effects will be a balance between the actions of valsartan on RAS and sacubitril on NEP.

Adverse Effects

The prevention of degradation of substance P and bradykinin by the inhibition of NEP with sacubitril has resulted in a lower incidence of cough and lesser incidence of angioedema of 0.45% by sacubitril/valsartan in patients with HF compared to the combination of NEP with enalapril where the incidence of cough was higher as well as the incidence of angioedema 2.17% in patients with hypertension, because bradykinin is degraded by both neprilysin and the ACE.[14,21] The most worrisome adverse effect of sacubitril blockade of NEP is the prevention of degradation of Aβ peptide and the possible increase in the incidence of Alzheimer's disease (AD) after its prolonged use for the treatment of hypertension,[22-25] since NEP has been touted as a possible therapeutic agent for AD.[23] In addition, hypertension has been blamed as a promoter of AD through its disruption of the structure and function of cerebral blood vessels leading to dementia and possibly to AD.[26] How these adverse neurologic effects of sacubitril/valsartan will play out long term is not clear at present.

Safety and Efficacy of Sacubitril/Valsartan as an Antihypertensive Agent

The efficacy of sacubitril/valsartan as an antihypertensive agent has been studied mostly in comparison with a single angiotensin II receptor type-1 blocker (ARB) **(Tables 1 and 2)**. Studies have demonstrated consistent BP reductions by sacubitril/valsartan that is superior to its competitors. The role of sacubitril/valsartan as add-on therapy in uncontrolled hypertension has also been validated in selected studies. However, data comparing the effects of sacubitril/valsartan to other drug classes (namely beta blockers, thiazide diuretics, and calcium channel blockers) are lacking. Patients with certain comorbidities, such as diabetics, chronic kidney disease, and the obese, are also poorly represented in the present literature.

SODIUM–GLUCOSE COTRANSPORTER 2 INHIBITORS

This new class of drugs consists of four members—canagliflozin, dapagliflozin, empagliflozin, and ertugliflozin—which were approved by the FDA and EMA for the treatment of type 2 diabetes mellitus

(T2DM). These drugs are safe and effective in lowering plasma glucose and in addition have significant beneficial effects in decreasing BP and reducing the incidence of CVD and HF.[37-46]

MECHANISM OF ACTION OF SGLT2 INHIBITORS

The plasma glucose is tightly controlled through an elaborate control system that involves intestinal absorption, glucose production, renal reabsorption, and utilization and excretion by a number of tissues in the body. The kidneys play an important role in glucose homeostasis, through glomerular filtration, proximal tubule reabsorption, and endogenous production of glucose, especially in times of low plasma glucose levels.[47,48] Under normal circumstances, the kidneys filter 160–180 g of glucose/day, which is almost totally reabsorbed by the kidney through an elaborate system of sodium–glucose cotransporters located in the proximal convoluted tubules.[47,48] Glucose reabsorption by the kidneys is facilitated through the sodium–glucose cotransporters 1 and 2 (SGLT1 and SGLT2) by the proximal tubule,

TABLE 1: Studies on sacubitril/valsartan in hypertension in Asia.

Author/study	Conditions	Age (years)	Ethnicity	Number of patients
Kario et al.[27] Multicenter, randomized, double-blind	• Office SBP ≥140 and <180 mm Hg • Office DBP ≥95 and <110 mm Hg	>18	Asian	389
Ito et al.[28] Multicenter, open label	• msSBP ≥140 and <180 mm Hg • eGFR ≥15 and <60 mL/min/1.73 m²	>20	Asian	32
Supasyndh et al.[29] Multicenter, randomized, double-blind	• Office SBP ≥150 and <180 mm Hg • Difference between msSBP at randomization and previous visit ≤15 mm Hg	>65	Asian	688
Supasyndh et al.[30] Multicenter, open-label	• Office SBP ≥140 and <180 mm Hg, and • Office DBP ≥95 and <110 mm Hg	>18	Asian	341
Wang et al.[31] Multicenter, randomized, double-blind	• Treatment naïve, msSBP ≥150 and <180 mm Hg • Previously treated, msSBP ≥145 and <180 mm Hg	>18	Asian	266
Wang et al.[20] Multicenter, randomized, double-blind	• Treatment naïve, SBP ≥140 and <180 mm Hg • Previously treated, SBP ≥120 and ≤160 mm Hg, and <180 mm Hg after washout	>18	Asian	72
Huo et al.[32] Multicenter, randomized, double-blind	• Treatment naïve, msSBP ≥150 and <180 mm Hg • Previously treated, msSBP ≥140 and <180 mm Hg, and ≥150 and <180 mm Hg after washout	>18	Asian	1,438

Contd...

Contd...

Intervention	Length of follow-up	Results
Sacubitril/valsartan 100 mg QD versus sacubitril/valsartan 200 mg QD versus 400 mg QD versus placebo	8 weeks	Sacubitril/valsartan was superior to placebo in reduction of clinic DBP, SBP, and pulse pressures across all doses
Initiate with sacubitril/valsartan 100 mg QD, followed by a stepwise optional dose titration to 200 and 400 mg	8 weeks	Geometric mean reduction in UACR was 15.1%; mean reduction in msSBP and msDBP was 20.5 ± 11.3 and 8.3 ± 6.3 mm Hg
Sacubitril/valsartan versus olmesartan, starting with 100 mg or 10 mg QD; doses were increased to sacubitril/valsartan 200 mg or olmesartan 20 mg at week 4 and then to 400 mg or 40 mg at week 10 if BP >140/90 mm Hg	14 weeks	Sacubitril/valsartan resulted in a greater reduction of msSBP than olmesartan only (−22.71 vs. −16.11 mm Hg, respectively; $p <0.001$)
Start with sacubitril/valsartan 200 mg QD, increased to 400 mg if msSBP ≥140 mm Hg or msDBP ≥90 mm Hg after 4 weeks; after 4 weeks, amlodipine 5–10 mg and hydrochlorothiazide 6.25–25 mg were added at any visit if msSBP >140 mm Hg or msDBP >90 mm Hg	12 months	Sacubitril/valsartan-based regimen significantly reduced msSBP and msDBP from baseline (−24.7 and −16.2 mm Hg), with 75.3, 90.6, and 87.6% response rates in overall
Sacubitril/valsartan 200 mg QD + amlodipine 5 mg QD versus amlodipine 5 mg QD	8 weeks	Sacubitril/valsartan with amlodipine led to greater reductions in 24-h SBP compared with amlodipine monotherapy from baseline (−13.9 vs. −0.8 mm Hg, $p < 0.001$)
Sacubitril/valsartan 400 mg or valsartan 320 mg QD for 4 weeks, followed by a washout period of 1–2 weeks, then crossed over and treated for 4 weeks	4 weeks in each treatment period	Sacubitril/valsartan was associated with a significant increase in natriuresis (adjusted treatment difference: 24.5 mmol/6 h, 50.3 mmol/24 h, both $p <0.001$) and diuresis (adjusted treatment difference: 291.2 mL/6 h, $p <0.001$; 356.4 mL/24 h, $p = 0.002$) on day 1, with greater reductions in office
Sacubitril/valsartan 200 mg QD versus sacubitril/valsartan 400 mg QD versus olmesartan 20 mg QD	8 weeks	Sacubitril/valsartan provided larger decreases in msSBP compared to olmesartan at week 8 (between-treatment difference: −2.33 mm Hg [95% CI: From −4.00 to −0.66 mm Hg], $p <0.05$ for noninferiority and superiority for 200 mg; −3.52 [from −5.19 to −1.84 mm Hg], $p <0.001$ for superiority for 400 mg)

(CI: confidence interval; DBP: diastolic blood pressure; msDBP: mean sitting diastolic blood pressure; msSBP: mean sitting systolic blood pressure; QD: once a day; SBP: systolic blood pressure; UACR: urine albumin-creatinine ratio)

TABLE 2: Global studies on sacubitril/valsartan in hypertension.

Author/study design	Conditions	Age (years)	Ethnicity	No of patients
Ruilope et al.[33] Multicenter, randomized, double-blind	• Treatment naïve, msDBP 95–109 mm Hg • Previously treated, msDBP 90–109 mm Hg after washout	18–75	Multiethnic; 87% white	1328
Izzo et al.[34] Multicenter, randomized, double-blind	• Office SBP ≥150 and <180 mm Hg • Office DBP ≥70 mm Hg	>18	Multiethnic; 68.4% white	907
Williams et al.[35] Multicenter, randomized, double-blind	• Treatment naïve, msSBP ≥150 and <180 mm Hg • Previously treated, msSBP ≥140 and <180 mm Hg, and ≥150 and <180 mm Hg after washout	>60	Multiethnic; 64.3% white	432
Cheung et al.[36] Multicenter, randomized, double-blind	• Treatment naïve, msSBP ≥150 and <180 mm Hg • Previously treated, msSBP ≥145 and <180 mm Hg after washout	>18	Multiethnic; 57.6% white	376

Interaction	Length of follow-up	Results
Sacubitril/valsartan 100 mg versus sacubitril/valsartan 200 mg versus sacubitril/valsartan 400 mg versus 80 mg valsartan versus 160 mg valsartan versus 320 mg valsartan versus 200 mg sacubitril versus placebo	13 weeks (8 weeks of treatment)	Sacubitril/valsartan significantly decreased msDBP compared to valsartan only (mean reduction: −2.17 mm Hg, 95% CI −3.28 to −1.06; $p < 0.0001$); 200 mg of sacubitril/valsartan was superior also to 160 mg valsartan (msDBP reduction −2.97 mm Hg, 95% CI −4.88 to −1.07, $p = 0.0023$), as was 400 mg sacubitril/valsartan to 320 mg valsartan (msDBP reduction −2.70 mm Hg, 95% CI −4.61 to −0.80, $p = 0.0055$).
Sacubitril/valsartan 400 mg QD versus free valsartan 320 mg QD with placebo or increasing doses of free sacubitril (50, 100, 200, or 400 mg QD)	8 weeks	Sacubitril/valsartan 400 mg resulted in greater reductions in sitting office SBP and 24-h ambulatory SBP than with valsartan 320 mg (−5.7 and −3.4 mm Hg, respectively, $p < 0.05$ each)
Sacubitril/valsartan 200 mg versus olmesartan 20 mg for 4 weeks, then doubled doses. If msSBP >140 mm Hg or msDBP >90 mm Hg after 12 weeks, amlodipine (2.5–5 mg) followed by hydrochlorothiazide (6.25–25 mg) were added every 4 weeks up to week 24	52 weeks	Sacubitril/valsartan resulted in greater reductions of central aortic systolic pressure than olmesartan at week 12 by a difference of −3.7 mm Hg ($p = 0.010$). At week 52, there were no differences between the BP parameters of the two groups; however, more patients required add-on antihypertensive therapy with olmesartan (47%) versus sacubitril/valsartan (32%; $p < 0.002$).
Addition of sacubitril/valsartan 200 mg QD to uncontrolled hypertension under olmesartan 20 mg QD	8 weeks	Addition of sacubitril/valsartan led to superior reductions in 24-h mean ambulatory systolic BP versus olmesartan alone (−4.3 mm Hg vs. −1.1 mm Hg, $p < 0.001$); sacubitril/valsartan was also superior for reductions in 24-h mean ambulatory DBP, and pulse pressures across all doses

(CI: confidence interval; DBP: diastolic blood pressure; msDBP: mean sitting diastolic blood pressure; msSBP: mean sitting systolic blood pressure; SBP: systolic blood pressure) with the SGLT2 having a high capacity and low affinity, while SGLT1 has a low capacity but a high affinity for glucose transport.[49-51] Their hypoglycemic effects are due to an increase in renal glucose excretion, and in volume contraction, which, in addition, leads to loss of calories and weight. These latter actions of SGLT2 inhibitors result in decrease of BP and CV adverse events in diabetic patients with hypertension and CVD.

Antihypertensive Effects of SGLT 2 Inhibitors

Several studies **(Table 3)** have shown BP-lowering effects of SGLT 2 inhibitors in patients with T2DM and hypertension.[37-42] The data from these studies suggests that there was modest reduction in SBP and DBP with SGLT2 inhibitors in diabetic patients whose mean BP was mildly elevated. There could be more antihypertensive effects in patients with stage 2 or resistant hypertension. More studies in patients with stage 2 or RHTN are required to show its optimal benefits.

Adverse Effects

Generally, SGLT2 inhibitors are well tolerated, but several adverse effects have been noted with their use. These are mainly due to increased diuresis and natriuresis, which could lead to hypovolemia and hypotension. Hypoglycemia due to glycosuria could

TABLE 3: Studies on antihypertensive effects of SGLT2i.

Author	Patients	Age (years)	Follow-up (weeks)
Weir et al.[37]	2,313	56	26
		56	26
Townsend et al.[38]	171	57	6
			6
Kinguchi et al.[39]	85	65	24
Tikkanen et al.[40]	60	60	12
	60	60	12
Baker et al.[41]	12,960	55	4–52
Liu et al.[42]	519	57	26
	510	58	26

SGLT2	Dose	SBP (mm Hg)	DBP (mm Hg)	ΔSBP (mm Hg)	ΔDBP (mm Hg)
Canagliflozin	100	129	78	−4.3	−2.5
Canagliflozin	300	129	78	−5.0	−2.4
Canagliflozin	100	140	79	−4.5	−3.8
Canagliflozin	300	140	79	−6.2	−3.2
Dapagliflozin	10	142	79	−4.4	−2.3
Empagliflozin	10	132	75	−3.4	−1.0
Empa	25	132	75	−4.2	−1.4
SGLT2s	Diff	130	78	−4.0	−1.6
Ertugliflozin	5	131	78	−4.6	−1.9
Ertugliflozin	15	131	78	−4.6	−1.7

predispose to diabetic ketoacidosis (DKA), hyperuricemia, and genital infections, especially in women. Another possible adverse effect of the SGLT 2 inhibitors is their interference with bone mineral metabolism, which might affect bone density and predispose to bone fractures.[52] Bone fractures have been reported only with canagliflozin, which has been shown to cause an increase in the serum collagen type 1 beta-carboxy telopeptide, a bone resorption marker, as well as in serum osteocalcin, a bone formation marker.[53] However, three recent meta-analyses have not confirmed the increased incidence of bone fractures with the SGLT 2 inhibitors compared to placebo.[54-56]

MINERALOCORTICOID RECEPTOR ANTAGONISTS

Spironolactone

In 2003, Nishizaka et al.[57] highlighted the importance of adding a low dose of spironolactone to the therapeutic scheme of patients with RHTN, with the aim of obtaining an additional reduction in BP in both black and Caucasian populations, regardless of aldosterone–renin ratio (ARR). Sartori et al.[58] conducted the first prospective study involving difficult-to-control hypertensive patients with high ARR and showed the importance of this ratio in the pathophysiology of RHTN, even in the absence of clinical manifestations, thus reinforcing the inclusion of aldosterone antagonists in the therapy of these patients. Lane et al.[59] evaluated resistant hypertensive patients, adding spironolactone (25–50 mg/day) to standard triple therapy. These authors observed an additional antihypertensive effect in this group of subjects, suggesting that the addition of spironolactone may be useful, even in the absence of an elevated ARR in RHTN. Other studies substantiated the importance of the addition of spironolactone in antihypertensive therapy of RHTN patients. However, the high incidence of gynecomastia and breast pain among patients taking this drug was significant.[59,60-63]

Eplerenone

A multicenter, double-blinded, placebo-controlled trial demonstrated that eplerenone was effective in reducing BP in subjects with mild–moderate HTN compared to a placebo. In addition, no clinically relevant safety issues were observed in eplerenone-treated subjects.[64] Selective aldosterone blockade with eplerenone was also useful as an add-on therapy in hypertensive patients who were inadequately controlled on either ACE inhibitors or ARBs alone.[65] Either alone or in combination with enalapril, eplerenone also proved to be effective in regression of target-organ damage, such as left ventricular hypertrophy (LVH) in hypertensive subjects and albuminuria in type-2 diabetic patients, but was found to be even better when combined with an ACE inhibitor.[66,67] Moreover, eplerenone reduces arterial stiffness, the collagen:elastin ratio, and circulating inflammatory mediators.[68] All these findings in HTN favor the use of eplerenone as the fourth drug to treat RHTN. The selective aldosterone antagonist eplerenone has also been explored in RHTN. This drug proved to be effective and well tolerated, with modest changes in serum potassium in this high-risk population. At the end of a 12-week active treatment period added to the complex medication regimen of RHTN subjects, the change from baseline in 24-hour mean BP was −12.2/−6 mm Hg ($p < 0.0001$).[57] Moreover, the addition of eplerenone enabled 39% of patients to achieve 24-hour average ambulatory BP (ABP) levels <135/85 mm Hg and a 63.5% success rate in achieving office systolic BP <140 mm Hg. Despite this, aldosterone and renin activity could not predict BP responses to eplerenone in this study population.[57] In addition, a randomized, open-label, parallel-controlled trial demonstrated that endothelial function assessed by flow-mediated vasodilation improved after 12 weeks of eplerenone, which seems to be a BP-independent effect.[69] Taken together, these findings suggest that eplerenone treatment not only reduces BP levels but also limits end-organ damage.

Aldosterone Antagonists in RHTN: Current Insights and Perspectives

Currently, mineralocorticoid receptor antagonists (MRAs) are not indicated to be used as first-, second-, or even third-line drugs in RHTN. On the contrary, due to the high prevalence of primary aldosteronism (PA) in RHTN, studies have shown relevant antihypertensive benefits of adding an MRA to the existing multidrug regimen.[60,70] Williams et al.[58] performed the first randomized controlled trial (the PATHWAY-2 study) comparing different antihypertensive treatments in a rigorous assessment of subjects with RHTN. In this study, spironolactone (25–50 mg/day) was clearly considered the most effective drug added to the three recommended drugs—an ACE inhibitor/angiotensin II-receptor blocker, plus a calcium-channel blocker, plus a thiazide-like diuretic in the treatment of RHTN. This trial is considered a milestone, since it overcame the limitations of previous observational and interventional studies, mainly because PATHWAY-2 was designed to use active comparators (widely used antihypertensive drugs), instead of just a placebo.[71] Moreover, a recent systematic review and meta-analysis has supported it by comparing MRAs with other fourth-line antihypertensive agents in patients with RHTN. MRAs reduced BP more effectively than the other fourth-line agents in randomized and nonrandomized studies.[72] It is well known that the effect of MRAs on BP reduction includes renal and extrarenal pathways. Treatment with MRAs has been shown to attenuate end-organ damage, mainly because of the prevention of nongenomic effects of aldosterone, which lead to increased arterial stiffness and oxidative stress. For instance, reduced cardiac hypertrophy was seen at 3- and 6-month follow-ups in RHTN subjects (with or without PA) taking spironolactone (added to the ongoing antihypertensive regimen at 25 mg/day and titrated to 50 mg/day at 4 weeks).[73] The BP-lowering effect and BP-independent effect contribute to place MRAs as very attractive drugs to treat the complex and multifactorial condition of RHTN (**Fig. 2**).

The most concerning adverse effect of MRA treatment is hyperkalemia.[74,75] Therefore, periodic monitoring of serum potassium and renal function is mandatory, especially in patients at high risk of developing this disorder (elderly patients with renal impairment or diabetes).[76] Taking concurrent pharmacotherapies associated with hyperkalemia, such as potassium supplements, other potassium-sparing diuretics, and nonsteroidal anti-inflammatory drugs, should be avoided. Furthermore, the concomitant use of an MRA with ACE inhibitors or ARBs requires special attention.[77,78] Because of this, experts have recommended MRAs for subjects with RHTN only with careful monitoring of serum potassium levels. Finally, it has been demonstrated that the combined use of spironolactone with a thiazide diuretic, such as chlorthalidone, at optimal doses not only provides greater efficacy but also

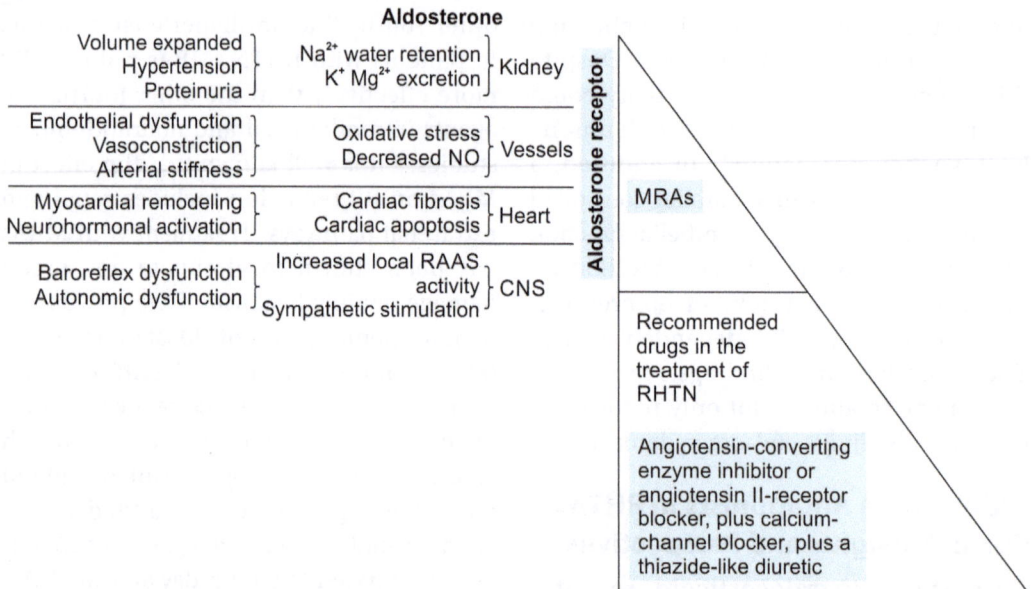

Fig. 2: Fourth-line antihypertensive agents in patients with RHTN. (CNS: central nervous system; MRAs: mineralocorticoid-receptor agonists; RAAS: renin–angiotensin–aldosterone system; RHTN: resistant hypertension)
Notes: MRAs compete for the binding sites of aldosterone, effectively decrease blood pressure, and attenuate end-organ damage, mainly because of preventing nongenomic effects of aldosterone, which lead to arterial stiffness and increased oxidative stress.

reduces the risk of spironolactone-induced hyperkalemia.[79]

Eplerenone in the treatment of RHTN still lacks data, but substantial efficacy and good tolerability have been demonstrated with modest changes in plasma potassium.[57]

The most recently developed MRA, finerenone, has not been studied in RHTN, although its pharmacokinetic profile is promising.[80]

A recent highly selective and potent aldosterone-synthase inhibitor—RO6836191—has the potential of being used in the clinical setting.[81]

Another aldosterone-synthase inhibitor—CYP11B2 (LC1699)—reduces both office and ABPM pressures in PA, but its development was discontinued because cortisol response to adrenocorticotropic hormone stimulation was significantly suppressed in 20% of patients.[82] These findings suggest that new compounds will be identified for future use to treat RHTN.[83]

Finally, thiazolidinedione agonists, which act on PPARγ receptors and are widely used in the treatment of type 2 diabetes, in addition to their known antiproliferative effects, can also suppress aldosterone production.[84] Therefore, they may potentially be useful in combination with conventional antihypertensive therapy for patients with RHTN who also have insulin resistance and type 2 diabetes. MRAs as spironolactone should be considered the fourth-line drug in the treatment of RHTN.[72,85-87] With the recent evidence, greater efforts are needed to increase the use of recommended antihypertensive drugs, including such MRAs as spironolactone, among patients with RHTN.

CENTRALLY ACTING AMINOPEPTIDASE A INHIBITORS

There is experimental as well as clinical evidence that the BP is regulated by both a central and a systemic RAS. In the brain the BP is regulated by the central RAS, which generates angiotensin III (Ang III) by the zinc-dependent aminopeptidase A (APA) by cleaving the N-terminal aspartate from angiotensin II (Ang II). Ang III has similar affinities to Ang II for the receptors A1 and A2 and is the active brain peptide for the central regulation of BP.[88,89] Ang III and Ang II are the main hormones for the central and systemic BP regulation and the CV system regulation.

Blocking the central RAS may have several benefits by decreasing the sympathetic tone and vascular resistance, the release of arginine-vasopressin (AVP), and the reduction of blood volume and systemic vascular resistance (SVS).[89-91] Some hypertensive patients have increased activity of the central RAS and low activity of the peripheral RAS, and these patients have been shown to be resistant to treatment with inhibitors of the peripheral RAS.[92]

Therefore, there is a need for the development of new and more effective drugs with both systemic and central action. Such drugs appear to be the inhibitors of central APA-A, and a specific and selective inhibitor of AMA-A (EC33 S-3-amino-4-mercapto butyl sulfonic acid) has been shown to inhibit the human, rat, and mouse AMA-A enzymes.[93]

An orally administered prodrug (EC33, firabastat) has been obtained by disulfide bridge-mediated dimerization of RB150/QGC001.[94] After oral administration, firibastat is cleaved in the brain by brain reductases to generate two active EC33 molecules, which inhibit the APA-A activity and the generation of Ang III.[93] Inhibition of brain APA-A has been shown to reduce the BP in various hypertensive animal models such as the DOCA-salt hypertensive rat, the spontaneously hypertensive rat,[94,95] and the hypertensive humans.[96,97]

In a pilot, phase IIA proof-of-concept crossover study, 34 patients with ambulatory SBP (ASBP) of 135/85 to <170/105 mm Hg, firibastat 250 mg twice daily for 1 week, uptitrated to 500 mg twice daily for additional 4 weeks, reduced the daily ASBP by 3 mm Hg and the office SBP by 5 mm Hg without affecting heart rate renin, angiotensin, aldosterone, or cortisol effect, suggesting a novel mechanism of antihypertensive action.[96]

In another multicenter, open-label, phase-II study,[97] 256 overweight or obese hypertensive patients with mean age of 58.3 years received firibastat 250 mg twice daily for 2 weeks and later 500 mg twice daily if their automated office BP (AOBP) was >140/90 mm Hg. Firibastat lowered the AOBP by 9.5/4.2 mm Hg ($p < 0.0001$) and 85% of patients did not require additional drugs for the treatment of their BP. Greater SBP response to firibastat was seen in obese patients (−10.2 mm Hg; $p < 0.0001$), in blacks (−10.5 mm Hg; $p < 0.0001$), and in patients who were not blacks (−8.9 mm Hg; $p < 0.0001$), and the AOBP response to firibastat was similar regardless of age, sex, or BMI. Additional long-term studies with a comparator antihypertensive drug are needed to establish the place of firibastat in the treatment of hypertension.

Adverse Effects

Firibastat was well tolerated with no changes in serum potassium or renal function. Only minor reversible adverse effects were noted with the most common being headaches (4%) and skin reactions (3%). No cough or angioedema were noted. The skin reactions (rashes) have been attributed to the molecular structure EC33, the active metabolite of firibastat containing a zinc-binding sulfhydryl group known to cause skin rashes.[98]

ENDOTHELIN RECEPTOR ANTAGONISTS

Endothelin was discovered by Hickey et al. in 1985 from bovine aortic endothelial cells as a potent vasoconstrictive substance,[99] and later in 1988, Yanagisawa et al.,[100] identified its structure and function and named it endothelin 1 (ET-1). Since then, two ET peptides have been identified comprising the ET system consisting of ET-1, ET-2, and ET-3, and they exert their vasoconstrictive actions through stimulation of their receptors, ET-A, ET-B, and ET-C.[101] Of the three ETs, ET-1 is the most abundant, located in the vascular system, and is mostly involved in the maintenance of vascular tone,[102] and BP.[103]

For the antagonism of the vasoconstrictive and hypertensive effects of ETs, ET receptor antagonists have been developed, which block the ET receptors, ET-A and ET-B. In this regard, bosentan is the first one developed with the dual receptor (ET-A/ET-B) receptor antagonism and tested for the treatment of patients with essential hypertension.[104] In this study, patients with DBP 95–115 mm Hg treated with bosentan 100–2,000 mg/day showed a DBP reduction of 6 mm Hg compared to placebo, which was similar to treatment with enalapril 20 mg/day.

Later, a more selective ET-A receptor antagonist, darusentan, was developed for the treatment of hypertension, which given in doses of 10, 30, and 100 mg/day reduced the DBP in a dose-response manner, by 3.7, 4.9, and 8.3 mm Hg, placebo subtracted.[105]

In another study of patients with resistant to treatment hypertension, darusentan, given in daily doses of 50, 100, and 300 mg for 14 weeks, reduced the BP by 12.7/10, 18/10, and 18/11 mm Hg, respectively ($p < 0.0001$) for all doses compared reduction with placebo of 9/5 mm Hg.[106]

Also, in another study of 849 patients with resistance to treatment hypertension on ≥3 antihypertensive drugs including a diuretic, darusentan was administered in daily doses of 50, 100, and 300 mg and was compared to guanfacine 1 mg/day, or placebo. After 14 weeks of treatment, darusentan was better than guanfacine in reducing the clinic SBP by 15 ± 14 compared to 12 ± 13 mm Hg with guanfacine ($p < 0.05$), but was not better than the placebo of 14 ± 14 mm Hg.[107] However, bosentan was better than placebo in reducing the 24-hour ASBP by –9 ± 12 mm Hg compared to placebo by –2 ± 12 mm Hg.

Also, the antihypertensive effects of the selective ET receptor antagonists were analyzed in a review and meta-analysis by Yuan et al.[108] in 4,898 hypertensive patients with other conditions, mean age of 59.8 years. In this meta-analysis, several ET selective inhibitors (atrasentan, avosentan, bosentan, darusentan, and tezosentan) were tested in various dosages and observation periods. The analysis of results showed that on average, all reduced the 24-hour ABP by 7.65/5.92 mm Hg compared to placebo but were associated with more side effects than placebo.

Besides essential hypertension, the ET receptor antagonists have also been tested in patients with pulmonary arterial hypertension (PAH) of different etiologies with conflicting results, with macitentan showing the most promising results.[109,110] Also, studies in patients with HFrEF and HFpEF have, been disappointing due to the nonimprovement in symptoms but increased incidence of adverse effects.[111,112]

In addition, phases II and III short-term studies with nonselective and selective endothelin receptor antagonists (ERAs) in patients with hypertension and renal failure with proteinuria have shown some promising results. In this regard, a long-term double-blind, placebo-controlled phase-III study (SONAR) in 4,711 completed patients with T2DM and renal failure (eGFR 25-75 mL/min/1.73 m^2) demonstrated a beneficial effect of atrasentan.[113] After a mean follow-up of 2.2 years, atrasentan 0.75 mg/day compared to placebo reduced the composite primary endpoint (doubling of serum creatinine, end-stage renal disease, chronic dialysis, kidney transplantation, or death from renal failure), hazard ratio (HR) 0.65 [95% confidence ratio (CI) 0.49-0.88, p = 0.0047). Anemia and fluid retention were more frequent in the atrasentan group.

In another dose–response, double-blind, active control phase 2 study, the dual ET (ETA/ETB) inhibitor aprocitentan was studied in 409 completed patients with hypertension.[114] The patients were randomized to aprocitentan 5, 20, 25, and 50 mg/day. Patients were randomized to aprocitentan vs placebo or lisinopril and were followed for 8 weeks. Aprocitentan in doses 10, 25, and 50 mg/day decreased the sitting unattended BP by 7.05/4.93, 9.90/6.99, and 7.58/4.95 mm Hg, respectively, versus placebo ($p \leq 0.014$), and by 4.8/3.81 mm Hg with lisinopril. Similar positive results were obtained with the 24-hour ABP measurements. Adverse effects with aprocitentan included a dose–response decrease in hemoglobin, hematocrit, albumin, and uric acid with an increase in plasma volume, but no change in body weight.

Adverse Events

Treatment with the various ERAs has been associated with several adverse effects as has been reported by a major review and meta-analysis of 4,894 patients.[115] The most common were anemia, relative risk/ratio 2.69 (95% CI 1.78-4.07); palpitation, RR 1.28 (95% CI 0.77-2.14); abdominal pain, RR 1.17 (95% CI 0.55-2.52); constipation, RR 1.36 (95% CI 0.88-2.11); peripheral edema, RR 1.44 (95% CI 1.20-1.74); flushing; RR 1.64 (95% CI 0.97-2.79), abnormal liver function, RR 2.38 (95% CI 1.36-4.18), sinusitis, RR 1.17 (95% CI 0.78-1.75); respiratory tract infection, RR 1.15 (95% CI: 0.78-1.75); dyspnea, RR 1.17 (95% CI 0.94-1.46); and respiratory failure, RR 1.84 (95% CI 0.78-4.34).

SOLUBLE GUANYLATE CYCLASE STIMULATORS

The soluble guanylate cyclase (sGC) is a major receptor of nitric oxide and a significant signaling enzyme in the transduction of the nitric oxide–cyclic guanosine monophosphate (NO-cGMP) signaling pathway, since impaired vascular NO-cGMP signaling is a key pathway in regulating vascular relaxation and is associated with the development of hypertension.[116] Thus, sGC stimulators have a unique mechanism of action by stimulating the NO/sGC/cGMP pathway and causing systemic vasodilation through modulation of the activity of downstream targets, such as protein kinase G1, decrease of intracellular calcium, membrane hyperpolarization, and inhibition of light chain phosphorylation.[116] The cGMP signaling cascade is an important regulator of CV homeostasis by regulating the vascular tone, as well as water and sodium handling and platelet aggregation. Due to its CV regulatory effects, NO through its cGC–cGMP signaling pathway has been at the center of attention.

They also have beneficial metabolic effects and a very good safety profile with mild adverse effects such as headache, dizziness, or orthostatic hypotension but no adverse effects on platelet function.

They have a long duration of action, which makes them suitable for once-a-day administration.

However, despite the tremendous progress regarding the impaired NO/sGC/cGMP signaling in a variety of diseases, drugs that stimulate its function do not appear to be in the current scope of the pharmacological industry for the treatment of hypertension.

Currently, only the Ironwood pharmaceutical's sGC stimulator IW-1973 [praliciguat (PRL)] is being tested in patients and animals with hypertension with promising results.[117-120]

In a phase-I randomized, placebo-controlled study, Hanrahan et al.[117] investigated the antihypertensive and safety effects of PRL in 44 normotensive healthy subjects with a mean age of 39 years. The participants were divided into three groups (G1–G3) of eight subjects each, who received the drug and G4 of 12 subjects who received a placebo; G1 subjects received 15 mg/day of the drug for 14 days and advanced to 30 mg/day for 7 more days; G2 subjects received 20 mg/day for 14 days and then 40 mg/day for additional 7 days; G3 subjects received 30 mg/day for 14 days and 40 mg/day for additional 7 days; And G4 subjects received a placebo for the duration of the study. At the end of the study (day 21), PRL reduced the BP in G1 subjects by 8.21/6.61 mm Hg, in G2 subjects by 6.29/3.98 mm Hg, in G3 subjects by 9.05/6.12 mm Hg, and placebo in G4 subjects by 4.81/1.67 mm Hg. The drug was well tolerated and there were no significant clinical or metabolic adverse effects noted except mild headache. Pharmacokinetically, the drug achieved a T_{max} within 2–4 h and had a $T_{1/2}$ of 123–173 h, achieving a steady state within 14–15 days, which makes it suitable for once-a-day administration.

The other study by Hanrahan et al.[118] was a phase IIA, double-blind, placebo-controlled trial of 26 patients with T2DM and hypertension mean age 62 years. The patients were divided in 3:5:5 ratio into three groups, placebo (G1, $n = 6$), PRL 40 mg/day (G2, $n = 10$) for days 1–14, or PRL 20 mg twice daily for days 1–7 and then 40 mg/day for days 8–14 (G3, $n = 10$). The BP was measured by ABP measurement (ABPM). Participants treated with PRL for 14 days had a least-square (LS) mean 24-hour ABPM SBP reduction, placebo-subtracted of –2 (95% CI –10 to 5) mm Hg, DBP of –4 (95% CI –9 to 1) mm Hg, and MAP of –5 (95% CI –10 to 1) mm Hg. In a post hoc analysis, patients with a baseline MAP >92 mm Hg treated with PRL had a greater LS mean in MAP by 14 mm Hg compared to placebo. In addition, PRL had beneficial metabolic effects on plasma glucose decrease by –0.7 mmol, plasma total cholesterol by –0.6 mmol, and plasma LDL cholesterol by –0.4 mmol and triglycerides by 0.2 mmol compared to placebo. Among the adverse effects of PRL treatment were hypoglycemia in five patients who were also treated with hypoglycemic drugs and gastrointestinal bleeding in one patient.

Frey et al.[119] investigated the acute antihypertensive effects of the experimental sGC stimulator BAY 63-2621 in randomized placebo-controlled study in 58 normal subjects. The subjects received BAY 63-2621 orally in solution, 0.25 mg ($n = 6$), 0.5 mg ($n = 5$), 1 mg ($n = 12$), 2.5 mg ($n = 6$), 5 mg ($n = 10$), or a matching placebo solution ($n = 11$) for 72 hours inside the hospital, and after 1 week later. Administration of the drug resulted in a mild but statistically significant decrease in DBP and MAP of −2.2 and −2.6 mm Hg, respectively, at 1-mg dose ($p = 0.035$); also, the 2.5-mg dose reduced the DBP and MAP by −2.4 and 3.2, respectively ($p = 0.0017$), and 5-mg dose also reduced the DBP and MAP by −3.4 and −3.8, respectively, from control ($p = 0.0025$). The drug was well tolerated with the exception of mild orthostatic hypotension in one subject noted with the 0.5-, 1.0-, and 2.5-mg doses. The drug was rapidly absorbed and reached a peak effect at 0.5–1.5 h and had a long-lasting effect with a half-life of 5–10 h.

The antihypertensive effects of sGC stimulators have also been tested in several animal hypertension models.[120-124]

REFERENCES

1. Egan BM. Hypertension in military veterans is associated with combat exposure and combat injury. J Hypertens. 2020;38(7):1255-6.
2. Lim SS, Vos T, F laxman AD, Danaei G, Shibuya K, Adair-Rohani H, et al. A comparative risk assessment of burden of disease and injury attributable to 67 risk factors and risk factor clusters in 21 regions, 1990–2010: A systematic analysis for the Global Burden of Disease Study 2010. Lancet. 2012;380:2224-60.
3. Franklin SS, Jacobs MJ, Wong ND, L'Italien GJ, Lapuerta P. Predominance of isolated systolic hypertension among middle-aged and elderly US hypertensives: Analysis based on National Health and Nutrition Examination Survey (NHANES) III. Hypertension. 2001;37(3):869-74.
4. Forouzanfar MH, Liu P, Roth GA, Ng M, Biryukov S, Marczak L, et al. Global burden of hypertension and systolic blood pressure of at least 110 to 115 mm Hg, 1990–2015. J Am Med Assoc. 2017;317(2):165-82.
5. Joffres M, Falaschetti E, Gillespie C, Robitaille C, Loustalot F, Poulter N, et al. Hypertension prevalence, awareness, treatment and control in national surveys from England, the USA and Canada, and correlation with stroke and ischaemic heart disease mortality: a cross-sectional study. BMJ Open. 2013;3(8):e003423.
6. Franklin SS, Gustin W, Wong ND, Larson MG, Weber MA, Kannel WB, et al. Hemodynamic patterns of age-related changes in blood pressure. The Framingham Heart Study. Circulation. 1997;96(1):308-15.
7. Lewington S, Clarke R, Qizilbash N, Peto R, Collins R; Prospective Studies Collaboration. Age-specific relevance of usual blood pressure to vascular mortality: a meta-analysis of individual data for one million adults in 61 prospective studies. Lancet. 2002;360(9349):1903-13.
8. Anchala R, Kannuri NK, Pant H, Khan H, Franco OH, Di Angelantonio M, et al. Hypertension in India: a systematic review and meta-analysis of prevalence, awareness, and control of hypertension. J Hypertens. 2014;32(6):1170-7.
9. Chow CK, Teo KK, Rangarajan S, Islam S, Gupta R, Avezum A, et al. Prevalence, awareness, treatment, and control of hypertension in rural and urban communities in high, middle, and low income countries. J Am Med Assoc. 2013;310(9):959-68.
10. Kearney PM, Whelton M, Reynolds K, Muntner P, Whelton PK, He J, et al. Global burden of hypertension: analysis of worldwide data. Lancet. 2005;365(9455):217-23.
11. Campbell NR, Brant R, Johansen H, Walker RL, Wielgosz A, Onysko J, et al. Increases in antihypertensive prescriptions and reductions in cardiovascular events in Canada. Hypertension. 2009;53(2):128-34.
12. Azizi M, Rossignol P, Hulot JS. Emerging drug classes and their potential use in hypertension. Hypertension. 2019;74(5):1075-83.
13. Burnet JC Jr. Vasopeptidase inhibition: a new concept in blood pressure management. J Hypertens Suppl. 1999;17(1):S37-43.
14. Kostis JB, Packer M, Black HR, Schmieder R, Henry D, Levy E. Omapatrilat and enalapril in patients with hypertension: The Omapatrilat Cardiovascular Treatment vs Enalapril (OCTAVE) trial. Am J Hypertens. 2004;17(2):103-11.

15. Nussberger J, Cugno M, Amstutz C, Pellacani A, Agostoni A. Plasma bradykinin in angio-edema. Lancet 1998;351(9117):1693-7.
16. Chen HH, Burnett JC Jr. Clinical applications of the natriuretic peptides in heart failure. Eur Heart J Suppl. 2006;8(Suppl. E):E18-25.
17. Lee CY, Burnett JC Jr. Natriuretic peptides and therapeutic applications. Heart Fail Rev. 2007;12(2):131-42.
18. de Bold AJ, Borenstein HB, Veress AT, Sonnenberg H. A rapid and potent natriuretic response to intravenous injection of atrial myocardial extract in rats. Life Sci 1981;28(1):89-94.
19. Rubatu S, Sciarretta S, Valenti V, Stanzione R Volpe M. Natriuretic peptides: An update on bioactivity, potential therapeutic use, and implications in cardiovascular diseases. Am J Hypertens. 2008;21(7):733-41.
20. Wang TD, Tan RS, Lee HY, Ihm SH, Rhee MY, Tomlinson B, et al. Effects of sacubitril/valsartan (LCZ696) on natriuresis, dieresis, blood pressure, and NT-pro-BNP in salt sensitive hypertension. Hypertension. 2017;69(1):32-41.
21. Campbell DJ. Neprilysin inhibitors and bradykinin. Front Med (Lausanne). 2018;5:257.
22. Chrysant SG, Chrysant GS. Sacubitril/valsartan: a cardiovascular drug with pluripotential actions. Cardiovasc Diagn Ther. 2018;8(4):543-8.
23. Nalvaeva NN, Belyaev ND, Kerridge C, Turner AJ. Amyloid-clearing proteins and their epigenetic regulation as a therapeutic target in Alzheimer's disease. Front Aging Neurosci. 2014;6:236.
24. Webster CI, Burrell M, Olsson LL, Fowler SB, Digby S, Sandercock A, et al. Engineering neprilysin activity and specificity to create a novel therapeutic for Alzheimer's disease. PLoS One. 2014;9(8):e104001.
25. Langenickel TH, Tsubouchi C, Ayalasomayajula S, Pal P, Valentin MA, Hinder M, et al. The effect of LZC696 (sacubitril/valsartan) on amyloid-β concentrations in cerebrospinal fluid in healthy subjects. Br J Clin Pharmacol. 2016;81(5):878-90.
26. Iadecola C, Yaffe K, Biller J, Biller J, Bratzke LC, Faraci FM, et al. Impact of hypertension on cognitive function: A scientific statement from the American Medical Association. Hypertension. 2016;68(6):e67-94.
27. Kario K, Sun N, Chiang FT, Supasyndh O, Baek SH, Inubushi-Molessa A, et al. Efficacy and safety of LCZ696, a first-in-class angiotensin receptor neprilysin inhibitor, in Asian patients with hypertension: A randomized, double-blind, placebo-controlled study. Hypertension. 2014;63(4):698-705.
28. Ito S, Satoh M, Tamaki Y, Gotou H, Charney A, Okino N, et al. Safety and efficacy of LCZ696, a first-in-class angiotensin receptor neprilysin inhibitor, in Japanese patients with hypertension and renal dysfunction. Hypertens Res. 2015;38(4):269-75.
29. Supasyndh O, Wang J, Hafeez K, Zhang Y, Zhang J, Rakugi H. Efficacy and safety of sacubitril/valsartan (LCZ696) compared with olmesartan in elderly asian patients (≥65 years) with systolic hypertension. Am J Hypertens. 2017;30(12):1163-9.
30. Supasyndh O, Sun N, Kario K, Hafeez K, Zhang J. Long-term (52-week) safety and efficacy of Sacubitril/valsartan in Asian patients with hypertension. Hypertens Res. 2017;40:472-6.
31. Wang J-G, Yukisada K, Sibulo A, Hafeez K, Jia Y, Zhang J. Efficacy and safety of sacubitril/valsartan (LCZ696) add-on to amlodipine in Asian patients with systolic hypertension uncontrolled with amlodipine monotherapy. J Hypertens. 2017;35(4):877-85.
32. Huo Y, Li W, Webb R, Zhao L, Wang Q, Guo W. Efficacy and safety of sacubitril/valsartan compared with olmesartan in Asian patients with essential hypertension: a randomized, double-blind, 8-week study. J Clin Hypertens (Greenwich). 2019;21(1):67-76.
33. Ruilope LM, Dukat A, Böhm M, Lacourcière Y, Gong J, Lefkowitz MP. Blood-pressure reduction with LCZ696, a novel dual-acting inhibitor of the angiotensin II receptor and neprilysin: a randomised, double-blind, placebo-controlled, active comparator study. Lancet. 2010;375:1255-66.

34. Izzo JL, Zappe DH, Jia Y, Hafeez K, Zhang J. Efficacy and safety of crystalline valsartan/sacubitril (LCZ696) compared with placebo and combinations of free valsartan and sacubitril in patients with systolic hypertension: the RATIO study. J Cardiovasc Pharmacol. 2017;69(6):374-81.
35. Williams B, Cockcroft JR, Kario K, Zappe DH, Brunel PC, Wang Q, et al. Effects of sacubitril/valsartan versus olmesartan on central hemodynamics in the elderly with systolic hypertension: the PARAMETER study. Hypertension. 2017;69(3):411-20.
36. Cheung DG, Aizenberg D, Gorbunov V, Hafeez K, Chen CW, Zhang J. Efficacy and safety of sacubitril/valsartan in patients with essential hypertension uncontrolled by olmesartan: A randomized, double-blind, 8-week study. J Clin Hypertens. 2018; 20(1):150-8.
37. Weir MR, Januszewicz A, Gilbert RE, Vijapurkar U, Kline I, Fung A, et al. Effect of canagliflozin on blood pressure and adverse events related to osmotic diuresis and reduced intravascular volume in patients with type 2 diabetes mellitus. J Clin Hypertens. 2014;16(12):875-82.
38. Townsend RR, Machin I, Ren J, Trujillo A, Kawaguchi M, Vijapurkar U, et al. Reductions in mean 24-h ambulatory blood pressure after 6-week treatment with canagliflozin in patients with type 2 diabetes mellitus and hypertension. J Clin Hypertens. 2016; 18:43-52.
39. Kinguchi S, Wakui H, Ito Y, Kondo Y, Azushima K, Osada U, et al. Improved home BP profile with dapagliflozin is associated with amelioration of albuminuria in Japanese patients with diabetic nephropathy: The Yokohama add-on inhibitory efficacy of dapagliflozin on albuminuria in Japanese patients with type 2 diabetes study (Y-AIDA study). Cardiovasc Diabetol. 2019;18(1):110.
40. Tikkanen I, Narko K, Zeller C, Green A, Salsali A, Broedl UC, et al. Empagliflozin reduces blood pressure in patients with type 2 diabetes and hypertension. Diabetes Care. 2015;38(3):420-8.
41. Baker WL, Smyth LR, Riche DM, Bourret EM, Chamberlin KW, White WB, et al. Effects of sodium-glucose co-transporter 2 inhibitors on blood pressure: A systematic review and meta-analysis. J Am Soc Hypertens. 2014;8(4):262-75.
42. Liu J, Pong A, Gallo S, Darekar A, Terra SG. Effect of ertugliflozin on blood pressure in patients with type 2 diabetes mellitus: a post hoc pooled analysis of randomized controlled trials. Cardiovasc Diabetol. 2019;18(1): 59.
43. Inzucchi SE, Zinman B, Wanner C, Ferrari R, Fitchett D, Hantel S, et al. SGLT-2 inhibitors and cardiovascular risk: Proposed pathways and review of ongoing outcome trials. Diab Vasc Dis Res. 2015;12(2):90-100.
44. Abdul-Ghani M, Del Prato S, Chilton R, DeFronzo RA. SGLT 2 inhibitors and cardiovascular risk: Lessons learned from the EMPA-REG OUTCOME study. Diabetes Care. 2016;39(5):717-25.
45. Zinman B, Wanner C, Lachin JM, Fitchett D, Bluhmki E, Hantel S, et al. Empagliflozin, cardiovascular outcomes, and mortality in type 2 diabetes. N Engl J Med. 2015; 373(22):2117-28.
46. Neal B, Perkovic V, Mahaffey KM, de Zeeuw D, Fulcher G, Erondu N, et al. Canagliflozin and cardiovascular and renal events in type 2 diabetes. N Engl J Med. 2017;377(7): 644-57.
47. Wiviott SD, Raz I, Bonaca MP, Bonaca MP, Mosenzon O, Kato ET, et al. Dapagliflozin and cardiovascular outcomes in type 2 diabetes. N Engl J Med. 2019;380(4):347-57.
48. Cannon CP, McGuire DK, Pratley R, Dagogo-Jack S, Mancuso J, Huyck S, et al. Design and baseline characteristics of the eValuation of ERTuglifozin efficacy and Safety CardioVascular outcomes trial (VERTIS-CV). Am Heart J. 2018;206:11-23.
49. Zelniker TA, Wiviott SD, Raz I, Im K, Goodrich EL, Bonaca MP, et al. SGLT2 inhibitors for primary and secondary prevention of cardiovascular and renal outcomes in type 2 diabetes: a systematic review and meta-analysis of cardiovascular outcome trials. Lancet. 2019;393(10166):31-9.

50. Gallo LA, Wright EM, Vallon V. Probing SGLT2 as a therapeutic target for diabetes: Basic physiology and consequences. Diab Vasc Dis Res. 2015;12(2):78-89.
51. Gerich JE. Role of the kidney in normal glucose homeostasis and in the hyperglycaemia of diabetes mellitus: therapeutic implications. Diabet Med. 2010;27(2):136-42.
52. Meir C, Schwartz AV, Egger A, Lecka-Czernik B. Effects of diabetes drugs on the skeleton. Bone. 2016;82:93-100.
53. Blevins TC, Farooki A. Bone effects of canagliflozin, a sodium-glucose cotransporter 2 inhibitor, in patients with type 2 diabetes mellitus. Postgrad Med. 2017;129(1):159-68.
54. Tang HL, Li DD, Zhang JJ, Hsu YH, Wang TS, Zhaiet SD, al. Lack of evidence for a harmful effect of sodiumglucose co-transporter 2 (SGLT2) inhibitors on fracture risk among type 2 diabetic patients: A network and cumulative meta-analysis of randomized controlled studies. Diabetes Obes Metab. 2016;18(12):1199-206.
55. Ruanpeng D, Ungprasert P, Sangtian J, Harindhanavudhi T. Sodium–glucose cotransporter 2 (SGLT2) inhibitors and fracture risk in patients with type 2 diabetes mellitus: A meta-analysis. Diabetes Metab Res Rev. 2017;33(6).
56. Azharuddin M, Adil M, Ghosh P, Sharma M. Sodium–glucose cotransporter 2 inhibitors and fracture risk in patients with type 2 diabetes mellitus: a systematic literature review and Bayesian network meta-analysis of randomized controlled trials. Diabetes Res Clin Pract. 2018;146:180-90.
57. Nishizaka MK, Zaman MA, Calhoun DA. Efficacy of low-dose spironolactone in subjects with resistant hypertension. Am J Hypertens. 2003;16(11 Pt 1):925-30.
58. Sartori M, Calo LA, Mascagna V, et al. Aldosterone and refractory hypertension: A prospective cohort study. Am J Hypertens. 2006;19(4):373-80.
59. Lane DA, Shah S, Beevers DG. Low-dose spironolactone in the management of resistant hypertension: A surveillance study. J Hypertens. 2007;25(4):891-4.
60. Gaddam KK, Pratt-Ubunama MN, Calhoun DA. Aldosterone antagonists: effective add-on therapy for the treatment of resistant hypertension. Expert Rev Cardiovasc Ther. 2006;4(3):353-9.
61. Pimenta E, Calhoun DA. Resistant hypertension and aldosteronism. Curr Hypertens Rep. 2007;9(5):353-359.
62. Jansen PM, Danser AH, Imholz BP, van den Meiracker AH. Aldosterone-receptor antagonism in hypertension. J Hypertens. 2009;27(4):680-91.
63. Das G, De P. Aldosterone-renin ratio in patients with resistant hypertension. QJM. 2010;103(11):897-9.
64. Weinberger MH, Roniker B, Krause SL, Weiss RJ. Eplerenone, a selective aldosterone blocker, in mild-to-moderate hypertension. Am J Hypertens. 2002;15(8):709-16.
65. Krum H, Nolly H, Workman D, He W, Roniker B, Krause S, et al. Efficacy of eplerenone added to renin-angiotensin blockade in hypertensive patients. Hypertension. 2002;40(2):117-23.
66. Pitt B, Reichek N, Willenbrock R, Zannad F, Phillips RA, Roniker B, et al. Effects of eplerenone, enalapril, and eplerenone/enalapril in patients with essential hypertension and left ventricular hypertrophy: The 4E-left ventricular hypertrophy study. Circulation. 2003;108(15):1831-38.
67. Epstein M, Williams GH, Weinberger M, Lewin A, Krause S, Mukherjee R, et al. Selective aldosterone blockade with eplerenone reduces albuminuria in patients with type 2 diabetes. Clin J Am Soc Nephrol. 2006;1(5):940-51.
68. Savoia C, Touyz RM, Amiri F, Schiffrin EL. Selective mineralocorticoid receptor blocker eplerenone reduces resistance artery stiffness in hypertensive patients. Hypertension. 2008;51(2):432-9.
69. Eguchi K, Kabutoya T, Hoshide S, Ishikawa S, Kario K. Add-on use of eplerenone is effective for lowering home and ambulatory blood pressure in drug-resistant hypertension. J Clin Hypertens (Greenwich). 2016;18(12):1250-7.

70. Ouzan J, Perault C, Lincoff AM, Carre E, Mertes M. The role of spironolactone in the treatment of patients with refractory hypertension. Am J Hypertens. 2002;15 (4 Pt 1):333-9.
71. Narayan H, Webb DJ. New evidence supporting the use of mineralocorticoid receptor blockers in drug-resistant hypertension. Curr Hypertens Rep. 2016; 18(5):34.
72. Sinnott SJ, Tomlinson LA, Root AA, Mathur R, Mansfield KE, Smeeth L, et al. Comparative effectiveness of fourth-line anti-hypertensive agents in resistant hypertension: A systematic review and meta-analysis. Eur J Prev Cardiol. 2017;24(3):228-38.
73. Gaddam K, Corros C, Pimenta E, Ahmed M, Denney T, Aban I, et al. Rapid reversal of left ventricular hypertrophy and intracardiac volume overload in patients with resistant hypertension and hyperaldosteronism: a prospective clinical study. Hypertension. 2010;55(5):1137-42.
74. Witham MD, Gillespie ND, Struthers AD. Hyperkalemia after the publication of RALES. N Engl J Med. 2004;351(23):2448-50.
75. Juurlink DN, Mamdani MM, Lee DS, Kopp A, Austin PC, Laupacis A, et al. Rates of hyperkalemia after publication of the Randomized Aldactone Evaluation Study. N Engl J Med. 2004;351(6):543-51.
76. McMurray JJ, Adamopoulos S, Anker SD, Auricchio A, Böhm M, Dickstein K, et al. ESC guidelines for the diagnosis and treatment of acute and chronic heart failure 2012. Eur J Heart Fail. 2012;14(8):803-69.
77. Pitt B, Bakris G, Ruilope LM, DiCarlo L, Mukherjee R. Serum potassium and clinical outcomes in the Eplerenone Post-Acute Myocardial Infarction Heart Failure Efficacy and Survival Study (EPHESUS). Circulation. 2008;118(16):1643-50.
78. Jessup M, Abraham WT, Casey DE, Feldman AM, Francis GS, Ganiats TG, et al. 2009 Focused update: ACCF/AHA guidelines for the diagnosis and management of heart failure in adults: a report of the American College of Cardiology Foundation/American Heart Association Task Force on Practice Guidelines. Circulation. 2009;119(14):1977-2016.
79. Epstein M, Calhoun DA. Aldosterone blockers (mineralocorticoid receptor antagonism) and potassium-sparing diuretics. J Clin Hypertensn (Greenwich). 2011;13(9):644-8.
80. Lentini S, Heinig R, Kimmeskamp-Kirschbaum N, Wensing G. Pharmacokinetics, safety and tolerability of the novel, selective mineralocorticoid receptor antagonist finerenone: Results from firstin-man and relative bioavailability studies. Fundam Clin Pharmacol. 2016;30(2):172-84.
81. Bogman K, Schwab D, Delporte ML, Palermo G, Amrein K, Mohr S, et al. Preclinical and early clinical profile of a highly selective and potent oral inhibitor of aldosterone synthase (CYP11B2). Hypertension. 2017; 69(1):189-96.
82. Calhoun DA, White WB, Krum H, Guo W, Bermann G, Trapani A, et al. Effects of a novel aldosterone synthase inhibitor for treatment of primary hypertension: Results of a randomized, double-blind, placebo- and active-controlled phase 2 trial. Circulation. 2011;124(18):1945-55.
83. Shibata H, Itoh H. Mineralocorticoid receptor-associated hypertension and its organ damage: Clinical relevance for resistant hypertension. Am J Hypertens. 2012;25(5):514-23.
84. Kashiwagi Y, Mizuno Y, Harada E, Shono M, Morita S, Yoshimura M, et al. Suppression of primary aldosteronism and resistant hypertension by the peroxisome proliferator-activated receptor gamma agonist pioglitazone. Am J Med Sci. 2013; 345(6):497-500.
85. Liu G, Zheng XX, Xu YL, Lu J, Hui RT, Huang XH. Effect of aldosterone antagonists on blood pressure in patients with resistant hypertension: a meta-analysis. J Hum Hypertens. 2015;29(3):159-66.
86. Dahal K, Kunwar S, Rijal J, Alqatahni F, Panta R, Ishak N, et al. The effects of aldosterone antagonists in patients with resistant hypertension: a meta-analysis of

randomized and nonrandomized studies. Am J Hypertens. 2015;28(11):1376-85.

87. Guo H, Xiao Q. Clinical efficacy of spironolactone for resistant hypertension: a meta-analysis from randomized controlled clinical trials. Int J Clin Exp Med. 2015; 8(5):7270-8.

88. Yang Y, Liu C, Lin YL, Li F. Structural insights into central hypertension regulation by human aminopeptidase A. J Biol Chem 2013;288(35):25638-45.

89. Marc Y, Llorens-Cortes C. The role of the brain renin–angiotensin system in hypertension: Implications for new treatment. Progr Neurobiol 2011; 95: 89-103

90. Keck M, De Almeida H, Compere D, Inguimbert N, Flahault A, Balavoine F, et al. NI956/QGC006, a potent orally active, brain-penetrating aminopeptidase A inhibitor for treating hypertension. Hypertension 2019;73(6):1300-7.

91. Boitard SE, Marc Y, Keck M, Mougenot N, Agbulut O, Balavoine F, et al. Brain renin-angiotensin system blockade with orally active aminopeptidase A inhibitor prevents cardiac dysfunction after myocardial infarction in mice. J Mol Cell Cardiol. 2019; 127:215-22.

92. Bakris G, Bursztyn M, Gavras I, Bresnahan M, Gavras H. Role of vasopressin in essential hypertension: Racial differences. J Hypertens. 1997;15(5):545-50.

93. Bolineau L, Frugiere A, Marc Y, Inguimbert N, Fassot C, Balavoine F, et al. Orally active aminopeptidase A inhibitors reduce blood pressure: a new strategy for treating hypertension. Hypertension. 2008; 51(5):1318-25.

94. Marc Y, Hamazzou R, Balavoine F, Flahault A, Llorens–Cortes C, et al. Central antihypertensive effects of chronic treatment with RB150: An orally active aminopeptidase A inhibitor in deoxycorticosterone acetate-salt rats. J Hypertens. 2018;36(3):641-50.

95. Marc Y, Gao J, Balavoine F, Michaud A, Roques BP, Llorens–Cortes C. Central antihypertensive effects of orally active aminopeptidase A inhibitors I spontaneously hypertensive rats. Hypertension. 2012; 60(2):411-18.

96. Azzizi M, Courand PY, Denolle T, Delsart P, Zhygalina V, Amar L, et al. A pilot double-blind randomized placebo-controlled crossover pharmacodynamic study of the centrally active aminopeptidase A inhibitor, firibastat, in hypertension. J Hypertens. 2019;37(8):1722-28.

97. Ferdinand KC, Balavoine F, Besse B, Black HR, Desbrandes S, Dittrich HC, et al. Efficacy and safety of firibastat, a first-in-class brain aminopeptidase A inhibitor, in hypertensive overweight patients of multiple ethnic origins. A phase 2, open-label, multicenter, dosetitrating study. Circulation. 2019;140(2):138-46.

98. Kitamura K, Aihara M, Osawa J, Naito S, Ikezawa Z. Sulfhydryl drug-induced eruption: a clinical and histological study. J Dermatol. 1990;17(1):44-51.

99. Hickey KA, Rubanyi G, Paul RJ, Highsmith RF. Characterization of a coronary vasoconstrictor produced by cultured endothelial cells. Am J Physiol. 1985;248(5 Pt 1): C550-6.

100. Yanagisawa M, Kurihara H, Kimura S, Tomobe Y, Kobayashi M, Mitsui Y, et al. A novel potent vasoconstrictor peptide produced by vascular endothelial cells. Nature. 1988;332(6163):411-15.

101. Dhaun N, Webb DJ. Endothelins in cardiovascular biology and therapeutics. Nat Rev Cardiol. 2019;16(8):491-502.

102. Haynes WG, Webb DJ. Contribution of endogenous generation of endothelin-1 to basal vascular tone. Lancet. 1994; 344(8926):852-4.

103. Haynes WG, Ferro CJ, O'Kane KP, Somerville D, Lomax CC, Webb DJ. Systemic endothelin receptor blockade decreases peripheral vascular resistance and blood pressure in humans. Circulation. 1996;93(10):1860-70.

104. Krum H, Viskoper RJ, Lacourciere Y, Budde M, Charlon V. The effect of an endothelin receptor antagonist, bosentan, on blood pressure in patients with essential hypertension. N Engl J Med. 1998;338(12):784-90.

105. Nakov R, Pfarr E, Eberle S. Darusentan: an effective endothelin A receptor antagonist for treatment of hypertension. Am J Hypertens. 2002;15(7 Pt 1):583-589.
106. Weber MA, Black HR, Bakris G, Krum H, Linas S, Weiss R, et al. A selective endothelin-receptor antagonist to reduce blood pressure in patients with treatment-resistant hypertension: a randomized, double-blind, placebo-controlled trial. Lancet. 2009;374(9699):1423-31.
107. Bakris GL, Lindholm LH, Black HR, Krum H, Linas S, Linseman JV, et al. Divergent results using clinic and ambulatory blood pressures. A report of a darusentan-resistant hypertension trial. Hypertension. 2010;56(5):824-30.
108. Yuan W, Cheng G, Li B, Li Y, Lu S, Liu D, et al. Endothelin-receptor antagonist can reduce blood pressure in patients with hypertension: a meta-analysis. Blood Press. 2017;26(3):139-49.
109. Pulido T, Adzerikho I, Channick RN, Delcroix M, Galiè N, Ghofrani HA, et al. Macitentan and morbidity and mortality in pulmonary arterial hypertension. N Engl J Med. 2013;369(9):809-18.
110. Belge C, Delcroix M. Treatment of pulmonary arterial hypertension with the dual endothelin receptor antagonist macitentan: Clinical evidence and experience. Ther Adv Respir Dis. 2019;13:1753466618823440.
111. Kaluski E, Cotter G, Leitman M, Milo-Cotter O, Krakover R, Kobrin I, et al. Clinical and hemodynamic effects of bosentan dose optimization in symptomatic heart failure patients with severe systolic dysfunction, associated with secondary pulmonary hypertension-a multi-center randomized study. Cardiology. 2008;109(4):273-80.
112. Zile MR, Bourge RC, Redfield MM, Zhou D, Baicu CF, Little WC, et al. Randomized, double-blind, placebocontrolled study of sitaxesartan to improve impaired exercise tolerance in patients with heart failure and preserved ejection fraction. JACC Heart Fail. 2014;2:123-30.
113. Heerspink HKL, Andress DL, Bakris G, Brennan JJ, Correa-Rotter R, Dey J, et al. Rationale and protocol of the study of diabetic nephropathy with AtRasentan (SONAR) trial: a clinical trial design novel to diabetic nephropathy. Diabetes Obes Metab. 2018;20(6):1369-76.
114. Verweij P, Danaietash P, Flamiom B. Ménard J, Bellet M. Randomized dose-response study of the new dual endothelin receptor antagonist aprocitentan in hypertension. Hypertension. 2020;75:956-65.
115. Wei A, Gu Z, Li J, Liu X, Wu X, Han Y, et al. Clinical adverse effects of endothelin receptor antagonists insights from meta-analysis of 4894 patients from 24 randomized double-blind placebo-controlled clinical trials. J Am Heart Assoc 2016;5(11):e003896.
116. Park M, Sandner P, Krieg T. cGMP at the centre of attention: Emerging strategies for activating the cardioprotective PKG pathway. Basic Res Cardiol. 2018;113(4):24.
117. Hanrahan JP, Wakefield JD, Wilson PJ, Mihova M, Chickering JG, Ruff D, et al. A randomized, placebo-controlled, multiple-ascending-dose study to assess the safety, tolerability, pharmacokinetics, and pharmacodynamics of the soluble guanylate cyclase stimulator praliciguat in healthy subjects. Clin Pharmacol Drug Devel. 2019;8(5):564-75.
118. Hanrahan JP, Seferovic JP, Wakefield JD, Wilson PJ, Chickering JG, Jung J, et al. An exploratory, randomized, placebo-controlled, 14 day trial of the soluble guanylate cyclase stimulator praliciguat in participants with type 2 diabetes and hypertension. Dabetologia. 2020;63(4):733-43.
119. Frey R, Muck W, Unger S, Unger S, Artmeier-Brandt U, Weimann G, et al. Single-dose pharmacokinetics, pharmacodynamics, tolerability, and safety of the soluble guanylate cyclase stimulator, BAY 63-2521: An ascending-dose study in healthy male volunteers. J Clin Pharmacol. 2008;48:926-34.
120. Shea CM, Price GM, Liu G, Sarno R, Buys ES, Currie MG, et al. Soluble guanylate cyclase stimulator praliciguat attenuates inflammation, fibrosis, and organ damage in the Dahl model of cardiorenal failure. Am J Physiol Renal Physiol. 2020;318: F148-59.

121. Tobin JV, Zimmer DP, Shea CM, Germano P, Bernier SG, Liu G, et al. Pharmacological characterization of IW-1973, a novel soluble guanylate cyclase stimulator with extensive tissue distribution, antihypertensive, anti-inflammatory, and antifibrotic effects in preclinical models of disease. J Pharmacol Exp Ther. 2018;365(3):664-75.
122. Sharovska Y, Kalk P, Lawrenz B, Lawrenz B, Godes M, Hoffmann LS, Wellkisch K, et al. Nitric oxide-independent stimulation of soluble guanylate cyclase reduces organ damage in experimental low-renin and high-renin models. J Hypertens. 2010;28(8):1666-75.
123. Geschka S, Kretschmer A, Sharkbvska Y, Evgenov OV, Lawrenz B, Hucke A, et al. Soluble guanylate cyclase stimulation prevents fibrotic tissue remodeling and improves survival in salt-sensitive Dahl rats. PloS One. 2011;6(7):e21853.
124. Zanfolin M, Faro R, Araujo EG, Guaraldo AMA, Antunes E, De Nucci G. Protective effects of BAY 41-2272 (sGC stimulator) on hypertension, heart, and cardiomyocyte hypertrophy induced by chronic L-NAME treatment in rats. Cardiovasc Pharmacol. 2006;47(3):391-5.

CHAPTER 40

Combination Therapy in Hypertension

A Muruganathan

INTRODUCTION

Hypertension (HTN) is a chronic, multifactorial disorder that leads to pathophysiological changes in target organs over time through various mechanisms. The recommended blood pressure (BP) threshold in uncomplicated conditions is below 140/90 mm Hg. However, achieving BP control with a single agent, acting through a specific mechanism, may not always be feasible. A meta-analysis of over 40 studies has demonstrated that combining two agents from different classes of antihypertensive drugs leads to a greater reduction in BP compared to increasing the dose of a single agent. Therapy involving two drugs, either separately or in fixed combinations with agents exhibiting complementary actions, has shown improvement in cardiovascular outcomes. This often includes combining a diuretic with a renin–angiotensin aldosterone system (RAAS) blocker. The choice of combination therapy depends on factors such as risk profile, presence of comorbidities such as diabetes and renal dysfunction, as well as individual patient tolerance to potential adverse effects.

RATIONAL COMBINATION THERAPY FOR HYPERTENSION: FOUR W'S[1,2]

There four W's of rational combination therapy for HTN are as follows: (1) When and where to implement combination therapy? (2) Why do we opt for combination therapy? (3) What and how to employ (principles of) combination therapy?

When to Implement Combination Therapy?

Combination therapy is recommended when BP remains uncontrolled with a single drug and becomes crucial in achieving the desired level. Even a modest reduction of 2 mm Hg in systolic blood pressure (SBP) can lead to a 7–10% decrease in the risk of cardiovascular events. Current HTN treatment guidelines acknowledge that a significant number of patients do not achieve adequate control with a single agent, warranting combination treatment with antihypertensive from different classes. This is particularly relevant if initial monotherapy fails to meet the BP goal, or if there are accompanying risk factors, target organ damage/complications, or concurrent diseases/conditions. For patients with stage-1 HTN, Combination Therapy is often the preferred approach. In cases of stage-2 HTN (defined as SBP ≥160 mm Hg or DBP ≥100 mm Hg), a more aggressive treatment approach is generally needed to attain the BP goal and mitigate the long-term complications of HTN. Consideration of combination therapy as initial treatment may be necessary when BP exceeds the goal by more than 20/10 mm Hg, as it doubles the risk of stroke, ischemic heart disease, and cardiovascular disease.

Why do We Use Combination Therapy?

Single-drug Regimen Limitations[3]

Monotherapy proves effective in only 25% of patients, with most drugs reducing SBP by 7–13 mm Hg and DBP by 4–8 mm Hg. The complexity of high BP arises from a multifactorial mechanism, and drugs may also trigger counter-regulatory responses. Mere dose escalation is unlikely to significantly enhance response and may heighten side effects. Identifying the optimal drug through substitution is time-intensive.

Advantages of Combination Therapy[2]

Combination therapy addresses a broader range of HTN phenotypes, resulting in a lower failure rate. Besides achieving higher rates of BP control, commencing treatment with combination therapy, as opposed to monotherapy, can expedite the attainment of the BP goal, thereby reducing the long-term risk of HTN-related complications. Swift normalization of BP may confer target organ protection, as delayed or ineffective therapy cannot reverse progressive organ damage. Smaller doses of individual drugs minimize side effects compared to a single drug at full dose. A single pill or once-daily administration also significantly improves medication adherence and cost-effectiveness.

Recent surveys indicate that patients on combination therapy exhibit lower dropout rates than those on any monotherapy. The tolerability profile of a drug can be enhanced by adding a second agent in some cases. For instance, the addition of an ACE inhibitor or ARB to a diuretic improves the tolerability of the diuretic by reducing the incidence and magnitude of hypokalemia.

Antihypertensive agents from different classes may have complementary effects, potentially offsetting adverse reactions from each other. For example, a diuretic can mitigate edema resulting from treatment with a calcium channel blocker. Adding an angiotensin-converting enzyme (ACE) inhibitor to a calcium channel blocker may reduce peripheral edema, presumably through venodilation. Compelling indications may necessitate the use of antihypertensives with different mechanisms of action.[1,3]

While antihypertensive drug classes and individual agents may have only minor variations in BP-reducing ability, the combined effect of two agents can be considerably more impactful. Thus, combining an ACE inhibitor with a diuretic lead to fully additive BP reduction, whereas adding the same ACE inhibitor to an angiotensin receptor blocker (ARB) results in an additional BP reduction of only 2–3 mm Hg.

A meta-analysis by Wald et al.[4] demonstrated that BP reduction achieved with drug combinations from two different classes is approximately five times greater than doubling the dose of one drug. The guidelines endorsed by the European Society of Cardiology (ESC)/European Society of Hypertension (ESH) advocate achieving adequate BP control through combination therapy with at least two or more antihypertensive drugs from different classes. Eighth Joint National Committee (JNC 8) recommendation 9 also supports the use of two or more drugs if necessary for HTN control.

Evidence for Combination Therapy

The evidence for combination therapy is listed in **(Fig. 1 and Table 1)**.

Guidelines: International Support for FDC

	ACC/AHA 2017	ESC/ESH 2013/2018	India 2013	China 2010	Thailand 2015	WHO HEARTS
Recommendations when to use two BP lowering drugs						
Not controlled on monotherapy	Yes	Yes	Yes	Yes	Yes	Yes
Initial treatment for selected patients e.g., >20/10 mm Hg from goal* and/or high CV risk	Yes	Yes	Yes	Yes	Yes	Yes
Recommendations when to use single pill combinations						
Recommended to substitute for separate pills to improve adherence	Yes	Yes	Yes	Yes	Yes	Yes

*Some referred to this as stage II HTN or marked BP elevation

- For patients needing >1 BP lowering drug, Fixed dose combination (FDC) is recommended

A
- ACC/AHA 2017– [ARB or ACEI] [Thiazide/Thiazide Like] [CCB]

Guidelines: Focus on 4 Combinations

	Example combinations*	Dose options (mg)
ACEI and thiazide or thiazide-like diuretics	Lisinopril and hydrochlorothiazide	10 mg and 12.5 mg; 20 mg and 12.5 mg; 20 mg and 25 mg
ARB and CCB	Telmisartan and amlodipine	40 mg and 5 mg; 80 mg and 5 mg; 80 mg and 10 mg
ACEI and CCB	Lisinopril and amlodipine	10 mg and 5 mg; 20 mg and 5 mg; 20 mg and 10 mg
ARB and thiazide or thiazide-like diuretics	Telmisartan and hydrochlorothiazide	40 mg and 12.5 mg; 80 mg and 12.5 mg; 80 mg and 25 mg

*Indicative components–similar clinical performance can be expected with other once-daily drugs from the same class (a "square box" application) to optimise choice.

B
- Each qualified with a **square box**
- Ensures pharmacological class therapeutic equivalence; provides choice to nations while focusing options

Figs. 1A and B: Two-drug fixed-dose combinations of antihypertensive drugs proposed for inclusion in WHO's essential medicines list.[5-10] (ACEI: angiotensin converting enzyme inhibitor; ARB: angiotensin receptor blocker; CCB: calcium channel blocker; NR: not reported)

Source A:
Indian guidelines on hypertension (IGH)-III, 2013, Journal of the Association of Physicians of India 2013; 61;6–36.
Mancia G, Fagard R, Narkiewicz K, et al. Journal of Hypertension. 2013;31:1281–35.
Whelton PK, Carey RM, Aronow WS, et al. Journal of the American College of Cardiology 2017:24430.
Jaffe MG, Frieden TR, Campbell NRC, eta al. J Clim Hypertens (Greenwich) 2018;20:829–36.
Source B:
Kishore SP, Salam A, Rodgers A, Jaffe MG, Frieden T. Lancet 2018:392:1072–88.
Salam A, Kanukula R, Esam H, et al. An application to include blood pressure lowering drug fixed dose combinations to the model essential medicines list for the treatment of essential hypertension in adults.

What and how to be Used in Combination Therapy?

Combination therapy can encompass fixed dose combinations or the sequential addition of drugs **(Figs. 2A and B)**. These combinations may be tailored based on the presence of comorbidities such as diabetes mellitus (DM), chronic renal failure (RF), heart failure (HF), thyroid disorders, and for specific population groups like the elderly and pregnant females.

Essential Considerations for Combination Therapy

The fundamental hemodynamic parameters crucial for BP regulation include intravascular volume, cardiac output (CO), and systemic vascular resistance. The RAAS and the sympathetic nervous system act as meticulous regulators, continuously fine-tuning and calibrating these parameters (**Fig. 3**).

Persistent HTN can develop only in response to an increase in CO or a rise in peripheral vascular resistance (**Fig. 4**).[11]

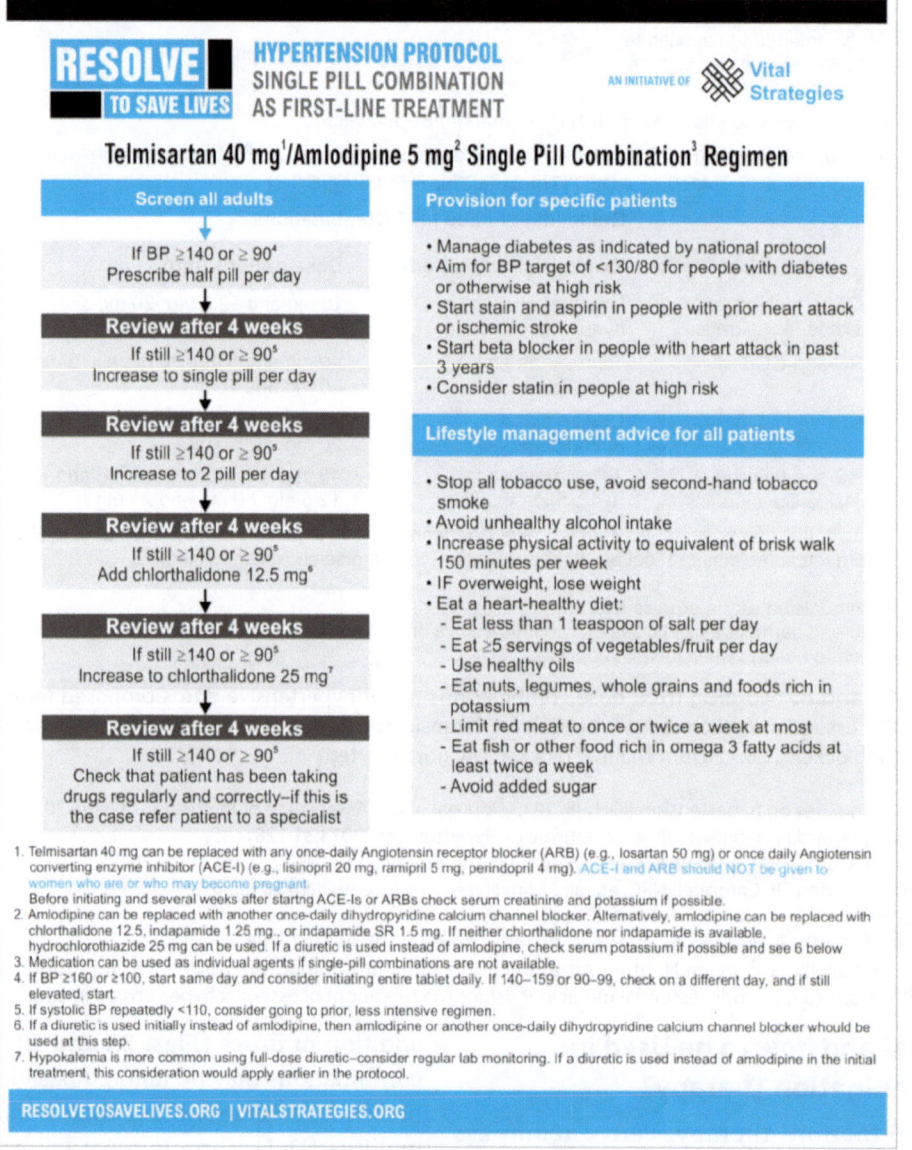

Fig. 2A

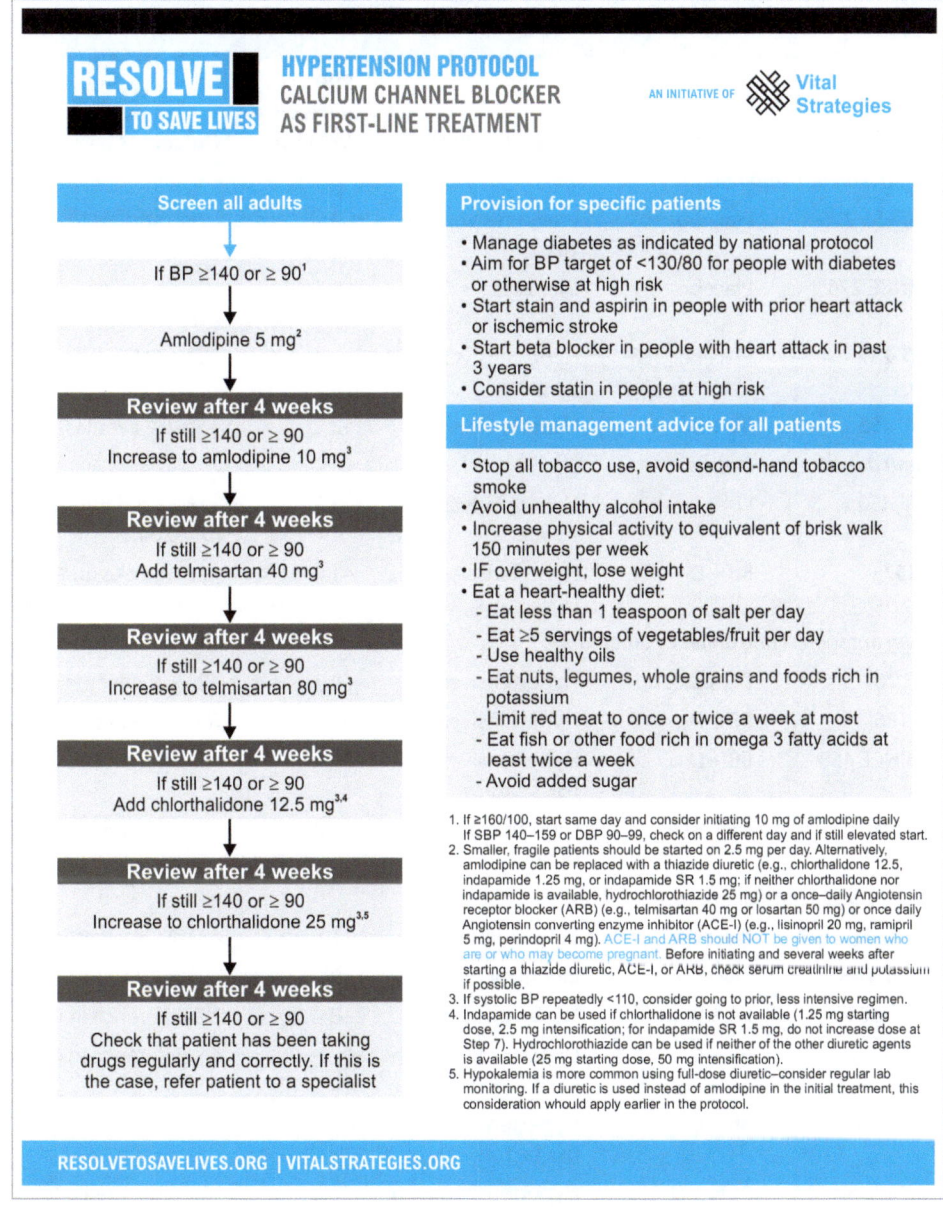

Fig. 2B

Figs. 2A and B: (A) Recommended single-pill combination hypertension treatment regimen; (B) Recommended single-agent hypertension treatment regimen.

■ PRINCIPLES OF COMBINATION

- Different mechanisms (CO + peripheral resistance)
- Same mechanism, different pathway (CO or peripheral resistance)
- Same mechanism, same pathway (CO or peripheral resistance)[12]

TABLE 1: Major drug combinations used in trials of antihypertensive treatment in a step-up approach or as a randomized combination.

Trial	Comparator	Type of patients	SBP difference (mm Hg)	Outcomes
ACEI and diuretic combination				
PROGRESS 296	Placebo	Previous stroke or TIA	−9	−28% strokes ($p < 0.001$)
ADVANCE 276	Placebo	Diabetes	−5.6	−9% micro-/macrovascular events ($p = 0.04$)
HYVET 287	Placebo	Hypertensives aged 80 years	−15	−34% CV events ($p < 0.001$)
CAPPP 455	BB + D	Hypertensives	+3	+5% CV events ($p =$ NS)
ARB and diuretic combination				
SCOPE 450	D + placebo	Hypertensives aged 70 years	−3.2	−28% nonfatal strokes ($p = 0.04$)
LIFE 457	BB + D	Hypertensives with LVH	−1	−26% stroke ($p < 0.001$)
Calcium antagonist and diuretic combination				
FEVER 269	D + placebo	Hypertensives	−4	−27% CV events ($p < 0.001$)
ELSA 186	BB + D	Hypertensives	0	NS difference in CV events
CONVINCE 458	BB + D	Hypertensives with risk factors	0	NS difference in CV events
VALUE 456	ARB + D	High-risk hypertensives	−2.2	−3% CV events ($p =$ NS)
ACEI and calcium antagonist combination				
SystEur 451	Placebo	Elderly with ISH	−10	−31% CV events ($p < 0.001$)
SystChina 452	Placebo	Elderly with ISH	−9	−37% CV events ($p < 0.004$)
NORDIL 461	BB + D	Hypertensives	+3	NS difference in CV events
INVEST 459	BB + D	Hypertensives with CHD	0	NS difference in CV events
ASCOT 423	BB + D	Hypertensives with risk factors	−3	−16% CV events ($p < 0.001$)
ACCOMPLISH 414	ACEI + D	Hypertensives with risk factors	−1	−21% CV events ($p < 0.001$)
BB and diuretic combination				
Coope&Warrender 453*	Placebo	Elderly hypertensives	−18	−42% strokes ($p < 0.03$)
SHEP 449	Placebo	Elderly with ISH	−13	−36% strokes ($p < 0.001$)
STOP 454	Placebo	Elderly hypertensives	−23	−40% CV events ($p = 0.003$)

Contd...

Contd...

Trial	Comparator	Type of patients	SBP difference (mm Hg)	Outcomes
STOP 2 460	ACEI or CA	Hypertensives	0	NS difference in CV events
CAPPP 455	ACEI + D	Hypertensives	–3	–5% CV events (p = NS)
LIFE 457	ARB + D	Hypertensives with LVH	+1	+26% stroke (p <0.001)
ALLHAT 448	ACEI + BB	Hypertensives with risk factors	–2	NS difference in CV events
ALLHAT 448	CA + BB	Hypertensives with risk factors	–1	NS difference in CV events
CONVINCE 458	CA + D	Hypertensives with risk factors	0	NS difference in CV events
NORDIL 461	ACEI + CA	Hypertensives	–3	NS difference in CV events
INVEST 459	ACEI + CA	Hypertensives with CHD	0	NS difference in CV events
ASCOT 423	ACEI + CA	Hypertensives with risk factors	+3	+16% CV events (p < 0.001)
Combination of two RAAS/ACEI + ARB or RAS blocker + Renin inhibitor				
ONTARGET	ACEI or ARB	High-risk patients	–3	More renal events
ALTITUDE 433	ACEI or ARB	High-risk diabetic	–1.3	More renal events

(ACEI: angiotensin-converting-enzyme inhibitor; ARB: angiotensin receptor blocker; BB: β-blocker; CA: calciumantagonist; CHD: coronary heart disease; CV: cardiovascular; D: diuretic; ISH: isolated systolic hypertension; LVH: left ventricular hypertrophy; NS: not significant; RAAS: renin–angiotensin aldosterone system; RAS: rennin angiotensin system; TIA: transient ischemic attack)

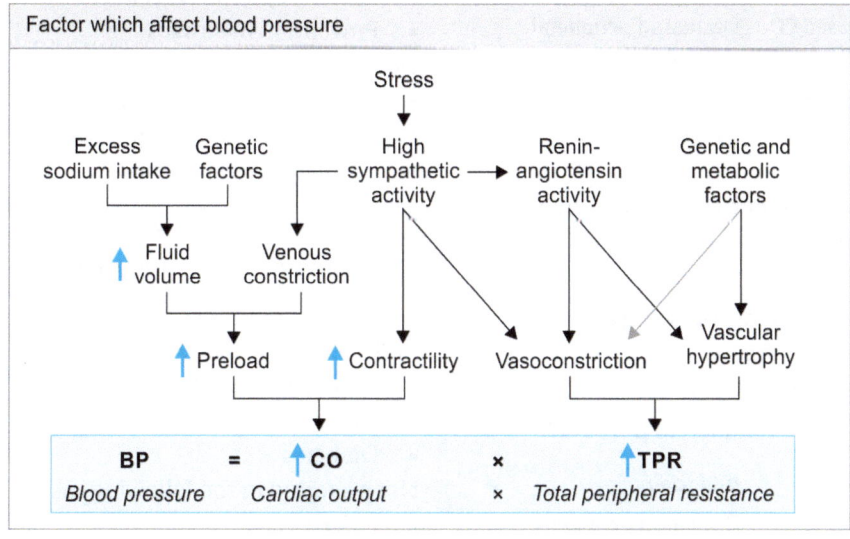

Fig. 3: Interplay of various factors affecting CO and peripheral resistance.

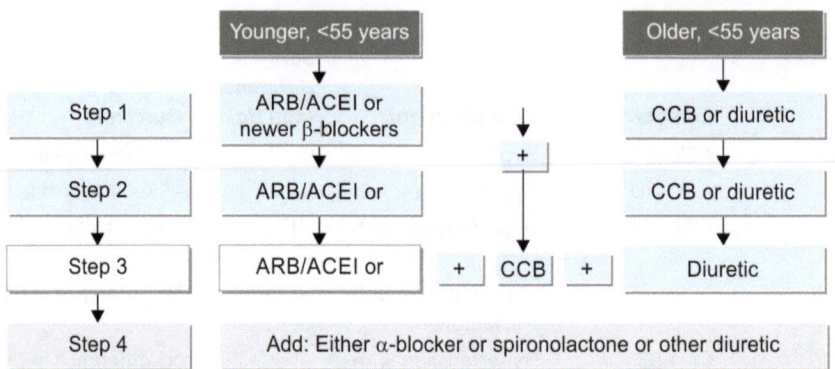

Fig. 4: Indian guidelines on hypertension III: Algorithm for recommended drug combination.

Different Mechanisms

a.

β-blockers	Calcium blocker [dihydropyridine (DHP)]
Decreased CO	Decreased peripheral resistance

Preferred in the following cases:
- Coronary artery disease (CAD); high BP
- Pregnancy; HTN

Not preferred in diabetic nephropathy; β-blockers and non-DHP calcium blockers not to be combined.

b.

β-Blockers	Angiotensin inhibitor
Decreased CO	Decreased peripheral resistance

Preferred in the following cases:
- Coronary artery disease; postmyocardial infraction
- Left ventricular (LV) dysfunction; heart failure (HF)
- Diabetes mellitus + CAD

Not preferred in the following cases:
- To achieve targets
- Renal failure

Not a good combination in pure HTN.

c.

β-Blockers	α-Blockers
Decreased CO	Decreased peripheral resistance

Preferred in the following cases:
- Accelerated high blood pressure (HBP) due to sympathetic over action
- Coronary artery disease + benign prostate hypertrophy
- Renal failure
- Renal + HF (carvedilol)

Not preferred in target organ protection.

d.

Diuretic	Calcium blocker (DHP)
Decreased CO	Decreased peripheral resistance

Preferred in the following cases:
- Isolated systolic HTN in elderly
- Prevention of strokes

Not preferred in the following cases:
- Target organ protection
- Diabetes mellitus; nephropathy
- Coronary artery disease

e.

Diuretic (K losing)	Angiotensin I
Decreased CO	Decreased Peripheral resistance

Preferred in the following cases:
- To achieve targets
- Heart failure, LV dysfunction
- Diabetes

Not preferred in the following cases:
- Elderly HTN
- Severe RF

Different Mechanism Summary

- β-Blockers + Calcium blockers
- β-Blockers + Angiotensin inhibitors
- β-blockers + α-Blockers
- Diuretic + Angiotensin inhibitors
- Diuretic + Calcium blockers

Same Mechanism, Different Pathways (Decreased Cardiac Output)

β-Blockers	Diuretic
Decrease contractility	Decrease preload

Preferred in uncomplicated HBP without target organ disease; not preferred in DM, metabolic syndrome, obese hypertensives.

Same Mechanism, Different Pathways (Decreased Peripheral Resistance)

a.

Angiotensin I	Calcium blockers
Vascular hypertrophy ↓	Vasoconstriction ↓

Preferred in the following cases:
- To achieve targets
- End-organ protection
- Diabetes mellitus; HBP + Nephropathy
- CAD (non-DHP)
- Obese, metabolic syndrome
- Prevent future DM

Not preferred in elderly HTN.

b.

Angiotensin I	A-Blockers
Vascular hypertrophy↓	Vasoconstriction↓

Preferred in the following cases:
- For effective BP lowering
- In cases where angiotensin I and calcium blockers cannot be combined
- With benign prostate hypertrophy
- Diabetes mellitus + Nephropathy

Not preferred in the elderly.

c.

Calcium blockers	α-Blockers
Decrease intracellular cardiac	Block α stimulation

Preferred in the following cases:
- Renal failure
- Benign prostatic hyperplasia (BPH)
- Bronchial asthma/peripheral vascular disease

Not preferred in the following cases:
1. Elderly
2. Coronary artery disease (CAD)
3. Diabetes mellitus

Same Mechanism, Different Pathways Summary

- β-Blockers + diuretic (CO)
- Calcium blockers + ANG inhibitors (peripheral resistance)
- Angiotensin inhibitors + α-blockers (peripheral resistance)
- Calcium blockers + α-blockers peripheral resistance)

Same Mechanism, Same Pathway

	CO
Diuretics	• Thiazide + loop diuretics • Thiazide + aldosterone inhibitors • Loop diuretics + aldosterone inhibitors
	Peripheral resistance
Calcium blockers	• DHP and non-DHP • [CAD, bronchial asthma, arrhythmia, and peripheral vascular disease (PVD)]
Angiotensin I	ACEI and ARB (nephropathy; chronic HF)

Other Combinations: Centrally Acting Drugs

α-Methyl dopa + hydralazine	Renal failure; Pregnancy
Clonidine + diuretics	Severe HTN, renal HTN
Reserpine + diuretics	Still some patients are taking!

Initial Combination Therapy Even in Stage I

CAD	β-blockers and ramipril
LV dysfunction	Specific β-blockers; ramipril
HF	Specific β-blockers, ACEI, and Aldo inhibitors
DM and CAD	Carvedilol; ramipril
Stroke (secondary prevention)	ACEI and indapamide
HF and RF (ACEI intolerance)	Hydralazine and nitrates

Combinations to be Avoided

β-blockers and diuretics	Diabetes
ACEI and ARB	Simple HTN
β-blockers and clonidine	Bradycardia
β-blockers and non-DHP Calcium blockers	Brady
β-blockers and ACE I or ARB	Simple HTN
ACEI, ARB, and Aldo inhibitors	Hyperkalemia

A combination therapy that includes B and D may have a higher risk of inducing new-onset diabetes compared to other combination therapies. It is important to note that the use of beta-blockers (B) should generally be reserved for special situations.

When considering the use of β-blockers (newer β-blockers, in this case), age is a significant factor to take into account:

- Younger individuals, typically those aged below 55 years, may have different considerations for β-blocker therapy.
- In contrast, older individuals, typically those aged 55 years and above, may require a more cautious approach when using β-blockers.

In summary, the decision to include β blockers in combination therapy should be made carefully, considering the potential risk of inducing new-onset diabetes, age-specific factors, and the presence of special situations that may warrant their use.[13]

Single-pill Combination versus Free Combination

Single pill (fixed-dose) combinations (SPCs) are often considered superior due to the following several key advantages:

- *Improved adherence:* The SPCs simplify treatment regimens and reduce pill burden, which can significantly enhance patient adherence. Studies have shown that patients receiving SPCs demonstrated a 26% improvement in adherence compared to those taking separate components.
- *Enhanced convenience:* The SPCs consolidate multiple medications into a single pill, making it more convenient for patients to manage their medication regimen.
- *Better efficacy and tolerability:* The SPCs are formulated to ensure compatibility between different components. This can lead to better overall efficacy and tolerability compared to combining individual medications.
- *Flexible dosage options:* The SPC formulations often offer a range of dosages for each individual component. This flexibility allows for easier dosage adjustment and titration to achieve optimal BP control.
- *Endorsement by guidelines:* The SPCs are currently recommended by international guidelines as the preferred strategy for combining BP-lowering drugs. This endorsement is based on the demonstrated benefits of improved adherence and simplified therapy.

In summary, SPCs offer a range of advantages over free combinations, including improved adherence, convenience, efficacy, and flexibility in dosage options. They are also supported by international guidelines

TABLE 2: Comparison between different HTN management strategies.

	Low-dose monotherapy	High-dose monotherapy	Free combination therapy	SPC therapy
Efficacy	–	+	++	++
Time to reach BP target	–	+	++	++
BP variability	–	–	+	+
Simplicity	+	+	–	+
Flexibility	+	+	+	+**
Compliance	+	+	–	+
Tolerability	+	–	+	++*

*Lower doses generally used in SPCs.
**An increasing number of single-pill combinations are available with a range of doses which is a potential advantage.
(BP: blood pressure; HTN: hypertension; SPC: single-pill combination)

as the preferred approach to combining BP-lowering medications **(Table 2)**.[14]

Combination of Two or More Drugs

If the target BP is not achieved with a two-drug combination at full doses, several options can be considered. Swapping to another two-drug combination or adding a third drug are viable approaches. It is advisable to prioritize selecting an agent from a different class than the initial two drugs in the combination therapy. The addition of a third drug may involve medications like spironolactone (with careful assessment of renal functions and potassium levels), minoxidil, hydralazine, carvedilol, and others, depending on the specific conditions being treated. Centrally acting drugs should be considered as a last resort due to their potential for side effects.[15]

Clinical trials indicate that to reach BP targets, around 24 to 32% of patients may require three or more drugs. A triple-drug combination, such as the calcium channel blocker amlodipine and the diuretic HCTZ combined with an ARB (valsartan or olmesartan), demonstrated statistically greater BP reduction compared to any of their component two-drug combinations. Combinations of an ACE inhibitor or ARB, a calcium channel blocker, and a diuretic represent a rational and effective treatment for a substantial percentage of patients. These combinations are favored in patients without conditions that necessitate the use of a drug from another class.

■ CONCLUSION

Combination therapy for HTN is endorsed by guidelines and widely accepted by healthcare providers. The strategic use of drug combinations is crucial in achieving more rapid BP control and more effective organ protection. The choice of combination therapy should be individualized based on risk factors and the presence of comorbidities. Physicians should not hesitate to initiate combination therapy if BP is not adequately controlled with a single agent.

■ REFERENCES

1. Shina SK. Monotherapy versus combination therapy for the initial treatment of hypertension. Journal of Clinical and Preventive Cardiology. 2020;9(2):78-83.

2. Atkins ER, Chow CK. Low-dose combination therapy for initial treatment of hypertension. Current Hypertension Reports. 2020;22:1-5.
3. Parati G, Kjeldsen S, Coca A, et al. Adherence to single-pill versus free-equivalent combination therapy in hypertension: a systematic review and meta-analysis. Hypertension. 2021;77(2):692-705.
4. Wald DS, Law M, Morris JK, Bestwick JP, Wald NJ. Combination therapy versus monotherapy in reducing blood pressure: meta-analysis on 11,000 participants from 42 trials. The American Journal of Medicine. 2009;122(3):290-300.
5. Indian guidelines on hypertension (IGH)-III, 2013, Journal of the Association of Physicians of India 2013; 61;6–36.
6. Manica G, Gagarrd R, Narkiewicz K, et al. Journal of Hypertension 2013;31:1281–35.
7. Whelton PK, Careyh RM, Arrow WS, et al. Journal of the American College of Cardiology 2017:24430.
8. Jaffe MG, Frieden TR, Campbell NRC, et al. J Clim Hypertens (Greenwich) 218;20:829–36.
9. Kishore SP, Salam A, Rodgers A, Jaffe MG, Frieden T. Lancet. 2018:292:1072–88.
10. Salam A, Kanukula R, Esam H, et al. An application to include blood pressure lowering drug fixed dose combinations to the model essential medicines list for the treatment of essential hypertension in adults.
11. Garjon J, Saiz LC, Azparren A, et al. First-line combination therapy versus first-line monotherapy for primary hypertension. Cochrane Database of Systematic Reviews. 2020(2).
12. Gradman AH, Basile JN, Carter BL, et al, American Society of Hypertension Writing Group. Combination therapy in hypertension. Journal of the American Society of Hypertension. 2010;4(2):90-8.
13. Kalra S, Kalra B, Agrawal N. Combination therapy in hypertension: An update. Diabetology and metabolic syndrome. 2010;2(1):1-1.
14. Gorostidi M, de la Sierra A. Combination therapy in hypertension. Advances in therapy. 2013;30:320-36.
15. Mallat SG, Itani HS, Tanios BY. Current perspectives on combination therapy in the management of hypertension. Integrated blood pressure control. 2013:69-78.

SECTION 10
Genetics and Hypertension

41. **Genetic Approaches to Hypertension: Reverence to Human Hypertension**
    Chamma Gupta, Abhishek Byahut, Bidita Khandelwal

CHAPTER 41

Genetic Approaches to Hypertension: Reverence to Human Hypertension

Chamma Gupta, Abhishek Byahut, Bidita Khandelwal

■ INTRODUCTION

Blood pressure (BP) is a highly variable, heritable trait that is regulated by multiple biological mechanisms and is dependent on environmental cues. Hypertension (HTN) is defined as a systolic blood pressure (SBP) of 140 mm Hg or more, or a diastolic blood pressure (DBP) of 90 mm Hg or more, or taking anti-HTN medication.[1] Diurnal variations in BP have been observed.[2] Globally, the World Health Organization (WHO) has reported more than 1 billion individuals between the ages of 30 and 79 years with HTN with two-thirds of them residing in low- and middle-income countries (LMIC). According to reports, HTN is the largest global cause of premature death. It is called a "silent killer" that has minimal impact on quality of life when it is mild with an estimated 46% of HTN individuals ignorant of their condition.[3] However, if untreated, can lead to a serious medical condition. An elevated level of BP might result in fatal atherosclerotic conditions such as myocardial infarction (MI), renal failure, and stroke. Hypertension continues to be a significant risk factor for cardiovascular, cerebrovascular, and renovascular diseases and the burden of the same is increasing.[4,5]

The majority of cases of high BP are idiopathic. It has long been hypothesized that consuming more salt intake as well as the patient's genetic capacity for a salt response is one of the modifiable factors in relation to the emergence of HTN. Age, obesity, sedentary lifestyle, lack of physical activity regimen, high alcohol intake, and obstructive sleep apnea are all common risk factors for HTN. However, none of these elements can entirely account for the onset and progression of the disease. Several "risk" genes and environmental variables interact to result in a complicated genetic condition known as HTN (genetic heritability: 30%).[6] This chapter explores the association of genetics with high BP.

■ PATHOGENESIS

Despite the discovery of numerous defects at the gene level as distinct causes, most cases of HTN are still caused by behavioral and external factors. The complexity of BP's etiology, wherein the inherited and the environmental cues interact with a plethora of physiological pathways, has been revealed through progressive advances in our comprehension of the ailment. Although the reported epidemiological data have advanced our understanding on response of external factors on BP, in particular to diet and exercise, it has been challenging to identify the specific function of heredity.

■ GENETIC ASSOCIATION OF HYPERTENSION

Pickering and associates were among the first researchers to establish the hereditary association of BP.[7] Studies have demonstrated that third-generation people are more likely to get the same disease if their grandparents or parents had higher BP.[8] These inherited types of HTN are caused by gain- or loss-of-function due to genetic alteration in the sympathetic, glucocorticoid, or mineralocorticoid pathways.[9] Inferential studies of a family history of HTN parents with affected individuals with elevated BP in various communities in Europe and North America provided more specific evidence of the role of hereditary variables on BP.[10] It is believed that a more complicated "triad" comprising the genome, epigenome, and microbiota influences the inheritance of HTN. Genetic investigations have suggested a large portion of hereditary effect on HTN to be located within noncoding regions of our DNA and functions via persistent epigenetic regulation or gene–gene interactions.[11]

With the advent of genomic era and the completion of human genome project (HGP), several bioinformatics tools and advanced technology including single-nucleotide polymorphism (SNP), exome sequencing, next-generation sequencing (NGS), genome-wide association studies (GWAS) and epigenome-wide association studies (EWAS) have unraveled the role of numerous BP loci and almost around 280 genetic variants involved and associated with the pathogenesis of high BP.[12] Although each SNP normally contributes very little to the SBP and DBP levels, there are reports as one of the recent study by Warren et al. that the combinatorial effect of many SNPs has a significant cumulative impact.[13]

Using multistage design, two approaches have been employed to understand the genetic association of BP. First, "linkage analysis and NGS" were used to identify the genes responsible for Mendelian forms of HTN, and rare variations with significant effects on BP were described. This strategy improved the understanding on pathophysiology of the specific disorder, paving the way to a specialized treatment. "Population studies employing GWAS" centered on family members, twins/siblings, and/or adopted child is the other approach that can detect polymorphisms caused by single gene, that can affect the likelihood of acquiring elevated BP.[14] Genome-wide association studies has found 16 novel loci associated with normal/high SBP and DBP. Six loci contain alleles which have initially been suspected to regulate BP (*GUCY1A3-GUCY1B3, NPR3-C5orf23, ADM, FURIN-FES, GOSR2, GNAS-EDN3*), while the additional 10 offer fresh insights into BP physiology. In contrast to other complex or renal disease, HTN, left ventricular wall thickness, stroke, and coronary artery disease (CAD) were all associated with a genetic risk score based on 29 genome-wide significant variations.[15]

Despite the fact that, a growing number of rare diseases have contributed to the detection of apparent and causative Mendelian mutations, research on twins and families have suggested that up to 30–50% of the variation in BP levels may be genetically determined. However, at the community scale, the smooth Gaussian distribution of BP indicates that these alterations are dubious to have any significant impact and that, instead, numerous heritable properties, each of minor profile, are susceptible to be causing high BP levels. The utmost prevalent form of HTN is a complicated feature with a polygenic base as well as environmental factors that may have an impact through epigenetic modifications that could potentially be passed down through generations. Premature start of this ailment is typically thought to be more particular and genetically determined than environmental or behavioral variables, similar to other features.[16-18]

MONOGENIC FORMS OF HYPERTENSION

Monogenic form of HTN is a hereditary syndrome, regulated by single or specific rare gene mutation following the Mendelian law of inheritance. The kidney and adrenal glands were found to be key regulators of BP levels by the finding of genes for monogenic types of HTN. The majority of these diseases are caused by mutations that either acquire or lose function and disrupt the sympathetic, glucocorticoid, or mineralocorticoid pathways.[16] When diagnosing HTN in children, it is crucial to keep these uncommon disorders in mind because the younger the kid, HTN is more likely to be brought on by a secondary cause. Over the past century, more and more disorders linked to monogenic HTN have been discovered. Further understanding of these disorders has been made possible by recent improvements in genomic sequencing methodology. Three different mechanisms contributing to the volume expansion caused by monogenic HTN are as follows:[19]

1. Increased sodium ion reabsorption by hyperactive channels;
2. Hyperstimulation of mineralocorticoid receptors (MR) as a result of changes in steroid synthesis;
3. Elevated mineralocorticoid synthesis.

Overall, 12 genes [*CYP11B1* (11-β hydroxylase), *CYP11B2* (aldosterone synthase), *WNK1, WNK4* (lysine-deficient protein kinase 1 and 4), *KLHL3* (kelch-like 3), *CUL3* (cullin 3), *SCNN1B, SCNN1G* (amilorid-sensitive sodium channel, β and γ subunit gene coding 2-subclasses of the ENaC sodium channel), *CYP17A1* (steroid 17-hydroxylase/17,20 lyase), *HSD11B2* (11-beta-hydroxy steroid dehydrogenase), *NR3C2* (MR), *KCNJ5* (potassium inwardly rectifying channel, subfamily J, member 5)] have been found, resulting in eight distinct Mendelian disorders that cause HTN. The different classified forms of monogenic syndromes in HTN are listed in **Table 1** with details on the affected gene, chromosome loci (Chr), mode of inheritance and genetic mechanism.

POLYGENIC (ESSENTIAL) FORM OF HYPERTENSION

Polygenic form of HTN, also known as essential hypertension (EH) is regulated by more than one gene. Numerous individual factors, such as polygenic traits and environmental factors including nutrition and exercise, frequently contribute to EH. The fundamental processes of EH is still unknown. Inherent constraints in all research studies of EH, such as genetic, phenotypic variation, sample biases, discrepancy in model assumption, and environmental problems, add to this genetic complexity. Recent research using animal models have shown the intricate genetic basis of BP quantitative trait loci (QTLs), complex QTL–QTL interactions, and potent genome underlying the polygenic HTN. A QTL is a single locus and single gene; therefore, identifying QTLs for polygenic HTN in people or animal models is similar to identifying the genes involved.[20,21]

Considering that the targeted gene is causation, rather than merely a marker gene, for BP management, the proposed gene in question should be linked to EH. The majority of these genes are associated with one of the following five physiological classes: The renin–angiotensin–aldosterone system (RAAS), sodium volume, adrenergic, vascular, and metabolic systems. Angiotensin-converting

TABLE 1: Genetic classification of HTN.[9,16,19,25]

Type	Disease	Gene(s)	Chr	Mode of inheritance and genetic mechanism
Monogenic				
Low renin level	Liddle syndrome	SCNN1B, SCNN1G	16p12.2	AD; GOF
	Congenital adrenal hyperplasia	CYP17A1	8q24.3	AR; LOF
	Apparent mineralocorticoid excess	HSD11B2	16q22.1	AR; LOF
	Gellers syndrome	NR3C2	4q31.23	AR
Normal aldosterone levels	Gordon syndrome (pseudohypoaldosteronism type II)	WNK1, WNK4	12p13.33	AD or AR; LOF
High aldosterone levels	Familial hyperaldosteronism type I (glucocorticoid-remediable aldosteronism)	CYP11B2	8q24.3	AD; GOF
	Familial hyperaldosteronism type II	CLCN2	3q27.1	AD
	Familial hyperaldosteronism type III	KCNJ5	11q	AD; LOF
	Familial hyperaldosteronism type IV	CACNA1H (calcium channel)	16p13.3	AD, GOF
Adrenergic/sympathetic excess	High metanephrine and normetanephrine levels: Familial pheochromocytoma	KIF1B (neoplasia of the adrenal medulla)	1p36.22	AD
Vascular smooth muscle proliferation	HTN and brachydactyly syndrome	PDE3A (phosphodiesterase)	12p12.2	AD, GOF
Polygenic				

Physiological classes	Gene(s) and genetic mechanism	Chr
RAAS	AGT alteration, M235T polymorphism in AGT, AG7, ACE, AT1R CYP11B2 alteration, T344C, A6457G variants in CYP11B2	1q42.2, 17q23.3, 8q24.3
G-Proteins or signal Transduction pathway	C825T alteration in G protein β3 subunit	12p13.31
Norandergenic system	ADRBI, β1 adrenergic receptor polymorphism, S49G, R389G, β2 receptor gene polymorphism-R16G, Q27G	5q32

(AR: autosomal recessive; AD: autosomal dominant; Chr: chromosome loci; GOF: gain of function; HTN: Hypertension; LOF: loss of function; RAAS: renin–angiotensin–aldosterone system) enzyme *(ACE)*, angiotensin *(AGT)*, *AT1R* (AGT II receptor I) *CYP11B2*, *GNB3* (G protein subunit *β3*), *MTHFR*, *NOS3* are some of the potential genes reported in a meta-analysis study for EH.[6,22] **(Table 1)**.

ASSOCIATION OF EPIGENETIC FACTORS WITH HYPERTENSION

Epigenetics comprises all heritable variations in the control of gene expression that do not result from changes to the DNA sequence.[23] Numerous variables, including environmental impacts throughout fetal development and childhood, chemical agent exposure, ageing, food, pharmaceuticals, and others, might affect epigenetic alterations.[24] Studies in the field of epigenetic changes sheds light on the fact that the modulation of BP readings cannot be fully elucidated by Mendel's inheritance alone and may also provide an explanation for a portion of the remaining heritability that GWAS was unable to account for. Histone modification in the DNA packaging, noncoding RNAs, chromatin conformation and DNA methylation have all lately gained attention as key participants in a number of pathophysiological processes, including the regulation of BP. This has boosted interest in the study of epigenetic alterations.[25]

By altering gene expression, epigenetic mechanisms help to regulate physiology and disease. Epigenetic alterations result from the interaction between DNA and environmental stimuli. In addition to genes, one epigenetic process called DNA methylation serve as a link between the inherited, external, and related factors that contribute to the illness condition. According to a study, there are ethnic disparities in the sites and locations that are differently methylated and are linked to BP.[26] A function for DNA methylation in the etiology of HTN has also been shown by candidate gene analysis in cell-line and animal research.[27] In numerous human investigations, differences in DNA methylation have been linked to changes in BP and the onset of HTN. *HSD11B2* is one of the candidate gene found to be associated to high BP in human by DNA methylation.[28] Based on the kind of pollutant and the exposed timeline, pregnant women exposed to air contaminants was linked to higher or lower DNA methylation in infant bloodstains and elevated SBP in 11-year-old children.[29]

It has been demonstrated that a number of therapies or genetic alterations that alter BP also alter histone modification (histone acetylation/methylation). Several long noncoding RNAs (lncRNAs) are also reported to be involve in the modulation of BP-relevant activities. For instance, angiotensin II treatment of rat vascular smooth muscle cells results in the variable expression of various lncRNA. Also, *rs9349379*, a common and intronic SNP, has been identified as the potential causative variant in a loci that has been linked to high BP and four other vascular ailments by genetic fine mapping research.[30]

PHARMACOGENOMICS

Ideally, drug response can be predicted using genetics. In an effort to give "the right dose of the right treatment to the right patient," pharmacogenomics aims to find genetic variations linked to a greater response to one pharmacological group than the other set.[31]

The SOPHIA research, which comprised 372 HTN patients receiving losartan monotherapy, is an illustration of this kind of investigation. The scientists found a strong correlation between four SNPs on the *CAMK1D* gene and BP effect using a whole-genome method. The calcium-dependent kinase *NURR1*, *ARF1*, *ATF2*, and *CREB* are all associated with the generation of aldosterone, and *CAMK1D* encodes for this kinase.[15]

FUTURE PROSPECTIVE AND TRANSLATION OF GENETIC FINDINGS

Further research is needed to determine whether the genetic findings from the GWAS have implications for novel HTN mechanisms and pathways, as well as potential treatment targets. The main issue is still that if we can simply use this genetic data to enhance patient care and treatment. Currently, the HTN therapies (anti-HTN drugs) are started much later in life, when end-organ damage has already begun, BP readings are already elevated, and arteries have stiffened. The conventional therapies do not account for the varying involvement of biological system in the etiology of high BP in a person. An individual' risk of acquiring HTN as well as the possible primary causal pathways could be determined by scanning the whole genome for identified variations linked to an elevated risk of HTN and combining this evidence into genetic risk scores. These insights form the cornerstone of "precision medicine," which focuses on locating high-risk, presymptomatic patients with specific disease processes and therapeutic responses.[32] This strategy might result to be efficacious in prevention of CVDs by:

1. Early screening of individuals at a higher risk earlier to the phenotype's development.
2. Proactive and tailored lifestyle modifications.
3. Logical and targeted choice of CVDs medications effective for affected individual.

Despite the fact that this is an appealing possibility, more crucial steps must be taken before considering the utility of DNA sequencing for precision medicine in HTN and its complications.

CONCLUSION

Hypertension is a multifactorial disorder with complex trait. This is a result of several modifiable as well as nonmodifiable factors including the high salt intake, sedentary lifestyle, obesity, hereditary, and environmental variables or due to inheritance of epigenetics. Studies in genetics and genomes have made significant contributions to our understanding of the pathogenesis of HTN. The two types of high BP are monogenic, that is, genetically inherited and polygenic, are caused by one and numerous gene variations, respectively. In addition to genes, epigenetic processes such as DNA methylation, chromatin remodeling, histone acetylation or methylation and noncoding RNA sequences may serve as a mediator between inherited, environmental, and related factors that contribute to HTN. Application of precision medicine strategies to these diseases may have considerable positive effects on the economy and public health. The morbidity and mortality linked to uncontrolled HTN can be reduced with the appropriate therapy. There is potential for early detection and better management of the many kinds of HTN with future improvements in genetic testing technologies and therapeutic choices.

REFERENCES

1. Whelton PK, Carey RM, Aronow WS, Casey DE, Collins KJ, Dennison HC, et al. 2017 ACC/AHA/AAPA/ABC/ACPM/AGS/APhA/ASH/ASPC/NMA/PCNA guideline for the prevention, detection, evaluation, and management of high blood pressure in adults. J Am Coll Cardiol 2018;71(19):e127-48.

2. Centers for Disease Control and Prevention. (2021). High blood pressure symptoms, causes, and problems. [Online] Available from: https://www.cdc.gov/bloodpressure/about.htm [Last accessed November, 2023].
3. World Health Organization. (2022). Hypertension. [Online] Available from: https://www.who.int/news-room/fact-sheets/detail/hypertension [Last accessed November, 2023].
4. Acelajado MC, Oparil S. Hypertension in the elderly. Clin Geriatr Med. 2009;25(3):391-412.
5. Kunes J, Zicha J. The interaction of genetic and environmental factors in the etiology of hypertension. Physiol Res. 2009;58(Suppl. 2):S33-42.
6. Agarwal A, Williams GH, Fisher NDL. Genetics of human hypertension. Trends in Endocrinol Metab. 20051;16(3):127-33.
7. Pickering GW. Relation between genetic and social factors and arterial pressure. Recenti Prog Med. 1961;30:397-416.
8. Kotchen TA, Cowley AW Jr, Liang M. Ushering hypertension into a new era of precision medicine. JAMA. 2016;315(4):343-4.
9. Burrello J, Monticone S, Buffolo F, Tetti M, Veglio F, Williams TA, et al. Is there a role for genomics in the management of hypertension? Int J Mol Sci. 2017;18(6):1131.
10. Mo R, Omvik P, Lund-Johansen P. The Bergen blood pressure study: Offspring of two hypertensive parents have significantly higher blood pressures than offspring of one hypertensive and one normotensive parent. J Hypertens. 1995;13(12 Pt 2):1614-7.
11. Padmanabhan S, Joe B. Towards precision medicine for hypertension: a review of genomic, epigenomic, and microbiomic effects on blood pressure in experimental rat models and humans. Physiol Rev. 2017;97(4):1469-528.
12. Patel RS, Masi S, Taddei S. Understanding the role of genetics in hypertension. Eur Heart J. 2017;38(29):2309-12.
13. Warren HR, Evangelou E, Cabrera CP, Gao H, Ren M, Mifsud B, et al. Genome-wide association analysis identifies novel blood pressure loci and offers biological insights into cardiovascular risk. Nat Genet. 2017;49(3):403-15.
14. Munroe PB, Barnes MR, Caulfield MJ. Advances in blood pressure genomics. Circ Res. 2013;112(10):1365-79.
15. Frau F, Zaninello R, Salvi E, Ortu MF, Braga D, Velayutham D, et al. Genome-wide association study identifies CAMKID variants involved in blood pressure response to losartan: the SOPHIA study. Pharmacogenomics. 2014;15(13):1643-52.
16. Ehret GB, Caulfield MJ. Genes for blood pressure: an opportunity to understand hypertension. Eur Heart J. 2013;34(13):951-61.
17. Dominiczak A, Delles C, Padmanabhan S. Genomics and precision medicine for clinicians and scientists in hypertension. Hypertension. 2017;69(4):e10-3.
18. Wang J, Gong L, Tan Y, Hui R, Wang Y. Hypertensive epigenetics: from DNA methylation to microRNAs. J Hum Hypertens. 2015;29(10):575-82.
19. Raina R, Krishnappa V, Das A, Amin H, Radhakrishnan Y, Nair NR, et al. Overview of monogenic or Mendelian forms of hypertension. Front Pediatr. 2019;7:263.
20. Deng AY. Genetic basis of polygenic hypertension. Human Molecular Genetics. 2007;16(Spec No. 2):R195-202.
21. Deng AY. Positional cloning of quantitative trait loci for blood pressure: how close are we? A critical perspective. Hypertension. 2007;49(4):740-7.
22. Lohmueller KE, Pearce CL, Pike M, Lander ES, Hirschhorn JN. Meta-analysis of genetic association studies supports a contribution of common variants to susceptibility to common disease. Nat Genet. 2003;33(2):177-82.
23. López-Jaramillo P, Camacho PA, Forero-Naranjo L. The role of environment and epigenetics in hypertension. Expert Rev Cardiovasc Ther. 2013;11(11):1455-7.
24. Raftopoulos L, Katsi V, Makris T, Tousoulis D, Stefanadis C, Kallikazaros I. Epigenetics, the missing link in hypertension. Life Sci. 2015;129:22-6.
25. Wise IA, Charchar FJ. Epigenetic modifications in essential hypertension. Int J Mol Sci. 2016;17(4):451.

26. Kazmi N, Elliott HR, Burrows K, Tillin T, Hughes AD, Chaturvedi N, et al. Associations between high blood pressure and DNA methylation. PLoS One. 2020;15(1):e0227728.
27. Rivière G, Lienhard D, Andrieu T, Vieau D, Frey BM, Frey FJ. Epigenetic regulation of somatic angiotensin-converting enzyme by DNA methylation and histone acetylation. Epigenetics. 2011;6(4):478-89.
28. Friso S, Pizzolo F, Choi SW, Guarini P, Castagna A, Ravagnani V, et al. Epigenetic control of 11 beta-hydroxysteroid dehydrogenase 2 gene promoter is related to human hypertension. Atherosclerosis. 2008;199(2):323-7.
29. Breton CV, Yao J, Millstein J, Gao L, Siegmund KD, Mack W, et al. Prenatal air Pollution exposures, DNA methyl transferase genotypes, and associations with newborn LINE1 and Alu methylation and childhood blood pressure and carotid intima-media thickness in the children's health study. Environmental Health Perspectives. 2016;124(12):1905-12.
30. Liang M. Epigenetic mechanisms and hypertension. Hypertension. 2018;72(6):1244-54.
31. Voora D, Ginsburg GS. Clinical application of cardiovascular pharmacogenetics. J Am Coll Cardiol. 2012;60(1):9-20.
32. Collins FS, Varmus H. A new initiative on precision medicine. N Engl J Med. 2015;372(9):793-5.

SECTION 11

Interventional Interventions in Hypertension

42. **Baroreceptor Stimulation and Hypertension**
    Anjan Lal Dutta, Soumik Chaudhuri

CHAPTER 42

Baroreceptor Stimulation and Hypertension

Anjan Lal Dutta, Soumik Chaudhuri

■ INTRODUCTION

Hypertension stands as a prominent cardiovascular risk factor worldwide and is the leading avoidable cause of death.[1] It poses a significant public health challenge. Recent estimates indicate that over 207 million individuals in India currently grapple with hypertension.[2] Globally, this number surpasses one billion, projected to escalate to 1.5 billion by 2025.[3] The evolution of diverse antihypertensive drug categories has substantially contributed to reducing cardiovascular events.[4] Despite growing awareness and implementation of hypertensive management over the last decades, perfection remains elusive.[5] This underscores the necessity for innovative and efficacious approaches.

Antihypertensive medications span various classifications, exerting distinct or synergistic effects. Nevertheless, even with optimal utilization of these agents, a subset of hypertensive patients (5–15%) experience uncontrolled blood pressure (BP).[6] This group is commonly termed "resistant hypertension." While 5–15% may seem modest in proportion, considering hypertension's widespread prevalence, the absolute count of resistant hypertensives becomes noteworthy. Consequently, the quest for alternative hypertension control methods has gained momentum in recent years. In the mid-20th century, interventional hypertension management gained traction but waned due to unfulfilled early promise. Scientific interest has gradually resurged over the past decade, focusing on two primary contenders: carotid baroreceptor stimulation and renal sympathetic denervation. The latter, however, faces controversy regarding efficacy. Future refinements may reshape this landscape.

Integral to BP homeostasis, the carotid baroreflex plays a pivotal role. These baroreceptors in the carotid sense intra-arterial BP, prompting adjustments in sympathetic tone in opposition. Elevated BP triggers baroreceptor activation, culminating in a notable decrease in sympathetic tone, whereas heightened sympathetic activity compensates for reduced BP. The carotid baroreflex was historically perceived as a "short-term buffer," tasked with regulating sudden and fleeting BP fluctuations near a "set-point." Its contribution to long-term BP management remained insufficiently elucidated.[7] Recent evidence, however, challenges this enduring notion, strongly suggesting that the carotid baroreflex system might have the potential to exert sustained and enduring effects on BP. This resurgence casts light on the interventional activation of the carotid baroreflex as a prospective avenue for the enduring management of resistant hypertension.

BAROREFLEX ARC ANATOMY

The central element of the arterial baroreflex system, the carotid baroreflex circuit, holds paramount significance. Despite the presence of baroreceptors in peripheral areas such as the heart, pulmonary vasculature, and the aortic arch, a wealth of compelling evidence underscores the pivotal role played by carotid baroreceptors in BP buffering.

Stretch-sensitive mechanosensors, the carotid baroreceptors, are located at the left and right carotid sinus. Afferent fibers in the carotid sinus nerve (a branch of cranial nerve IX; Glossopharyngeal) convey information from the carotid baroreceptors, with associated sensory cell bodies residing in the petrosal ganglia. Aortic arch baroreceptors transmit their afferent signals through the aortic depressor nerve (a branch of cranial nerve X; vagus), and their sensory cell bodies are situated in the nodose ganglia.

The journey of these afferent signals leads them to the nucleus tractus solitaris (NTS), positioned in the dorsal medulla, serving as a pivotal "reception center" for impulses originating from arterial baroreceptors. These signals subsequently travel to the caudal ventrolateral medulla (CVLM), which functions as the transformative "conversion center." Here, excitatory signals sourced from peripheral baroreceptors undergo processing and conversion into efferent inhibitory signals. These inhibitory signals then proceed to the rostral ventrolateral medulla (RVLM), the master "coordinating center." It is from the RVLM that sympathetic outflow emanates, coursing through interomediolateral cell columns within the spinal cord, ultimately reaching effector organs such as blood vessels and the heart. This orchestration effectively governs sympathetic tone within the vasculature.[8]

A comprehensive visualization of the integrated baroreceptor system is depicted in the accompanying **Figure 1**.

Figure 1 illustrates the fundamental framework of the central amalgamation of arterial baroreceptor input. The key components are designated as follows: Nucleus tractus solitaris, CVLM, RVLM, nucleus ambiguus (NA), cardiac output (CO), stroke volume (SV), mean arterial pressure (MAP), total peripheral resistance (TPR), and heart rate (HR).

BAROREFLEX SENSITIVITY: EXPLANATION AND SIGNIFICANCE

Baroreflex sensitivity (BRS) serves as a surrogate indicator of cardiovascular health, reflecting the autonomic response to changes in arterial pressure. Various assessment methods exist, encompassing both noninvasive techniques (such as computer-assisted spectral imaging, oscilloscopy, Valsalva maneuver, and lower body negative pressure chamber approaches) and invasive ones (including muscle sympathetic nerve activity or MSNA).[9]

Alterations in BP incite compensatory adjustments in HR, mediated through the baroreflex. This relationship can be graphed, as depicted in **Figure 2**. The curve exhibits a sigmoidal pattern, with the linear segment analyzed via regression to ascertain the slope and BRS. A high BRS indicates a more pronounced reduction in HR in response to an elevation in pressure. Conversely, a low BRS manifests as a flattened slope, suggesting minimal HR response to changes in MAP.

Diminished BRS (characterized by a flattened slope) is evident in several conditions, including obesity, aging, hypertension, diabetes, and coronary artery

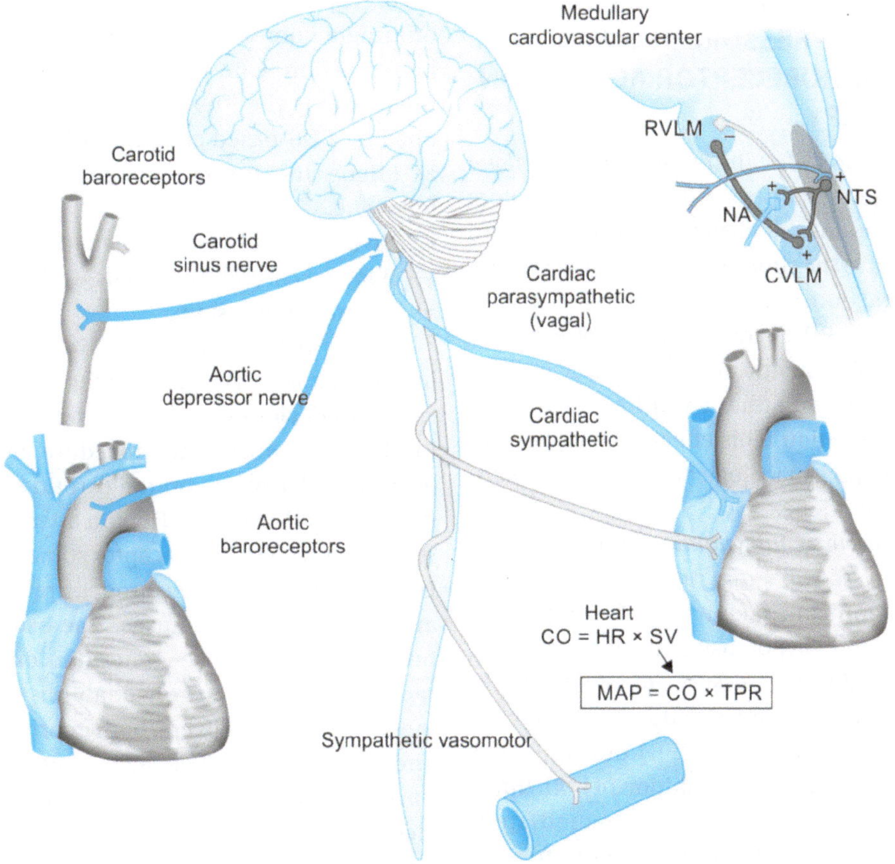

Fig. 1: Fundamental framework of the central amalgamation of arterial baroreceptor input. (CO: cardiac output; CVLM: caudal ventrolateral medulla; HR: heart rate; MAP: mean arterial pressure; NA: nucleus ambiguus; NTS: nucleus tractus solitaris; RVLM: rostral ventrolateral medulla TPR: total peripheral resistance; SV: stroke volume)

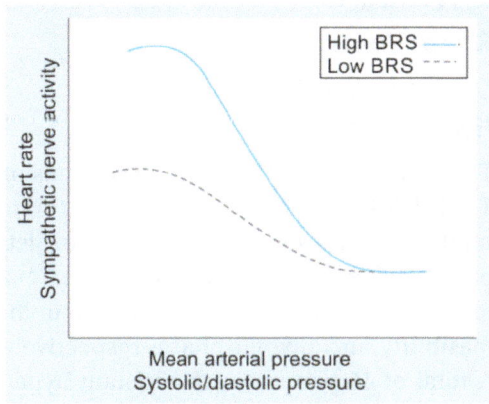

Fig. 2: Baroreflex sensitivity. (BRS: baroreflex sensitivity)

disease. Notably, these conditions are associated with poorer prognoses.[10] Following a myocardial infarction, reduced BRS may predict the likelihood of fatal arrhythmias and cardiac mortality.[11] Similarly, in congestive heart failure, diminished BRS is indicative of a high risk of sudden cardiac death.[12]

Remarkably, consistent physical exercise can enhance BRS and thus safeguard against age-related deterioration in baroreflex function. This enhancement exhibits a "dose-dependent" relationship, underscoring the progressively beneficial impact of regular exercise.

MECHANISMS UNDERLYING BLOOD PRESSURE REDUCTION VIA BARORECEPTOR ACTIVATION THERAPY

- *Inhibition of central sympathetic outflow:* Activation of physiological baroreceptors in response to elevated arterial pressure leads to the suppression of central sympathetic outflow, resulting in a decrease in HR and BP. Chronic baroreceptor activation consistently and sustainably inhibits central sympathetic outflow, leading to BP reduction. This effect extends beyond mere pharmacological adrenergic mechanisms alone.[12]
- *Impact on renal sympathetic nerve activity, renin secretion, and renal hemodynamics:* A significant factor contributing to the long-term hypotensive effects of BAT is the inhibition of pressure-dependent renin release. The modest reduction in glomerular filtration rate (GFR) during BAT is influenced by the inhibition of both direct and indirect (angiotensin-mediated) effects of renal nerves on sodium reabsorption. Consequently, BAT offers notable clinical advantages for hypertensive patients with sympathetic activation and a renin-angiotensin-aldosterone system amenable to neural modulation.[13]
- *Influence on cardiac autonomic activity:* Baroreceptor activation therapy (BAT) restores cardiac BRS and enhances HR variability. Diminished parasympathetic activity contributes to impaired cardiac BRS and HR variability, both of which are improved through Baroreceptor Activation devices.[14]

BARORECEPTOR ACTIVATION THERAPY: THE DEVICE

Recent technological advancements have reignited scientific exploration of baroreceptor activation devices, potentially offering a compelling solution for resistant hypertension. One pioneering endeavor in this realm is the implantable device developed by a US-based company, CVRx, known as Rheos. Its components encompass the following:
- An implantable pulse generator (IPG)
- Bilateral carotid sinus leads
- Programmer system.

The subsequent-generation devices include Barostim Neo and MobiusHD. A typical Rheos device implantation site is depicted in **Figure 3**. During the procedure, optimal electrode placement on the carotid sinus is guided by reductions in HR and arterial pressure upon carotid baroreceptor stimulation.[15] Once confirmed, the electrodes are secured around the carotid sinuses. The externally programmable pulse generator employs radiofrequency control, enabling adjustments in current delivery, both intermittently and continuously. The second-generation Barostim Neo, featuring a miniaturized electrode, is less invasive and is implanted on only one side.

THE EVIDENCE FOR BARORECEPTOR ACTIVATION THERAPY

Rheos Trials

Device-based Therapy in Hypertension Trial

The Device-based Therapy in Hypertension Trial (DEBuT-HT) was a multicenter non-randomized trial designed to assess the safety of baroreflex activation therapy (BAT).[16,17] A total of 16 and 17 centers participated in the feasibility and pivotal phase, respectively. A total of 45 patients with resistant hypertension were enrolled in this trial, and the primary inclusion criteria included resistant hypertension. Subsequently, some of these

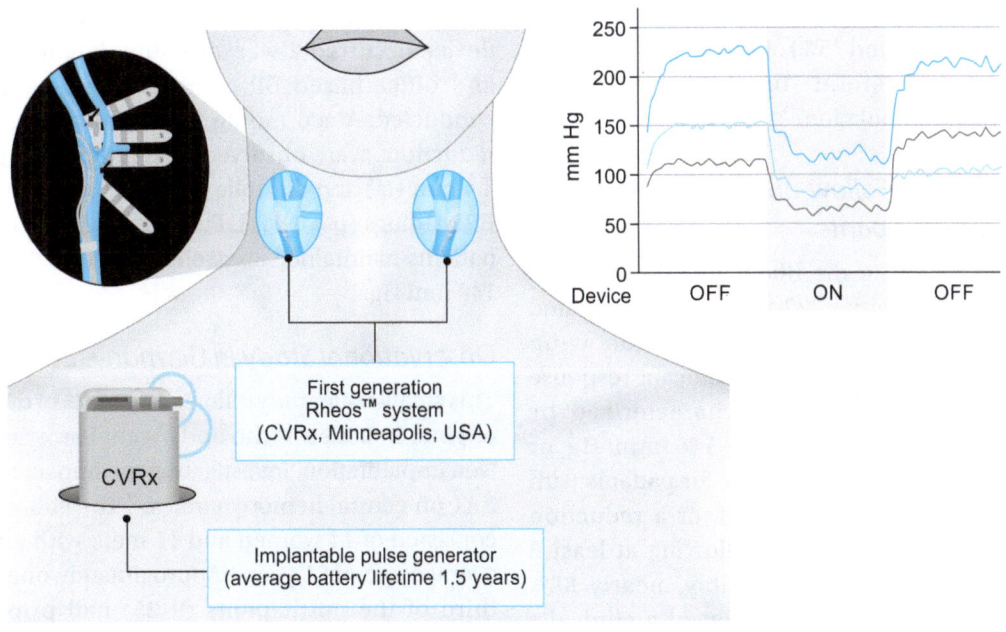

Fig. 3: Typical implantation of a Rheos device.

TABLE 1: Office-based BP response in the DEBuT-HT trial.				
Number of patients	Time	Systolic reduction of BP (mm Hg)	Diastolic reduction of BP (mm Hg)	p-value
37	3 months	21 ± 4	12 ± 2	<0.001
26	1 year	30 ± 6	20 ± 4	<0.001
17	2 years	33 ± 8	22 ± 6	<0.002

(BP: blood pressure)

patients were monitored and followed up for up to two years. Throughout the follow-up periods, mean office-based BP consistently decreased compared to baseline values. The specifics of this response are detailed in **Table 1**.

The DEBuT-HT trial highlighted promising reductions in office-based BP over the follow-up duration, demonstrating the potential effectiveness of BAT in managing resistant hypertension.

Rheos Pivotal Trial

This double-blind randomized controlled trial encompassed 265 participants afflicted with resistant hypertension, divided into two groups at a ratio of 2:1. Group A ($n = 181$) underwent immediate device activation (1 month after implant), while group B's ($n = 84$) device activation was delayed for 7 months postimplant. Results at 6 months revealed that 42% of group A patients achieved a systolic BP below 140 mm Hg (measured via office-based BP), in contrast to 24% in group B. By the 1-year mark, both groups had undergone activated BAT for either 12 or 6 months. Surprisingly, over 80% of patients experienced a reduction in systolic BP by at least 10 mm Hg, and approximately half of the study's cohort achieved systolic BP at or below 140 mm Hg. Notably, a substantial portion (around 75%) of participants received unilateral carotid stimulation instead of bilateral stimulation.[18]

Long-term Follow-up of Rheos Pivotal Trial Participants

Subsequent to the Rheos pivotal trial, 276 out of the initial 322 patients participated in a comprehensive long-term follow-up assessment. A clinically significant response to BAT treatment was characterized by sustained systolic BP of 140 mm Hg or lower (130 mm Hg or lower for patients with diabetes or renal disease), or a reduction of 20 mm Hg or more following at least 6 months of BAT. Remarkably, nearly 88% of patients ($n = 244$) achieved a clinically significant response. The BP measurements were conducted using office-based assessments. Among patients initially demonstrating a clinical response, over 55% sustained BP reductions throughout the average follow-up period of 28 months.[18]

Barostim Neo Trials

Barostim Neo Trial (XR-1 Verification Study)

This single-group trial aimed to evaluate the effectiveness and safety of the Barostim Neo device (formerly, XR-1). The study enrolled 30 patients across seven centers, mainly located in Europe (six centers). Resistant hypertension was defined as resting systolic BP over 140 mm Hg despite the use of at least three antihypertensive drugs, including a diuretic. The participants included 14 males and 16 females, primarily middle-aged and obese (average age: 57 years), taking an average of six hypertension medications. Baseline BP averaged at 171.7 (±20.2) mm Hg systolic/99.5 (± 13.9) mm Hg diastolic. Activation of the Barostim Neo device occurred 2 weeks postimplantation, and office-based BP measurements were conducted. At a 6-month follow-up, average reductions were observed in systolic (26.0 ± 4.4 mm Hg) and diastolic (12.4 ± 2.5 mm Hg) BP readings ($p < 0.001$). Furthermore, 43% of patients maintained a systolic PB at or below 140 mm Hg.

Observational Study in Germany (2015)

This small-scale study followed up on 25 of the original 30 patients who underwent Barostim Neo implantation, investigating the impact of BAT on central hemodynamics.[19] The cohort consisted of 14 women and 11 men, with an average age of 61 years. Approximately one-third of the participants (9/25) had prior renal denervation and many were obese. After 6 months of BAT therapy, measured in an office setting, average peripheral BP decreased from 109.9 (± 20.4) to 97.3 (± 18.5) mm Hg ($p < 0.01$). Additionally, central aortic systolic BP exhibited a significant reduction, declining from 147.2 (± 27.8) to 130.2 (± 25.2) mm Hg ($p < 0.01$).

Barostim Neo Pivotal Trial

This ongoing randomized-controlled multi-center trial seeks to establish the efficacy and safety of the Barostim Neo system in managing resistant hypertension. The study plans to enroll over 300 patients in the United States. The primary efficacy endpoint is a systolic BP reduction of 12.5 mm Hg, with a superiority margin of at least 5 mm Hg for the Barostim Neo treatment group (BAT plus optimal medical management) compared to the control group (optimal medical management only). The conclusive demonstration of whether Barostim Neo treatment can effectively reduce morbidity or mortality is still pending.[20]

MobiusHD Devices

Controlling and Lowering Blood Pressure with MobiusHD First-in-Man at Six European Centers Study

The controlling and lowering blood pressure with MobiusHD first-in-Man at six European centers (CALM FIM EUR) prospective open-label study was conducted at six European centers. Eligible participants were individuals with resistant hypertension (systolic BP cutoff of ≥160 mm Hg), despite being on at least three antihypertensive agents, one of which was a diuretic. The MobiusHD devices were unilaterally implanted in the internal carotid artery. Notably, the primary endpoint for this study at 6 months was safety, focusing on the incidence of serious adverse events. Efficacy, including changes in both office and 24-h ambulatory BP, was considered a secondary endpoint.[21] Over the period between December 2013 and February 2016, thirty patients were successfully implanted with the device. The participants had an average age of 52 years, an equal distribution of sexes, and were using an average of 4.4 antihypertensive drugs. By the 6-month mark, there were five serious adverse events, occurring in four patients: Hypotension, wound infection, aggravated hypertension, and intermittent claudication. The efficacy endpoints are summarized in **Table 2** (*Note: Unfortunately, without access to the actual data and formatting capabilities, the authors are unable to provide specific numerical values or detailed formatting for* **Table 2**).

The CALM-FIM EUR study primarily aimed to assess the safety of the MobiusHD devices, while secondary endpoints explored their efficacy in terms of BP changes. For precise numerical values and comprehensive results, referring to the original study publications or relevant medical sources is advisable.

TABLE 2: Efficacy of the CALM-FIM EUR study.

	Office BP	Ambulatory BP
Mean systolic BP	184 mm Hg	166 mm Hg
Reduction in systolic BP at 6 months	24 mm Hg (13–34)	21 mm Hg (14–29)
p-value	0.0003	<0.0001
Mean diastolic BP	109 mm Hg	100 mm Hg
Reduction in diastolic BP at 6 months	12 mm Hg (6–18)	12 mm Hg (7–16)
p-value	0.0001	<0.0001

(BP: blood pressure)

In patients with resistant hypertension, the application of baroreceptor amplification through IPG or endovascular methods (such as the MobiusHD device) has demonstrated a significant capacity to effectively lower BP levels while maintaining an acceptable safety profile. However, before definitive guidelines can be established, the need for randomized and double-blinded studies is evident.

ADVERSE EFFECTS OF BARORECEPTOR ACTIVATION THERAPY

Procedural adverse effects encompass wound site infections and complications, temporary and permanent hypoglossal nerve damage, surgical complications, and chronic pain in the glossopharyngeal nerve region. Some patients report a sensation of tingling in the neck, which tends to diminish over time. In a few cases, patients may experience hypertensive crises and even strokes related to BAT.[22] Notably, post-1 year of BAT, the assessment of renal function reveals a mild increase in serum creatinine and an insignificant reduction in estimated glomerular filtration rate (e-GFR), suggesting that BAT does not appear to significantly affect kidney function.[23]

CONCLUSION

Baroreceptor Activation Therapy has demonstrated promising initial outcomes by achieving and sustaining a consistent and safe reduction in BP levels among patients with resistant hypertension. Concerns about safety, observed with the first-generation Rheos devices, have been addressed through the more compact and advanced Barostim Neo device. The customizable and fully reversible nature of this therapy makes it an appealing therapeutic approach, with high patient compliance compared to drug regimens. The management of resistant hypertension has historically posed challenges, with these patients at heightened risk due to uncontrolled arterial hypertension. A combination of conventional drug therapies, lifestyle adjustments, and innovative interventions like Baroreceptor Activation holds significant promise. Ongoing randomized controlled trials will inevitably shape the future role of BAT in hypertension management.

REFERENCES

1. Mills KT, Bundy JD, Kelly TN, Reed JE, Kearney PM, Reynolds K, et al. Global disparities of hypertension prevalence and control: A systematic analysis of population-based studies from 90 countries. Circulation. 2016;134(6):441-50.
2. Gupta R, Xavier D. Hypertension: The most important noncommunicable disease risk factor in India. Indian Heart J. 2018; 70(4):565-72.
3. Kearney PM, Whelton M, Reynolds K, Muntner P, Whelton PK, He J, et al. Global burden of hypertension: analysis of worldwide data. Lancet. 2005;365(9455):217-23.
4. Pierdomenico SD, Lapenna D, Bucci A, Di Tommaso R, Di Mascio R, Manente BM, et al. Cardiovascular outcome in treated hypertensive patients with responder, masked, false resistant, and true resistant hypertension. Am J Hypertens. 2005;18(11):1422-8.
5. Egan BM, Zhao Y, Axon RN. US trends in prevalence, awareness, treatment, and control of hypertension, 1988-2008, JAMA. 2010;303(20):2043-50.
6. Papadopoulos DP, Papademetriou V. Resistant Hypertension: Diagnosis and Management. J Cardiovasc Pharmacol Ther. 2006;11(2):113-8.
7. Cowley AW Jr, Liard JF, Guyton AC. Role of baroreceptor reflex in daily control of arterial blood pressure and other variables in dogs. Circ Res. 1973;32(5):564-76.
8. Thrasher TN. Unloading arterial baroreceptors causes neurogenic hypertension. Am J Physiol Regul Integr Comp Physiol. 2002;282(4):R1044-53.
9. Benarroch EE. The arterial baroreflex: Functional organization and involvement in neurologic disease. Neurology. 2008;71(21): 1733-8.
10. Lanfranchi PA, Somers VK. Arterial baroreflex function and cardiovascular variability: Interactions and implications. Am J Physiol Regul Integr Comp Physiol. 2002;283(4):R815-26.
11. La Rovere MT, Pinna GD, Raczak G. Baroreflex sensitivity: Measurement and clinical implications. Ann Noninvasive Electrocardiol. 2008;13(2):191-207.
12. Lohmeier TE, Hildebrandt DA, Dwyer TM, Iliescu R, Irwin ED, Cates AW, et al. Prolonged activation of the baroreflex decreases arterial pressure even during chronic adrenergic blockade. Hypertension. 2009;53(5):833-8.
13. DiBona GF, Kopp UC. Neural control of renal function. Physiol Rev. 1997;77(1):75-197.
14. Reed MJ, Robertson CE, Addison PS. Heart rate variability measurements and the prediction of ventricular arrhythmias. Quart J Med. 2005;98(2):87-95.
15. Tordoir JHM, Scheffers I, Schmidli J, Savolainen H, Liebeskind U, Hansky B, et al. An implantable carotid sinus baroreflex activating system: Surgical technique and

short-term outcome from a multi-center feasibility trial for treatment of resistant hypertension. Eur J Vasc Endovasc Surg. 2007;33(4):414-21.
16. Alnima T, Scheffers I, De Leeuw PW, Winkens B, Jongen-Vancraybex H, Tordoir JHM, et al. Sustained acute voltage-dependent blood pressure decrease with prolonged carotid baroreflex activation in therapy-resistant hypertension. J Hypertens. 2012;30(8):1665-70.
17. Scheffers IJ, Kroon AA, Schmidli J, Jordan J, Tordoir JJM, Mohaupt MG, et al. Novel baroreflex activation therapy in resistant hypertension: Results of a European multi-center feasibility study. J Am Coll Cardiol. 2010;56(15):1254-8.
18. Bakris GL, Nadim MK, Haller H, Lovett EG, Schafer JE, Bisognano JD, et al. Baroreflex activation therapy provides durable benefit in patients with resistant hypertension: Results of long-term follow-up in the Rheos Pivotal Trial. J Am Soc Hypertens. 2012;6(2):152-8.
19. Wallbach M, Lehnig LY, Schroer C, Helms HJ, Lüders S, Patschan D, et al. Effects of baroreflex activation therapy on arterial stiffness and central hemodynamics in patients with resistant hypertension. J Hypertens. 2015;33(1):181-6.
20. Hoppe UC, Brandt MC, Wachter R, Beige J, Rump LC, Kroon AA, et al. Minimally invasive system for baroreflex activation therapy chronically lowers blood pressure with pacemaker-like safety profile: Results from the Barostim neo trial. J Am Soc Hypertens. 2012;6(4):270-6.
21. Spiering W, Williams B, van der Heyden J, van Kleef M, Lo R, Versmissen J, et al. Endovascular baroreflex amplification for resistant hypertension: A safety and proof-of-principle clinical study. Lancet. 2017;390(10113):2655-61.
22. Bisognano JD, Bakris G, Nadim MK, Sanchez L, Kroon AA, Schafer J, et al. Baroreflex activation therapy lowers blood pressure in patients with resistant hypertension: Results from the double-blind, randomized, placebo-controlled Rheos pivotal trial. J Am Coll Cardiol. 2011;58(7):765-73.
23. Alnima T, De Leeuw PW, Tan FE, Kroon AA, et al. Renal responses to long-term carotid baroreflex activation therapy in patients with drug-resistant hypertension. Hypertension. 2013;61(6):1334-9.

SECTION 12: Guidelines and Meta-analysis

43. Comparison of Various Guidelines in Hypertension: Which is Best for India?
    Anant Ramkishanrao Munde, Sadanand R Shetty

CHAPTER 43

Comparison of Various Guidelines in Hypertension: Which is Best for India?

Anant Ramkishanrao Munde, Sadanand R Shetty

BACKGROUND

Hypertension (HTN) is the leading cause of cardiovascular (CV) mortality and morbidity worldwide with more than a billion people in the world living with HTN.[1,2] It is of particular importance in Asia as more than half of the world's population with HTN live in Asia and is expected to rise further as the population ages and with increasing obesity in the region.[3,4] There is hardly any doubt in today's clinical practice that treatment of HTN is very effective in reducing CV mortality and morbidity.

However, there is a wide disparity in awareness, treatment, and control rates between high-income and low-to-middle-income countries many of which are in Asia.[5,6] Guidelines on the management of HTN have been developed by various professional bodies and institutions primarily address the issues of diagnosis, treatment, and control in order to rationalize and improve the management of HTN. While initial guidelines were developed in the United States (US) and Europe and used by many practitioners, many Asian countries have more recently produced their own national guidelines.

CHRONOLOGY OF HYPERTENSION GUIDELINES

The United States Guidelines

The US was the first to introduce guidelines on the management of HTN in 1977 developed by the Joint National Committee (JNC) an organization established in 1972 through the US National Institute of Health. Subsequently, updates were done periodically. In the JNC VII in 2003, instead of the previous classification of what was termed "normal" and "borderline" blood pressure (BP), the term pre-HTN was introduced for the first time to replace these two categories of BP, that is, pre-HTN for systolic blood pressure (SBP) between 120 and 139 mm Hg and/or diastolic blood pressure (DBP) between 80–89 mm Hg. This itself raised a lot of discussions then but surprisingly no further updates or changes were forthcoming until 14 years later in November 2017 when instead of the JNC, it was the professional societies led by the American Society of Cardiology, American Heart Association who were tasked with issuing an update to the JNC VII. As history tells us a major and, in some ways, controversial change in 2017, guidelines were in the threshold for the diagnosis of HTN where any BP ≥130/80 mm Hg is deemed to receive a diagnosis of HTN. Consequently, the target of control for most adults was also lowered to a BP of <130/80 mm Hg.[7]

European Guidelines

It was several years later in 2003 that the European Society of Hypertension (ESH) released their first guidelines on the management of HTN. New updates were published in 2007, 2013, and the latest in August 2018. Unlike the US guidelines, the ESH in their latest update did not alter the threshold for the diagnosis of HTN but instead retained it as a BP of ≥140/90 mm Hg. However, their new recommended target BP for control of <130/80 mm Hg for most adults and most of the associated clinical conditions such as stroke and coronary artery disease (CAD) was strangely lower than their diagnostic threshold.[8]

A revolutionary departure from their previous guidelines was the recommendation for the use of combination drugs as initial therapy in patients with HTN. This was in part driven by the new and more stringent BP target of <130/80 mm Hg and also by the ample evidence that most patients need 2 or more drugs even to achieve the previous higher target of <140/90 mm Hg.

The exceptions to combination therapy as initial therapy as recommended by the ESH-European Society of Cardiology (ESC) are to consider use of monotherapy in low-risk grade 1 HTN (SBP <150 mm Hg), or in very old (≥80 years) or frailer patients. The American Heart Association/American College of Cardiology (AHA-ACC) guidelines recommend initiation of combination therapy for those with stage 2 HTN and an average BP >20/10 mm Hg above their BP target. However, because the US' definition of stage 2 HTN is a BP ≥140/90 mm Hg, effectively this is similar to the ESC-ESH's recommendations of using combination therapy as initial therapy in patients with HTN. For their stage 1 HTN, that is BP 130–139/80–89 mm Hg, monotherapy is recommended. All other guidelines, on the contrary, continue to recommend monotherapy as initial therapy for patients with HTN, except when the BP is ≥160/100 mm Hg whence dual therapy can be considered as initial therapy.

International Guidelines

To improve the management of HTN, the International Society of Hypertension (ISH) published in 2014 with the American Society of Hypertension Clinical Practice Guidelines for the Management of Hypertension in the Community. Subsequently, ISH was developed and issued for the first time in 2020 as a worldwide practice guidelines.[9] Recognizing that there are disparities of resources between high- and low- to middle-income countries, the ISH tailored recommendations as essential and optimal standards of care in a practical format that is easy-to-use particularly in low, but also in high resource settings by clinicians, but also nurses and community health workers, as appropriate. The International Consortium on Health Outcome Measurement (ICHOM) has also recommended standards of care in low- and middle-income countries that would be appropriate for use in South East and East Asia countries.[10]

Asian Guidelines

Low- and middle-income regions often follow guidelines from high-income regions closely, as their resources and health systems to develop and implement local guidelines remain challenging. However, more recently several countries in Asia particularly the low-middle-income countries with large populations but low treatment and control rates have developed their national guidelines. Except for a few countries such as Cambodia, most South East Asian countries do have their national guidelines **(Table 1)** shows the year of their latest guidelines, and as can be seen, almost everyone except Singapore released an updated guideline after 2017, the year the latest US guidelines were released.[11-27]

DIFFERENCES AND SIMILARITIES

Although guidelines were developed based on existing evidence and using the same evidence base, there were still differences in their recommendations particularly on the diagnostic BP threshold. There were also differences in the recommendations for the use of out-of-office BP measurements, the target BP for control and initiation of drug therapy, and the use of combination therapy, in particular, the single-pill combination. However, there were also many similarities.

The differences and similarities from the angle of the diagnostic BP threshold, BP categories, recommendations for overall CV risk assessment, use of out-of-office BP measurements, initiation of anti-HTN therapy (for all adults, adults with increased CV risk, older adults and adults with specific indications), and the recommended target of BP control in the various groups are discussed in the following sections.

DIAGNOSTIC BP THRESHOLD FOR HYPERTENSION AND HYPERTENSION CATEGORIES

The US guidelines created a lot of controversies and discussions when they lowered the threshold for the diagnosis of HTN to a SBP of ≥130 mm Hg and/or a DBP ≥80 mm Hg in 2017.[28] However, almost all other guidelines following the release of the US guidelines including the ESH, ISH, and many of the Asian guidelines retained the diagnostic threshold of ≥140/90 mm Hg **(Table 1)**.[11] Changes also occurred in the HTN categories. The US guidelines no longer had a stage 3 HTN group, only classifying a BP of between 130/80 and 140/90 as stage 1 and anything above 140/90 as stage 2 HTN. The ESH retained the three grades of HTN, while for the Asian guidelines, all except Korea retained three categories of HTN **(Table 1)**. Like the US guidelines, the ISH opted for two categories of HTN only. When it comes to what is deemed "normal" BP, the guidelines differed considerably. The US because of the new lower diagnostic threshold for HTN now considers an SBP of <120 mm Hg and DBP of <80 mm Hg as normal while many of the Asian guidelines considered these levels as optimal and SBP of 120–129 and/or DBP of 80–85 as "normal" The ESH, on the contrary, deemed SBP 120–129 and/or DBP <80 mm Hg as normal while the ISH used SBP <130 mm Hg and DBP <85 mm Hg as "normal" BP **(Table 1)**. One of the reasons for the lower diagnostic BP threshold proposed by the US was attributed to the available and consistent epidemiological evidence as well as several meta-analyses which showed that a BP of between 130–139/80–90 mm Hg already carries a 1.5–2 times the risk of coronary and stroke events compared to SBP below 120 mm Hg. Because of this increased CV risk even at BP lower than the conventional HTN BP threshold of ≥140/90 mm Hg, it was felt to be important to identify those at increased risk so that preventive measures are in place early, especially as it is known BP rises with increasing age. The concern with adopting this lower BP threshold is that many more people will now be labeled as "hypertensive" which by itself carries its own psychological, economic, and social issues. However, to be fair to the US, they do not recommend that all such individuals with BP in the range 130–139/80–89 mm Hg be treated pharmacologically but to implement lifestyle changes and only be given drugs if associated with atherosclerotic cardiovascular disease events (ASCVD) or target organ damage or the overall CV risk is greater than 10%. Although the prevalence of HTN will be increased from 31.9 to 45% an increase of 13.7%, the extra

TABLE 1: Blood pressure categories UK, European, International, and Asian HTN guidelines.

BP category (mm Hg)	AHA/ACC 2017	ESC/ESH 2018	ISH 2020	CHL 2018	HK 2018	India 2019	Indonesia 2019	JSH 2019
SBP <120 and DBP <80	Normal	Optimal		Normal	Optimal	Optimal	Optimal	Normal
SBP: 120–129 and DBP <80	Elevated							High normal
SBP 120–129 and DBP 80–84		Normal			Normal	–	Normal	
SBP 120–139 and DBP 80–89				High normal				
SBP <130 and/or DBP <85			Normal			Normal		
SBP 130–139 and/or DBP 80–89	Grade 1							Elevated
SBP 130–139 and/or DBP 85–89		High normal	High normal		High normal	High normal	High normal	
SBP 140–159 and/or DBP 90–99	Grade 2	Grade 1	Grade 1	Grade 1 (mild)	Grade 1	Stage 1	Grade 1	Grade 1
SBP 160–179 and/or DBP 100–109	Grade 2	Grade 2	Grade 2	Grade 2 (moderate)	Grade 2	Stage 2	Grade 2	Grade 2
SBP ≥180 and/or DBP ≥110	Grade 2	Grade 3	Grade 2	Grade 3 (severe)	Grade 3	Stage 3	Grade 3	Grade 3
SBP ≥140 and DBP <90	NA	ISH	ISH	ISH	ISH	ISH	ISH	ISH
CV risk assessment	Yes	Yes	Yes	Yes	Yes	Yes	Yes	Yes

Contd...

CHAPTER 43: Comparison of Various Guidelines in Hypertension: Which is Best for India?

Contd...

BP category (mm Hg)	KSH 2018	Malaysia 2018	Pakistan 2018	Philippines 2018	Singapore 2017	Taiwan 2015, 2017	Thailand 2019	Vietnam 2018
SBP <120 and DBP <80	Normal	Optimal	Optimal	Normal		Normal	Optimal	Optimal
SBP: 120–129 and DBP <80	Elevated							
SBP 120–129 and DBP 80–84	–	Normal	Elevated			Pre-HTN	Normal	Normal
SBP 120–139 and DBP 80–89				Elevated	Normal			
SBP <130 and/or DBP <85								
SBP 130–139 and/or DBP 80–89	Pre-HTN	At risk	Pre-HTN					
SBP 130–139 and/or DBP 85–89					High normal		High normal	High normal
SBP 140–159 and/or DBP 90–99	Grade 1	Stage 1 (mild)	Stage 1	Stage 1	Grade 1	Stage 1	Stage 1	Grade 1
SBP 160–179 and/or DBP 100–109	Grade 2	Stage 2 (moderate)	Stage 2	Stage 2	Grade 2	Stage 2	Stage 2	Grade 2
SBP ≥180 and/or DBP ≥110	Grade 2	Stage 3 (severe)	Stage 3	Stage 2	Grade 3	Stage 3	Stage 3	Grade 3
SBP ≥140 and DBP <90	ISH	ISH	ISH	ISH	ISH	ISH	ISH	ISH
CV risk assessment	Yes	Yes	Yes	Yes	Yes	Yes	Yes	Yes

(AHA/ACC: American Heart Association/American College of Cardiology; BP: blood pressure; CHL: Chinese Hypertension League; CV: cardiovascular; DBP: diastolic blood pressure; ESC/ESH: European Society of Cardiology/European Society of Hypertension; HK: Hong Kong; ISH: International Society of Hypertension; JSH: Japanese Society of Hypertension; KSH: Korean Society of Hypertension; NA: not available; SBP: systolic blood pressure) number of people needing pharmacological agents will only be increased by 1.9% from 34.3 to 36.2%.[29] Perhaps another reason is because of the Systolic Blood Pressure Intervention Trial (SPRINT) study which showed that hypertensives treated more intensively to achieve a lower BP target of <120/80 mm Hg benefitted more reduction in CV mortality and morbidity than a BP of <140/90 mm Hg.[30] However, patients with SBPs of <143.5 mm Hg in the HOPE-3 study did not benefit from BP-lowering drugs compared to those with baseline SBP >143.5 mm Hg.[31] A further important point to note is that the HOPE-3 was a primary prevention trial of patients with intermediate CV risk while the SPRINT patients were of high CV risk highlighting that the treatment threshold and goal BP may be different for individuals with different CV risk.

GLOBAL CARDIOVASCULAR RISK ASSESSMENT

Although earlier JNC editions on the management of HTN did include statements about the increased risk of CV mortality and morbidity in HTN individuals with other CV risk factors such as smoking, presence of diabetes, hyperlipidemia, there were no recommendations about overall/global CV risk assessment until JNC VI in 1997 where a new table describing risk stratification were added. Cardiovascular risk was stratified into three groups moving from lower to higher risk, where group A were HTN patients with no other CV risk factors and with no target organ damage or clinical cardiovascular disease (CVD); group B patients with at least one CV risk factor but no diabetes, or target organ damage or clinical CVD; and group C HTN patients with target organ damage or CVD and/or diabetes, with or without other CV risk factors were added. These groups stratified by risk served as a guide as to when to initiate anti-HTN therapy and that it is not just based on the absolute BP reading alone but on the presence or the absence of other CV risk factors. In the latest US guidelines, a formal approach to stratify CV risk was introduced where it was recommended that an overall CV risk assessment be done and an absolute value of risk be assigned to certain patients. This was of particular importance in those without coexisting ASCVD or diabetes, as their recommendation in this group of patients is that a BP between 130–139/80–89 mm Hg and with a CV risk of 10% using the pooled Cohort risk calculator or greater should be treated pharmacologically.

The 2018 ESH guidelines stratified CV risk by categories of low, moderate, high, or very high-risk factoring in the HTN stages according to BP levels, presence of CV risk factors, hypertension-mediated organ damage (HMOD), or comorbidities.

Similar to the ESH, the ISH stratified CV risk by BP levels according to additional risk factors, HMOD, and previous CVD but has only 3 instead of 4 categories, that is, low, medium, or high.

Almost all the Asian guidelines also recommend performing an overall CV risk assessment **(Table 1)**. Most Asian countries except for Thailand do not have their own country's risk prediction chart nor have they validated existing risk calculation tools. Hence, most guidelines did not specifically recommend the use of any CV risk assessment tools but adopted and recommended the risk categories recommended by ESH for overall CV risk assessment. While the Malaysian guidelines' risk stratification table differs slightly from the ESH's and is recommended for use, the Framingham General CVD prediction tool has been validated and found to work well especially as the background CV risk of Malaysia mirrors that at the height of the CV epidemic in the US around the 1950s.[32]

While there are differences in the risk categories, on a clinical and practical level, most guidelines recommend drug therapy as soon as the CV risk is high and some like the Malaysia guidelines even at medium CV risk.

USE OF OUT-OF-OFFICE BP MEASUREMENTS

The benefits of out-of-office BP measurements are well known. Besides being better predictors of CV mortality and morbidity than office BP, they are needed to identify white coat hypertension (WCH), masked and resistant HTN as well as to monitor BP control. The use of HBPM has been shown to lead to lower BPs, better adherence, and patient satisfaction.

The use of out-of-office BP measurements, using ambulatory blood pressure monitoring (ABPM) measurements or home blood pressure measurement (HBPM) to confirm the diagnosis of HTN, was first recommended by the National Institute for Health and Clinical Excellence (NICE) of the United Kingdom in 2011 and retained in their recent update in 2019. This created quite a lot of concern especially as many low-to middle-income countries in Asia do not have ABPM and not many patients have HBPM.[5] The rationale for recommending this was that many individuals found to have an elevated BP in the office/clinic may have a normal BP while out of the office/clinic, a situation called WCH. Identifying those with WCH translates to cost savings and adverse effects for the individuals for unnecessary drug treatment.

Not all the recent guidelines subscribed to this recommendation as the diagnosis of HTN is still based on office/clinic measurements although out-of-office BP measurements are encouraged to help in confirming the diagnosis. Furthermore, most Asian countries do not have their own HBPM consensus to guide practitioners on its appropriate use but Asian consensus and insights on the use of HBPM and ABPM have recently been published to aid practitioners in Asia in the interim.[33-36]

Although the US lowered their diagnostic office BP threshold to ≥130/80 mm Hg, their diagnostic for both HBPM and day ABPM threshold is also ≥130/80 mm Hg, and this is puzzling as it has been shown that HBPM tends to be around 5 mm Hg lower than office readings. However, the US did lower their ABPM threshold for the 24-h and night by 5 mm Hg. On the contrary, the ESC/ESH, ISH, and Asian countries retained their previous thresholds for out-of-office BP levels **(Table 2)**.

While NICE recommends out-of-office BP measurements for confirming a diagnosis of HTN, it does not recommend that titration of treatment to reach the BP target be based on HBPM. This is primarily because there is very little or at least no good evidence yet that treating HTN based on HBPM results in a better reduction in CV mortality or morbidity compared to using the conventional clinic BPs, which are backed up by numerous clinical outcome trials.

TABLE 2: Thresholds for diagnosing HTN based on clinic and out-of-office (HBPM and ABPM) BP for US, Europe, and Asia.

	ACC/AHA	ESC/ESH	ISH	Asia
Clinic	130/80	140/90	140/90	140/90
Home	130/80	135/85	135/85	135/85
ABPM: Daytime	130/80	135/85	135/85	135/85
Nighttime	110/65	120/70	120/70	120/70
24-h average	125/75	130/80	130/80	130/80

(ABPM: ambulatory blood pressure monitoring; ACC/AHA: American College of Cardiology/American Heart Association; BP: blood pressure; ESC/ESH: European Society of Cardiology/European Society of Hypertension; HBPM: home blood pressure measurement; HTN: Hypertension; ISH: International Society of Hypertension)

The latest US guidelines have also recommended wider use of out-of-office BP measurements and like NICE recommends it for confirming and titration of BP-lowering medication. ESH recommends out-of-office, measurements to confirm diagnosis but only when it is logistically and economically feasible. ISH recognizes that out-of-office BP measurements may not be feasible in most low-to-middle countries and has recommended out-of-office measurements as optimal and not essential.

In general, all the Asian guidelines have in their latest guidelines recommended wider use of out-of-office BP measurements, and to confirm the diagnosis if feasible. However, while all the guidelines do recommend and encourage the use of HBPM, the recommendation except for Japan is still to use office/clinic BPs to titrate medication while HBPM acts as a complement to management. In Japan, anti-HTN treatment based on HBPM is strongly recommended (recommendation grade 1 evidence level B).[17]

INITIATION AND CHOICE OF ANTIHYPERTENSIVE MEDICATIONS

There is universal agreement across all the guidelines that anti-HTN drugs be given if the BP is ≥160/90 mm Hg regardless of the CV risk. In such instances, a combination of two agents can be initiated except in those ≥75 years old. There is also agreement among almost all guidelines, except the US and Hong Kong guidelines, that for BPs between 140–159/90–99 mm Hg treatment with pharmacological agents should be based not on the BP alone but on the overall CV risk as well **(Table 3)**. For these guidelines, the recommendation for those with this level of BP and with medium or higher risk, anti-HTN agents are recommended. In contrast, the AHA/ACC recommends anti-HTN drugs for those with a BP ≥140/90 mm Hg without considering the overall CV risk. Because Hong Kong does not factor in CV risk, the indication for treatment is to start when BP is ≥160/100 mm Hg and only to start treatment for those with BP 140–159/90–99 mm Hg when lifestyle modifications fail after 6 months.

For the US guidelines, the recommendation is that all BPs ≥140/90 mm Hg (i.e., their stage 2) should be treated with BP-lowering medication. For those with BP between 130–139/80–89 (their stage 1), the recommendation is that anti-HTN medication should be prescribed if there is any ASCVD or the overall CV risk is ≥10%.[28] On the contrary, the European and Asian guidelines recommend pharmacological agents in individuals with a BP between 130–139/80–89 mm Hg only if their CV risk is high or very high. The ESH differ somewhat in their recommendation of initial therapy, where a combination of two drugs are recommended except for those with low-risk stage 1 HTN (BP 140–159/90–99 mm Hg) or in the very old (≥80 years) or frailer patients.[8]

In terms of choice of first-line anti-HTN drugs, the US recommends calcium channel blockers (CCBs), diuretics (Dus), angiotensin-converting enzyme inhibitor (ACE-I), and angiotensin receptor blocker (ARB) omitting β-blockers (BBs). The ESC/ESH, on the contrary, recommends all five classes including BB as possible first-line drugs. ISH, recognizing limited resources in low-to-middle-income countries, recommends any class of drugs that is available as long as they are evidence-based in relation to morbidity/mortality prevention and benefit the population being treated. Similar to the US, in general, the Asian countries' recommendation for first-line monotherapy

CHAPTER 43: Comparison of Various Guidelines in Hypertension: Which is Best for India?

TABLE 3: Initiation and choice of anti-HTN drugs.

Indications	AHA/ACC	ESC/ESH	ISH	Hong Kong	Japan
BP ≥130/80 mm Hg	Treat if ASCVD is positive or CV risk is ≥10%	Consider treatment in very high-risk with CVD, especially CAD	Treat if ASCVD is positive or DM or CKD or HMOD	Treat if ASCVD is positive or DM or CKD, CAD	Treat if high risk and LSC insufficient after 1 month
BP 140–159/90–99 mm Hg	Drug treatment	Immediate treatment in high or very high-risk with CVD, CKD, or HMOD	Immediate treatment in high risk or with CVD, CKD, DM, or HMOD	Consider starting if LSC is insufficient after 6 months or if HMOD is present	• Low/moderate risk treatment if LSC is insufficient after 1 month • High-risk immediate drug treatment
BP ≥160/110 mm Hg	Drug treatment	Immediate drug treatment	Immediate treatment in all patients		Immediate drug treatment
First-line drug	DU, CCB ACE-I, ARB	DU, CCB-ACE-I, ARB, BB	Any of DU, CCB-ACE-I, ARB, BB if available	DU, CCB-ACE-I, ARB	DU, CCB-ACE-I, ARB

Indications	Korea	Singapore	Taiwan	Upper middle income (China, Indonesia, Malaysia, Thailand)	Lower middle income (India, Pakistan, Philippines, Vietnam)
BP ≥130/80 mm Hg	LSC or treat if ASCVD is positive or CAD DM or CKD	–	Treat if DM or CHD or CKD	Drug treatment if ASCVD is positive, DM, HMOD	Drug treatment if ASCVD is positive, DM, HMOD
BP 140–159/90–99 mm Hg	Treat if RF ≥1, or DM or CVD or CKD or HMOD	Drug treatment	Drug treatment	Immediate drug treatment if very high risk, ASCVD is positive, DM, or CKD	Immediate drug treatment if very high risk, ASCVD is positive, DM, or CKD
BP ≥160/110 mm Hg	Immediate drug treatment	Immediate treatment	Drug treatment	Immediate drug treatment	Immediate drug treatment
First-line drug	DU, CCB ACE-I, ARB, BB	DU, CCB ACE-I, ARB, BB	Depends on indication but all 5 classes can be used	DU, CCB-ACE-I, ARB	DU, CCB ACE-I, ARB, BB except Pakistan: ACE-I, ARB, CCB

(ACE-I: angiotensin-converting enzyme inhibitor; AHA/ACC: American Heart Association/American College of Cardiology; ARB: angiotensin receptor blockers; ASCVD: atherosclerotic cardiovascular disease; BP: blood pressure; CAD: coronary artery disease; CCB: calcium channel blocker; CHD: coronary heart disease; CV: cardiovascular; CVD: cardiovascular disease; BB: β-blocker; DM: diabetes mellitus; DU: diuretic; ESC/ESH: European Society of Cardiology/European Society of Hypertension; HMOD: hypertension-mediated organ damage; ISH: International Society of Hypertension; LSC: lifestyle changes) includes DU, CCB, ACE-I, and ARB except for China, Indonesia, India, Korea, Singapore, and Thailand which also recommend BB as first-line as well **(Table 3)**.

For special groups of HTN patients, for example, HTN and CAD, HTN, and stroke, again there is universal agreement about the class of anti-HTN. In general, most of these patients require at least two drugs as their BP target is also lower, and almost all the combinations include an ACE-I or ARB with a CCB or DU Japan recommends for adults of age below 75 years and in special groups, a lower clinic BP target of less than 130/80 mm Hg and home BP Less than 125/75 mm Hg while for those ≥75 years old, a higher target of clinic BP <140/90 and home BP <135/85 mm Hg is recommended **(Table 3)**.

■ BP TARGET FOR CONTROL

The US recommends a lower BP target of <130/80 mm Hg as they use BP ≥130/80 mm Hg for the definition of HTN. This target applies to all groups of HTN patients regardless of their CV risk **(Table 4)**.

Although the ESH guidelines retained the diagnostic threshold as BP ≥140/90 mm Hg, their target for all groups of HTN in <65 years is surprisingly <130/80 mm Hg but not going to SBP of <120 mm Hg except in those with chronic kidney disease (CKD). In those ≥65 years old, the target is 130–139/70–79 mm Hg if tolerated.

The ISH's recommended target is similar to ESH. The guidelines have made very clear recommendations about drug choice for special groups **(Table 4)**. The recommendations of drug choice for each special group are very similar, mostly recommending renin-angiotensin system (RAS) blockers as the base and in combination with CCBs or Dus or as clinically indicated, for example, in patients with CAD, it is universal a BB is also recommended besides the RAS blockers.

Most guidelines did not make any specific recommendation for individuals with metabolic syndrome and HTN. The only exception is Taiwan who recommends ACE-I or ARB and not Dus or BBs unless clearly indicated for other existing comorbidities and India who recommends an ACE-I or ARB.[25]

Multiple sclerosis (MS) is very prevalent even in Asia and will increase with the epidemic of increasing obesity. Hence, it is important that future guidelines make specific commendations for such a situation.

For Asian countries, again all the countries except Japan recommend for patients with HTN BP <140/90 mm Hg as their target of control and lower targets of <130/80 mm Hg if tolerated. Japan's target is similar to the US' target, which is for <130/80 mm Hg for all HTN patients including those in the special groups.

Most Asian countries recommend the lower targets of <130/80 mm Hg for the special group of patients with HTN, with certain countries opting for the interim target of <140/90 (e.g., China), but going lower to <130/80 if tolerated. The classification of the elderly to varies somewhat in Asian countries but in general, the recommendation of target control is <140/90 mm for those under 75 years old and <150/90 mm Hg for those 75 years or older. Japan, on the contrary, recommends for adults <75 years a lower clinic BP target of <130/80 mm Hg and home BP <125/75 mm Hg, while for those ≥75 years, a higher target of clinic BP <140/90 and home BP <135/85 mm Hg is recommended but still 10 mm Hg lower than other Asian countries **(Table 4)**.

Of interest is the time frame to reach BP control. Studies have shown that early treatment can reduce left ventricular

CHAPTER 43: Comparison of Various Guidelines in Hypertension: Which is Best for India?

TABLE 4: Target for BP control and recommended anti-HTN drugs in special groups.*

	AHA/ACC 2017	ESC/ESH 2018	ISH 2020	CHL 2018	HK 2018	India 2019	Indo 2019	Japan 2019
Target BP mm Hg	<130/80	SBP 130 DBP 7079	<140/90	<140/90	<140/90	<130/80	SBP ≤130 DBP 70–79	<130/80
HTN + CAD	<130/80	SBP 130 DBP 70–79	<130/80	<140/90	NR	NR	SBP ≤130 DBP 70–79	<130/80
HTN + CVA	<130/80	SBP 130 DBP 70–79	<130/80	<140/90	NR	NR	SBP ≤130 DBP 70–79	<130/80 HBPM <125/75
HTN + HF	<130/80	SBP 130 DBP 70–79	<130/80 but not <120/70	<130/80	NR	<130/80	NR	SBP <130 DBP is not <80
HTN + UA	<130/80	<130–139/ 70–79	<130/80	NR	NR	NR	NR	<130/80
HTN + CKD	<130/80	SBP <140–130 If tolerated DBP 70–79	<130/80	• UAE is negative, <140/90 • UAE is positive, <130/80	V130/80	NR	SBP <140–130 if tolerated DBP 70–79	Office <130/80 HBPM <125/75
HTN + DM	<130/80	SBP 130 DB? 70–79	<130/80	<130/80	<130/80	NR	SBP ≤130 DBP 70–79	Office <130/80 HBPM <125/75
HTN + MS	NR	NR	NR	NR	NR	NR	NR	NR
HTN ≥65 years	<130/80	130–139/ 70–79	<140/90	<140/90	NR	130–140/ 80–90	SBP 130–139	<130/80
HTN ≥75 years					NR	130–140/ 80–90	SBP 130–139	Office <140/90 HBPM <135/85
HTN ≥80 years		130–139/ 70–79		<150/90	NR	130–140/ 80–90		

Contd...

Contd...

Drug choice in special groups	AHA/ACC 2017	ESC/ESH 2018	ISH 2020	CHL 2018	HK 2018	India 2019	Indo 2019	Japan 2019
HTN + CAD	BB RAS, CCB	RAS+BB/CCB or DU	RAS CCB DU	BB CCB+ACE DU	ACE BB, CCB	BB	BB/CCB + ARB/DU or BB/DU + CCB or BB + DU	BB CCB
HTN + CVA	DU RAS	RAS + CCB/DU	RAS CCB DU	CCB RAS DU	ACE BB, CCB	CCB	NR	CCBs, RAS DU
HTN + HF	RAS BB DU MRA (non-DHP CCB)	RAS, BB and MRAs	RAS, BB and MRA	RAS BB MRA	ACE DU	BB	RAS + DU + BB	RAS BB MRA + CCB DU
HTN + UA	RAS	RAS + CCB/DU	RAS + CCB DU	RAS+CCB DU	ACE	RAS	NR	NR
HTN + CKD	RAS	RAS + CCB/DU	RAS + CCB DU (loop)	RAS + CCB/DU	ACE	RAS ESRD α-B, central acting	RAS + CCB/DU	• Protein is positive, RAS • Protein is negative, RAS CCB DU
HTN + DM	DU, RAS CCB	RAS + CCB/DU	RAS ± CCB/DU	RAS+CCB DU			RAS + CCB/DU	• Alb is positive, RAS • Alb is negative, BB/DU + CBB/DU
HTN + MS	NR	NR	NR	NR	NR	RAS	NR	NR
HTN ≥65 years	DU CCB RAS						NR	
HTN ≥75 years		DU CCB RAS	DU CCB RAS	DU CCB RAS	CCB DU	CCB DU	NR monotherapy	CCB RAS DU
HTN ≥80 years								

Contd...

CHAPTER 43: Comparison of Various Guidelines in Hypertension: Which is Best for India?

Contd...

	Korea 2018	Malaysia 2018	Pakistan 2018	Philippines 2018	Singapore 2017	Taiwan 2015, 2017	Thailand 2019	Vietnam 2018
Target BP (mm Hg)	<140/90	<140/90	≤140/90	<130/80	<140/90	<140/90	120–130/70–79	<130/80
HTN + CAD	<130/80	<130/80	<130/80	NR	NR	<130/80	120–130/70–79	SBP 130 DBP 70–79
HTN + CVA	<130/80 lacunar stroke	<140/80	<130/80 lacunar stroke	<130/80	<130/80	Individualized	<140/90 120–130/70–79	SBP 130 DBP 70–79
HTN + HF	<130/80	<140/90	NR	NR	NR	NR	<130/80	SBP 130 DBP 70–79
HTN + UA	<130/80	• Proteinuria <1 g <140/90 • Proteinuria >1 g <130/80	NR	NR	<130/80	<120/NR	NR	<130–139/70–79
HTN + CKD	• UAE is negative, <140/90 • UAE is positive <130/80	• Proteinuria <1 g <140/90 • Proteinuria >1 g <130/80	<130/80	<130/80	<140/90 If + DM <130/80	• UAE is negative, <140/90 • UAE is positive, <130/80	120–130/70–79	SBP <140–130 If tolerated DBP 70–79
HTN + DM	<140/85, complicated <130/80	<140/90 If high-risk DM <130/80	<130/80	<130/80	• UAE is negative, <140/80 • UAE is negative, <130/80	<130/80	120–130/70–79	SBP 130 DBP 70–79
HTN + MS	NR	NR	NR	NR	NR	NR	NR	NR
HTN ≥65 years	<140/90	<140/90	NR	NR	NR	<140/90	130–139/70–79	SBP 130 DBP 70–79
HTN ≥75 years			NR	NR				
HTN ≥80 years		SBP <150	<150/90	<140/90	<150/90	<150/90	120–130/70–79	

Contd...

Contd...

	Korea 2018	Malaysia 2018	Pakistan 2018	Philippines 2018	Singapore 2017	Taiwan 2015, 2017	Thailand 2019	Vietnam 2018
HTN + CAD	BB CCB	BB RAS	BB, ACE	BB	BB, RAS	BB, RAS, CCB	BB RAS	RAS + BB CCB/DU
HTN + CVA	DU, RAS or DU + RAS	<140/90 If lacunar stroke <130/80	NR	RAS CCB, DU	DU CCB RAS BB	RAS, DU CCB	ACE-i+DU	RAS+CCB/DU Diuretic
HTN + HF	BB RAS MRA	BB RAS MRA	DU BB RAS MRA	BB DU	RAS, DU, BB, MRA	DU/loop DU BB RAS, MRA	RAS BB	RAS, BB and MRA
HTN + UA	NR	RAS + non-DHP CCB	NR	RAS CCB	RAS	RAS	RAS	RAS + CCB/DU
HTN + CKD	RAS if albuminuria	RAS + non-DHP CCB BP not to target DHP	RAS	RAS DU Non-DHP CCB	RAS	RAS loop DU	Any drug classes	RAS + CCB/DU
HTN + DM	RAS	RAS	RAS	RAS DU CCB	RAS CCB	RAS direct renin inhibitor	RAS CCB	DU, RAS CCB
HTN + MS	RAS CCB BB DU + RAS	NR	NR	NR	NR	RAS	NR	NR
HTN ≥65 years								
HTN ≥75 years	RAS CCB DU	DU CCB	DU CCB RAS	EAS, CCB, DU	CCB DU	NR	NR	DU CCB RAS
HTN ≥80 years								

(ACC/AHA: American College of Cardiology/American Heart Association; ACE: angiotensin-converting enzyme inhibitor; Alb: albuminuria; BB: β-blocker; BP: blood pressure; CAD: coronary artery disease; CCB: calcium channel blocker; CKD: chronic kidney disease; CVA: cerebrovascular accident; DBP: diastolic blood pressure; DHP: dihydropyridine; DM: diabetes mellitus; DU: diuretic; ESRD: end-stage renal disease; ESC/ESH: European Society of Cardiology/European Society of Hypertension; HTN: hypertension; HBPM: home blood pressure measurement; HF: heart failure; ISH: International Society of Hypertension; MRA: mineralocorticoid receptor antagonist; MS: multiple sclerosis (MS); NR: no recommendation; RAS: renin-angiotensin system inhibitors [includes ACE and angiotensin receptor blocker (ARB)]; SBP: systolic blood pressure; UA: unstable angina; UAE: urinary albumin excretion)
*Blood pressure, diastolic blood pressure, and systolic blood pressure measurements are presented in mm Hg.

hypertrophy significantly within 6 months of treatment. Separation of stroke incidence can also be seen within 6 months of better BP lowering in clinical outcome trials. However, most guidelines except for China, Indonesia, Japan, Malaysia, and Pakistan do not clearly specify the time frame to reach control **(Table 4)**. Again, this aspect may need to be highlighted more in future guidelines.

TARGET BLOOD PRESSURE IN ELDERLY

While the diagnostic BP threshold for the elderly remains the same as that for younger individuals, that is, ≥140/90 mm Hg by all guidelines and ≥130/80 mm Hg by the US guidelines, the target BP for control in the elderly varies considerably between the guidelines and varies according to different ages used **(Table 4)**. This is in part due to the various definitions of elderly. As a consequence, the recommendations for treatment of HTN in the elderly are complicated by these various definitions of "elderly" or "older" people used in randomized control trials where "older" was defined as >60 years of age in the earliest trials, then as 65, 70, and, finally, 75 or 80 years. Furthermore, many clinical trials did not include patients older than 75 years, and if they did, it was patients who were already on anti-HTN treatment prior to entering into the study.

In their recommendations for the treatment of HTN in the elderly, the ESH categorizes the elderly as two separate groups, that is the "old" as those ≥65 years and "very old" as those aged ≥80 years. Drug therapy is recommended in the old and very old when the BP is ≥140/90 mm Hg and ≥160/90 mm Hg, respectively. However, although the BP treatment threshold is higher for the very old, the target BP is the same at 130–139/70–79 mm Hg, if tolerated, for both the old and very old **(Table 4)**.

The US does not differentiate between the old and the very old, and their recommendation is a target of below 130/80 mm Hg, if tolerated, for anyone ≥65 years old.

The ISH, similar to the Americans, does not separate the elderly by different age groups but considers anyone aged ≥65 years as elderly. They are however more "conservative" than the Europeans and Americans as their BP target in anyone aged ≥65 years is higher at a BP of below 140/80 mm Hg.

Several of the Asian guidelines do differentiate between the "old" and the "very old" elderly but their recommended BP targets of <140/90 mm Hg for the old and below 150/90 mm Hg for the very old are higher than that of the American and European's recommendation of <130/80 and 130–139/70–79 mm Hg, respectively. While several Asian guidelines do make recommendations of BP targets for those aged ≥80 years, they actually did not make any specific recommendation for BP targets in those aged between 65–79 years. Presumably, their BP targets for those <80 years old would be the same as younger adults. On the contrary, several Asian guidelines while making recommendations for BP target for those aged ≥65 years do not make any specific recommendations in those aged ≥80 years, perhaps implying that the target is the same as for those aged 65–79 years **(Table 4)**.

CONCLUSION

In summary, the main difference between the guidelines is the new definition of HTN where the US is the only one with a lower diagnostic BP threshold of ≥130/80 mm Hg. This leads to differences in treatment initiation and BP target of control. The main objective of the

US guideline is to lower the burden of HTN-related disease, and they are trying to do this by identifying at-risk individuals earlier with their lower BP levels for diagnosis of HTN. On the contrary, the ESH and the Asian guidelines are more conservative and more focused on individuals and less on epidemiological issues. It would be interesting to see in the future which strategy will have a greater impact on the reduction of CV mortality and morbidity safely and cost-effectively.

■ REFERENCES

1. World Health Organization. Global status report on non-communicable diseases 2010. Available from: https://appsw hoint/ iris/ bitst ream/handle/10665/ 44579/ 97892 40686 458_engpd f;jsessionid =23A81 CA64B 5CF06 71EA0 F439C 19CDB 49?sequence=1. [Last accessed October, 2020].
2. World Health Organization. Global health observatory data raised blood pressure. Available from: https://wwwwh oint/ gho/ncd/risk_factors/blood_pressure_ prevalence_text/en/ [Last accessed October, 2020].
3. Kearney PM, Whelton M, Reynolds K, Muntner P, Whelton PK, He J. Global burden of hypertension: analysis of worldwide data. Lancet 2005;365(9455):217-23.
4. NCD Risk Factor Collaboration (NCD-RisC). Worldwide trends in blood pressure from 1975 to 2015: a pooled analysis of 1479 population-based measurement studies with 19·1 million participants. Lancet. 2017;389(10064):37-55.
5. Chia Y-C, Buranakitjaroen P, Chen C-H, Divinagracia R, Hoshide S, Park S, et al. Current status of home blood pressure monitoring in Asia: Statement from the HOPE Asia Network. J Clin Hypertens. 2017; 19:1192-201.
6. Mills KT, Bundy JD, Kelly TN, Reed JE, Kearney PM, Reynolds K, et al. Global disparities of hypertension prevalence and control: a systematic analysis of population-based studies from 90 countries. Circulation. 2016;134(6):441-50.
7. Whelton PK, Carey RM, Aronow WS, Casey DE Jr, Collins KJ, Himmelfarb CD, et al. 2017 ACC/AHA/AAPA/ABC/ACPM/AGS/ APhA/ASH/ASPC/NMA/PCNA Guideline for the prevention, detection, evaluation, and management of high blood pressure in adults: Executive summary: A report of the American College of Cardiology/ American Heart Association Task Force on Clinical Practice Guidelines. Hypertension. 2018;71(6):1269-324.
8. Williams B, Mancia G, Spiering W, Rosei EA, Azizi M, Burnier M, et al. 2018 ESC/ ESH guidelines for the management of arterial hypertension. Eur Heart J. 2018;39(33):3021-104.
9. Unger T, Borghi C, Charchar F, Khan NA, Poulter NR, Prabhakaran D, et al. 2020 International Society of Hypertension global hypertension practice guidelines. Hypertension. 2020;75(6):1334-57.
10. Zack R, Okunade O, Olson E, Salt M, Amodeo C, Anchala R, et al. Improving hypertension outcome measurement in low- and middle-income countries. Hypertension. 2019;73(5):990-7.
11. Joint Committee for Guideline Revision. Chinese guidelines for prevention and treatment of hypertension: a report of the revision committee of Chinese guidelines for prevention and treatment of hypertension. J Geriatr Cardiol. 2019;16(3):182-241.
12. Wang J-G, Chia Y-C, Chen C-H, Park S, Hoshide S, Tomitani N, et al. What is new in the 2018 Chinese hypertension guideline and the implication for the management of hypertension in Asia? J Clin Hypertens (Greenwich). 2020;22(3):363-368.
13. Primary Care Office, Department of Health, Hong Kong SAR Government. Hong Kong reference framework for hypertension care for adults in primary care settings. Revised edition; 2018. Available from: https://www. pco.gov.hk/english/resource/professionals_ hypertension_pdf.html [Last accessed October, 2020].

14. Lim MK, Ha SCN, Luk KH, Yip WK, Tsang CSH, Wong MCS. Update on the Hong Kong reference framework for hypertension care for adults in primary care settings: Review of evidence on the definition of high blood pressure and goal of therapy. Hong Kong Med J. 2019;25(1):64-7.
15. Shah SN, Munjal YP, Kamath SA, Wander GS, Mehta N, Mukherjee S, et al. Indian guidelines on hypertension-IV (2019). J Hum Hypertens. 2020;34(11):745-58.
16. Indonesian Society of Hypertension Consensus on Management of Hypertension. Konsensus Penatalaksanaan Hipertensi. 2019. Available from: http://faber.inash.or.id/upload/pdf/article_Update_konsensus_201939.pdf [Last accessed October, 2020]
17. Umemura S, Arima H, Arima S, Asayama K, Dohi Y, Hirooka Y et al. The Japanese Society of Hypertension Guidelines for the Management of Hypertension (JSH 2019). Hypertens Res. 2019;42(9):1235-481.
18. Hoshide S, Kario K, Tomitani N, Kabutoya T, Chia Y-C, Park S, et al. Highlights of the 2019 Japanese Society of Hypertension Guidelines and perspectives on the management of Asian hypertensive patients. J Clin Hypertens. 2020;22(3):369-77.
19. Kim HC, Ihm S-H, Kim G-H, Kim JH, Kim K-I, Lee H-Y, et al. 2018 Korean Society of Hypertension guidelines for the management of hypertension: Part 1 – Epidemiology of hypertension. Clin Hypertens. 2019;25:16.
20. Malaysian clinical practice guidelines on the management of hypertension 2018. 5th ed. http://wwwacadmedorgmy/index cfm?&menui d=67. Accessed October 25, 2020.
21. Pakistan Hypertension League. Third national guideline for the prevention, detection, evaluation and management of hypertension. Available from http://wwwphlpkorg/guideline/3rd%20Hypertension%20Guideline%202018%20PHL pdf [Last accessed October, 2020].
22. Philippines clinical practice guideline for adult hypertension: Prevention, screening, counseling and management. 2018. Available from: https://www.mahealthcare.com/pdf/practice_guidelines/Hypertension.pdf. [Last accessed October, 2020].
23. Singapore Ministry of Health. Hypertension clinical practice guidelines 1/2017. Available from: https://www.moh.gov.sg/docs/librariesprovider4/guidelines/cpg_hypertension-summary-card—nov-2017.pdf [Last accessed October, 2020].
24. Tay JC, Sule AA, Chew EK, Tey JS, Lau T, Lee S, et al. Ministry of health clinical practice guidelines: Hypertension. Singapore Med J. 2018;59(1):17-27.
25. Chiang C-E, Wang T-D, Ueng K-C, Lin T-H, Yeh H-I, Chen C-Y, et al. 2015 Guidelines of the Taiwan Society of Cardiology and the Taiwan Hypertension Society for the management of hypertension. J Chin Med Assoc. 2015;78(1):1-47.
26. Thai Hypertension Society. Guidelines in the treatment of hypertension. http://www.thaihypertension.org/guideline.html. [Last accessed October, 2020].
27. Vietnam National Heart Association/Vietnam Society of Hypertension. Guidelines for diagnosis and treatment of arterial hypertension in adults. Available from: https://www.slideshare.net/tshuynt/2018-vnhavsh-guidelines-for-diagnosis-and-treatment-of-hypertension-in-adults. [Last accessed October, 2020].
28. Whelton PK, Carey RM, Aronow WS, Casey DE Jr, Collins KJ, Himmelfarb CD, et al. 2017 ACC/AHA/AAPA/ABC/ACPM/AGS/APhA/ASH/ASPC/NMA/PCNA Guideline for the prevention, detection, evaluation, and management of high blood pressure in adults: A report of the American College of Cardiology/American Heart Association Task Force on Clinical Practice Guidelines. J Am Coll Cardiol. 2018;71(19):e127-e248.
29. Muntner P, Carey RM, Gidding S, Jones DW, Taler SJ, Wright JT Jr, et al. Potential US population impact of the 2017 ACC/AHA high blood pressure guideline. Circulation 2018;137(2):109-18.
30. Wright JT Jr, Williamson JD, Whelton PK, Snyder JK, Sink KM, Rocco MV, et al. A randomized trial of intensive versus

standard blood-pressure control. N Engl J Med. 2015;373(22):2103-16.
31. Lonn EM, Bosch J, López-Jaramillo P, Zhu J, Liu L, Pais P, et al. Blood-pressure lowering in intermediate-risk persons without cardiovascular disease. N Engl J Med. 2016;374(21):2009-20.
32. Chia Y-C, Jenkins C, Tang SY. 318 Validation of the Framingham general cardiovascular risk prediction score in a multi-ethnic primary care cohort. J Hypertens. 2012; 30(Suppl. 1):e93.
33. Shin J, Kario K, Chia YC, Turana Y, Chen C-H, Buranakitjaroen P, et al. Current status of ambulatory blood pressure monitoring in Asian countries: a report from the HOPE Asia Network. J Clin Hypertens (Greenwich). 2020;22(3):384-90.
34. Wang J-G, Bunyi ML, Chia YC, Kario K, Ohkubo T, Park S, et al. Insights on home blood pressure monitoring in Asia: Expert perspectives from 10 countries/regions. J Clin Hypertens (Greenwich). 2021;23(1):3-11.
35. Park S, Buranakitjaroen P, Chen CH, Chia Y-C, Divinagracia R, Hoshide S, et al. Expert panel consensus recommendations for home blood pressure monitoring in Asia: The Hope Asia Network. J Hum Hypertens. 2018;32(4):249-58.
36. Kario K, Shin J, Chen C-H, Buranakitjaroen P, Chia Y-C, Divinagracia R, et al. Expert panel consensus recommendations for ambulatory blood pressure monitoring in Asia: the HOPE Asia Network. J Clin Hypertens. 2019;21(9):1250-83.

SECTION 13: Miscellaneous

44. **Lipid and Hypertension**
    Aditi Parimoo, Sadanand R Shetty

45. **Role of Vitamin D$_3$ and Hypertension**
    Rajesh Kumar Jha, Srishti Jha

46. **Telemedicine and Its Role in the Management of Resistant Hypertension**
    Anant Ramkishanrao Munde, Sadanand R Shetty

47. **Adherence to the Treatment for Hypertension**
    Michaela M Watts, Fraz A Mir

48. **Navigating Dilemmas in the Management of Hypertension: A Perpetual Challenge**
    Alok Kumar Singh, Sadanand R Shetty

49. **Hypertension Clinic and Hypertension Center**
    A Muruganathan

CHAPTER 44

Lipid and Hypertension

Aditi Parimoo, Sadanand R Shetty

■ INTRODUCTION

Hypertension is one of the traditional risk factors for cardiovascular disease and has been associated with other risk factors such as diabetes, dyslipidemia, obesity, and chronic kidney disease.[1] The coexistence of hypertension and dyslipidemia in patients with coronary artery disease led to the hypothesis that the two may be causally related to each other. Many cross-sectional studies have linked the two together.[2,3] In this review, we will try to examine this association.

■ PATHOPHYSIOLOGICAL BASIS

Several mechanisms have been proposed to explain this relationship. Dyslipidemia causes endothelial dysfunction and subsequent loss of physiological vasomotor activity which has been hypothesized to cause hypertension. This in turn has been related to the overexpression of AT-I overexpression.[4] Dyslipidemia has also been related to insulin resistance and sympathetic overactivity, which may lead to hypertension.[5] Dyslipidemia also leads to decreased distensibility of large elastic arteries which may in turn reduce the Windkessel effect and increase systolic BP.[6] Finally, physical inactivity promotes dyslipidemia and obesity and the release of adipocytokines which in turn cause insulin resistance and physical inactivity.[7]

■ CURRENT EVIDENCE

The Physicians' Health Study was a randomized, double-blind, placebo-controlled trial of aspirin and β-carotene in the primary prevention of cardiovascular disease and cancer. Among the baseline characteristics that were examined among the study participants, the study demonstrated that higher plasma levels of total cholesterol, non-high-density lipoprotein (non-HDL) cholesterol, and total cholesterol/HDL were independently associated with a subsequent increased risk of incident hypertension in apparently healthy men and that higher levels of HDL cholesterol were associated with a decreased risk of hypertension.[8]

Laaksonen DE et al. also examined the role of dyslipidemia in causing hypertension in a population-based study.[9] The authors examined the association of dyslipidemia with incident hypertension over a period of 7 years in men who did not have hypertension at baseline. An increase in serum cholesterol levels was associated with an increased risk of new-onset hypertension independent of the features related to metabolic syndrome. The concentration of LDL cholesterol, the triglyceride content of HDL cholesterol, and apolipoprotein B levels were associated positively with incident hypertension whereas high levels of HDL cholesterol were protective.[8] Zhi-Rong Guo et al. examine the relationship between dyslipidemia and hypertension in a similar prospective study in the Chinese population. In their study, they observed that high levels of total cholesterol and non-HDL cholesterol were associated with incident hypertension, whereas HDL levels were protective.[10] All these studies concluded that the effects of dyslipidemia leading to hypertension were independent of their effects on insulin resistance and diabetes.

Moreover, the coexistence of the two risk factors has more than additive effects on causing cardiovascular disease.[11] Ayoade OG et al. attempted to examine the patterns of dyslipidemia associated with hypertension.[12] They conducted a cross-sectional study among known hypertensives and observed that overall, 60% of individuals in their cohort had dyslipidemia with the most common abnormalities being high total cholesterol, high LDL levels, high triglycerides, and low HDL in descending order. Moreover, women seemed to have higher levels of lipoproteins as compared to their male counterparts in the study.[12]

These studies have indicated that treatment of dyslipidemia may serve to delay the onset of hypertension and subsequent cardiovascular disease in at-risk individuals. Moreover, treatment of two risk factors as compared to treating hypertension alone has a more significant effect on cardiovascular risk reduction as indicated by the INTERHEART study.[13]

THERAPY

Concomitant management of dyslipidemia and hypertension is therefore essential for optimal reduction of atherosclerotic cardiovascular disease (ASCVD) risk. Guidelines of the European Society of Cardiology/European Society of Hypertension recommend lifestyle modification as the first line of management and include alcohol moderation, regular exercise, particularly aerobic exercise, and weight control.[14] Drug therapy for hypertension with thiazide diuretics and nonselective β-blockers has also been known to cause adverse effects on the lipid profile. These factors must be taken into consideration while treating both disorders concomitantly.[15]

Whether treatment of dyslipidemia confers a beneficial effect on the management of hypertension, indirect evidence from several clinical trials has been obtained.[16] One of the first studies demonstrating that statin therapy for dyslipidemia improved BP control in patients was the Brisighella Heart Study (BHS) group.[17] Statins upregulate endothelial nitric oxide synthase and downregulate the expression of AT-I receptors. They also seem to inhibit intracellular effects of AT-I-receptor activation and delay hypertension-induced vascular effects.[18]

CONCLUSION

The optimal medical management of both dyslipidemia and hypertension is essential to reduce the cumulative ASCVD risk. Dyslipidemia itself seems to be contributory to hypertension and hence, adequate lipid-lowering therapy is mandated to improve BP control in patients.

REFERENCES

1. Reaven GM, Lithell H, Landsberg L. Hypertension and associated metabolic abnormalities: the role of insulin resistance and the sympathomimetic system. N Eng J Med. 1996:334(6):374.
2. Oparil S, Zaman MA, Calhoun DA. pathogenesis of hypertension. Ann Intern Med. 2003;139(9):761-76.
3. Haffner SM, Miettinen H, Gaskill SP, Stern MP. Metabolic precursors of hypertension: the San Antonio Heart Study. Arch Intern Med. 1996;156(17):1994-2000.

4. Nickenig G. Central role of AT(1)-receptor in atherosclerosis. J Hum Hypertens. 2002;16(Suppl 3):S26-33.
5. Egan DM. Insulin resistance and the sympathetic nervous system. Curr Hypertens Rep. 2003;5(3):247-54.
6. Westerhof N, lankhaar JW, Westerhof BE. The arterial Windkessel. Med Biol Eng Comput. 2009;47(2):131-41.
7. McGill JB, Haffner S, Rees TJ, Sowers JR, Tershakovec AM, Weber M. Progress and controversies: treating obesity and insulin resistance in the context of hypertension. J Clin Hyperetns (Greenwich). 2009;11(1):36-41.
8. Halperin RO, Sesso HD, Ma Jing, Buring JE, Stampfer MJ, Gaziano JM, et al. Dyslipidemia and the risk of incident hypertension in men. Hypertension. 2006;47(1):45-50.
9. Laaksonen DE, Niskanen L, Nyyssonen K, Lakka TA, Laukkanen JA, Salonen JT, et al. Dyslipidemia as a predictor of hypertension in middle-aged men. Eur Heart J. 2008; 29(20):2561-8.
10. Guo ZR, Hu XS, Wu M, Zhou MH, Zhou ZY. A prospective study on the association between dyslipidemia and hypertension. Zhonghua Liu Xing Bing Xue Za Zhi. 2009;30(6):554-8.
11. Dalal JD, Padmanabhan NC, Jain P, Patil S, Vasnawala H, Gulati A, et al. Lipitension: Interplay between dyslipidemia and hypertension. Indian J Endocrinol Metab. 2012;16(2):240-5.
12. Ayoade OG, Umoh I, Amadi ZC. Dyslipidemia and associated risk factors among Nigerians with hypertension. Dubai Med J. 2020;3(4):155-61.
13. Yusuf S, Hawken S, Ounpuu S, Dans T, Avezum A, Lanas F, et al. INTERHEART Study. Investigators effect of potentially modifiable risk factors associated with myocardial infarction in 52 countries (the INTERHEART Study): Case-control study. Lancet. 2004;364(9438):937-52.
14. ESH/ESC Task Force for the Management of Arterial Hypertension. 2018 Practice Guidelines for the management of arterial hypertension of the European Society of Hypertension and the European Society of Cardiology. J Hypertens. 2019;37(2):456.
15. Borghi C, Fogacci F, Agnoletti D, Cicero AFG. Hypertension and dyslipidemia combined therapeutic approaches. High Blood Press Cardiovasc Prev. 2022;29(3):221-30.
16. Strazzullo P, Kerry SM, Barbato A, Versiero M, D'Elia L, Cappuccio FP et al. Do statins reduce blood pressure? A meta-analysis of randomized, controlled trials. Hypertension. 2007;49(4):792-98.
17. Borghi C, Dormi A, Veronesi M, D'Elia L, Cappuccio FP, Brisighella Heart Study Working Party. Brisighella Heart Study Working Party Association between different lipid-lowering treatment strategies and blood pressure control in the Brisighella Heart Study. Am Heart J. 2004;148(2):285-92.
18. Briasoulis A, Aggarwal V, Valachis A, Messerli FH. Antihypertensive effects of statins: A meta-analysis of prospective controlled studies. J Clin Hyperetns. 2013; 15(5):310-20.

Role of Vitamin D$_3$ and Hypertension

Rajesh Kumar Jha, Srishti Jha

CHAPTER 45

INTRODUCTION

Hypertension, a global health enigma, stands prominently as a major risk factor in the pathogenesis of cardiovascular diseases, contributing significantly to the global burden of morbidity and mortality. The interface of vitamin D$_3$ (cholecalciferol) with cardiovascular health, and specifically its potential modulatory effects on blood pressure, has been the subject of extensive scientific scrutiny. This chapter aims to dissect the intricate relationship between vitamin D$_3$ and hypertension, assimilating a broad spectrum of clinical trial outcomes and evidence-based medical insights. It encompasses a rigorous examination of epidemiological patterns, detailed physiological mechanisms, pathophysiological constructs, clinical presentations, and strategic management approaches.

PHYSIOLOGY OF VITAMIN D$_3$

Vitamin D$_3$, a secosteroid hormone, is synthesized in the skin under ultraviolet B radiation and obtained through dietary sources. It undergoes two hydroxylations: First, in the liver forming 25-hydroxyvitamin D [25(OH)D], and subsequently in the kidneys generating 1,25-dihydroxyvitamin D [1,25(OH)2D], the physiologically active form. This active metabolite is instrumental in calcium and phosphorus homeostasis and exerts a significant influence on cardiovascular dynamics. It modulates the renin–angiotensin–aldosterone system (RAAS), a critical regulatory axis in vascular tone and fluid balance.[1] Vitamin D$_3$'s role extends beyond RAAS modulation. It influences endothelial and smooth muscle cell function, contributing to vascular homeostasis. Vitamin D receptors (VDR) in cardiovascular tissues suggest its direct role in cardiovascular health.[2]

EPIDEMIOLOGY OF HYPERTENSION AND VITAMIN D DEFICIENCY

Globally, hypertension is prevalent in over a billion individuals and is influenced by genetic, environmental, and lifestyle factors. Vitamin D deficiency, characterized by serum 25(OH)D levels below 20 ng/mL, is widely prevalent, especially in areas with limited sunlight exposure. Epidemiological studies have consistently shown an inverse relationship between vitamin D levels and hypertension risk. A landmark epidemiological study, "Effect of vitamin D supplementation on blood pressure" demonstrated a significant inverse correlation between serum 25(OH)D levels and hypertension incidence.[3] Seasonal variations in blood pressure correlate with changes in vitamin D levels, further supporting its potential role in hypertension. Geographical studies indicate higher hypertension rates in high-latitude regions with less sunlight.[4]

Elderly individuals and those with chronic kidney disease (CKD) often have vitamin D deficiency and hypertension. Studies suggest that vitamin D therapy may have specific benefits in these populations.

■ PATHOPHYSIOLOGY

Vitamin D deficiency can lead to hypertension through various mechanisms:
- *The RAAS activation:* Vitamin D deficiency results in an upregulated RAAS, leading to increased vascular resistance and hypertension.[5]
- *Endothelial dysfunction:* Inadequate vitamin D levels are associated with impaired endothelial function, reducing nitric oxide synthesis and increasing arterial stiffness.[6]
- *Inflammatory pathways:* Vitamin D insufficiency correlates with increased inflammatory markers, contributing to vascular inflammation and hypertension.[7]
- *Cardiac dysfunction:* Vitamin D affects cardiac function. It regulates myocardial calcium levels, influencing contractility and contributing to blood pressure regulation.[8]

■ CLINICAL FEATURES

Hypertension typically presents without symptoms initially. Chronic hypertension can lead to pathological alterations such as hypertensive heart disease, including left ventricular hypertrophy, accelerated atherosclerosis, microvascular damage, CKD, and cerebrovascular changes, potentially culminating in myocardial infarction, stroke, and end-organ failure.[9]

■ CLINICAL TRIALS

Following are the vitamin D supplementation trials:
- *Vitamin D and omega-3 trial (VITAL):* This trial assessed the effects of vitamin D3 supplementation on cardiovascular health and hypertension, revealing a non-significant reduction in blood pressure among participants.[10]
- *Randomized evaluation of calcium or vitamin D (RECORD):* This study found no significant impact on blood pressure with vitamin D supplementation in an older adult population.[11]
- *VITAL study subgroup analyses:* Subgroup analyses revealed nuances in Vitamin D's effect on different populations, suggesting personalized approaches might be more effective.[10]
- *Other trials:* Studies such as D2d (diabetes vitamin D) and the vitamin D–RAAS study offer further insights but also indicate the complexity of the relationship.[12]

Research continues to explore genetic factors influencing vitamin D metabolism and its impact on hypertension. Novel therapeutic interventions targeting VDR and vitamin D metabolism are under investigation.[13]

A meta-analysis in the *Journal of the American College of Cardiology* (2023) concluded that vitamin D supplementation may lower blood pressure in individuals with vitamin D deficiency, but the clinical significance is uncertain.[14]

■ MANAGEMENT STRATEGIES

Current clinical guidelines recommend the cautious use of vitamin D supplementation in hypertension management, particularly in individuals with confirmed vitamin D deficiency. Monitoring of blood pressure response is crucial.[15] Management strategies should be individualized, considering factors such as baseline vitamin D status, comorbidities, and lifestyle. Vitamin D supplementation should be tailored based on serum 25(OH)D levels, with regular monitoring.[16]

Pharmacotherapy

Antihypertensive medication regimens remain the cornerstone of hypertension management, considering potential interactions with vitamin D metabolism.[17]

Lifestyle Modifications

Dietary modifications, regular physical activity, and weight management are essential in managing hypertension, synergizing with pharmacotherapy.[18]

■ CONCLUSION

The relationship between vitamin D3 and hypertension is complex and multifactorial. Epidemiological evidence suggests a correlation between vitamin D deficiency and increased hypertension risk, but the results from clinical trials on vitamin D supplementation are mixed. The current management paradigm involves a multipronged approach, incorporating lifestyle modifications, potential vitamin D supplementation, and conventional antihypertensive therapies. Ongoing research is critical in elucidating this relationship and optimizing treatment strategies ("Vitamin D and Health," National Institutes of Health, 2023)[19].

■ REFERENCES

1. Holick MF. Vitamin D Deficiency. N Engl J Med. 2007;357(3):266-81.
2. Norman PE, Powell JT. Vitamin D and cardiovascular disease. Circ Res. 2014;114(2):379-93.
3. Pilz S, Gaksch M, Kienreich K, Grubler M, Verheyen N, Fahrleitner-Pammer A, et al. Effects of vitamin D on blood pressure and cardiovascular risk factors: a randomized controlled trial. Hypertension. 2015;65(6):1195-201.
4. Rostand SG. Ultraviolet light may contribute to geographic and racial blood pressure differences. Hypertension. 1997;30 (2 Pt 1): 150-6.
5. Forman JP, Giovannucci E, Holmes MD, Bischoff-Ferrari HA, Tworoger SS, Willett WC, et al. Plasma 25-hydroxyvitamin D levels and risk of incident hypertension. Hypertension. 2007;49(5):1063-9.
6. Zittermann A, Schleithoff SS, Koerfer R. Vitamin D and vascular calcification. Curr Opin Lipidol. 2007;18(1):41-6.
7. Michos ED, Melamed ML. Vitamin D and cardiovascular disease risk. Curr Opin Clin Nutr Metab Care. 2008;11(1):7-12.
8. Belenchia AM, Tosh AK, Hillman LS, et al. Correcting vitamin D insufficiency improves insulin sensitivity in obese adolescents: a randomized controlled trial. Am J Clin Nutr. 2013;97:774-81.
9. Kaplan NM. Kaplan's Clinical Hypertension, 9th edition. Philadelphia, USA: Williams & Wilkins; 2005, p. 528.
10. Manson JE, Cook NR, Lee IM, ChristenW, Bassuk SS, Mora S, et al. Vitamin D Supplements and prevention of cancer and cardiovascular disease. N Engl J Med. 2019;380(1):33-44.
11. Witham MD, Nadir MA, Struthers AD. Effect of vitamin D on blood pressure: a systematic review and meta-analysis. J Hypertens. 2009; 27(10):1948-54.
12. Pittas AG, Dawson-Hughes B, Sheehan P, Ware JH, Knowler WC, Aroda VR, et al. Vitamin D supplementation and prevention of type 2 diabetes. N Engl J Med. 2019; 381(6):520-530.
13. Dominguez LJ, Farruggia M, Veronese N, Barbagallo M. Vitamin D Sources, Metabolism, and Deficiency: Available Compounds and Guidelines for Its Treatment. Metabolites. 2021;11(4):255.
14. Barbarawi M, Kheiri B, Zayed Y, Barbarawi O, Dhillon H, Swaid B, et al. Vitamin D Supplementation and Cardiovascular Disease Risks in More Than 83 000 Individuals in 21 Randomized Clinical Trials: A Meta-analysis. JAMA Cardiol. 2019;4(8):765-76.
15. Whelton PK, Carey RM, Mancia G, Kreutz R, Bundy JD and Williams B. Harmonization

of the American College of Cardiology/ American Heart Association and European Society of Cardiology/European Society of Hypertension Blood Pressure/Hypertension Guidelines: Comparisons, Reflections, and Recommendations. Circulation. 2022; 146:868-877
16. Holick MF. Vitamin D: a d-lightful solution for health. J Investig Med. 2011;59(6):872-80.
17. Williams B, Mancia G, Spiering W, RoseiEA, Azizi M, Burnier M, et al. 2018 ESC/ESH guidelines for the management ofarterial hypertension: The Task Force for the management of arterial hypertension of the European Society of Cardiology and the European Society of Hypertension. Eur Heart J. 2018;36(10):1953-2041.
18. Appel LJ, Brands MW, Daniels SR, Karanja N, Elmer PJ, Sacks FM, et al. Dietary approaches to prevent and treat hypertension: Ascientific statement from the American Heart Association. Hypertension. 2006;7(2):296-308.
19. Office of Dietary Supplements - Vitamin D. (n.d.). https://ods.od.nih.gov/factsheets/VitaminD-HealthProfessional/.

CHAPTER 46

Telemedicine and Its Role in the Management of Resistant Hypertension

Anant Ramkishanrao Munde, Sadanand R Shetty

■ INTRODUCTION

Telemedicine, a groundbreaking approach for conducting remote clinical assessments and providing mental health support, first emerged in the mid-20th century.[1,2] since then, its scope has expanded to encompass telehealth and mobile health (mHealth) applications, particularly through video visits.[3]

One significant factor contributing to the growing gap in life expectancy between rural and urban areas is the limited access to healthcare services.[4] Extending telemedicine services, both in primary care and specialized consultations, holds great potential for benefiting patients residing in remote regions. Telemedicine stands as a promising tool for enhancing healthcare accessibility, empowering patients, shaping their attitudes and behaviors, and ultimately ameliorating their medical conditions. Given the rise in life expectancy and improved survival rates from cardiovascular events, leading to a greater burden on population health, its utilization is projected to increase significantly in the near future for managing both acute and chronic diseases.

The prominence of telemedicine surged during the coronavirus disease 2019 (COVID-19) pandemic. Bringing hypertensive patients into clinics for routine blood pressure (BP) checks during such a crisis posed a serious risk, particularly for older adults or those with underlying medical conditions. The imperative for social distancing and restricted mobility, essential for controlling the COVID-19 pandemic, underscored and exacerbated the urgent requirement for telemedicine as the primary means to manage various chronic conditions, including hypertension.

■ DEFINITIONS AND OVERVIEW

Telehealth encompasses the broad utilization of electronic information and telecommunication technologies to facilitate healthcare, which may encompass a range of services from health education to population health management.[5] While telehealth can operate in a consultative model, where clinicians use digital health tools to communicate, it is more commonly employed to facilitate communication between clinicians and patients. This interaction can occur through live video sessions, as well as via remote monitoring devices and mobile technology.

Telemedicine, a subset of telehealth, has a more specific definition. It refers to the exchange of medical information between different locations through electronic communications, to enhance a patient's clinical health status during a remote clinical service.[6] Increasingly, mobile wireless technologies, often referred to as "mobile health" or "mHealth," are harnessed to deliver both telemedicine and telehealth services.

To conduct telemedicine effectively, both audio and visual components are imperative. It can be delivered in real-time through live, two-way audio–visual interactions between patients and providers (referred to as "synchronous" telemedicine), or by storing and forwarding data and images for later use (known as "asynchronous" telemedicine). Asynchronous telemedicine complements both traditional face-to-face ("in-person") care and synchronous telemedicine approaches. For instance, it can be utilized for screening diabetic retinopathy,[7] conducting dermatologic evaluations,[8] or employing remote patient monitoring devices for managing chronic diseases.[9]

PREPARING FOR THE TELEMEDICINE VISIT

Prior to the telemedicine appointment, it is crucial to make necessary preparations to anticipate and address patient expectations, and to ensure that the required technology for a successful telemedicine visit is operational and easily accessible. This includes verifying technological prerequisites, obtaining informed consent, discussing reimbursement and co-pay responsibilities, and establishing privacy expectations. Providers should also ready their workspace for an efficient video visit, and conduct thorough tests of audio and video connections. The use of a laptop or desktop computer is recommended to minimize camera movement. While the physical examination may be more focused and limited, it should still encompass a comprehensive visual assessment of the patient throughout the telemedicine encounter.

TELEMONITORING

Data generated by remote patient monitoring devices (such as glucometers, BP monitors, scales, oximeters, and noninvasive ventilation equipment for sleep apnea) can be transmitted to the healthcare provider, and in some instances, automatically integrated into the patient's electronic medical record. This information equips the provider with valuable insights to monitor and fine-tune therapy, which may include adjustments to medication regimens and offering guidance on behavioral modifications.

TELEMEDICINE CLOSED-LOOP HEALTHCARE MODEL

Presently, the predominant method of delivering telemedicine services is through the Internet, often facilitated by mobile devices, and operates within a closed-loop healthcare model, also known as the Internet of Medical Things (IoMT), as illustrated in the accompanying **Figure 1**.

ROLE OF TELEMEDICINE IN THE MANAGEMENT OF RESISTANT HYPERTENSION

The global prevalence of hypertension is estimated to affect around 1.4 billion individuals, and by 2025, as shown in **Figure 2**, it is projected to surpass 1.6 billion.[1] The cardiovascular (CV) risks associated with elevated BP have been recognized since the inception of the Framingham Heart Study in 1948.[2-4,10] The consistent correlation between BP levels and the risk of adverse events in vital organs such as the brain, heart, and kidneys has been extensively documented.[2-6] In general, every 20 mm Hg rise in systolic blood pressure (SBP) doubles the risk of CV-related mortality.[5]

From 1988 to 1994, there was an observed rise in the prevalence of hypertension across various gender and ethnic groups in the United States, with non-Hispanic black

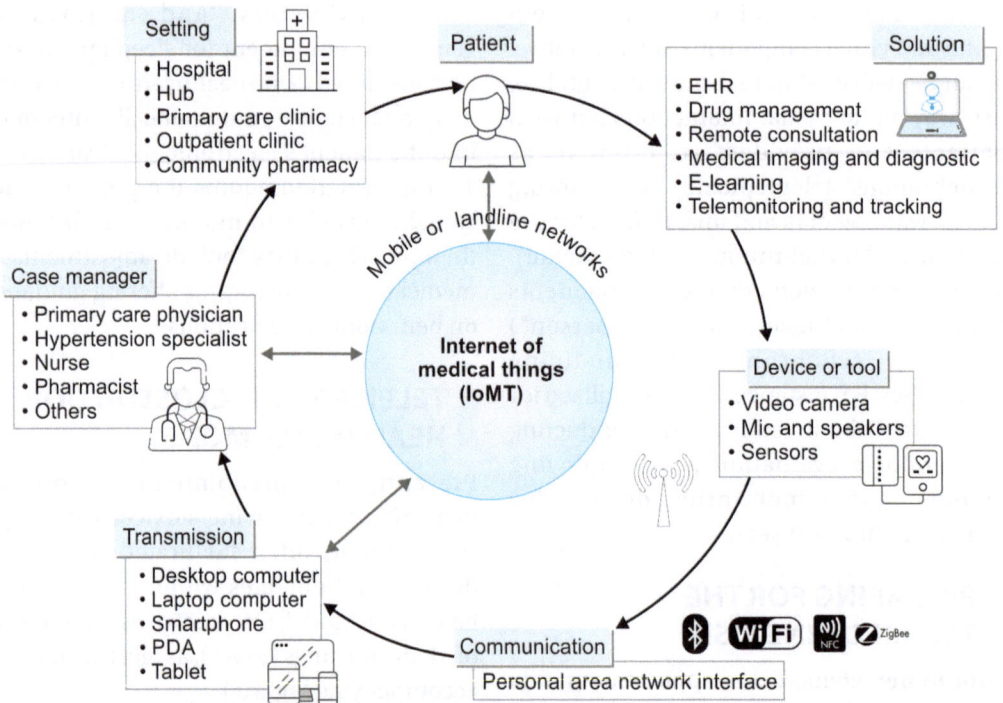

Fig. 1: Basic Telehealth Services and their workflow. (EHR: electronic health record; Mic: microphone; NFC: near-field communication; PDA: personal digital assistant)

women exhibiting the highest prevalence (42.9%) between 2007 and 2012. Throughout this period, 82.7% were aware of their hypertensive status, 76.5% were actively receiving treatment, but only 54.1% achieved BP control.

In India, approximately 33% of urban and 25% of rural populations suffer from hypertension. Among them, 25% of rural and 42% of urban individuals are aware of their hypertensive condition. Merely 25% of rural and 38% of urban hypertensive patients receive treatment, and only one-tenth of rural and one-fifth of urban Indian hypertensive population have their BP under control.[6]

Currently, there exist over 125 distinct medications, nearly all of which are available in generic form, spanning eight different antihypertensive drug classes aimed at reducing BP. Additionally, there are more than 15 fixed-dose, single-pill combination agents. Despite this extensive array of treatment options, BP control remains less than optimal in numerous regions worldwide.[2,4,7-9] The global prevalence of true resistant hypertension stands at approximately 10%.

Given that hypertension is the most prevalent and significant risk factor for cardiovascular disease on a global scale, it represents an ideal target for telemedicine, particularly telemonitoring.[11] However, while telemedicine has demonstrated its efficacy in improving BP control compared to standard care, its precise role in everyday clinical practice remains somewhat unclear.[12] Although most guidelines mention it in the context of differentiating white coat or masked hypertension, there are currently

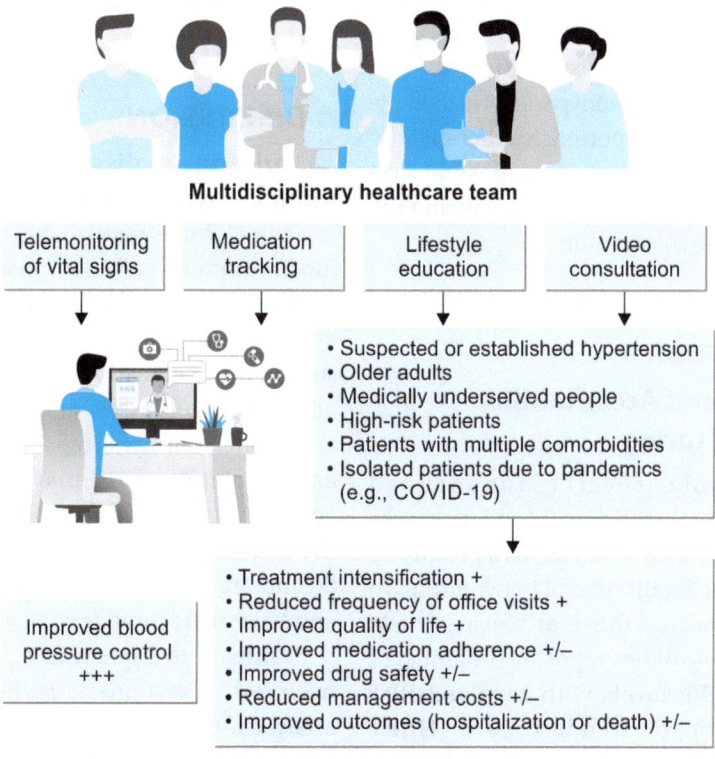

Fig. 2: Telemedicine and its effectiveness in BP control.

no specific recommendations addressing the broader integration of telemedicine into general hypertension management, with the partial exception of the 2017 Hypertension Clinical Practice Guidelines, which suggest that telehealth strategies can serve as valuable adjuncts to interventions proven to lower BP in adults with hypertension.[13]

■ RESISTANT HYPERTENSION

Resistant hypertension is defined by the 2018 American Heart Association (AHA) scientific statement, the 2017 American College of Cardiology (ACC)/AHA hypertension guideline, and the 2018 European Society of Cardiology and European Society of Hypertension (ESC/ESH) statement as persistently elevated BP that remains above target levels despite concurrent use of three antihypertensive agents from distinct classes.[13-16] In cases where tolerated, one of these agents should be a diuretic, and all medications should be prescribed at the maximum recommended (or maximally tolerated) antihypertensive doses.[14] Patients whose BP is controlled with four or more medications should also be classified as having resistant hypertension.

■ APPARENT, TRUE, AND PSEUDORESISTANT HYPERTENSION

For individuals who initially seem to exhibit resistant hypertension according to the aforementioned definition, it is imperative to discern whether the hypertension is

genuinely resistant. The five most common causes of pseudoresistance are as follows:
1. Inaccurate measurement of BP.
2. Poor adherence to antihypertensive therapy.
3. Suboptimal antihypertensive therapy.
4. Inadequate adherence to lifestyle and dietary approaches aimed at reducing BP.
5. White coat hypertension.

SCIENTIFIC EVIDENCE FROM STUDIES

Feasibility and Acceptability of Telemonitoring

Findings from several randomized trials indicate that home blood pressure telemonitoring (HBPT) stands as a promising tool for enhancing BP control in hypertensive patients, especially those at elevated risk. The majority of studies reported a significant reduction in BP levels with regular HBPT in comparison to standard care. HBPT interventions demonstrated a high level of acceptance among patients, leading to an improvement in their quality of life. Moreover, they were associated with lower medical costs compared to standard care, despite potential technology-related expenses. Patients requiring continuous monitoring of multiple vital signs and stringent BP control, such as those with high-risk chronic conditions (such as ischemic heart disease or heart failure, diabetes, etc.), as well as nonadherent patients, are likely to derive particular benefits from HBPT. Overall, HBPT can be a beneficial choice, especially when establishing a network among healthcare professionals (including doctors, nurses, and pharmacists) is essential for enhancing the screening and management of hypertension and its associated comorbidities, ultimately leading to effective cardiovascular disease prevention within the community.

PROOF OF EFFICACY

See **Table 1**.

DISCUSSION

As previously discussed, determining whether hypertension is truly resistant is crucial for effective management. The most common causes of pseudoresistance include inaccurate BP measurements, poor adherence to antihypertensive therapy, suboptimal medication regimens, inadequate adherence to lifestyle and dietary changes, and white coat hypertension. Telemedicine and telemonitoring play a vital role in addressing many of these issues by enabling the tracking of vital signs, including BP, and facilitating communication between patients and healthcare providers.

Tables 1 to 3 provide a comprehensive overview of systematic reviews and meta-analyses, demonstrating the superiority of telemedicine in hypertension management compared to standard care. These studies consistently show significant reductions in BP levels, improved adherence to antihypertensive medications, enhanced quality of life, and reduced healthcare costs and hospitalizations. Notably, the benefits were particularly pronounced in patients with higher baseline BP, obesity, diabetes, prior stroke, and among individuals of Black ethnicity. However, some subgroups, such as those with coronary artery disease (CAD), chronic kidney disease (CKD), pregnancy, and underprivileged individuals, showed less significant effects.

Telemonitoring of BP, along with the tracking of additional vital and nonvital signs, coupled with effective communication between patients and case managers (often nurses or pharmacists supervised by clinicians) through various digital platforms,

TABLE 1: Systematic reviews and meta-analyses demonstrating the efficacy of telehealth in hypertension management compared to usual care.

Author	Type of intervention	Type of subjects	Setting	Number of studies (comparison)	Number of subjects
Omboni and Guarda[17]	BP exchanged through landline or mobile telephone/modem transmission or internet + patient education + case manager	Hypertensive patients (1 study in obese and 1 in people with diabetes mellitus only)	Mainly general practices or community clinics	12 RCTs	4,389
Agarwal et al.[18]	BP telemonitoring	Hypertensive patients	Mainly community and general practice	7 RCTs	1,510
Verberk et al.[19]	BP exchanged through landline or mobile telephone/modem transmission or internet + patient education + case manager	Hypertensive patients	Mainly general practices or community clinics	9 RCTs	2,501
Omboni et al.[20]	BP exchanged through landline or mobile telephone/modem transmission or internet + patient education + case manager	Hypertensive patients (1 study, only obese; 2 studies, only patients with diabetes mellitus)	Mainly general practices or community clinics	23 RCTs	7,037
Zullig et al.[21]	Home BP monitoring and nurse telephone call + behavioral modification and medication management	Hypertensive patients (stroke or TIA)	Community or hospital	7 RCTs	2,081
Liu et al.[22]	Internet-based lifestyle interventions and BP measurement during a face-to-face visit	Mainly hypertensive patients (also obese, diabetics, and postmenopausal women)	Mainly community and general practice	11 RCTs (2 not RCTs)	2,221
Niznik et al.[23]	Pharmacist-led telephonic clinics, pharmacist management of BP through web communication, electronic messaging (email), or telemonitoring + education	Hypertensive patients (±CKD)	Pharmacies	7 RCTs	3,336

Contd...

Contd...

Author	Type of intervention	Type of subjects	Setting	Number of studies (comparison)	Number of subjects
Tucker et al.[24]	Web or phone feedback plus education, counseling, or tele-counseling.	Hypertensive patients	Primary care, outpatients, and community	18 RCTs	9,175
Xiong et al.[25]	mHealth interventions (apps, SMS, voice calls, or emails used as reminders and health education and lifestyle-related recommendations, digital medicines, wireless BP monitoring, and electronic medication tray)	Hypertensive patients	Primary care or community clinics, hospitals	16 RCTs 1 non-RCT 4 before and after studies without a control group	4,017
Choi et al.[26]	Data transmitted by telephone, internet, mobile phones, or email	Hypertensive patients	Urban	27 RCTs	9,435
Ma et al.[27]	eHealth interventions (interactive wireless communication by smartphone, computer, and personal digital assistance tools, self-care behavioral change, or education dissemination)	Hypertensive patients	Mainly community and general practice	14 RCTs	3,998
Lu et al[28]	mHealth interventions (mobile phones or wearable sensors) transmitting data to care providers	Hypertensive patients	Mainly community and general practice	11 RCTs	4,271
Omboni et al.[29]	BP exchanged through mobile phone, telephone, modem, internet or email + patient education + pharmacist management	Hypertensive patients	Community pharmacies	4 RCTs	1,565

Contd...

Contd...

Author	Type of intervention	Type of subjects	Setting	Number of studies (comparison)	Number of subjects
Alessa et al.[30]	mHealth interventions (smartphone app + email, SMS, voice calls used as contact or health education and lifestyle-related recommendations, electronic medication device, wireless BP monitoring)	Patients with hypertension, metabolic syndrome, obstructive sleep apnea, and obesity	Primary care or community clinics, outpatient clinics, hospitals	• 9 RCTs • 5 nonrandomized studies	2,402
Luo et al.[31]	A BP telemonitoring + telephone follow-up or interactive video consultation + education program	Patients with hypertension and CKD stage III	Community and outpatient clinics	3 RCTs	680

Publication year (range)	Quality of studies or publication bias	Median length (range) of follow-up, wk	Outcomes assessed	Summary of main results
1996–2010	• 12 acceptable • Low publication bias	24 (8–240)	• BP changes • Rate of BP control • Number of antihypertensive drugs	• Office (but not ambulatory) BP was reduced significantly more in patients randomized to the intervention • Office BP control (percentage of patients at target) was better in the telemedicine group • The intervention was associated with a significantly increased use of antihypertension medications
1996–2008	No publication bias	24 (8–48)	BP changes	Greater SBP reduction was observed compared with usual care in subjects using telemonitoring than in those performing self-BP monitoring without remote transmission and counseling
1996–2010	Low publication bias	26 (8–52)	BP changes	• Larger office BP reduction in the intervention group • The difference in the effect size of the intervention is larger if treatment is not modified

Contd...

Contd...

Publication year (range)	Quality of studies or publication bias	Median length (range) of follow-up, wk	Outcomes assessed	Summary of main results
1996–2011	• 23 acceptable • Low publication bias (except for cost analysis)	24 (8–240)	• BP changes • Rate of BP control • Number of antihypertensive drugs • Adherence to treatment • Number of office visits • Healthcare costs • Quality of life • Adverse events	• Significantly improved office BP changes and control with the intervention • Larger prescription of antihypertensive medications in the intervention • No difference in adherence to treatment and the number of office consultations • Intervention is cost-effective if only medical costs are considered (excluding the costs for the technology) • Improved physical component of quality of life • No difference in the risk of adverse events
2009–2013	Very poor (only descriptive review and few studies included)	12 (6–24)	• BP changes • Rate of BP control • Adherence to treatment	• Larger BP reduction in the intervention group in 2 studies, no effect in 3 studies • Improved BP control with the intervention (2 studies) • More medication changes in the intervention group (1 study) • No difference in medication adherence (1 study)
2004–2012	• No publication bias for SBP • Low publication bias for DBP	14 (8–48)	BP changes	• Internet based lifestyle intervention significantly reduced BP • The greatest SBP reduction was observed for interventions that lasted at least 6 months, used ≥5 behavior change techniques or delivered health messaged proactively

Contd...

Contd...

Publication year (range)	Quality of studies or publication bias	Median length (range) of follow-up, wk	Outcomes assessed	Summary of main results
2008–2014	Not evaluated	48 (24–72)	• BP changes • Rate of BP control • Morbidity and mortality	• Significant decrease in BP with pharmacist intervention compared with usual care • Larger proportion of patients with controlled BP in the intervention group • No differences in deaths, hospitalizations • Number of days spent in the hospital, emergency department visits, or skilled nursing facility admissions
2007–2014	Low risk of bias	43 (4–72)	• BP changes • Rate of BP control	• Self-monitoring of BP with counseling or tele-counseling or with web/phone feedback plus education is associated with a significantly larger BP reduction and a higher proportion of patients at a target than usual care • Results are consistent at both 6 and 12 months • Trend to attenuation of the effect for patients followed up for >1 year. The effect is more consistent in people on fewer BP medications and with higher baseline BP
2000–2017	• 6 good • 7 fair • 8 poor	12 (4–48)	Medication adherence	12 of the 21 studies found improvements in the patients' medication adherence
1996–2017	Low risk of bias	24 (8–52)	• BP changes • Rate of BP control	• Office (but not ambulatory) BP was reduced significantly more in patients randomized to the intervention • Office BP control (percentage of patients at target) was better in the telemedicine group • The intervention was more effective in smaller cities compared with larger cities • The intervention was similar regardless of the medically underserved areas

Contd...

Publication year (range)	Quality of studies or publication bias	Median length (range) of follow-up, wk	Outcomes assessed	Summary of main results
2008–2017	• 14 good • Low risk of bias	24 (12–96)	• Physical outcomes (BP, body weight, and cholesterol) • Self-care behavioral outcomes (medication adherence, sodium intake, healthy diet, physical activity, smoking, and alcohol consumption) • Psychosocial wellbeing (anxiety, stress, depression, and quality of life)	• The intervention significantly reduced office BP and significantly decreased the proportion of patients with inadequate BP control and their body weight • The sodium intake was reduced significantly more in patients randomized to the intervention • The effectiveness of the intervention on self-care behavioral change and psychosocial wellbeing is insufficient
2007–2019	• 4 high • 7 low • Low publication bias	48 (4–72)	BP changes	• The intervention was associated with a significantly larger BP reduction • No significant differences in BP reduction were observed between trials of shorter and longer duration • Trials with more frequent BP measurement weekly had a larger effect on DBP than those with less frequent measurements • The magnitude of BP reduction was larger among subjects with inadequate baseline BP control than among those with adequate baseline BP control

Contd...

Contd...

Publication year (range)	Quality of studies or publication bias	Median length (range) of follow-up, wk	Outcomes assessed	Summary of main results
2008–2018	Not evaluated	96 (24–216)	• BP changes • Rate of BP control • Cost-effectiveness	• BP reductions and proportions of patients at target following a pharmacist' intervention were significantly larger than those in the usual care group • The benefit of the pharmacist's intervention was markedly reduced or abolished months after its withdrawal • Improved BP control was achieved at a relatively low cost compared with the usual care (3 studies)
2012–2017	• 2 good • 4 fair • 8 poor	24 (8–52)	BP changes	• The majority (10 of 14) of studies demonstrated a positive effect on SBP, whereas the others showed a neutral effect • Apps that are incorporating more comprehensive functionalities are likely to be more effective
2011–2014	• 3 moderate quality • 3 low risk of bias	24 (24–48)	• BP changes • Creatinine changes • eGFR changes	• SBP was reduced by the intervention and DBP increased, with no statistically significant difference compared with usual care • BP control rates were not significantly improved • Serum creatinine was nonsignificantly decreased, and eGFR was maintained at baseline levels

(App: application; BP: blood pressure; CKD: chronic kidney disease; DBP: diastolic blood pressure; eGFR: estimated glomerular filtration rate; RCT: randomized controlled studies; SBP: systolic blood pressure; SMS: short message system; TIA: transient ischemic attack)

TABLE 2: Summary of the evidence for benefits of telemedicine in hypertension management compared with usual care.[32]

Type of outcome	Effect	Strength of evidence
BP reduction	Increased	Moderate
BP control	Improved	High
Use of antihypertensive medications	Increased	Low
Adherence to antihypertensive treatment	Improved	Very low
Frequency of office consultations	Reduced	Low
Quality of life or psychosocial wellbeing	Improved	Low
Drug safety	Improved	Very low
Costs	Reduced	Very low
Deaths or hospitalizations	Reduced	Very low

TABLE 3: Effectiveness of telemedicine on different subgroups of hypertensive patients.[32]

Significant effects	Nonsignificant effects or insufficient evidence
Patients with higher BP	Patients with CAD
Obese patients	Patients with CKD
Patients with previous stroke	Patients in developing countries
Diabetic patients	Pregnant women
Blacks (living in medically underserved areas)	

(CAD: coronary artery disease)

proves to be the most effective telemedicine approach. Proactive interventions driven by healthcare professionals yield the most substantial benefits.

With the advent of mobile apps, there is potential for more direct patient involvement in self-management, possibly under the guidance of a multidisciplinary clinical team. However, the sustainability and long-term clinical effectiveness of these interventions require further investigation, as few studies have explored benefits beyond the 12-month mark. Some evidence suggests that positive effects persist even after interventions are discontinued, but determining optimal schedules for long-term care postachievement of BP control remains an area of ongoing research. Understanding the ideal frequency and duration of intervention (e.g., monthly, quarterly, or biannually BP monitoring) is crucial, given that hypertension is a chronic and enduring condition.

■ BENEFITS OF TELEMEDICINE

- Strengthening the physician-patient relationship through telemedicine can lead to improved BP control and reduced cardiovascular risk.
- Telemedicine has the potential to influence patients' attitudes and behaviors, promoting self-management and ultimately enhancing their overall medical condition.
- Telemedicine enables physicians and healthcare facilities to extend their services beyond physical locations, reaching a larger number of patients, including older adults and underserved populations (e.g., those in remote or economically disadvantaged areas), resulting in time and cost savings.
- It offers a means of providing care in situations where face-to-face contact is challenging, such as during infectious disease outbreaks (e.g., COVID-19), periods of isolation (as seen in natural disasters), instances of disability, or due to geographical barriers.

- Rapid communication with specialists is facilitated in cases of acute symptoms or sudden spikes in BP.
- Telemedicine grants hypertensive patients access to diagnostic procedures that may not be readily available in remote areas, such as ambulatory BP monitoring or electrocardiogram facilities.

BARRIERS AND CHALLENGES

- The dissemination and adoption of telehealth strategies in the daily practice of healthcare professionals and patients have been impeded by factors including incomplete evidence on clinical efficacy and economic benefits from randomized studies, technological limitations, high costs of devices, diversity in solutions and technologies, insufficient infrastructure and standards, inadequate reimbursement, as well as concerns regarding privacy and security.
- Cultural barriers, including limited informatics skills, lack of motivation, and inadequate understanding of the clinical utility of telemedicine, present significant challenges to its routine use, both from the perspective of healthcare providers and patients.

CONCLUSION

- Telemedicine emerges as a valuable strategy for providing effective care to hypertensive patients and enhancing their overall management.
- Existing evidence substantiates its applicability in cases of apparent or pseudo resistant hypertension. Nevertheless, further scientific validation is required to ascertain its efficacy in true resistant hypertension and within specific subgroups.

- Despite its potential, several barriers impede the seamless integration of telemedicine into the routine clinical management of hypertensive patients. Notably, it is often viewed as an adjunct to existing care rather than an integral tool seamlessly integrated into current care delivery. Overcoming these challenges will be crucial for realizing the full potential of telemedicine in hypertension management.

REFERENCES

1. Egan BM. Hypertension in military veterans is associated with combat exposure and combat injury. J Hypertens. 2020;38(7):1255-56.
2. Lim SS, Vos T, F laxman AD, Danaei G, Shibuya K, Adair-Rohani H, et al. A comparative risk assessment of burden of disease and injury attributable to 67 risk factors and risk factor clusters in 21 regions, 1990–2010: A systematic analysis for the Global Burden of Disease Study 2010. Lancet. 2012;380(9859):2224-60.
3. Franklin SS, Jacobs MJ, Wong ND, et al. Predominance of isolated systolic hypertension among middle-aged and elderly US hypertensives: Analysis based on National Health and Nutrition Examination Survey (NHANES) III. Hypertension. 2001; 37:869-74.
4. Forouzanfar MH, Liu P, Roth GA, Ng M, Biryukov S, Marczak L, et al. Global burden of hypertension and systolic blood pressure of at least 110 to 115 mm Hg, 1990–2015. J Am Med Assoc. 2017; 317(2):165-82.
5. Lewington S, Clarke R, Qizilbash N, et al. Age-specific relevance of usual blood pressure to vascular mortality: a meta-analysis of individual data for one million adults in 61 prospective studies. Lancet. 2002;360(9349):1903-13.
6. Anchala R, Kannuri NK, Pant H, Pant H, Khan H, Franco OH, et al. Hypertension in India: a systematic review and meta-analysis of prevalence, awareness, and

control of hypertension. J Hypertens. 2014;32(6):1170-77.
7. Chow CK, Teo KK, Rangarajan S, Islam S, Gupta R, Avezum A, et al. Prevalence, awareness, treatment, and control of hypertension in rural and urban communities in high-, middle-, and low-income countries. J Am Med Assoc. 2013;310(9):959-68.
8. Kearney PM, Whelton M, Reynolds K, Muntner P, Whelton PK, He J, et al. Global burden of hypertension: analysis of worldwide data. Lancet. 2005;365(9455):217-23.
9. Campbell NR, Brant R, Johansen H, Walker RL, Wielgosz A, Onysko J, et al. Increases in antihypertensive prescriptions and reductions in cardiovascular events in Canada. Hypertension. 2009;53(2):128-34.
10. Joffres M, Falaschetti E, Gillespie C, Robitaille C, Loustalot F, Poulter N, et al. Hypertension prevalence, awareness, treatment and control in national surveys from England, the USA and Canada, and correlation with stroke and ischaemic heart disease mortality: A cross-sectional study. BMJ Open. 2013;3(8):e003423.
11. GBD 2015 Risk Factors Collaborators. Global, regional, and national comparative risk assessment of 79 behavioural, environmental and occupational, and metabolic risks or clusters of risks, 1990-2015: A systematic analysis for the Global Burden of Disease Study 2015. Lancet. 2016; 388(10053):1659-724.
12. Omboni S. Connected health in hypertension management. Front Cardiovasc Med. 2019; 6:76.
13. Whelton PK, Carey RM, Aronow WS, Casey DE, Collins KJ, Himmelfarb CD, et al. 2017 ACC/AHA/AAPA/ABC/ACPM/AGS/APhA/ASH/ASPC/NMA/PCNA guideline for the prevention, detection, evaluation, and management of high blood pressure in adults: A report of the American College of Cardiology/American Heart Association Task Force on Clinical Pr. Circulation. 2018:138(17):e484-94.
14. Carey RM, Calhoun DA, Bakris GL, Brook RD, Daugherty SL, Dennison-Himmelfarb CR, et al. Resistant hypertension: detection, evaluation, and management: a Scientific Statement from the American Heart Association. Hypertension. 2018;72(5):e53-90.
15. Williams B, Mancia G, Spiering W, Rosei EA, Azizi M, Burnier M, et al. 2018 ESC/ESH Guidelines for the management of arterial hypertension. Eur Heart J. 2018; 39(33):3021-104.
16. Omboni S, Ferrari R. The role of telemedicine in hypertension management: focus on blood pressure telemonitoring. Curr Hypertens Rep. 2015;17(4):535.
17. Omboni S, Guarda A. Impact of home blood pressure telemonitoring and blood pressure control: a meta-analysis of randomized controlled studies. Am J Hypertens. 2011; 24:989-98.
18. Agarwal R, Bills JE, Hecht TJ, Light RP. Role of home blood pressure monitoring in overcoming therapeutic inertia and improving hypertension control: a systematic review and meta-analysis. Hypertension. 2011;57(1):29-38.
19. Verberk WJ, Kessels AG, Thien T. Telecare is a valuable tool for hypertension management, a systematic review and meta-analysis. Blood Press Monit. 2011;16(3):149-55.
20. Omboni S, Gazzola T, Carabelli G, Parati G. Clinical usefulness and cost effectiveness of home blood pressure telemonitoring: Meta-analysis of randomized controlled studies. J Hypertens. 2013;31(3):455-67.
21. Zullig LL, Melnyk SD, Goldstein K, Shaw RJ, Bosworth HB. The role of home blood pressure telemonitoring in managing hypertensive populations. Curr Hypertens Rep. 2013;15(4):346-55.
22. Liu S, Dunford SD, Leung YW, Brooks D, Thomas SG, Eysenbach G, et al. Reducing blood pressure with Internet-based interventions: a meta-analysis. Can J Cardiol. 2013;29(5):613-21.
23. Niznik JD, He H, Kane-Gill SL. Impact of clinical pharmacist services delivered via telemedicine in the outpatient or ambulatory care setting: a systematic review. Res Social Adm Pharm. 2018;14(8):707-17.

24. Tucker KL, Sheppard JP, Stevens R, Bosworth HB, Bove A, Bray EP, et al. Self-monitoring of blood pressure in hypertension: a systematic review and individual patient data meta-analysis. PLoS Med. 2017;14(9): e1002389.
25. Xiong S, Berkhouse H, Schooler M, Pu W, Sun A, Gong E, et al. Effectiveness of mHealth interventions in improving medication adherence among people with hypertension: a systematic review. Curr Hypertens Rep. 2018;20(10):86.
26. Choi WS, Choi JH, Oh J, Shin IS, Yang JS. Effects of remote monitoring of blood pressure in management of urban hypertensive patients: a systematic review and meta-analysis. Telemed J E Health. 2020;26(6):744-59.
27. Ma Y, Cheng HY, Cheng L, Sit JWH. The effectiveness of electronic health interventions on blood pressure control, self-care behavioural outcomes and psychosocial well-being in patients with hypertension: a systematic review and meta-analysis. Int J Nurs Stud. 2019;92:27-46.
28. Lu X, Yang H, Xia X, Lu X, Lin J, Liu F, et al. Interactive mobile health intervention and blood pressure management in adults. Hypertension. 2019;74:697-704.
29. Omboni S, Tenti M, Coronetti C. Physician–pharmacist collaborative practice and telehealth may transform hypertension management. J Hum Hypertens. 2019;33(3):177-87.
30. Alessa T, Hawley MS, Hock ES, De Witte L. Smartphone apps to support self-management of hypertension: Review and content analysis. J Med Internet Res. 2019; 7(5):e13645.
31. Luo L, Ye M, Tan J, Huang Q, Qin X, Peng S, et al. Telehealth for the management of blood pressure in patients with chronic kidney disease: A systematic review. J Telemed Telecare. 2019;25(2):80-92.
32. Omboni S, McManus RJ, Bosworth HB, Chappell LC, Green BB, Kario K, et al. Evidence and recommendations on the use of telemedicine for the management of arterial hypertension: An international expert position paper. Hypertension. 2020;76(5):1368-83.

CHAPTER 47

Adherence to the Treatment for Hypertension

Michaela M Watts, Fraz A Mir

■ INTRODUCTION

Case History

A 48-year-old woman with apparently resistant hypertension was prescribed multiple antihypertensive agents. These comprised ramipril 10 mg once daily, bisoprolol 10 mg once daily, amlodipine 10 mg od, spironolactone 25 mg once daily, indapamide 2.5 mg once daily, doxazosin XL 4 mg once daily, and methyldopa 250 mg three times a day.

She attended the hypertension clinic in the morning and underwent "directly-observed therapy," that is, nurse-led administration of her prescribed medication and measurement of her blood pressure response. Her baseline average seated blood pressure was 168/102 mm Hg, with a heart rate of 96 bpm.

High-performance liquid chromatography-tandem mass spectrometry (HPLC–MS) of a urine sample taken immediately prior to her directly-observed therapy revealed that none of the prescribed drugs was detectable.

Her 24-h ambulatory blood pressure monitoring following stepwise administration of ramipril 10 mg, amlodipine 10 mg, and indapamide 2.5 mg revealed a daytime average of 134/78 mm Hg (nighttime average 115/69 mm Hg).

As the population ages and life expectancy increases, more people are living with several long-term conditions, including hypertension, that are being managed with an increasing number of medicines. Maintaining a careful balance gets more difficult for people and health professionals, particularly when also trying to reduce health inequalities in the population.

Medicines are the most common intervention in healthcare. However, it has been estimated that between 30 and 50% of medicines prescribed for long-term conditions are not taken as intended.[1] Typically, adherence rates of 80% or more are needed for optimal therapeutic efficacy.

Optimizing a person's medicines is important to ensure a person is taking their medicines as intended and can support the management of long-term conditions, comorbidities, and polypharmacy. Medicines optimization is defined as "a person-centered approach to safe and effective medicines use, to ensure people obtain the optimal benefits from their medications."[2] Medicines optimization applies to patients who may or may not take their medicines effectively. Shared decision making is a fundamental part of evidence-based medicine, seeking to use the best available evidence to guide decisions about the care of the individual patient, taking into account their needs, preferences, and values.[3]

A critical part of shared decision making is about health professionals understanding the person's desired level of inclusion in decision making about their medicines. It is often difficult for the person and the health professional to decide whether the medicines being taken are appropriate and the decision may be different for each person.

We know as clinicians that the use of the same and appropriate terminology is fundamental to understanding the patient's medicines-taking behavior. Compliance has been commonly used and implies that the patient complies with the doctor's orders; however, most doctors no longer wish to practice medicine in such a paternalistic way.

Concordance is a complex concept that is preferred but not practical in everyday general practice; it covers the process of incorporating patient beliefs and preferences in the decision-making process and includes wider supportive care for the patient. On the contrary, "adherence" describes the extent to which the patient's behavior matches advice from the prescriber and will be the term used predominantly in this chapter.

In response to the scale of the problem in the UK, National Institute for Health and Care Excellence (NICE) developed guidelines (Medicines adherence: Involving patients in decisions about prescribed medicines and supporting adherence CG76 2009)[4] with recommendations about how healthcare professionals can help patients to make informed decisions by facilitating the involvement of patients in the decision to prescribe, and how they can support patients to "adhere" to the prescribed medicine.

Adherence encompasses numerous health-related behaviors that extend beyond simply taking prescribed drugs. Defining adherence as to the extent to which the patient follows medical instructions is a helpful starting point. However, the term "medical" may be insufficient in describing the range of interventions used to treat chronic hypertension. In addition, the term "instructions" implies that the patient is passive, an acquiescent recipient of expert advice rather than an active collaborator in treatment. Adherence to any regimen reflects behavior of one type or another. Seeking medical attention, filling prescriptions, taking medications as prescribed, attending follow-up appointments, following a diet, and/or executing lifestyle changes including moderation in alcohol consumption and smoking cessation are all examples of therapeutic behaviors.

Therefore, the definition of adherence (to long-term therapy) is the extent to which a person's behavior corresponds with shared decision making with a healthcare provider and seems appropriate.

Five Interacting Dimensions Affecting Adherence (Table 1)

The common belief that patients are solely responsible for "adhering" to their therapy is misleading and most often reflects a misunderstanding of how other factors affect people's behavior and capacity to adhere to their treatment. "Therapy" includes all treatment modalities—non-pharmacological and pharmacological. Adherence is a multifactorial phenomenon determined by the interplay of five sets of factors or "dimensions," of which patient-related factors are just one determinant.[5]

Socioeconomic-related Factors

Socioeconomic status has not consistently been found to be an independent predictor of adherence; however, in developing countries, low socioeconomic status may put patients in the position of having to choose between competing priorities including demands to direct their limited resources to meet the needs of other family members, such as children or parents for whom they care.

Some other factors reported to have a significant effect on adherence are illiteracy,

TABLE 1: Adherence and treating hypertension.

Factors	Factors affecting adherence	Interventions to improve adherence
Socioeconomic-related factors	(–) Poor socioeconomic status, illiteracy, unemployment, limited drug supply, and high cost of medication	Family preparedness, patient health insurance, uninterrupted supply of medicines, sustainable financing, affordable prices, and reliable supply systems
Healthcare team/health system-related factors	(–) Lack of knowledge and training for healthcare providers on managing chronic diseases, inadequate relationship between healthcare provider and patient, lack of knowledge and inadequate time for consultations, and lack of incentives and feedback on performance (+) Good relationship between patient and physician	Training in the education of patients on the use of medicines; good patient–physician relationship; continuous monitoring and reassessment of treatment; monitoring adherence; nonjudgemental attitude and assistance; uninterrupted ready availability of information; rational selection of medications; training in communication skills; delivery, financing, and proper management of medicines; pharmaceuticals: developing drugs with better safety profile, participation in patient education programs and developing instruments to measure adherence for patients
Condition-related factors	(+) Understanding the perceptions about hypertension	Education on the use of medicines
Therapy-related factors	• (–) Complex treatment regimens; duration of treatment; low drug tolerability, adverse effects of treatment • (+) Monotherapy with simple dosing schedules; less frequent dose; fewer changes in antihypertensive medications; newer classes of drugs with fewer side effects: angiotensin II antagonists and calcium channel blockers	Simplification of regimens
Patient-related factors	• (–) Inadequate knowledge and skill in managing the disease symptoms and treatment, no awareness of the costs and benefits of treatment, nonacceptance of monitoring; patients' understanding of risk and communication about it from healthcare provider • (+) Perception of the health risk related to the disease, active participation in monitoring, participation in management of disease	Behavioral and motivational intervention, good patient-physician relationship, self-management of disease and treatment, self-management of side effects, memory aids, and reminders

(+), factors having a positive effect on adherence; (–), factors having a negative effect on adherence.
Source: Sabaté E. Adherence to long-term therapies: Evidence for action. 2003 World Health Organization, Geneva, Switzerland. Available from http://www.who.int/chronic_ conditions/adherencereport/en/ [Last accessed November, 2023][5]

low level of education, unemployment, lack of effective social support networks, unstable living conditions, a long distance from the treatment center, costly transportation, premium charges for medication particularly in privately funded healthcare systems, changing environmental situations, culture and lay beliefs about illness and treatment, and family dysfunction.

Healthcare Team and System-related Factors

A good patient–prescriber relationship may improve adherence. However, there are many factors that have a negative effect. These include poorly developed health services, poor medication distribution systems, lack of knowledge and training for healthcare providers on managing chronic diseases such as hypertension, overworked healthcare providers, short consultations, the poor capacity of the system to educate patients about their condition and provide them with timely follow-up, and lack of knowledge on adherence and of effective intervention for improving it. One point of notable interest is the fact that patients involved in research trials tend to adhere more to treatment and as a consequence have better outcomes too. Recreating such high adherence levels in routine clinical practice remains elusive. Hypertension is hugely common in the Indian population and rather than drug treatment for all, population-level public health measures are required; for example, stopping smoking, weight loss, exercising, salt, alcohol and carbohydrate consumption reduction, etc.

Condition-related Factors

Condition-related factors represent particular illness-related demands faced by the patient. Some strong determinants of adherence are those directly related to the severity of symptoms. In general, hypertensive patients have little or no symptoms which increases the difficulty in convincing the patient that they need life-long treatment. This is particularly the case when medications used to treat hypertension cause side-effects. The severity of the disease and the availability of effective treatments are also factors. Their impact depends on how they influence patients' risk perception, the importance of following treatment, and the priority placed on adherence. Unless patients understand the risks they face from nonadherence, they are unlikely to engage in a successful process of adherence.

Therapy-related Factors

There are many therapy-related factors that can affect adherence. Most notable are those related to the complexity of the medical regimen, previous treatment failures, and/or side effects (discussed above), frequent changes in treatment, and the immediacy of beneficial effects.

Vrijens et al.[6] explored the characteristics of dosing history in nearly five thousand patients prescribed once-a-day antihypertensive medications. **Figure 1** demonstrates the time course of adherence/compliance parameters, described as "execution/persistence." By around 6 months, only about two-thirds of patients were still taking their medication; even few were taking it as prescribed originally. The resulting shortfalls in drug exposure that these dosing errors may create could be a common cause of low rates of blood pressure control and high variability in responses to prescribed antihypertensive drugs.

Randomized trials have shown that a polypill combining a statin with one or more antihypertensive drugs and aspirin

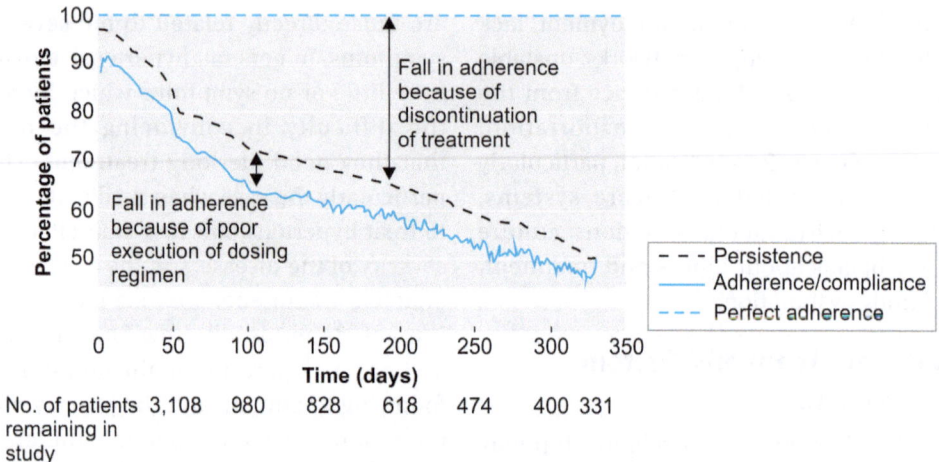

Fig. 1: Time course of adherence/compliance parameters (execution, persistence) Vrijens et al.[6]

improves treatment adherence rates and safely reduces cardiovascular risk factors in patients with established cardiovascular disease.[7] However, in contrast to conditions such as HIV, asthma, and migraine, for which combination treatments have gotten collective approval, the idea of a polypill for cardiovascular disease prevention, while seemingly popular among patients, has proved to be less so among specialist physicians. The reasoning behind this includes negative perceptions about the lack of flexibility in dosing and also concerns about the loss of autonomy in clinical decision making. Until recently there has been little enthusiasm from pharmaceutical companies to develop polypills because of perceived low financial margins, despite there being a huge target population. The tide seems to be turning, however, with the recent approval of a polypill that contains aspirin, ramipril, and atorvastatin in more than 30 countries across both Latin America and Europe. The availability and use of an affordable polypill would be universally welcome to help achieve the World Health Organization target of reducing the number of deaths from noncommunicable diseases by 25% by 2025.

Patient-related Factors

Patient-related factors represent the resources, knowledge, attitudes, beliefs, perceptions, and expectations of the patient. Patients' knowledge and beliefs about their hypertension, motivation to manage it, confidence in their ability to engage in illness-management behaviors including lifestyle choices, and expectations regarding the outcome of treatment and the consequences of poor adherence, interact to influence adherence behavior.[8]

In 2005, a study reviewed the qualitative research on drug taking in a wide range of medical conditions and found that patients often actively decided not to take drugs (intentional nonadherence) rather than unintentionally omitting them.[9] A systematic review of qualitative research looking at people's perspectives on hypertension and drug taking, found that many participants in the individual studies perceived stress to be the primary cause and exacerbating factor of (their) hypertension. These participants widely described symptoms that they perceived to be caused by hypertension, especially headaches, palpitations, and dizziness. Contrary to the conclusions of individual studies, these participant-reported symptoms were found to be consistent among different ethnic and geographical groups. Participants intentionally adjusted their drug dose, took drugs sporadically, and stopped altogether, often without seeking medical advice beforehand. Reasons given for reducing their treatments included a perception that their blood pressure had improved because of a reduction in symptoms and that they felt the drugs were unnecessary when they were under less stress, they had a dislike of taking drugs, worried about risks of addiction or tolerance, and also side effects.

Patient-related factors reported to affect adherence are as follows:
- Forgetfulness
- Psychosocial stress
- Anxieties about possible adverse effects
- Low motivation
- Inadequate knowledge and skill in managing their disease and treatment × Lack of self-perceived need for treatment
- Lack of perceived effect of treatment
- Negative beliefs regarding the efficacy of the treatment
- Lack of perception of the health risks related to hypertension
- Misunderstanding of medication instructions
- Lack of engagement in monitoring of their blood pressure
- Low treatment expectations
- Low attendance at follow-up appointments
- Anxiety over the complexity of the drug regimen
- Feeling stigmatized by the disease

Perceptions of personal need for medication are influenced by symptoms, expectations, and experiences, and by illness cognitions. Concerns about medication typically arise from beliefs about side effects and disruption of lifestyle, and from more abstract worries about the long-term effects.

■ ADHERENCE AND HYPERTENSION

We live in a rapidly changing environment. Throughout the world, health is being forged by the same powerful forces: An aging worldwide population, rapid urbanization, and global increase in unhealthy lifestyles. Increasingly, we are seeing that both wealthy and resource-poor countries are facing the same health issues. One of the most striking examples of this significant shift is the fact that noncommunicable diseases, such as cardiovascular disease, cancer, diabetes, and chronic lung diseases, have overtaken infectious diseases as the world's leading cause of death.[10] Indeed, the biggest modifiable risk factor and threat to human life globally is now thought to be hypertension.

It is well known that high blood pressure increases the risk of ischemic heart disease 3–4-fold and of overall cardiovascular risk by 2–3-fold. The incidence of stroke increases approximately threefold in patients with borderline hypertension and approximately eightfold in those with definite hypertension. It has been estimated that 40% of cases of acute myocardial infarction or stroke are attributable to known hypertension. Clinical trials have demonstrated that the treatment of mild-to-moderate hypertension can reduce the risk of stroke by 30–43% and myocardial infarction by 15%.

Despite the wide availability of effective treatments, both pharmacological and nonpharmacological studies have shown that in many countries less than a quarter of patients who are treated for hypertension achieve optimum blood pressure levels. About a third of urban and a quarter of rural Indians are hypertensive. However, of these, only 25% of rural and 42% of urban Indians are aware that they are hypertensive. Those being treated are 25 and 38%, respectively. Only one-tenth of rural and one-fifth of urban Indians have their blood pressure under control.[11]

Poor adherence has been identified as the cause of failure to control hypertension in up to two-thirds of patients. Usually, most patients start with lifestyle modifications including losing weight, smoking cessation, reduction in alcohol consumption, eating fresh fruits, and vegetables high in potassium, regular exercising, etc. There is good evidence to show that taken together, these interventions can reduce blood pressure significantly. The challenge, of course, is to maintain such a healthy lifestyle in the long term.[12] Even so, lifestyle modifications should be reiterated regularly, regardless of whether or not the patient is on antihypertensive medications.

In addition to the prevention of death, stroke, and myocardial infarction, other costly consequences of untreated hypertension can also be prevented or minimized by effective treatment.[13,14] Examples of the benefits of treatment include reduction in risk of cardiac failure, reduction in the incidence of dementia, preservation of renal function, and prevention of blindness in diabetic patients with hypertension. It is apparent that in many countries, poorly controlled blood pressure represents not only a significant health burden but consequently, an important economic liability. It is clear, therefore, that improving adherence could represent both an important potential source of health and economic advancement.[15,16]

ASSESSING AND TACKLING ADHERENCE: THE CAMBRIDGE PERSPECTIVE

Patients do not always take their medicines exactly as prescribed and healthcare professionals are often unaware of how patients take their medicines. The purpose of assessing adherence is not only to monitor patients but also to find out whether the patient needs more information and support around taking their medications. In years gone by, "tagging" medicines with measurable drugs (e.g., barbiturates) was acceptable ethically. In the current era, antihypertensive drugs can be detected in blood and urine samples, the latter by employing high-performance liquid chromatography-tandem mass spectrometry (HPLC-MS/MS). However, the use of such techniques can risk undermining the clinician–patient relationship and it is important that the clinician informs the patient prior to the sample collection. The clinician should consider assessing nonadherence by directly asking the patient if they have missed any doses of medicine recently. To make it easier for the patient to report nonadherence, the question should be asked in a way that does not apportion blame. Clinicians should explain to the patient the reason why they are being asked the question. It is useful to ask about a specific period such as "in the past week." It is also useful to ask the patient about their medicine-taking behaviors such as reducing the prescribed dose, stopping and starting medicines, or taking "medicine holidays." Also, the physician can consider using records of prescription reordering, pharmacy patient medication records, and return of any unused medicines to identify potential nonadherence.

As the evidence supporting interventions to increase adherence is largely inconclusive, one should only use interventions to overcome the practical problems associated with patient nonadherence when and if a specific need is identified; the intervention should be tailored to the needs of the individual. Interventions might include suggesting that patients record their medicine taking or keeping a "diary," encouraging patients to monitor their condition; for example, regular recording of blood pressures at home, and simplifying the dosing regimen; for example, combination and once-daily medications. For the elderly or those less physically able, the use of liquid preparations, alternative packaging for the medicine, or using a multicompartment medicines system should be considered.

As mentioned already, while hypertensive patients largely have no symptoms, side effects from antihypertensive drugs are not uncommon. They can be enough of an irritation for some patients to stop some or all of their treatment.[17] Of all modern antihypertensive agents, angiotensin receptor blockers have the most favorable side effect profile and are most likely to be tolerated. If nonadherence remains the case it should be discussed how the patient would like to deal with side effects; discussion of the benefits, disadvantages, and long-term effects with the patient to allow them to make an informed choice. Do they understand and appreciate the concept and level of risk to their health because of nonadherence? The clinician should consider adjusting the dosage of the medication: Often patients can tolerate smaller doses of multiple agents rather than increased doses of just one or two; consideration for switching to another medicine with a different range of side effects can also be effective. Contemplate what other strategies might be used (for example, timing of medicines). Asking patients if prescription costs are a problem for them and if they are, consider possible options to reduce costs (e.g., in the UK, it is possible to purchase a prepayment annual certificate).

■ DIRECTLY OBSERVED THERAPY

Suboptimal adherence to antihypertensive medication is an underestimated contributing factor in apparent treatment-resistant hypertension. Resistant hypertension supposedly has a prevalence of approximately 10%.[18] Such patients have a higher cardiovascular risk and consequently a poorer cardiovascular prognosis. In the experience of the authors, once secondary causes have been excluded, truly resistant hypertension is much rarer and constitutes a minority of patients. One strategy being increasingly employed to assess concordance in the field of hypertension, and thereby exclude resistant hypertension, is directly observed therapy (DOT). This is adapted from the approach applied so successfully in the treatment of tuberculosis. Patients are observed taking their antihypertensive medications under direct supervision at a "DOT" clinic. At the DOT clinic visit, patients are asked to attend first thing in the morning unmedicated. They are fitted with a 24-h ambulatory blood pressure monitor for ease of repeated measurement and each of their antihypertensive drugs, at currently prescribed doses, are administered by a healthcare professional using a step-wise algorithm (Fig. 2).

Typically, the treatment guidance from the British Hypertension Society/National Institute of Clinical Excellence is followed. This is derived, in part, from research conducted in Cambridge. The patient then remains in the clinic under observation for 4-6 h. Ambulatory blood pressure monitoring readings continue for the next

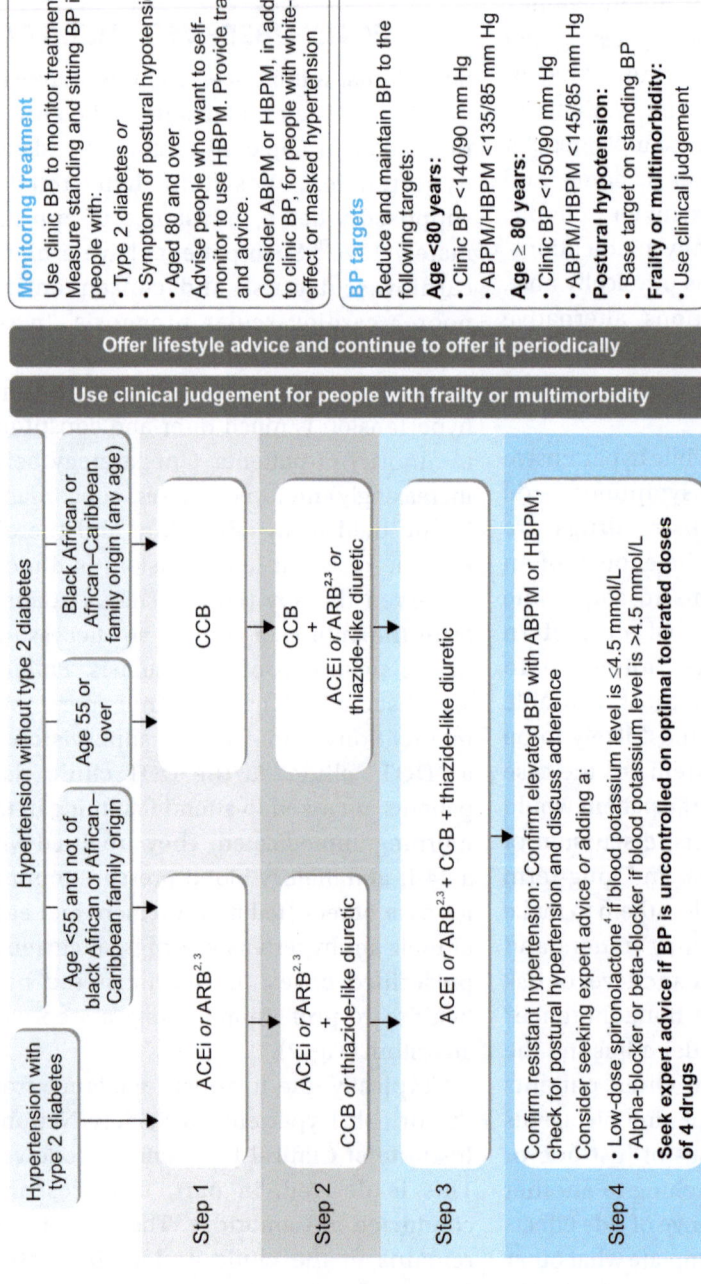

Fig. 2: Choice of antihypertensive drug, monitoring treatment and BP targets. (ABPM: ambulatory blood pressure; ACEi: ACE inhibitor; ARB: angiotensin-II receptor blocker; BP: blood pressure; CCB: calcium-channel blocker; HBPM: home blood pressure monitoring)

Source: National Institute for Health and Care Excellence (NICE). Hypertension in adults: diagnosis and management. 2022. Available from www.nice.org.uk/guidance/ng136

24 h. Comparisons are then made between pre- and post-DOT clinics. Results from studies suggest that up to 50% of patients undergoing DOT with apparently treatment-resistant hypertension are shown to be nonadherent to treatment.[19] Hence, the DOT clinic can be an effective method of identifying truly resistant hypertensive patients.

■ CONCLUSION

Adherence to medical therapeutics is one of clinical medicine's most demanding challenges. It requires time and patience, excellent communication, and a functional relationship between clinician and patient. Concordance in the area of hypertension is even more arduous given the asymptomatic nature of the condition and the side effects of antihypertensive agents. As discussed, a variety of methods can be employed to both assess and tackle patient adherence to therapy and thereby identify truly "resistant hypertensives." Nonadherence to therapy is an important cause of suboptimal blood pressure control but for now, there are few practical tools that exist to accurately and routinely detect it. The use of a simple urine-based assay to evaluate the prevalence of nonadherence to pharmacological anti-hypertensive treatment, that is, HPLC-MS/MS urine analysis could be used to exclude nonadherence and therefore better stratify further investigations and interventions. The Leicester group in 2014 found that out of a cohort of 208 hypertensive patients referred with inadequate blood pressure control at least 25% were found to be totally or partially nonadherent to their prescribed antihypertensive treatment. Moreover, they found there was a linear relationship between blood pressure and the numerical difference in detected/prescribed antihypertensive medications.[20]

Implications for Clinicians and Education about Hypertension

Some of the evidence discussed in this chapter adds gravity to the criticism of educational interventions that assume poor adherence to treatment is due to patients' deficiencies or failings, either in their knowledge or remembering to take drugs. The participants in some of the qualitative studies reviewed did not simply have a knowledge deficit but they held alternative explanations for their hypertension; many participants consciously chose to avoid taking their prescribed medications.

This may explain in part why educational interventions that simply aim to inform patients about the "current" or "conventional" medical view have proved to be ineffective. In the future, to deal with these problems, clinicians and any educational interventions must recognize and integrate patients' concerns and viewpoints. Patients should be given an honest and accurate depiction of the likely benefits and adverse effects of their prescribed treatments. Safety of long-term use of drugs should be discussed; including that treatment is not thought to accumulate or "build up" in the body or to cause a physical dependence or addiction. Fears about addiction or treatment tolerance and resistance could be further tackled by informing patients that they are unlikely to experience adverse effects if they decide to stop, no matter how long they have taken the treatment. This is at odds with existing educational interventions, which seek to emphasize the importance of continuous uninterrupted tablet taking.

The possibility of symptoms and patients' experiences should be acknowledged. Patients should be told that people with hypertension will often report symptoms but that they have not been found to be a reliable indication of variations in their blood pressure levels. Patients should be informed that their risk of cardiovascular disease is increased regardless of whether they have symptoms, and that treatment can effectively prevent cardiovascular disease. Stress should be placed in the context of other modifiable and nonmodifiable risk factors for hypertension and cardiovascular disease; however, it should be noted that relieving stress alone is unlikely to normalize blood pressure and that antihypertensive treatment is recommended at times of both high and low stress.

Nonintentional factors, for example, "forgetting" and "being busy," were cited by many patients as reasons for nonadherence. However, there is some evidence from randomized controlled trials that reminder interventions may be beneficial. Indeed, a number of trials exploring the effects of mobile phone apps, self-administration techniques as well as nurse involvement are ongoing. The corollary seems to be that the greater the number and intensity of "interventions," the better the adherence to treatment. Finally, in the recent literature, there was an absence of robust evidence that educational interventions for hypertension need to be tailored to a particular cultural or ethnic group; it is more important to take into account of common understandings and experiences across the world. However, tailoring management to the individual and their personal needs remains paramount.

■ REFERENCES

1. World Health Organization. World Health Report, 2003: Shaping the Future. World Health Organization: Geneva, 2003.
2. National Institute for Health and Care Excellence. Medicines optimisation: the safe and effective use of medicines to enable the best possible outcomes, NICE guideline [NG5], 2015. Available from https://www.nice.org.uk/guidance/ng5 [Last accessed November, 2023].
3. Elwyn G, Coulter A, Laitner S, Walker E, Watson P, Thomson R. Implementing shared decision making in the NHS. BMJ. 2010;341:c5146.
4. National Institute for Health and Care Excellence. Medicines adherence: involving patients in decisions about prescribed medicines and supporting adherence, Clinical guideline [CG76], 2009. Available from https://www.nice.org.uk/guidance/cg76 [Last accessed November, 2023].
5. Sabaté E. Adherence to long-term therapies: Evidence for action. 2003 World Health Organization, Geneva, Switzerland. Available from http://www.who.int/chronic_conditions/adherencereport/en/ [Last accessed November, 2023].
6. Vrijens B, Vincze G, Kristanto P, Urquhart J, Burnier M. Adherence to prescribed anti-hypertensive drug treatments: Longitudinal study of electronically compiled dosing histories. BMJ. 2008;336(7653):1114-7.
7. Tomaszewski M, White C, Patel P, Masca N, Damani R, Hepworth J, et al. High rates of non-adherence to antihypertensive treatment revealed by high-performance liquid chromatography-tandem mass spectrometry (HPLC-MS/MS) urine analysis. Heart 2014;100(11):855-61.
8. Luscher TF, Vetter H, Siegenthaler W, Vetter W. Compliance in hypertension: facts and concepts. J Hypertens. 1985;3(1):S3-9.
9. Pound P, Britten N, Morgan M, Yardley L, Pope C, Daker-White G, et al. Resisting medicines: A synthesis of qualitative studies of medicine taking. Soc Sci Med. 2005;61(1):133-55.
10. GBD 2019 Risk Factors Collaborators. Global burden of 87 risk factors in 204 countries and territories, 1990–2019: A systematic analysis for the Global Burden of Disease Study 2019. Lancet. 2020;396:1223-49.
11. Anchala R, Kannuri NK, Pant H, Khan H, Franco OH, Di Angelantonio E, et al. Hypertension in India: A systematic review and meta-analysis of prevalence, awareness, and control of hypertension. J Hypertens. 2014;32(6):1170-7.

12. Morisky DE, Levine DM, Green LW, Shapiro S, Russell RP, Smith CR. Five-year blood pressure control and mortality following health education for hypertensive patients. Am J Public Health. 1983;73(2):153-62.
13. Singer RB. Stroke in the elderly treated for systolic hypertension. J Insur Med.1992; 24(1):28-31.
14. Thompson DW, Furlan AJ. Clinical epidemiology of stroke. Neurol Clin. 1996;14(2): 309-5.
15. Forette F, Seux ML, Staessen JA, Thijs L, Babarskiene MR, Babeanu S, et al. The prevention of dementia with antihypertensive treatment: New evidence from the Systolic Hypertension in Europe (Syst-Eur) study. Arch Intern Med. 2002;162(18):2046-52.
16. Bergström J, Alvestrand A, Bucht H, Gutierrez A. Progression of renal failure in man is retarded with more frequent clinical follow-ups and better blood-pressure control. Clin Nephrol. 1986;25(1):1-6.
17. Andrade JP, Vilas–Boas F, Chagas H, Andrade M. Epidemiological aspects of adherence to treatment of hypertension. Arq Bras Cardiol. 2002;79(4):375-84.
18. Judd E, Calhoun DA. Apparent and true resistant hypertension: definition, prevalence and outcomes. J Hum Hypertens. 2014;28(8): 463-8.
19. Hameed MA, Cappuccio F, Padmanabhan S, Dasgupta I. J Human Hypertension. 2016; 30:633-56.
20. Tomaszewski M, White C, Patel P, Masca N, Damani R, Hepworth J, et al. High rates of non-adherence to antihypertensive treatment revealed by high-performance liquid chromatography-tandem mass spectrometry (HPLC-MS/MS) urine analysis. Heart. 2014;100 (11):855-61.

Navigating Dilemmas in the Management of Hypertension: A Perpetual Challenge

Alok Kumar Singh, Sadanand R Shetty

INTRODUCTION

Hypertension (HTN) is a major modifiable cardiovascular (CV) risk factor, contributing significantly to CV disease burden and disability worldwide, but certain issues regarding diagnostic cut-off of HTN, which drug should be used as the first choice and which guideline to follow and so many questions pose dilemmas to the treating physician on a daily basis when they encounter a patient with HTN in the clinic. In this chapter, we will discuss the point of confusion and dilemma that every physician faces on a daily basis and even international and national guidelines have divergence of recommendations on them.

WHAT SHOULD BE THE CUTOFF FOR DIAGNOSIS OF HYPERTENSION?

It is difficult to believe that only about 50 years ago, HTN was considered an essential condition to survive and need not be treated. However, after the discovery of thiazide diuretics in the 1960s, the landmark multicenter VA cooperative study phase 1[1] of the trial examined active treatment (hydrochlorothiazide, reserpine, and hydralazine) versus placebo in 143 veterans with severe HTN [diastolic blood pressure (DBP), 115–129 mm Hg] and achieved an average fall of blood pressure (BP) by 43/30 mm Hg in the treated group over the average follow-up of 1.5 years. The results of this trial showed clear morbidity and mortality benefits of drug treatment of HTN. The VA cooperative study phase 2[2] examined the benefit of active treatment versus placebo in moderately severe HTN (DBP 90–115 mm Hg) patients. Using the same drug treatment as in the first VA cooperative study, this study achieved an average fall in diastolic BP by 19 mm Hg in the treatment group. The results showed significant morbidity and mortality benefits over the mean period of 3.8-year follow-up. These two studies established the following two facts beyond doubt: (1) Treatment of BP above 90 mm Hg of DBP is beneficial and (2) the second severe form of HTN derives more and relatively early benefit after drug treatment.

After VA cooperative study, another landmark study was hypertension detection and follow-up (HDFP)[3] in 1979, which demonstrated the benefit in mortality and morbidity by aggressive, goal-directed BP treatment with stepwise incremental therapy as opposed to more casual BP management without trying to reach a target BP. The drugs utilized in this study were chlorthalidone (CTDN), reserpine, K-sparing diuretics, methyldopa, hydralazine, and guanethidine. The cut-off of HTN in HDFP was DBP 90 mm Hg.

The VA cooperative study phase 1, followed by the phase 2 study, established for the first time that diastolic HTN >90 mm Hg was treatable with available drugs and reduced stroke, CHF, and mortality. The HDFP study further confirmed the finding of the VA cooperative study and established that BP treatment target to diastolic goal of 90 gave much better CV outcome results than usual BP treatment. Both MRC[4] and EWHPE[5] confirmed this finding for younger and older patients, respectively, in the non-US population. A hypertension optimal treatment (HOT)[6] study established that lowering the diastolic BP goal <90 (85 or 80) does not add any further CV or mortality benefits. So, these landmark studies have established the cutoff of DBP as 90 mm Hg.

However, isolated systolic HTN accounting for majority of hypertensive population, especially in elderly, was not considered treatable until 1991, when systolic hypertension in elderly program (SHEP)[7] study was completed and showed tremendous benefits of treating systolic BP (SBP) over 160 mm Hg using only simple drugs such as small dose CTDN with the addition of atenolol if needed. The average BP achieved in the active treatment arm was 143/65 mm Hg (155/72 in the control group). In this study, for the first time, a SBP cutoff of 140 mm Hg was taken. These trials established conclusively that treatment of HTN, whether systolic or diastolic HTN treatment, is beneficial with simpler drugs such as hydrochlorothiazide, CTDN, reserpine, hydralazine, K-sparing diuretics, methyldopa, and guanethidine.

The first Joint National Committee on Prevention, Detection, and Treatment of High Blood Pressure (JNC report) was issued in 1977.[8] Prior to JNC 5,[9] recommendations for drug therapy were based on DBP, reflecting the design of studies completed before 1988. Based on the results of contemporary clinical trials, JNC 5 emphasized the importance of systolic HTN for the first time. As in JNC 4,[10] the BP goal was <140/90 mm Hg in JNC 5 but the HTN was classically defined as 140/90 mm Hg and above for the first time in JNC 5.[9]

After the JNC 5 guideline, ACCORD[11] study showed no significant difference in outcome with systolic blood pressure (SBP) 140 versus 120 in diabetics. However, the most recent SPRINT[12] study with a somewhat similar protocol to that in ACCORD but in the nondiabetic population showed an almost one-quarter reduction in all-cause mortality and a one-third reduction of CV events with SBP goal of 120 mm Hg. Based on the result of SPRINT, the American College of Cardiology/American Heart Association (ACC/AHA)[13] have revised the HTN cutoff as 130/80. However, the European Society of Cardiology/European Society of Hypertension (ESC/ESH)[14] and other societies such as ISH[15] have retained the cutoff as 140/90 mm Hg because of the conflicting results of ACCORD and SPRINT as well as the method of BP which was different in SPRINT from the rest of the previous randomized clinical trials.

Basically, all recent dilemmas regarding the diagnostic cut-off of BP were started after the recommendation of recent ACC/AHA guidelines, which based their recommendation on SPRINT trial outcome data without highlighting the fact that the method of BP measurement was entirely different from previous landmark trial in SPRINT trial. All other landmark trials were based on office BP measurement, whereas in SPRINT trial automated out-of-office blood pressure measurement (AOBP) technique was used. Unattended systolic BP measured using an AOBP device as in SPRINT is on average 10 mm Hg lower than the office sphygmomanometer or oscillometric value.[16]

■ WHICH DRUG IS BETTER?

Apart from diagnostic cutoff, another question that always poses a dilemma to a physician's mind is which drug is better.

If we see historically in the landmark trial like VA cooperative, HDFP studies have used simple and cheap drugs such as hydrochlorothiazide, CTDN, reserpine, hydralazine, K-sparing diuretics, methyldopa, and guanethidine and demonstrated the mortality benefit, so controlling the BP is more important in contrast to the fact which drug to be used. The Antihypertensive and lipid-lowering treatment to prevent heart attack trial (ALLHAT)[17] in 2002, the largest antihypertensive trial till date, tried to resolve the question of superiority of any of the newer class of antihypertensive drugs such as angiotensin-converting enzyme inhibitor (ACEI), calcium channel blocker (CCB), and α-blocker give better CV outcomes than the older drugs such as thiazide-like diuretic CTDN. The predefined primary outcome of this trial was fatal coronary heart disease or nonfatal myocardial infarction (MI) combined. Secondary outcomes included all-cause mortality, fatal and nonfatal stroke, coronary artery disease, peripheral vascular disease, heart failure (HF), end-stage renal disease, and cancer. The ALLHAT included over 40,000 high-risk hypertensive patients (aged 55 years or older) who were followed up for over 5 years (with the exception of the doxazosin treatment arm, which was discontinued prematurely due to a higher incidence of HF). There was no difference in the primary outcome of combined fatal congenital heart disease (CHD) or nonfatal or fatal MI, and the secondary outcomes of all-cause mortality, end-stage renal disease, peripheral vascular disease, or cancer, between the three treatment groups. So, if we see the result in totality, there was no real difference between the comparator drugs.

On subgroup analysis, it has been found that lisinopril had a 10% higher incidence of combined cardiovascular disease (CVD), a 15% higher incidence of stroke, and a 19% higher incidence of HF than CTDN, whereas amlodipine had a 38% higher incidence of HF compared to CTDN. This can be explained by the fact that the SBP in the lisinopril group was higher by 2 mm Hg compared to CTDN for the 5-year observation period. It is important to note that the addition of atenolol was allowed to all three classes of drugs (CTDN, amlodipine, and lisinopril) if BP is not on target. The ALLHAT study also showed that the use of thiazide drugs (CTDN) did not increase the incidence of MI or mortality over other classes of drugs (CCB, ACEI, or AB). It also showed incidence of CHF was higher with the use of CCB, and ACEI than with CTDN.

The AASK[18] study was done in African-Americans with CKD and showed that tight BP control over usual BP control did not affect CKD progression, but the use of ACEI caused superior renoprotection over CCB. The ASCOT[19] study showed the superiority of the combination of ACEI and CCB over β-blocker (BB) and thiazide [hydrochlorothiazide (HCTZ)] in preventing CV outcomes. CAFE,[20] a substudy of ASCOT, showed that BB failed to lower central aortic BP as opposed to peripheral BP. HYVET[21] study showed that treatment of HTN in very elderly (>80 years) is even more beneficial than in any other age group. ACCOMPLISH[22] study showed the superiority of a combination of ACEI and CCB over ACE and thiazide (HCTZ but not CTDN) for CV outcomes.

So, if we see in totality, then it is more important to control BP rather than the choice of antihypertensive drug. Our point of view on this issue is that most patients of HTN ultimately will require more than one drug for the control of BP and majority hypertensive patients have associated comorbidities so in that case some drugs score over others such as in the presence of coronary artery disease, HF, migraine and thyrotoxicosis BB are the preferred choice, whereas in a patient with chronic kidney disease and HF ACE inhibitors are a preferred choice. So, when choosing an antihypertensive drug, the level of BP and comorbidities plays an important role.

■ HOW MUCH LOW TO GO?

For perfusion of the vital organs such as the brain, kidney, and heart, a minimum BP is required. Increasing BP is a risk factor for CV diseases and lowering BP is beneficial in reducing CV events but how much low to go is still not well settled. The ACCORD study showed that in diabetics, lowering the BP target to 120 systolic over the conventional 140 added no further reduction in CV or renal outcomes. The SPRINT study showed significant mortality and CV benefits in a group with a systolic BP treatment goal of 120 compared to the goal of 140 in nondiabetic patients. Now, most of the guidelines recognize the fact if the patient can tolerate it without any side effects, then we should target for 130/80 mm Hg BP in most of the population. Older frail patients' BP should be lowered slowly and a close watch for any side effects is required.

■ CONCLUSION

Hypertension is the most common modifiable risk factor for the prevention of CV diseases. Because of divergent ethnicity and multiple guidelines, lot of dilemmas come into the mind of treating physicians. We must take evidence and guideline in totality and try to individualize the best treatment for the indexed patient.

■ REFERENCES

1. Veterans Administration Cooperative Study Group on Antihypertensive Agents. Effects of treatment on morbidity in hypertension. Results in patients with diastolic blood pressures averaging 115 through 129 mm Hg. JAMA. 1967;202(11):1028-34.
2. Veterans Administration Cooperative Study Group on Antihypertensive Agents. Effects of treatment on morbidity in hypertension. II. Results in patients with diastolic blood pressure averaging 90 through 114 mm Hg. JAMA. 1970;213(7):1143-52.
3. Hypertension Detection and Follow-Up Program Cooperative Group. Five-year findings of the hypertension detection and follow-up program. I. Reduction in mortality of persons with high blood pressure, including mild hypertension. JAMA. 1979;242(23):2562-71.
4. Medical Research Council Working Party. MRC trial of treatment of mild hypertension: Principal results. Br Med J (Clin Res Ed). 1985;291(6488):97-104.
5. Amery A, Birkenhager W, Brixko P, Bulpitt C, Clement D, de Leeuw P, et al. Influence of antihypertensive drug treatment on morbidity and mortality in patients over the age of 60 years. EWPHE results: Sub-group analysis based on entry stratification. J Hypertens Suppl. 1986;4(6):S642-7.
6. Hansson L, Zanchetti A, Carruthers SG, Dahlöf B, Elmfeldt D, Julius S, et al. Effects of intensive blood pressure lowering and low dose aspirin in patients with hypertension: Principal results of the hypertension optimal treatment (HOT) randomized trial. Lancet. 1998;351(9118):1755-62.
7. SHEP Cooperative Research Group. Prevention of stroke by antihypertensive drug treatment in older persons with isolated systolic hypertension. Final results of the systolic hypertension in the elderly program (SHEP). JAMA. 1991;265(24):3255-64.
8. Joint National Committee on Detection, Evaluation, and Treatment of High Blood Pressure. Report of the Joint National Committee on Detection, Evaluation, and Treatment of High Blood Pressure: A cooperative study. JAMA. 1977;237(3):255-61.
9. Joint National Committee on Detection, Evaluation, and Treatment of High Blood

Pressure. The fifth report of the Joint National Committee on Detection, Evaluation, and Treatment of High Blood Pressure (JNC V). Arch Intern Med. 1993;153(2):154-83.
10. Joint National Committee on Detection, Evaluation, and Treatment of High Blood Pressure. The 1988 report of the Joint National Committee on Detection, Evaluation, and Treatment of High Blood Pressure. Arch Intern Med. 1988;148(5):1023-38.
11. ACCORD Study Group. Effects of blood pressure control in type 2 diabetes mellitus. N Engl J Med. 2010;362(17):1575-85.
12. SPRINT Research Group. A randomized trial of intensive versus standard blood-pressure control. N Engl J Med. 2015;373(22):2103-16.
13. Whelton PK, Carey RM, Aronow WS, Casey DE Jr, Collins KJ, Himmelfarb CD, et al. 2017 ACC/AHA/AAPA/ABC/ACPM/AGS/APhA/ASH/ASPC/NMA/PCNA guideline for the prevention, detection, evaluation, and management of high blood pressure in adults: A report of the American College of Cardiology/American Heart Association Task Force on Clinical Practice Guidelines. J Am Coll Cardiol. 2018;71(19):e127-e248.
14. Williams B, Mancia G, Spiering W, Rosei EA, Azizi M, Burnier M, et al., 2018 ESC/ESH guidelines for the management of arterial hypertension: the task force for the management of arterial hypertension of the European society of Cardiology and the European Society of hypertension: the task force for the management of arterial hypertension of the European society of Cardiology and the European Society of Hypertension. J Hypertens. 2018;36(10):1953-2041.
15. Unger T., Borghi C, Charchar F, Khan NA, Poulter NR, Prabhakaran D, et al., 2020 International Society of Hypertension global hypertension practice guidelines. J Hypertens. 2020;38(6):982-1004.
16. Wohlfahrt P, Cifkova R, Krajcoviechova A, Sulc P, Bruthans J, Linhart A, et al. Unattended automated office blood pressure measurement. Does it differ from office blood pressure? Insight from a random population sample. J Hypertens. 2019;37(Suppl. 1):E67.
17. ALLHAT Officers and Coordinators for the ALLHAT Collaborative Research Group. Major outcomes in high-risk hypertensive patients randomized to angiotensin-converting enzyme inhibitor or calcium channel blocker vs diuretic: The antihypertensive and lipid-lowering treatment to prevent heart attack trial (ALLHAT). JAMA. 2002;288(23):2981-97.
18. Staessen J, Bulpitt C, Clement D, De Leeuw P, Fagard R, Fletcher A, et al. Relation between mortality and treated blood pressure in elderly patients with hypertension: report of the European working party on high blood pressure in the elderly. BMJ. 1989;298(6687):1552-6.
19. Dahlof B, Sever PS, Poulter NR, Wedel H, Beevers DG, Caulfield M, et al. Prevention of cardiovascular events with an antihypertensive regimen of amlodipine adding perindopril as required versus atenolol adding ben-droflumethazide as required, in the Anglo Scandinavian cardiac outcomes trial-blood pressure lowering arm (ASCOT-BPLA): A multicentre randomised controlled trial. Lancet. 2005;366(9489):895-906.
20. Williams B, Lacy PS, Thom SM, Cruickshank K, Stanton A, Collier D, et al. Differential impact of blood pressure lowering drugs on central aortic pressure and clinical outcomes principal results of the conduit artery function evaluation (CAFE) study. Circulation. 2006:113(9):1213-25.
21. Beckett NS, Peters R, Fletcher AE, Staessen JA, Liu L, Dumitrascu D, et al. Treatment of hypertension in patients 80 years of age or older. N Engl J Med. 2008;358(18):1887-98.
22. Jamerson K, Weber MA, Bakris GL, Dahlöf B, Pitt B, Shi V, et al. Benazepril plus amlodipine or hydrochlorothiazide for hypertension in high-risk patients. N Engl J Med. 2008;359(23):2417-28.

CHAPTER 49

Hypertension Clinic and Hypertension Center

A Muruganathan

■ INTRODUCTION

Hypertension continues to be a significant global health concern, impacting millions of individuals across continents. Inadequate prevention and control efforts at the community level have resulted in substantial mortality and morbidity associated with hypertension. The direct correlation between blood pressure (BP) levels and adverse cardiovascular (CV) outcomes places hypertensive individuals at a heightened risk of CV events.

Hypertension accounts for more than 5.8% of total global deaths, 1.9% of years of life lost, and 1.4% of disability-adjusted life years. A recent study from India, involving 1.3 million adults aged 18 years and above, reported a prevalence of hypertension in 25.3% of individuals. Given this widespread prevalence, routine screening for hypertension in asymptomatic adults becomes imperative.

Despite being a condition that can often be effectively treated, hypertension frequently goes undiagnosed and is inadequately managed. Despite the availability of effective nondrug therapies and powerful medications, treatment outcomes are frequently suboptimal, largely due to issues with patient compliance. Consequently, the prevention and control of hypertension within the community remains a pivotal challenge. The establishment of a dedicated hypertension clinic, tailored to meet the needs of hypertensive patients, can play a significant role in addressing this challenge.

■ WHAT IS HYPERTENSION CLINIC?

The concept of a small outpatient clinic specializing in creating hypertension awareness, screening, and management, run by an experienced physician, is a valuable and targeted approach to addressing the growing prevalence of hypertension.

■ ORGANIZING OR BUILDING A SETUP

Setting up a specialized hypertension clinic requires careful attention to various aspects to ensure that it stands out from other healthcare facilities providing hypertension care **(Fig. 1)**.

The following list details the outline of the key features and facilities that could be incorporated into such a clinic:
- *Medical director/physician*: The clinic should be overseen by a physician with at least 10 years of experience in hypertension management, ensuring a high level of expertise in the field who can be named as a "hypertensionologist."
- *Comprehensive BP measurement*: The clinic should utilize good-quality, validated BP monitors and automated BP monitors if possible to ensure accurate

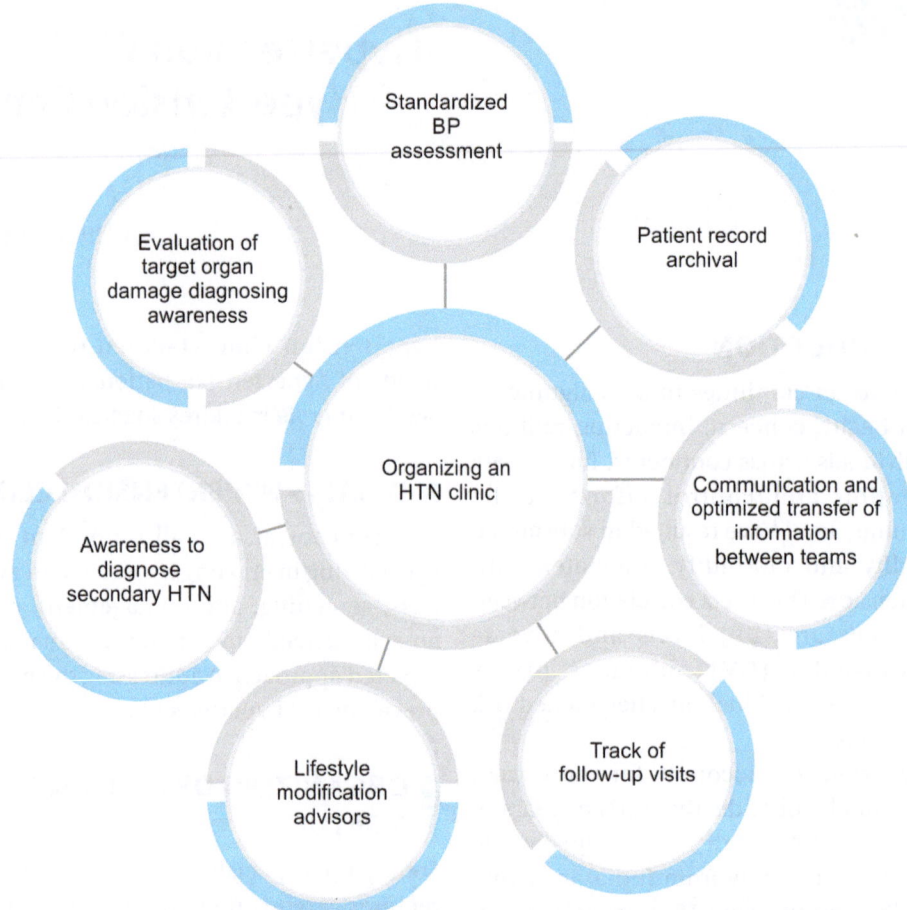

Fig. 1: Schematic diagram highlighting various components to involved in organizing a hypertensive clinic. (BP: blood pressure; HTN: hypertension)

measurements. The emphasis should be on proper techniques for measuring BP, and training programs for staff to maintain consistency.
- *Trained nursing staff*: Trained nurses should be part of the clinic staff to assist in BP measurement, patient education, and overall patient care.
- *Diet and exercise counselors*: Incorporate diet and exercise counselors who can provide personalized lifestyle recommendations to patients, including guidance on healthy eating habits and suitable physical activities.
- *Home BP monitor promotion*: Actively promote the use of home blood pressure monitor (HBPM) promotion monitors among patients for self-monitoring. Educate patients on proper usage and encourage regular reporting of home readings for better management; HBPM would help to diagnose white-coat hypertension and masked hypertension.
- *Ambulatory BP monitoring*: Equip the clinic with ambulatory BP monitoring (ABPM) facilities for more comprehensive and continuous monitoring, especially for patients with suspected white-coat

hypertension, masked hypertension, nocturnal hypertension, or those requiring 24-hour monitoring.
- *Variety of cuff sizes*: Provide different cuff sizes to accommodate patients of varying body sizes, with a specific focus on ensuring accurate measurements for obese individuals. This helps in addressing the diverse needs of the patient population.
- *Electrocardiogram machine*: Include an electrocardiogram (ECG) machine to assess cardiac health and identify any underlying heart conditions that may be contributing to hypertension.
- *Patient education programs*: Conduct regular educational programs for patients, focusing on the importance of BP control, medication adherence, lifestyle modifications, the importance of follow-up, and the benefits of home monitoring.
- *Telemedicine services*: Implement telemedicine services for remote consultations, follow-ups, ongoing support, and enhancing accessibility for patients who may face challenges with in-person visits.
- *Continuing medical education for staff*: Arrange regular continuing medical education (CME) sessions for practitioners, junior doctors, and staff members to keep them updated on the latest guidelines, research findings, and advancements in hypertension management.
- *Laboratory facilities*: Integrate basic laboratory facilities within the clinic to conduct essential tests, including lipid profiles, renal function tests, and electrolyte assessments, supporting a more comprehensive evaluation of patients.
- *Fundoscope*: Equip the clinic with fundoscopy to facilitate examination of the retina, aiding in the assessment of hypertensive retinopathy and potential complications related to elevated BP.
- *Echocardiogram (optional)*: Optionally include an echocardiogram machine to assess cardiac structure and function, especially in cases where there is a suspicion of cardiac involvement or secondary hypertension.
- *Simplified protocols*: Develop and implement simplified protocols for hypertension management based on the latest clinical guidelines. These protocols should cover diagnosis, treatment initiation, medication adjustments, and lifestyle recommendations.
- *Proper data maintenance: Electronic health records (EHR)*: Implement an efficient electronic records system for proper data maintenance. This helps in tracking patient histories, treatment plans, and outcomes, contributing to better continuity of care and data-driven decision-making.
- *Diagnostic clues for secondary hypertension*: Recognize the importance of clinical examination and patient history in identifying potential clues for secondary hypertension. Experienced physicians should be attuned to signs that may prompt further investigation into underlying causes of high BP.
- *Referral system to hypertension specialty center*: Establish a seamless referral system to a hypertension specialty center for cases requiring more specialized care, complex diagnostic assessments, or that may involve secondary hypertension. This ensures that patients receive the appropriate level of care when needed.
- *Multidisciplinary collaboration*: Encourage collaboration with specialists in related fields, such as nephrology, endocrinology, and cardiology, to provide

a multidisciplinary approach to patient care when necessary.
- *Collaboration with local communities*: Establish partnerships with local communities to increase awareness about the clinic's services, encourage regular health checkups, and facilitate community engagement.
  - Foster a sense of community and support among patients by organizing regular engagement activities and support groups. This can enhance patient motivation, adherence to treatment plans, and overall well-being.
- *Communication and information transfer*
  - Establish effective communication channels for the seamless exchange of information between the clinic, the patient, primary care, and other specialist medical teams.
  - Utilize telemedicine to enhance compliance, including home BP monitoring, reminders and appointments for patients, and communication for unattended appointments.
  - Explore alternative models of continuing care, such as "shared care" with general practice or "intermediate care" with specialist nurse teams specializing in BP, diabetes, lipids, etc.
- *Regular quality audits*: Conduct regular quality audits to assess the clinic's performance, adherence to protocols, and patient satisfaction. This continuous improvement process ensures that the clinic maintains high standards of care.
- *Community health outreach programs*: Extend the clinic's impact through community health outreach programs, including health camps, educational sessions, and screenings, to raise awareness about hypertension and its management.
- *Counseling services*: Integrate counseling services, including mental health support, as stress and mental well-being can significantly impact hypertension. This holistic approach addresses the broader health needs of patients.
- *Follow-up monitoring:* By incorporating these additional features, the hypertension clinic becomes a comprehensive healthcare facility capable of offering specialized care, addressing potential secondary hypertension causes, and promoting a holistic approach to patient well-being. This model facilitates collaboration with Hypertension specialty centers, ensuring that patients receive optimal care throughout their hypertension management journey.

NEED FOR A HYPERTENSION CLINIC IN INDIA

As the Indian population continues to grow rapidly, so does the number of hypertensive patients. This increasing burden of hypertension is straining our healthcare resources and economy, leading to a rise in complications and a decline in the overall quality of life. It is imperative to implement effective and timely treatment strategies to mitigate hypertensive complications and enhance the well-being of affected individuals.

The primary objective of a hypertension clinic is to offer expert medical advice and specialized care for patients with hypertension. However, there are several additional aims that a BP service provided through a clinic can fulfill, all of which hold significant importance for the healthcare system. The specific structure and organization of a hypertension clinic may vary depending on its unique objectives, which can differ among clinics and local healthcare systems and may evolve over time. We have to develop and train more physicians to become hypertension specialists (hypertensionologists) who can tackle various issues of the management of hypertension.

WHO CAN RUN A HYPERTENSION CLINIC?

Doctors overseeing a hypertension clinic should be experts in the management of hypertension, ideally with extensive experience in this field. They can be supported by various medical and paramedical staff to carry out a range of activities related to the diagnosis and management of hypertension. Additionally, professional societies such as American College of Cardiology/American Heart Association (ACC/AHA) European Society of Cardiology (ESC), International Society of Hypertension (Indian Society of Hypertension, Association of Physcians of India, Indian Medical Association), Hypertension Society of India (HSI), API, and medical universities can offer specialized courses in the comprehensive management of hypertension, which can serve as valuable resources for individuals looking to establish and run a hypertension clinic. These courses must provide essential knowledge and skills necessary for effective hypertension management within a clinic setting.

WHAT IS HYPERTENSION CENTER? (FLOWCHART 1)

A hypertension center is a specialized tertiary care center dedicated to the diagnosis, treatment, and management of hypertension, often employing a multidisciplinary approach. It comprises a team of experts under one roof which includes general physician, nephrologist, cardiologist, neurologist, endocrinologist, dietitian, physiotherapist, and social counselor who collaborate to deliver comprehensive

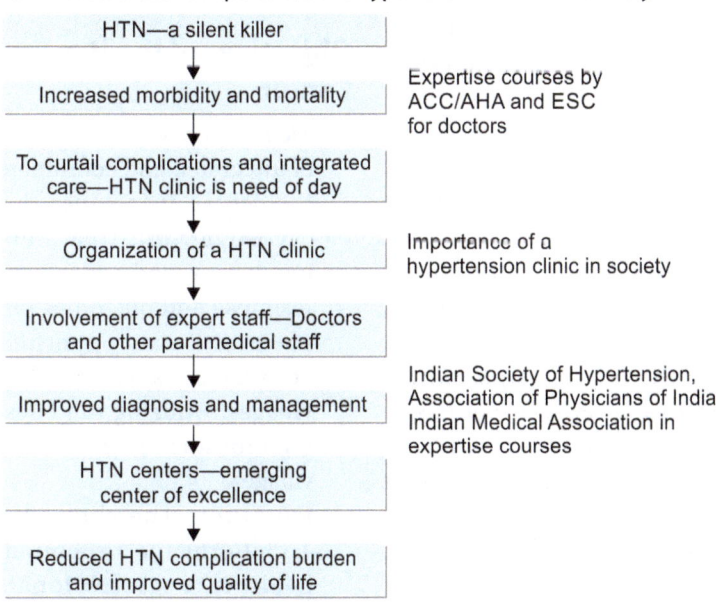

Flowchart 1: Importance of a hypertension center in society.

care for individuals with high BP. These team members may also be involved in primary care or work within institutions or hospitals, but they possess specific interests and expertise in the field of hypertension. Teams associated with hypertension centers are often recognized for their high-quality scientific work in both research and clinical management. They are equipped to diagnose not only primary hypertension but also secondary hypertension, with the necessary facilities at their disposal.

It is highly advisable to create a written protocol outlining the purpose, structure, and functioning of each hypertension center. This protocol serves as a valuable tool for standardizing the operations of hypertension clinics across India, ensuring consistency and excellence in the care provided.

Facilities offered by Hypertension Centers

- Provide a high standard of expertise and facilities for accurate BP measurement.
- Offer round-the-clock emergency services for hypertensive patients.
- Possess the capability to assess total CV risk by evaluating established indicators of organ damage.
- The center should have state-of-the-art equipment, infrastructure to deal with all hypertension emergencies/complications, and to diagnose secondary hypertension.
- House well-equipped ambulances equipped with both basic and advanced life support systems.
- *Establish a network of hypertensive patients:* Create a network of hypertensive patients to enhance the accuracy of diagnosis and improve the management of hypertension. This network can also serve as a platform for sharing experiences and insights.
- *Participation in multicenter clinical research:* Engage the clinic in multicenter clinical research activities to contribute to the advancement of hypertensive research and gain valuable insights into cutting-edge treatments and interventions.
- *Ongoing training and guidance for staff:* Provide regular training and guidance to staff members to ensure they are well equipped to conduct various diagnostic procedures accurately and efficiently. Certified and highly qualified staff can significantly enhance the clinic's reputation and effectiveness in treating hypertension.
- *Dietary and exercise advice:* Offer comprehensive dietary and exercise advice as integral components of hypertension management. Educate patients on the importance of making dietary changes to lower BP, prevent hypertension development, and reduce the risk of related complications.
- Implement rehabilitation programs to support patients in their journey toward better BP control.

Objectives of the Hypertension Center

- *Medical service*: This involves the delivery of integrated and coordinated care within the center. It includes the assessment, investigation, treatment, on-going monitoring, and evaluation of therapeutic response and outcomes for hypertensive patients. Create opportunity screening at various festivals, melas, and distant villages. Utilizing the latest technology, telemonitoring the center can adopt villages.
- *Education*: The clinic should serve as a platform for structured training for healthcare professionals, including

doctors, nurses, and other relevant staff. Patient education is also crucial, aiming to enhance their understanding of pertinent health issues and promote long-term compliance with treatment.
- *Referral center*: The clinic should function as a center of excellence capable of receiving patients with complex, secondary, and complicated forms of hypertension who have been referred by primary care physicians.
- *Research*: The center should actively participate in recruiting patients for clinical trials and facilitating the follow-up of patients involved in long-term research studies. Collaboration with other centers of excellence and regulatory authorities is essential in this endeavor. Develop periodical updates and protocols and disseminate them to practitioners.
- Conduct audits of drug use, effectiveness, and outcomes.

CONCLUSION

The imperative for comprehensive hypertension care is more pressing than ever. Adapting treatments to align with emerging and international standards is paramount. This transformation can be spearheaded by the expertise found in hypertension clinics, where the highest level of consultative care can be delivered, ultimately enhancing hypertensive care and overall quality of life. We need more and more hypertension specialty centers where the patient can be given comprehensive treatment with the support of other specialties. Furthermore, these clinics and centers can serve as hubs for disseminating knowledge through clinical research endeavors and educational programs.

Index

Page numbers followed by *b* refer to box, *f* refer to figure, *fc* refer to flowchart, and *t* refer to table

A

Acebutolol 162, 221, 279
Acetylcholine 207
Acute coronary
    syndrome 124, 282
Adenosine
  triphosphatase 29, 36, 52
  triphosphate 278, 291, 304
Adenylyl cyclase 304
Adherence 405, 409
Adipogenesis 62
Adiponectin 207
Adrenergic stimuli 49
Adrenocorticotropic
    hormone 207
  stimulation 312
Adrenomedullin 47
Aerobic exercise 198
  frequency of 199
Air pollution 202, 204, 205
  exposure 204
  levels 203
Albumin 315
Albuminuria 310, 374
Alcohol
  cessation of 172
  consumption reduction 407
Aldosterone 19, 49
  antagonists 120, 123, 130, 131, 182, 273, 311
  renin ratio 310
  synthase 341
    inhibitor 312
Aldosteronism, primary 311
Alpha-blockers 118, 119, 156, 158, 182, 217, 218, 221, 286, 288
  classification of 286
  selective 286
Alpha-methyldopa 129
Alpha-receptor agonists 288
Alpha-receptor
    antagonists 286-288
  benefits of 287
  effects of 287
  side effects of 288
Alzheimer's disease 305
Ambulatory arterial stiffness
    index 95
Ambulatory blood pressure 310
  monitoring 77, 81, 83, 87, 94-97, 97*t*, 113, 185, 187, 206, 215, 257, 367, 411, 422
    database, meta-analysis
      of 191
    importance of 94, 96
    inflations of 96
    interpretation of 96
    monitors 87
    report 96
American Academy of Family
    Physicians 225
American College of Cardiology 14, 114, 168, 174, 181, 207, 225, 282, 362, 365, 367, 374, 391, 417, 425
  Hypertension
    guideline 391, 417
American College of
    Physicians 225
American Heart Association 14, 57, 114, 168, 174, 181, 207, 225, 362, 365, 367, 374, 391, 417, 425
  guidelines 184
Amiloride 31, 219, 273, 341
Amlodipine 118, 123, 126, 191, 192, 219, 267, 270, 418
  effects of 191
Androgenetic alopecia, treatment
    of 291
Aneroid 113
Anesthesia, induction of 179
Aneurysm
  aortic 244
  cerebral 176
Angina pectoris 6, 282
Angioedema 255
Angioplasty 243
Angiotensin 18, 19, 28, 29, 49, 203, 255, 295, 305, 313, 333, 343
Angiotensin-aldosterone
    system 64
Angiotensin-converting enzyme 9, 18, 28, 30, 118, 148, 153, 157, 162, 181, 217, 220, 230, 255, 256, 260, 271, 275, 282, 300, 304, 326
  inhibitors 172, 190, 209, 217, 220, 255-257, 263, 327, 331, 368, 374, 418
    development of 9
    typical 177
Angiotensin-receptors 18, 19, 66, 305
  activation of 203
  blockers 30, 118, 120, 148, 153, 157, 172, 181, 190, 209, 220, 229, 260, 263, 275, 282, 326, 327, 331, 368
Anticonvulsants therapy 164
Antidepressants 154
Antihypertensive 164
  agent 305, 411
  doses 391
  drugs 103, 191, 303, 311, 327*t*, 390, 407, 411, 418, 419
  major 103
  effects 305, 309, 309*t*
  medications 162, 181, 286, 290, 368, 413
  therapy 96, 151, 300, 310, 392
    choice of 103
  treatment 156, 190, 191, 330*t*
    effectiveness of 188
    important focus of 187
Antinuclear antibody, formation
    of 292
Antipsychiatric drugs 110
Aorta 98*f*
  coarctation of 237, 238, 297

paracoarctation of 238
transverse 238
Aortic coarctation 113, 155
Aortic dissection 147, 148, 176, 244
Aortic waveform 101*f*
Apnea-hypopnea index 247
Arachidonate 69
Arachidonic acid 68
Aranidipine 269
Arginine-vasopressin 313
Arrhythmias 110, 118
  cardiac 283
Arterial baroreceptor input, central amalgamation of 351
Arterial blood pressure, simultaneous readings of 175
Arterial pulse 5, 240
  examination of 110
Arterial stiffness 101, 103, 187, 198
Arterial tree 99
Arteries 99
  brachiocephalic 240
  diseases of 6
  functions of 6
  large 99
  peripheral 110, 116
  subclavian 237
Arteriolar relaxation 292
Arterioles 99, 296
Arteriosclerosis 140
Asanas 3
Aspirin 408
  low-dose 163
Association of Physcians of India 425
Astrocytes 60
Atenolol 119, 120, 191, 221, 279
Atherosclerosis, accelerated 202
Atherosclerotic obstructive epicardial coronary artery disease 297
Atrasentan 314
Atrial fibrillation 111, 126, 157
Atrial natriuretic peptide 17, 21, 64, 305
Augmentation
  index 99
  pressure 99
Auscultatory blood pressure monitoring 88
Automated office blood pressure 77, 113, 313
Automated out-of-office blood pressure measurement 417
Autonomic nervous system 19, 24, 207, 247
Autoregulatory mechanisms, normal functioning of 138
Avosentan 314
Azelnidipine 270, 271
Azilsartan 220, 260
  medoxomil 261

B

Barbiturates 410
Barnidipine 270
Baroreceptor
  activation therapy 157, 158*fc*, 352
    adverse effects of 355
  stimulation 349
Baroreflex
  activation therapy 352
  arc anatomy 350
  sensitivity 350, 351
Barostim neo
  pivotal trial 354
  system 354
  treatment group 354
  trial 354
Baseline
  death rate 87
  laboratory tests 165
Basic telehealth services 390*f*
B-cells 60
Benazepril 220, 257
Benidipine 269, 270, 271
Benzothiazepine 268
Benzthiazide 273
Beta-activation 28
Beta-adrenergic receptors 278
  blockers 190, 279
  classification of 279*t*
Beta-adrenoceptor blockers
  classification of 279*t*
  mechanism of 278*f*
  various properties of 281*t*
Beta-blockers 103, 118-120, 122, 124, 130, 156, 158, 182, 191, 217, 218, 221, 229, 271, 278, 282, 283, 305, 331, 368, 374,
contraindications of 280
pharmacokinetics of 280
pharmacological actions of 279
side effects of 281
use of 334
Beta-hydroxy steroid dehydrogenase 341
Beta-natriuretic peptide 305
Beta-oxidation 73
Beta-spectrins 35
Betaxolol 221, 279
Biannually blood pressure monitoring 400
Bicuspid aortic valve 238
  congenital 116
Bifascicular block 129, 130*f*
Biomechanical stress 295
Biphasic P waves 298
Birmingham hypertension clinic 153*f*
Bisoprolol 120, 221, 279, 282, 404
Blindness, cortical 147
Blood 3
  flow 290
  sugar
    fasting 228
    postpartum 228
  vessels 95, 199, 280
  types of 290
Blood pressure 3, 13-15, 17, 21, 57, 57*t*, 65, 69, 77, 90, 94, 96, 113, 114, 145, 151, 152, 174, 204, 213, 215, 215*t*, 225, 255, 260, 267, 283, 292, 303, 325, 335, 339, 349, 352, 353, 355, 361, 365, 367, 374, 399, 410, 413, 421, 422
  apparatus 111
  categorization of 14*t*
  central systolic 100
  characteristic trait of 174
  circadian rhythms, assessment of 187
  continuous nature of 184
  control
    apparent lack of 152
    centers 184
    compliance of 90
    improvement of 90
  diastolic 13, 14, 79, 83, 95, 100, 113, 145, 161, 167, 176, 179, 181, 197, 202, 207,

215, 224, 225, 307, 308, 339, 361, 365, 374, 399, 416
dynamic nature of 184
electrical devices of 90
fall of 416
fluctuations 189
inaccurate measurement of 392
independent effect 311
intraoperative 179
levels 118, 300, 414
lower 290
lowering of 141, 197, 355
  therapy, effect of 298
measurement 78, 79, 88, 111
  accurate 161
  clinic 95, 175
  correct methodology of 77
  evolution of 4
  landscape of 99
  methods 113
  single 188
  techniques 80f, 83
monitoring 88, 180, 188, 288, 389
nocturnal dipping of 95, 96
normal 181
patterns, abnormal 188
rapidly reduce 292, 293
reduction 176, 292
regulation 68, 72
routine 388
safe levels of 182
several measurements of 181
sudden out of control of 109
systolic 13, 14, 77, 83, 87, 95, 98, 111, 113, 145, 161, 167, 176, 181, 182, 186, 197, 204, 207, 214, 215, 224, 225, 303, 307, 308, 325, 339, 361, 389, 399, 417
target 375
telemonitoring of 392
trends, longitudinal assessment of 91
variability 89, 184, 185, 188, 189, 190
  concept of 192
  consequences of 189
  phenotypes 190
  reduction 191
  short-term 186
variations 189

Body mass index 16, 209, 214
Bone morphogenetic proteins 49
Bonnet's sign 139
Bosentan 314
Brachial artery 100, 101f
Brachial blood pressure
  assessment 98
  measurement 98
Brachial-ankle pulse wave velocity 209
Bradycardia 122, 126, 129, 230
Bradykinin 255, 305
  enzymatic degradation of 304
Brain 64
  damage 189
  natriuretic peptide 64
Breathing 205
Bright's disease 6
British Hypertension Society 411
Broad P waves 298
Bumetanide 219

C

Calcium 38
  antagonist 126, 331
  blockers 333
  channel 52, 55
    antagonists 210
    blockers 55, 154, 156-158, 190, 192, 217, 219, 229, 267, 268, 305, 327, 368, 374, 418
    distribution of 268, 268f
    generalized structure of 53f
    pharmacology of 268, 268f
    role of 52
    types of 54fc
  ions 52
  randomized evaluation of 385
Canagliflozin 305
Candesartan 191, 220, 260, 261
Capacitance vessels 290
Capillaries 296
Captopril 220, 257
Carbohydrate consumption reduction 407
Carbon monoxide 202
Carbonic anhydrase inhibitors 273
Carboxy-terminal telopeptide 49
Cardiac cycle 99
Cardiac death, sudden 297
Cardiac dysfunction 62, 385

Cardiac function 296
  altered 295
Cardiac magnetic resonance imaging 299
Cardiac output 16, 17, 273, 328, 350, 351
Cardiac sympathetic system 153
Cardiac troponin, high-sensitive 209
Cardiomyocytes 296
  growth 295
Cardiorenal disease 218
Cardioselective beta-blocker 149, 279, 283
Cardiovascular complications risk factor 181
Cardiovascular disease 13, 20, 87, 167, 175, 189, 227, 326, 414, 419
  atherosclerotic 363, 382
  burden and disability worldwide 416
  diagnosis of 186
  global burden of 87
  higher risk of 95
  hypertensive 7
  increased risk of 89
  management of 186
  prevention 392
  risk of 199, 414
Cardiovascular events 95, 210
Cardiovascular extracellular matrix regulation, serum markers of 49
Cardiovascular hemodynamics 305
Cardiovascular issues 292
Cardiovascular manifestations, result of 174
Cardiovascular risk 87, 103, 188, 203, 204
  reduction 289
Cardiovascular system 99, 203, 249
Carotid
  approach 101f
  artery 100, 101f
    disease 299
    direct applanation tonometry of 101f
  baroreflex activation 222
  intima-media thickness 103, 209
  pulses 100
  waveform 101f

Carvedilol 120, 124, 218, 279, 282, 288, 335
Caudal ventrolateral medulla 350, 351
Celiprolol 279
Cell
 adhesion molecules 39
 membrane, role of 35
Central arteriovenous anastomosis 158
Central blood pressure 98, 101, 101f, 102t, 103
 experiences 98
 implications of 103
 measurement of 98, 103
Central natriuretic peptide 305
Central nervous system 18, 60, 248, 280, 312
Central pressure 100, 101f, 103
 assessment 99
Central sympathetic outflow 286
 inhibition of 352
Centrally acting aminopeptidase A inhibitors 313
Cerebral small vessel disease 189, 190
Cerebral vascular accident 124, 126
Cerebral vasculature 248
Cerebrovascular accidents 114, 147, 374
Cerebrovascular disease 187, 202
Cerebrovascular dysfunction 189
Chemokine synthesis 61
Chemokinesis 60
Chemoreceptors, activation of 203
Chemoreflex circuits 19
Chemotactic cytokines 60
Chest leads 118
Chinese Hypertension League 365
Chlorothiazide 273
Chlorthalidone 156, 217, 219, 261, 273, 416
Cholesterolemia 257
Choroid nerve 139
Chromatography-tandem mass spectrometry 410
Chromosome loci 341, 342
Chronic hypertension 141, 161, 165, 405
 management of 287
Chronic hypertensive, parental care for 165

Chronic kidney disease 22, 90, 111, 120, 129, 151, 184, 189, 215, 220, 276, 283, 287, 370, 374, 381, 385, 392, 399, 419
 progression 418
Chronic obstructive pulmonary disease 116, 118, 122
Cilnidipine 267, 270, 271
Circadian hemodynamic rhythms 246
Clinic blood pressure, normal 188
Clinical cardiovascular disease 366
Clonidine 120, 129, 221, 288
 patch 221
Clopamide 273
Closed-loop healthcare model 389
Coarctation
 congenital 244f
 stenting 243
Coffee, consumption of 94
Collagen amino-terminal peptide 49
Collagenases 43
Combination therapy 230, 268, 325, 326, 327, 328
 advantages of 326
Combined cardiovascular disease 418, 237
Community Health Outreach Programs 424
Community outreach programs 91
Comorbidities 22, 118, 207
Compensatory tone, loss of 137
Comprehensive blood pressure measurement 421
Compression, proximal 146
Computed tomography 147, 216, 240, 241
 aortogram 242t
Confidence interval 168, 176, 209, 246
Conivaptan 276
Connective tissue growth factor 49
Consecutive blood pressure measurements 186
Contemporary clinical trials, results of 417
Continuous Doppler across coarct segment 241

Continuous positive airway pressure 247, 250f
Cor pulmonale 122
Coronary artery disease 20, 22, 110, 119, 124, 170, 184, 228, 279, 332, 340, 362, 374, 392, 400
 risk of 118
Coronary blood flow 296
Coronary hypoperfusion 210
Coronavirus disease 2019 388, 400
 pandemic 388
Corticosterone 214
Cortisol 207
 metabolism of 214
Cotton-wool spots 138
Cranial nerve, branch of 350
C-reactive protein 58
Critical health issues, range of 184
C-type natriuretic peptide 64, 65
Cuff sphygmomanometry 100
Cushing's syndrome 109, 110, 155, 228
 features of 113
Cyanide toxicity 293
Cyclic adenosine monophosphate 21, 70, 278, 304, 305, 315
 stimulation of 290
Cyclooxygenase 59, 68, 69, 110
 isoenzyme 69
Cystatin C 208
Cystoid macular edema 141
Cytochrome P450 72
 enzymes 203
 role of 72
Cytokines 49, 58, 62
 inflammatory 203
 release 58
 role of 57, 59f
Cytoskeleton 39
 role of 37

D

Dangerous ventricular arrhythmias 132
Dapagliflozin 305
Darusentan 314
Daytime sleepiness 110
Deep breathing exercises 3
Deep symmetrical T inversion 125
Dendroaspis natriuretic peptide 65

Device-based therapy 352
Diabetes mellitus 3, 42, 96, 161, 163, 283, 305, 327, 332, 374
 external features of 114
 polydipsia of 110
Diabetic ketoacidosis 310
Diabetic nephropathy 256, 262
Diabetic renal disease, progression of 229
Diabetic retinopathy, screening 389
Diastolic blood pressure 13, 14, 79, 83, 95, 100, 113, 145, 161, 167, 176, 179, 181, 197, 202, 207, 215, 224, 225, 307, 308, 339, 361, 365, 374, 399, 416
 control 214
 goal 417
 load 95, 96
 overestimation of 113
 premature recording of 78
 values 95
Diastolic dysfunction 296, 299
Diastolic hypertension 87, 416
 treatment 417
Diathesis, high-pressure 6
Diazoxide 292
 intravenous administration of 292
 result of 292
Digital health platforms 91, 392
Dihydropyridines 126, 149, 219, 267, 268, 374
Dihydroxyvitamin D 384
Diltiazem 120, 126, 129, 219, 267
Direct renin inhibitors 221
Direct vasodilators 221, 290
Directly observed therapy 404, 411
 clinic 411
 visit 411
Directly relax blood vessels 294
Disability-adjusted life years 227
Discoid 40
Diuretics 229, 273, 274t, 331, 368, 374
 sites of action of 276f
 therapy 219t
Doppler scan 241
Doxazosin 221, 418
 gastrointestinal therapeutic system, effect of 287

Drugs
 classes of 418
 individual class of 229
 interactions 282
 score 418
 therapy 84fc, 85fc, 198, 417
Dual angiotensin receptor-neprilysin inhibitor 303
Dual antiplatelets 124
Ductal aorta junction 237
Ductal tissue 237
 theory 238
Ductus arteriosus 237
Dynamic resistance exercise 199
Dysgeusia 255
Dyslipidemia 209, 227, 283, 381

E

Ear coordination 78
Echocardiogram 109, 423
Echocardiography 238, 241, 298
Eclampsia 164
Edema 122
 acute pulmonary 149
 peripheral 315
 pulmonary 163
Efonidipine 267, 271
Eicosanoids 68, 69, 72
 multiple roles of 68
 types of 68
Eicosapentaenoic acid 68
Eighth Joint National Committee 326
Ejection fraction 282, 296
Elastin 45
Electrocardiogram 118, 119f, 120, 120f, 121f, 122, 122f-125f, 127f-133f, 165, 180, 228, 241, 298, 423
 criteria 118
 machine 423
Electrolytes, serum 180
Electronic health records 423
Elevated arterial blood pressure, cardiac effects of 295
Elschnig's spots 138, 139f
Embryology 237
Empagliflozin 305
Enalapril 220, 257
Enamelysin 43
Encephalopathy, hypertensive 147
End diastolic wall thickness 299
Endarteritis, infective 239

Endocarditis 239, 244
Endocrine system 249
Endoplasmic reticulum 53
End-organ damage 176
 features of 150
End-organ dysfunction 145
Endothelial adhesion 60
Endothelial cell 71
 migration 65
Endothelial derived relaxing factor 17
Endothelial dysfunction 19, 385
Endothelial nitric oxide synthase 38, 61
Endothelial progenitor cells 20, 71
Endothelin 17, 21, 49, 305, 314
 receptor antagonists 314, 315
Endothelium 60, 296
 dependent processes 290
 derived relaxing factors 73
 function 198
 mediated nitric oxide release 186
Enteropathy 262
Environmental pollution 202
Environmental protection agency 204
Epigenome-wide association studies 340
Epinephrine 278
Epiretinal membrane formation 141
Eplerenone 30, 220, 273, 310
Epoxyeicosatrienoic 72
Eprosartan 220, 261
Ertugliflozin 305
Esmolol 124, 279
Essential hypertension 6, 13, 16, 35, 36, 38, 40, 137, 165, 286, 341
 development of 17h
Estimated glomerular filtration rate 355, 399
Ethacrynic acid 219
European Medicines Agency 304
European Society of Cardiology 14, 114, 174, 225, 280, 326, 362, 365, 367, 374, 391, 417
 guidelines 111
European Society of Hypertension 14, 88, 114, 225, 280, 326, 361, 365, 367, 391, 417

Evidence-based medicine, fundamental part of 404
Excess thiocyanate, accumulation of 293
Exercise 197, 198, 205
　augments vasodilation endothelium-dependent 198
　frequency of 200
　intensity of 200
　programs 198
　regular 198
　types of 200
Extracellular matrix 42, 44, 46t, 48, 296
　metalloproteinase inducer 48
　regulation 45
Extracellular space 29
Eye examinations, regular 141

F

Fascicular block 129
Fatty acid levels 280
Felodipine 219
Fenoldopam 293, 294
Fetal anomalies 255
Fetal hydrops 163
Fibrillar collagens 45
Fibrillary waves 127
Fibrinogen 39, 203
Fibrinoid necrosis 146
Fibroblasts 60, 296
　growth factor 49
Fibroelastosis, endocardial 239
Fibronectin 39, 45
Fibrosis 153
Fingers, tar staining of 114
Finndiane study 170
Finn-home study 176
Fluctuations
　over time 185
　temporary telemonitoring of 185
Fluid retention 290, 291
Flushing 291
Food and Drug Administration 9, 260, 303
Fosinopril 220, 257
Fourth-line antihypertensive agents 311, 312f
Framingham Heart Study 213, 295, 299, 303, 389

Fundamental hemodynamic parameters 328
Fundoscope 423
Furosemide 219

G

Gaseous air pollutants 202
Gastrointestinal therapeutic system 267
Gelatinase 43, 45
Genetics 337
　findings 344
Genome-wide association studies 340
German antihypertensive efficacy and safety 287
Gestation, multiple 163
Gestational hypertension 161, 162
　management of 162
　plus proteinuria 166
Ghrelin 207
Glaucoma 141
Gliflozins 273
Global cardiovascular risk assessment 366
Glomerular filtration rate 287, 306, 352
Glomerulonephritis, chronic 208
Glucagon-like peptide-1 305
Glucocorticoid 340
Glucometers 389
Glucose 306
　intolerance 167, 292
　solution 293
　transport 309
Glycerol 273
Glycophorin A 35
Goldblatt type phenomenon 239
G-protein coupled transmembrane protein receptors 68
Granular lymphocytes, large 60
Guanethidine 417
Guanfacine 218, 221
Guanosine-5'-triphosphate 304
Guanylylcyclase 293
Gunn's sign 139

H

Hair growth, excessive 291
Haptotaxis 60

Hard
　exudates 139
　pulse disease 4
Headache 291
Health complications, hypertension-related 200
Healthcare 389
　professionals 400, 426
　training 91
　system 424
　team 407
Heart 203
　block, complete 111
　disease 197
　　congenital 418, 224
　　coronary 90, 167, 331
　　hypertensive 176, 295, 296, 299
　　ischemic 13, 151, 295, 392
　　failure 118, 129, 151, 176, 179, 184, 280, 282, 295, 304, 328, 392, 418
　　congestive 30, 239, 256, 273
　　diastolic 180
　　hypertensive 149
　　with reduced ejection fraction 115, 304
　functions of 6
　rate 350, 351
　valve disease 297
HELLP syndrome 164, 165
Hematocrit 315
Hematoma, intracranial 147
Hematopoiesis 59
Hematopoietins 62
Hemianopia, homonymous 147
Hemodynamic theory 238
Hemoglobin 315
Hemorrhage 139
　cerebral 148, 190, 239
　flame-shaped 139, 147
　intracranial 244
　retinal 139, 140
Hepatocyte growth factor 49
Hepta-helical chemokine 60
High blood pressure 167, 202
　accelerated 332
　outside clinical setting 184
　prevalence of 184
　protocol 276t
　treatment of 145
High clinic blood pressure 174

High-performance liquid
chromatography-
tandem mass
spectrometry 404
Home blood pressure
  levels 95*t*
  measurement 90, 367
  monitoring 77, 82, 83, 87, 88,
    91, 97*t*, 113, 184, 189,
    422
    advantages of 88, 91
    cost-effectiveness of 91
    devices, accessibility of 92
    limitations of 88
    promotion 422
    use of 83, 87, 90
  telemonitoring 392
  variability 191
Hormone 55
  antidiuretic 29
Human genome project 340
Hyaline 40
Hybrid sphygmomanometer 78
Hydralazine 118, 119, 121, 162,
  166, 182, 218, 221, 290,
  291, 335, 416-418
Hydrochlorothiazide 217, 261,
  273, 416, 418
  combination therapy 191
Hydroflumethiazide 273
Hydroxyeicosatetraenoic
  acid 72, 73
Hydroxyheptadecatrienoate 69
Hydroperoxyeicosatetraenoic
  acid 71
Hydroxysteroid
  dehydrogenase 214
Hydroxyvitamin D 384
Hyperaldosteronism 109, 120,
  122, 130
Hypercalcemia 133*f*
Hypercholesterolemia
  external features of 114
  familial 110
Hyperinsulinemia 167
Hyperkalemia 120, 129, 131*f*, 132*f*,
  255
  features of 121*f*
Hyperparathyroidism 133, 133*f*
Hyperpiesia 6
Hypertension 3, 6, 13, 14*f*, 20, 27,
  42, 43, 45, 48, 49, 52, 55,
  57, 59*f*, 64, 71, 73, 84*fc*,
  85*fc*, 95*t*, 96, 97, 109,
110, 113, 114, 118, 124,
126, 126*fc*, 129, 130, 132,
133*fc*, 137, 151, 156*b*,
161, 167, 168, 171, 172*fc*,
175, 176, 197, 202, 224,
226, 244, 246, 247, 249,
256, 260, 261, 267, 273,
274*t*, 278, 286-288, 290,
306*t*, 308, 325, 332*f*, 335,
337, 339, 339*f*, 342, 343,
347, 349, 361, 363, 381,
384, 408, 409, 413, 416,
422, 423
  age-standardized prevalence
    of 15*f*
  apparent treatment-resistant
    151, 411
  arterial 4
  asymptomatic 149
  burden of 167
  cardiac consequences of 22*f*
  categories 363
  center 421, 425, 426
    in Society, importance
      of 425*fc*
    objectives of 426
  chronic 141, 161, 165, 405
  chronic prepregnancy 161
  classification of 114*t*
  clinic 421, 425
    need for 424
  clinical
    manifestations of 176
    practice guidelines 391
  complications of 20, 21,
    109, 325
  consequences of 20, 170
  control of 151, 421
  cutoff 417
  detection 416
  diagnosis of 91, 215*t*, 416
  diagnostic cut-off of 416
  disorder 161
    pathogenesis of 161
  drugs treatment of 416
  earlier onset of 22
  epidemiology of 14, 384
  essential 6, 13, 16, 35, 36, 38,
    40, 137, 165, 286, 341
  etiopathophysiology of 16
  evaluation of 107
  fast facts on 14
  genetic
    association of 339
  classification of 342*t*
  gestational 161, 162
  grade of 113
  growing prevalence of 421
  guidelines, chronology of 361
  high prevalence of 151
  high pulse pressure 111
  infrequent occurrence of 175
  interventional management
    of 218
  isolated systolic 192, 225, 331,
    332, 417
  labile 175-177
  long-standing 165
  malignant 7, 138, 151
  management 170, 393*t*, 400*t*,
    401, 416
    general 391
    strategies 335
  mediated organ damage 109,
    110, 114, 366
    recognition of 109
  mild 90
  moderately severe 416
  molecular basis of 33
  monogenic forms of 341
  nocturnal 206, 208-210
  nonadherence secondary 198
  objective treatment 90
  optimal treatment 417
  paradoxical 243
  pathogenesis of 21*t*
  perioperative 179
  polygenic form of 341
  postpartum 165
  pre-existing 163
  pregnancy-induced 161, 162
  prevalence of 15*t*, 167, 168
  prevention of 170, 277
  previous history of 179
  primary 16
  prognostic stratification of 99
  pseudoresistant 175, 214, 391
  pulmonary 122, 122
    arterial 314
    venous 248
  refractory 151, 152, 152*b*, 153
  renovascular 113
  resistant 151, 152*f*, 154, 154*b*,
    155*fc*, 157, 158, 198, 213,
    215*t*, 216*t*, 219*t*, 226,
    290, 303, 312, 391
  secondary 16, 137, 155*t*, 165,
    216, 235, 423

severe 90, 162, 291
  intraoperative 182
Society of India 425
systemic 198
systolic 417
treatment of 91, 153, 229*t*, 277, 287, 314, 404, 417
trial 352
uncomplicated 282
worldwide responsibility of 197
Hypertensionologist 421, 425
Hypertensive clinic 422*f*
Hypertensive crisis 145
  development of 145*b*
Hypertensive disorders, classification of 161
Hypertensive emergency 145, 288, 290
  manifestations of 147*b*
  treatment of 293
Hypertensive encephalopathy 147
  symptoms of 146
Hypertensive heart disease 176, 295, 296, 299
  molecular basis of 295
  structural basis of 295
Hypertensive population, majority of 417
Hypertensive therapy 92
Hypertensive vasculopathy, diagnosis of 176
Hypertrichosis 291
Hypertrophy 297
  cardiac 188
  myocardial 153
Hypocalcemia 132*f*, 309
Hypo-high-density lipoprotein 257
Hypokalemia 121*f*, 130, 131*f*
Hypokinesis 60
Hypotension 291
Hypothyroidism 122
Hypoxemia, nocturnal 210
Hypoxic pulmonary vasoconstriction 248

I

Imidazoline-1 receptor 288
Immune system 57
Implantable pulse generator 352
Inaccurate blood pressure measurement 392

methods 187
Indapamide 118, 126, 156, 191, 219, 273, 404
  treatments 191
Indian Council of Medical Research 168
Indian Society of Hypertension 425
Indirect noninvasive methods 102*t*
Indoplasmic reticulum, membranes of 52
Inducible nitric oxide synthase 59
Infarction, postmyocardial 279
Inflammation 57
  systemic 203
Inflammatory pathways 385
Infra-hisian complete heart block 129*f*
Infrared photoplethysmography 186
Inhibitor 229
Inositol 1,4,5
  phosphate 68, 70
  trisphosphate 53
Insulin 207
  like growth factor 1 49
  resistance 257
  role of 38
  sensitivity 287
Intensity 199
Intensive care unit 148
Interferon 58
  alpha 60
  beta 60
  gamma 59, 60
Interleukin 49, 58, 60, 61, 203
  alpha 203
International Diabetes Federation 169
International Society of Hypertension 14, 362, 365
  Global Hypertension Practice Guidelines 151
Interventional therapy 157, 157*f*
Intima-media thickness 176
Intracardiac lesions 244
Intracellular calcium 38
  effect of 38
  regulators 269
Intravascular fluid overload 179
Intravenous sodium nitroprusside 182

Intrinsic sympathomimetic activity 281, 282
Invasive cardiac catheterization 101*f*
Irbesartan 220, 260, 262
Ischemia 146
  cardiac 179
  myocardial 181, 297
Isosorbide 273
Isradipine 219, 267

J

Japanese Society of Hypertension 365
Jet peak velocity 299
Joint National Committee 167, 276*t*, 282, 361
Journal of American College of Cardiology 385
Jugular venous
  pressure 111
  pulse 240

K

Keith-Wagener-Barker classification 140
Kidney 249, 306
  disease 228
    chronic 22, 90, 111, 120, 129, 151, 163, 184, 189, 215, 220, 276, 283, 287, 370, 374, 381, 385, 392, 399, 419
  transplantation 315
Korean Society of Hypertension 365
Korotkoff's sounds 77, 78
K-sparing diuretics 129, 416, 417, 418

L

L- and N-type calcium channels 270
Labetalol 162, 166, 218, 221, 288, 279
Labile hypertension 175-177
  consequences of 175
  origins of 175
Lacidipine 267
Lactate
  curves 199
  dehydrogenase 148

Lactic acidosis 293
Laminin 39, 45
Laplace's law 198, 207
Late gadolinium enhancement 299
Left anterior fascicular block 130*f*
Left bundle branch block 129
Left ventricular
 dysfunction 120, 122, 256, 263, 282
 end-diastolic pressure 297
 hypertrophy 19, 22, 114, 118, 188, 198, 214, 297, 298, 310, 331
  mass 103, 298
   index 209
  strain 298
Leptin 207
Lercanidipine 267
Leukotrienes 68, 69, 71, 72
Light chain phosphorylation 315
Light reflex
 accentuation of 138
 widening of 138
Limb leads 118
Lipid 228, 381
Lipoprotein
 high-density 167, 280
 low-density 287
 non-high-density 381
Lipoxins 68, 72
Lisinopril 220, 257, 418
Lithium 36
Liver
 dysfunction 163
 enzymes, elevated 164
 function, abnormal 315
Long-acting calcium channel blockers 148
Long-acting thiazide-like diuretic 153, 154
Loop diuretics 123, 131, 181, 219, 229
Losartan 220, 262
Low therapeutic response rates 23
Lower limb 297
 blood pressure 297
 pulse, absence of 110
Low-fat dairy products 171
Low-voltage QRS 122
L-type calcium channel modulators 269
Lupus syndrome, drug-induced 291

Lymph 3
Lymphocytes 40
Lysine-deficient protein kinase 341
Lysosomal membranes 52
Lysosome 53

M

Macroangiopathy 163
Macrophages 58, 60
Macular degeneration, age-related 141
Macular star formation 140
Madhumeha 3
Magnetic resonance 155
 imaging 147, 241
Malignancy 116
Malignant ventricular premature depolarization 126
Malondialdehyde 69
Mannitol 273
Manual blood pressure monitoring 77
Manual cuff inflation 88
Marfan syndrome 176
Masked hypertension 83, 89, 152, 174, 226
Mast cells 61
Maternal blood pressure, close monitoring of 165
Matrilysins 43
Matrix metalloproteinases 42, 43, 45, 47*f*, 48
 activator protein 48
 regulation 45
 targets of 48
Mean arterial pressure 350, 351
Medicine, yellow emperor's classic of 4
Membrane stabilizing activity 281
Mental status, altered 148
Mercapto-butyl sulfonic acid 313
Mercury 113
Meta-analysis, meta-regression of 204
Metabolic syndrome 167, 170, 171, 283
 clinical diagnosis of 169*t*
 features of 113
 prevalence of 169
Metabolic systems 341
Metalloelastase 43
Metalloproteinase, tissue inhibitors of 45

Methylation 344
Methyldopa 221, 404, 417, 418
Meticulous physical examination 109
Metolazone 219, 273
Metoprolol 124, 162, 221, 279
 tartrate 221
mHealth 388
Mibefradil 267
Microalbuminuria, persistent 137
Microphone 390
Microtubules 39
Microvascular damage 385
Mild hypertension 90
 study, treatment of 287, 300
Mineralocorticoid receptor 29, 30, 341
 agonists 312
 antagonists 217, 220, 310, 311
Minoxidil 221, 291, 335
 cardiac effects of 292
 dosage of 291
 therapy, complication of 292
Mitigating target-organ damage 184
Mitogen-activated protein kinases 73
Mitral annular velocity 299
Mitral regurgitation 115
 murmurs of 116*f*, 298
 severe 238
Mitral valve 238
Mobile health 388
Mobile technology 388
Moexipril 220, 257
Molar pregnancy 163
Monckeberg's medial calcification 145
Monoamine oxidase 16, 154
Monocytes 58, 60, 61
 chemotactic protein 59
Monophosphate 71
Monotherapy 326
Morning blood pressure surge 96, 187
Moxonidine 218, 221, 288
Multiple sclerosis 370
 diagnosis of 169
Murmurs 115
 abdominal 113
Muscle fibers 295
Myocardial function 296
Myocardial infarction 225, 339, 410
 nonfatal 418

Myocardial perfusion, impaired 295
Myocardium 296t

N

Naadi method 4
Nadolol 221
National Cholesterol Education Program Expert Panel 169
National Health and Nutrition Examination Survey 227
National Institute for Health and Care Excellence 174, 405
National Institute for Health and Clinical Excellence 88, 217, 284, 367, 411
Natriuretic peptides 49, 64, 65, 304
　receptor 65, 304
　therapeutic role of 66
Near-field communication 390
Nebivolol 218, 221, 279
Neck veins 180
Nephropathy 189, 332
　hypertensive 299
Neprilysin 66, 304
　inhibitor 66
　　new combination of 304
Neural crest cells, role of 237
Neurotransmitter
　exocytosis of 55
　release, inhibition of 286
Neutral endopeptidase, inhibitor of 303
Neutropenia 255
New York Heart Association 263
Next-generation sequencing 340
Nicardipine 149, 182, 219, 267, 270
Nicotinamide adenine dinucleotide phosphate 203
　oxidase subunits 204
Nifedipine 119, 122, 126, 162, 219, 267
Nilvadipine 269
Nisoldipine 219
Nitric oxide 17, 19, 21, 198, 203, 315
　effect of 38
　generation of 290

Nitrogen dioxide 202
Nitroglycerine 149, 182
Nitrous oxide 202
Nocturnal fluid redistribution 248
Nocturnal hypertension 206, 208-210
　diagnosis of 207
　pathophysiology of 207
Noncommunicable diseases 226, 408
Nondihydropyridines 219
Nondrug therapies 421
Non-hispanic black 389
Noninvasive ventilation equipment 389
Nonmethane hydrocarbons 202
Nonpharmacological therapy 154
Nonrapid eye movement 246
Nonselective alpha-blockers 286
Nonselective beta-blockers 149, 279
Non-ST elevated myocardial infarction 283
Nonsteroidal anti-inflammatory drugs 16, 110, 154
Norepinephrine 278
N-terminal aspartate 313
N-terminal pro-brain natriuretic peptide 209, 263
N-type calcium channels 267
Nucleus
　ambiguus 350, 351
　tractus solitaris 19, 350, 351
Nutrition examination survey 213

O

Obesity 3, 161, 247
　central 16, 257
　excessive 88
Obstructive sleep apnea 210, 246, 247
　syndrome 246
　treatment of 249, 250f
Office blood pressure
　measurement 80, 152f
　monitoring 87, 113, 184
Office hypertension, cross-classification of 83f
Olmesartan 220, 261, 262, 335
Optic nerve 139, 140
Optic neuropathy, anterior ischemic 141
Oral beta-blockers 162

Organ
　damage 184
　systems, involvement of 248
Organic mercurials 273
Organum vasculosum 248
Orthopedic diseases 116
Oscillometry, cuff-based 101f
Oscilloscopy 350
Osler's maneuver 146
Osmotic diuretics 273
Osteogenesis 62
Out-of-office
　blood pressure measurements, use of 367
　hypertension, cross-classification of 83f
Oxidative stress, systemic 203
Ozone gases 202

P

Palpitation 110, 291
Papilledema 139f
Paracrine 65
Paraganglioma 147, 155
Parenchymal renal disease 109
Percutaneous coronary intervention, primary 124
Perindopril 119, 124, 192, 220, 257
Peripheral arterial disease 111, 184
Peripheral dopamine-1 receptors 149
Peripheral sympathetic nerve terminals 286
Peripheral vascular
　pressure 70f
　resistance 16, 17, 19, 21, 290, 328
Peripheral vessels 116
Personal digital assistant 390
Pharmacogenomics 343
Pharmacological therapies 155, 181
Pharmacotherapy 386
Phenoxybenzamine 221
Phenylalkylamine 268, 269
Pheochromocytoma 113, 122, 147, 149, 155
Phosphatidylinositol 38
Phosphatidylserine 38
Phospholipase A2 69, 72
Physiotherapist 425
Pindolol 162, 221

Placebo-controlled study 316
Plasma
  glucose 306
  renin activity 240
Platelet 35, 40
  aggregation, promotion of 286
  cell structure 39f
  derived growth factor 49
  lipid bilayer, general diagram of 39f
  membrane 38, 40
    structural alterations of 40
  transfusion 165
Pleiotropic cytokine 61
Polycystic kidney 109, 113
Polypeptides atrial 64
Polypharmacy 226
Polythiazide 273
Polyunsaturated fatty acid 68
Poor blood pressure measurement technique 151
Posterior reversible leukoencephalopathy syndrome 147
Postural hypotension 288
  higher risk of 288
Potassium
  levels 335
  sparing diuretics 182, 219, 273
Potent aldosterone-synthase 312
Praliciguat 316
Pranayama 3
Prazosin 221
Preeclampsia 162, 166
  development of 163
  family history of 163
  late complication of 164
  mild 163
  occurrence of 163
  postpartum 165
  prevention of 163
  severe 163
Pregnancy 161, 165
  frequently encountered renal complication of 162
  hypertension 162t
Prehypertension 96
Preoptic nucleus 248
Pressure loads 188
Presynaptic alpha-receptor agonists 286
Priapism 288

Procollagen carboxy-terminal peptide 49
Proinflammatory cytokines 59, 61
Propranolol 120, 162, 221, 279
Prostacyclin 70f
Prostaglandin 68-73, 242
  receptors 73
  synthase 71
Prostanoids 69, 70, 72f
  nitric oxide 49
Prosthetic patch aortoplasty 243
Protein
  acute-phase 203
  kinase
    A 70
    C 73
    G pathway 293
Proteinuria 163, 176
  nephrotic-range 255
Proximal tubule 306
  reabsorption 306
Pseudohypertension 145, 226
Pseudopodal 40
Pseudoresistant hypertension 175, 214, 391
  prevalence 151
Psychiatric diseases 110
Psychiatric disorders 116
Public awareness campaigns 91
Pulse
  pressure 98
  volume plethysmography 102
  wave velocity 100, 176

Q

Quantitative trait loci 341
Quinapril 220

R

Radial artery 98f, 100
  applanation tonometry of 101f
  palpable 146
Radial pulses 100
Rakta dhatu 3
Rakta-poornata 3
Ramipril 119, 124, 220, 257, 404, 408
Ramipril Global Endpoint Trial 218, 264
Randomized controlled
  studies 399
  trials 13, 14

Rapid eye movement 246
Rash 255, 314
Rational combination therapy 325
Reactive oxygen species 19, 58, 98, 203
Red blood cell 35, 38
  deformability 36, 36f
  membrane 35, 38
  structure of 36f
Red thrombus 124
Reflex tachycardia 148, 287
Regional nerve blocks 182
Regular blood pressure monitoring 162
Regular physical activity, benefits of 197
Regurgitation, aortic 111, 115, 116, 240
Remote hypertension monitoring program 166
Renal denervation 157, 218
Renal disease, end-stage 189, 374, 418
Renal failure 147, 176, 255, 315, 332
  chronic prepregnancy 62, 327
Renal function
  careful assessment of 335
  impaired 180
  tests 423
Renal health 189
Renal hemodynamics 352
Renal insufficiency 163, 292
Renal parenchymal disease 155
Renal sympathetic
  denervation 157, 158fc
  nerve activity 352
Renal theory 239
Renin secretion 352
Renin–angiotensin–aldosterone
  pathway 176
  stimulation 161
  system 16-18, 21, 24, 27, 28fc, 29, 62, 64, 72, 146, 152, 186, 197, 207, 239, 248, 255, 260, 275, 283, 312, 325, 331, 341, 342, 370, 384
  activation 385
  blocker 154, 156, 158
  inhibitor of 291, 303
  mechanism of 28
Renovascular disease 228

Reserpine 416
Resistant hypertension 151, 152*f*, 154, 154*b*, 155*fc*, 157, 158, 198, 213, 215*t*, 216*t*, 219*t*, 226, 290, 303, 312, 391
   management of 154, 156*f*, 388, 389
   multifactorial condition of 311
   optimal treatment trial 156
   pathology of 152
   treatment of 291, 311
Respiratory failure 315
Respiratory system 248
Respiratory tract 280
   infection 315
Retinal arteriolar emboli 141
Retinal arteriole, macroaneurysm of 141
Retinal artery occlusion 141
Retinal pigment epithelium 138
Retinal vein occlusion 141, 141*f*
Retinopathy 137, 176
   diabetic 137, 141
   hypertensive 137, 140, 141, 299
Rheos pivotal trial 157, 352, 353
Rhythm abnormalities 297
Right bundle branch block 130*f*
Right ventricular hypertrophy 122
Rostral ventrolateral medulla 248, 350, 351
Ryanodine receptors 52

S

Sacubitril 303, 304
   actions of 304*f*
   blockade, adverse effects of 305
   mechanism of action of 304
Salt
   dietary intake of 94
   intake, low 156
Salus's sign 139
Sarcoplasmic reticulum 52
Scheie classification 140
Secondary hypertension 16, 137, 155*t*, 165, 216, 235, 423
   causes of 16*t*
Seizures, eclamptic 164
Sensitive potassium 291
   channel openers 291
Serotonin-acetylcholine pathways 203

Serum creatinine 165, 208, 228
   doubling of 315
Serum lactate dehydrogenase 163
Severe acute respiratory syndrome coronavirus 2 271
Severe preeclampsia 163
   features of 163
Short message system 399
Short-acting calcium antagonists 122, 124
Sildenafil 123
Single anti-hypertension drug therapy 162
Single-agent hypertension treatment regimen 329*f*
Single-nucleotide polymorphism 73, 340
Single-pill combination 334, 335
   agents 303, 390
   hypertension treatment regimen 329*f*
Sinus
   bradycardia 128*f*
   node 111
   tachycardia 123
Skeletal muscle 280
Skin reactions 313, 314
Sleep
   apnea 122, 123, 226, 246
   disordered breathing, terminology of 247
   insufficiency 248
Smoking, cessation of 172
Smooth muscle
   contraction, stimulation of 286
   relaxation of 286, 290
Snake venom metalloproteinases 46
Sodium 36, 38, 306
   excretion of 293
   glucose cotransporter 273, 306
      inhibitors 305
   nitroprusside 293
      higher doses of 293
   overload, high 198
   retention 65
   volume 341
Soft exudates 140
Solitary tract 248
Soluble guanylate cyclase 315
   stimulators 315
Sotalol 279

Sphincters, contraction of 286
Sphygmograph 5
Sphygmomanometer 175, 417
Spironolactone 30, 156, 217, 220, 273, 310, 404
   addition of 310
ST elevated myocardial infarction 283
Standard triple therapy 310
Status epilepticus, nonconvulsive 147
Stenosis, aortic 111
Stevens–Johnson syndrome 292
Stop hypertension 171
Stress, psychosocial 409
Stretching exercises 3
Stroke 90
   hemorrhagic 176
   higher risk of 187
   prevention of 332
   vascular 176
   volume 350, 351
Stromelysins 43
Subclavian flap aortoplasty 243
Suboptimal antihypertensive therapy 392
Sulfur dioxide 202
Superoxide 203
Surgery, complications of 243
Sympathectomy, surgical 7
Sympathetic nervous system 16, 20, 21, 65, 152, 198
Sympathetic tone 179, 198
Sympathomimetics 154
Syncope 110
Systolic blood pressure 13, 14, 77, 83, 87, 95, 98, 111, 113, 145, 161, 167, 176, 181, 182, 186, 197, 204, 207, 214, 215, 224, 225, 303, 307, 308, 325, 339, 361, 389, 399, 417
   ambulatory 313
   intervention trial 224, 366
   load 95, 96
   values, simultaneous 95
Systolic dysfunction 296, 299
   sign of 115
Systolic function, conventional measures of 296
Systolic hypertension 417
   false diagnoses of 87
   treatment 417

T

Tachycardia 122
   supraventricular 270
Target organ
   damage 135, 176, 208, 228
      signs of 140
      disease 118
T-cells 60
Telehealth 388
   services 388
Telemedicine 91, 388, 391f
   advantages of 91
   benefits of 400, 400t
   closed-loop healthcare
      model 389
   effectiveness of 400t
   encounter 389
   full potential of 401
   grants hypertensive 401
   role of 389
   services 388, 423
Telmisartan 119, 220, 260, 262
Terazosin 221, 287
Tezosentan 314
T-helper cell 60
Theophylline 273
Thiazides 229, 273, 418
   diuretics 131, 156, 158, 217,
      219, 229, 272, 305
   drugs, use of 418
Thiocyanate 293
   accumulation 293
Thrombocytopenia 163, 292
Thrombolytic therapy 149
Thrombotic thrombocytopenic
      purpura 147
Thrombotic vascular disease 163
Thromboxane 68-72
   polymorphism 73
   receptor 71
Thyroid 110
   disorders 109, 328
   dysfunction 155
Tibial artery 99
Timolol 221, 279
Tiredness 110
Tissue Doppler imaging 299
T-lymphocytes 58, 60
Tolvaptan 276
Torsemide 219
Trandolapril 220, 257
Transcutaneous pressure
      transducers 100, 101f

Transforming growth factor 59
   beta 19, 48, 61
Transient ischemic attack 110,
      331, 399
Triamterene 31, 219, 273
Tricuspid regurgitation 299
Troponin, high-sensitivity 261
True resistant hypertension,
      pathophysiology of 310
Tubule transport systems 276f
Tumor
   necrosis factor 59
      alpha 49, 58, 61, 161, 203
   suppression 62
T-wave 126fc
   inversion 119
Twenty four-hours ambulatory
      blood pressure 411
Tyrosine kinase 73, 161

U

University of Alabama
   Classification of
   Hypertension 153f
Unstable angina 283
Urban Indian Hypertensive
   Population 390
Uric acid 208
Urinalysis 228
Urinary bladder neck 287
Urinary tract infection 109
Urine 293
   albumin-creatinine ratio 307
   culture 165
   pregnancy test 148
U-tube 4

V

Vagal C-fibers 256
Valsalva maneuver 350
Valsartan 220, 260, 262, 303,
      304, 335
   efficacy of 191
   mechanism of action of 304
Valvuloplasty 243
Vascular damage
   higher prevalence of 187
   indicative of 138
   vicious cycle of 146
Vascular disease, atherosclerotic
      256
Vascular endothelial growth
      factor 48

   inhibitors 154
Vascular endotheliosis 163
Vascular smooth muscle
   cells 43, 71
   proliferation 65
Vascular system 314
Vascular tone, sympathetic
      modulation of 186
Vasculature 60, 203
Vasoactive substances 20, 21t
Vasoconstriction, induction
      of 286
Vasodilation 278
Vasodilator 218
Vasopressin 207
   receptor antagonists 276
Venous pulse, examination of 111
Ventricular septal defect 239
Verapamil 120, 126, 219, 267
Vessel wall 296
Veterans Administration Study
      Group 8
Vigorous diuretic therapy 131
Vision
   blurring of 147
   impaired 110
Visual symptoms 163
Vital study subgroup analyses 385
Vitamin
   C 164
   D 385, 386
      deficiency 384
      randomized evaluation
         of 385
      receptors 384
   D_3 384
      physiology of 384
      role of 384
   E 164
Volatile organic carbons 202
Voltage-gated channel
   structure of 53
   types of 54
von Willebrand factor 39

W

Wagener–Barker grade 147
Weight reduction 156
White coat 94
   effect 187
      detection of 84fc
   hypertension 89, 91, 94, 174,
      180, 226, 367, 392, 422
      assessment 83

detection of 85*fc*
development of 175
management of 177
reaction 88
syndrome 174
World Health Organization 171, 202, 339
World Hypertension League 9

X

Xipamide 273
X-ray chest 180

Z

Zinc 44*f*
 binding sulfhydryl group 314
 dependent aminopeptidase A 313
ion 44*f*
Zymogen activation 45
 cascade of 47*f*
 matrix metalloproteinases cascade of 47*f*